Emergency
medicine

The principles of practice

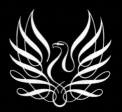

Emergency medicine

The principles of practice

Edited by

Gordian W O Fulde

MB BS, FRACS, FRCS (Edin), FRCS/RCP (A&E) (Edin), FACEM

Director, Emergency Department
St Vincent's Hospital, Sydney

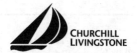

CHURCHILL LIVINGSTONE

Sydney   Edinburgh   London   New York
Philadelphia   St Louis   Toronto

ELSEVIER

Churchill Livingstone
is an imprint of Elsevier

Elsevier Australia
30–52 Smidmore Street, Marrickville, NSW 2204

This edition © 2004 Elsevier Australia
(a division of Reed International Books Australia Pty Ltd)
ACN 001 002 357

First edition 1988
Reprinted 1989
Second edition 1992
Reprinted 1994
Third edition 1998
Reprinted 2000

Coventry University

National Library of Australia Cataloguing-in-Publication Data

Emergency medicine : the principles of practice.

    4th ed.
    Includes index.
    ISBN 0 7295 3747 1.

    1. Emergency medicine. I. Fulde, Gordian W. O.

616.025

Publisher: Vaughn Curtis
Cover, internal design and typesetting by Toni Darben
Edited and project-managed by Carol Natsis
Proofread by Kate Ormston-Jeffery
Indexed by Max McMaster
Printed and bound in Australia by Ligare

Since the first edition of this book in 1988 and following editions in 1992 and 1998, emergency medicine has fortunately continued to advance. In this edition much new information, many new approaches and extensive refinements of existing clinical management have been incorporated. Again, current and respected practising clinicians have been chosen as authors for their clinical expertise and experience, so that they can compact their knowledge into the pocket-sized format. As healthcare resources continue to be stretched, the first hours of a patient's illness or initial contact with healthcare providers are even more critical to the outcome. The aim of this book is to help with this initial contact. Any suggestions for improving this will be very much appreciated: please send them to gfulde@stvincents.com.au.

Gordian Fulde

Acknowledgments

Once again I am very grateful to the busy clinician authors for their excellent contributions. Also, the support and stimulation from many doctors, nurses, students and other professionals who use this book and have helped with ideas are greatly appreciated.

How do I adequately thank my wife, Lesley, for her unfailing encouragement and support, let alone all that proofreading?

Even my daughters Sascha and Tiffany helped in their special ways.

Jodie Gueguen and Jo-Anne Pratt typed, collated, chased up details and much more; I sincerely thank them.

I thank the Commonwealth Serum Laboratory for permission to use their table on tetanus prophylaxis.

Gordian Fulde

Disclaimer
Every effort has been made to ensure that all the information contained in this book is correct and accurate. However, the publisher, editor and authors accept no responsibility for the clinical decisions, management or dosages given. The final responsibility rests with the treating doctor.

CONTENTS

Contents

Contents

Contents

Judy Alford MB BS (UWA)
Staff Specialist, Emergency Medicine, St Vincent's Hospital, Sydney, NSW.

Michael Ardagh MB ChB, FACEM, DCH, PhD
Professor of Emergency Medicine, Christchurch School of Medicine, New Zealand.

Glenn Arendts MB BS, FACEM
Staff Specialist, Emergency Medicine, St George Hospital, Sydney, NSW; Conjoint Lecturer, University of New South Wales, Sydney.

Neil Ballard MB BS (Adelaide), FACEM
Staff Specialist, Emergency Medicine, St Vincent's Hospital, Sydney, NSW; Staff Specialist, Retrieval Medicine, St George Hospital, Sydney, NSW.

Nicholas J Brennan MB BS (Hons), FRACP
Director, Department of Geriatric Medicine, St Vincent's Hospital, Sydney, NSW.

Phillip C Brenner MB BS, FRACS
Urologist, St Vincent's Clinic, Sydney, NSW; Conjoint Lecturer, University of New South Wales, Sydney.

Anthony F T Brown MBChB, FRCP, FRCS(Ed), FFAEM, FACEM
Associate Professor and Senior Staff Specialist, Department of Emergency Medicine, Royal Brisbane Hospital, QLD; Member, Court of Examiners, Australasian College for Emergency Medicine.

David A Brown MB BS (Hons), PhD, FRACP, FRCPA
NH&MRC Travelling Fellow, The Burnham Institute, La Jolla, CA, USA; Centre for Immunology, St Vincent's Hospital, Sydney/ University of New South Wales, Sydney.

Gary Browne MD, MB BS, FRACP, FACEM
Director, Emergency Department, Royal Alexandra Hospital for Children, Westmead, NSW; Member, Court of Examiners, Australasian College for Emergency Medicine.

Phillip Chang FRACS
Visiting Medical Officer, Department of Otolaryngology/Head & Neck Surgery, St Vincent's Hospital, Sydney, NSW.

Fiona Chow MB BS, FACEM
Staff Specialist, Emergency Medicine, St Vincent's Hospital, Sydney, NSW.

Bill Croker MB BS, BMedSci, FACEM
Emergency Physician, Nepean Hospital, Penrith, NSW; Emergency Physician, The Sanitarium Hospital, Wahroonga, NSW; Member, Court of Examiners, Australasian College for Emergency Medicine.

Shane Curran MB BS, BMedSci, FACEM
Staff Specialist, Emergency Physician, Calvary Hospital, Canberra, ACT; Lecturer, Emergency Medicine, School of Rural Health, University of New South Wales, Sydney.

Linda Dann MB BS, FANZCA, FACEM
Director, Emergency Medicine, Bankstown-Lidcombe Hospital, NSW; Member, Court of Examiners, Australasian College for Emergency Medicine.

Michael R Delaney MB BS, FRACO, FRACS
Visiting Ophthalmic Surgeon, St Vincent's Hospital, Sydney, NSW; Clinical Lecturer in Ophthalmology, University of NSW.

Anthony J Dodds MB BS (Hons), FRACP, FRCPA
Director, Clinical Haematology and Blood Stem Cell Transplantation; Chairman, SYDPATH, St Vincent's Pathology, St Vincent's Hospital, Sydney, NSW; Senior Lecturer, Faculty of Medicine, University of New South Wales, Sydney.

Martin Duffy MB BS, FACEM
Staff Specialist, Emergency Medicine, St Vincent's Hospital, Sydney, NSW; Senior Conjoint Lecturer, Emergency Medicine, University of New South Wales, Sydney.

Steve Dunjey MB BS, FACEM
Staff Specialist, Emergency Medicine, Royal Perth Hospital, Perth, WA; Clinical Senior Lecturer, Emergency Medicine, University of Western Australia, Crawley, WA; Member of the Court of Examiners, Australasian College for Emergency Medicine.

Robert Edwards MB BS, FACEM
Senior Staff Specialist, Emergency Medicine, Westmead Hospital, NSW; Staff Specialist, Emergency Medicine, Sydney Aeromedical Retrieval Service.

Bruce Fasher MB BS, DRCOG, DCH, FRCP(L), FRACP
Paediatric Physician, Emergency Department, Royal Alexandra Hospital for Children, Westmead, NSW.

Andrew Finckh MB BS, BA, FACEM
Staff Specialist, Emergency Medicine, St Vincent's Hospital, Sydney, NSW.

Peter Foltyn BDS(Syd)
Consultant Dentist, Dental Department, St Vincent's Hospital, Sydney, NSW.

S Lesley Forster MB BS(NSW), MHP, FRACMA, DipIndRel&LabLaw(Syd), FAFPHM
Director, Medical Administration and Clinical Support, St Vincent's Hospital, Sydney, NSW.

Gordian W O Fulde MB BS, FRCS(Edin), FRACS, FRCS(A&E)(Edin), FACEM
Director, Emergency Department, St Vincent's Hospital, Sydney, NSW; Associate Professor in Emergency Medicine, University of New South Wales, Sydney; Member, Senior Court of Examiners, Australasian College of Emergency Medicine.

Christopher F Gavaghan MB BS, FACEM
Director, Emergency Medicine, Lismore Base Hospital, NSW; Medical Director, Northern Region Helicopter Service, NSW; Retrieval Consultant, Ambulance

Service of NSW; Member Board of Examiners, Australasian College for Emergency Medicine.

Paul L Gaudry MB BS, FACEM
Director of Emergency Services, Western Sydney Area Health Service, NSW; Honorary Secretary, Australasian College for Emergency Medicine; Member of the Court of Examiners, Australasian College for Emergency Medicine.

Paul Gee FACEM, MB ChB, Dip Obs, BHB
Staff Specialist, Emergency Medicine, Christchurch Hospital, New Zealand.

Mark Gillett MB BS, DipRACOG, FRACGP, FACEM
Staff Specialist, Emergency Department, Royal North Shore Hospital, Sydney, NSW; Clinical Lecturer, University of Sydney; State Censor (NSW/ACT), Australasian College for Emergency Medicine; Member of the Court of Examiners, Australasian College for Emergency Medicine and Royal Australian College of General Practice.

Anthony J Grabs MB BS(Qld), FRACS (Gen&Vasc)
Director, Trauma Service, St Vincent's Hospital, Sydney, NSW; Lecturer in Surgery, St Vincent's Hospital, Sydney, University of New South Wales.

Salie Greengarten MB BS(Syd), MRCP(UK)
General Practitioner, Sydney, NSW.

John L Harkness MB BS, FRCPA, FASM, DCP(Lond)
Head, Division of Microbiology, St Vincent's Hospital, Sydney, NSW; Senior Lecturer, Faculty of Medicine, University of New South Wales, Sydney.

Ken Hillman MB BS, FRA, FANZCA, FFICANZCA
Professor of Intensive Care, University of New South Wales, Sydney; Director, The Simpson Centre for Health Service Research, Liverpool Hospital, NSW; Co-Director, Division of Critical Care, Liverpool Hospital, NSW.

Anna Holdgate MB BS, FACEM
Deputy Director, Emergency Medicine, St George Hospital, Sydney, NSW; Conjoint Lecturer, University of New South Wales, Sydney; Member of the Court of Examiners, Australasian College for Emergency Medicine.

Beaver Hudson RMN, RN
Clinical Nurse Consultant, Emergency Consultation Liaison Psychiatry, St Vincent's Hospital, Sydney, NSW

Sue Ieraci MB BS, FACEM
Area Adviser, Emergency Medicine, South Western Sydney Area Health Service; Staff Specialist, Emergency Medicine, Bankstown Hospital, NSW; Lecturer in Emergency Medicine, University of New South Wales, Sydney.

Frank Isaacs MB BS (Hons), FACD
Visiting Dermatologist, St Vincent's Hospital, Sydney, NSW.

George Jelinek MD, DipDHM, FACEM
Professor and Chairman, Emergency Medicine, University of Western Australia and Sir Charles Gairdner Hospital, Nedlands, WA; Editor-in-Chief, *Emergency Medicine* Journal; Member of the Court of Examiners, Australasian College for Emergency Medicine.

Diane King MB BS, FACEM
Director, Emergency Medicine, Flinders Medical Centre, Adelaide, SA; Divisional Director, Emergency and Perioperative Medicine, Flinders Medical Centre, Adelaide, SA; Senior Lecturer, Emergency Medicine, Flinders University, Adelaide, SA; Vice President and SAINT Councillor, Australasian College for Emergency Medicine; Member of the Court of Examiners, Australasian College for Emergency Medicine.

David J Lewis-Driver MB BS (Hons), FACEM, FRACGP, MRACMA
Director, Emergency Medicine, Logan Hospital, QLD; Senior Lecturer, Department of Anaesthesiology and Critical Care, University of Queensland, Brisbane; Member Fellowship Examination Committee, Australasian College for Emergency Medicine; Member of the Court of Examiners, Australasian College for Emergency Medicine.

Sally McCarthy MB BS, FACEM, MBA
Director, Emergency Medicine, Prince of Wales Hospital, Sydney, NSW; Senior Lecturer, Emergency Medicine, University of New South Wales, Sydney.

Mary McCaskill MB BS, BSc(Med), Dip Paeds, FACEM
Paediatric Emergency Physician, Royal Alexandra Hospital for Children, Westmead, NSW.

Thomas McDonagh MB BS, FACEM
Staff Specialist, Emergency Department, North West Regional Hospital, Burnie, Tasmania; Lecturer, Emergency Medicine, University of Tasmania.

Dr Greg McDonald MB BS, FACEM
Director of Emergency Care, Sydney Adventist Hospital; Member of the Court of Examiners, Australasian College for Emergency Medicine.

Michael Novy MB BS, FACEM
Staff Specialist, Emergency and Retrieval Medicine, St George Hospital, Sydney, NSW.

Nirmal Patel MD, MB BS (Hons), FRACS
Otolaryngology/Head & Neck Surgeon, Department of Otolaryngology, New York University, New York, NY.

Ronald Penny AO, DSc, MD, MB BS, FRACP, FRCPA
Emeritus Professor of Medicine, University of New South Wales; Senior Clinical Adviser, New South Wales Health Department; Consultant, HIV Medicine and Clinical Immunology, St Vincent's Clinic, Sydney, NSW.

Sarah Pett BSc (Hons), MB BS (Hons), DTM&H, MRCP (UK)
Lecturer, National Centre in HIV Epidemiology and Clinical Research, University of New South Wales, Sydney; Immunology and Infectious Diseases Clinical Service, St Vincent's Hospital, Sydney, NSW.

Susan Phin MB BS, FRACP
Emergency Paediatrician, Royal Alexandra Hospital for Children, Westmead, NSW.

Paul Preisz MB BS, FACEM
Deputy Director, Emergency Department, St Vincent's Hospital, Sydney, NSW; Lecturer, Emergency Medicine, University of New South Wales, Sydney; Member, Court of Examiners, Australasian College for Emergency Medicine.

Donald S Pryor MB BS, MD, FRACP
VMO Neurologist, St George Hospital, Sydney, NSW; Conjoint Senior Lecturer, University of New South Wales, Sydney.

John R Raftos MB BS (Hons), FACEM
Director of Emergency Services, Sutherland Hospital, Caringbah, NSW; Staff Specialist, Emergency Medicine, St Vincent's Hospital, Sydney, NSW.

Drew Richardson MB BS (Hons), FACEM, MRACMA
NRMA-ACT Road Safety Trust Chair of Road Trauma and Emergency Medicine, Australian National University, Canberra, ACT; Senior Staff Specialist, Emergency Department, The Canberra Hospital, Canberra, ACT; Associate Professor, Emergency Medicine, Canberra Clinical School and University of Sydney; Member, Court of Examiners, Australasian College for Emergency Medicine.

John B Roberts MB BS, FACEM
Director, Emergency Department, Port Macquarie Base Hospital, NSW; Senior Lecturer, University of New South Wales, Sydney; Member, Court of Examiners, Australasian College for Emergency Medicine.

Patricia A Saccasan-Whelan MB BS, FACEM
Director, Emergency Department, Goulburn Base Hospital, NSW; Goulburn NSW Disaster Coordinator, Southern Area Health Service, NSW.

E S Seelan MB BS, FRANZCR
Managing Radiologist, Mayne Health Diagnostic Imaging, Miranda, NSW; Former Director of Radiology, Sutherland Hospital, Caringbah, NSW.

Joanne Sheedy Bachelor of Applied Science (Physiotherapy), Graduate Diploma Health Research Methods; Trauma Service Manager, St Vincent's Hospital, Sydney, NSW.

David H Sonnabend MD, BS, BSc(Med), FRACS, FAOrthA
Head, Department of Orthopaedics and Traumatic Surgery, Royal North Shore Hospital, NSW; Professor of Orthopaedics and Traumatic Surgery, University of Sydney.

Geoffrey Stubbs MB BS, FRACS, FAOrthA, ARSM
Consultant Orthopaedic Surgeon, The Canberra Hospital; Calvary Hospital; John James Hospital, Canberra, ACT; Lecturer in Anatomy, USYDGMP.

John Vinen MB BS, MHP, FACEM
Head, Department of Emergency Medicine, Royal North Shore Hospital, Sydney, NSW; Member, Court of Examiners, Australasian College for Emergency Medicine.

Jeff Wassertheil CS&J, MB BS, MClinEd, MRACMA, MACLM
Head, Emergency Medicine Academic Stream, Southern Clinical School, Monash University, Faculty of Medicine, Nursing and Health Sciences; Associate Professor/Director, Emergency Medicine, Peninsula Health, Frankston, Victoria; Deputy Chief Medical Coordinator, Medical Displan, Victoria.

Christopher Weatherall MB BS (Hons I), BSc(Med) (Hons I)
Senior Registrar, Department of Immunology, Allergy and Infectious Diseases, St George Hospital, Sydney, NSW.

Contributors

Anthony J Whelan MB BS, FRACP
Physician, Goulburn Base Hospital, NSW.

Alex Wodak MB BS, FRACP, FAFPHM, ChAM, MRCP
Director, Alcohol and Drug Service, St Vincent's Hospital, Sydney, NSW; Senior Lecturer, School of Public Health and Community Medicine, School of Medicine, National Drug and Alcohol Research Centre, Centre for HIV Epidemiology and Clinical Research, University of New South Wales, Sydney.

Allen Yuen MB BS (Hons), FRACGP, FACEM
Director, Emergency Medicine, Epworth Hospital, VIC; Senior Examiner, Australasian College for Emergency Medicine; Associate, Department of Medicine, Monash University, Melbourne.

1 Cardiopulmonary resuscitation

Paul Preisz and Gordian W O Fulde

Cardiopulmonary resuscitation is one of the most difficult areas in clinical medicine and outcomes are often said to be extremely poor, especially in patients with unwitnessed out-of-hospital cardiac arrest. While many accepted practices do not yet have a strong evidence base a number of principles can now reasonably be supported. Early intervention is essential, and in general terms every minute that passes without cardiac output leads to a dramatic worsening of prognosis.

Basic life support (BLS) needs to be early and effective and should be supplemented by advanced life support (ALS) as soon as possible. In particular, direct current (DC) cardioversion should be performed urgently in those patients with a rhythm disturbance that is likely to be responsive. Even if the underlying rhythm is unclear, early cardioversion should be performed in patients with possible ventricular fibrillation or any tachyarrhythmia with significantly compromised cardiac output. Resuscitation should never be withheld, except in those cases where there is no doubt that it is not in a patient's best interests and a full and well-documented discussion with the patient and the patient's family has already taken place.

Cardiopulmonary resuscitation (CPR) includes basic life support and advanced life support. The aim of CPR is to re-establish cardiac output and spontaneous ventilation. A standardised approach allows teaching of the required skills and improves the likelihood that appropriate steps are taken under the stressful circumstances of a life-threatening emergency, even if those involved rarely perform CPR. Therapy to reverse the primary illness should be urgently considered while resuscitation is being performed.

Despite the difficulties in performing research in this area the body of evidence is growing and new concepts are under investigation—such as circulatory support alone (chest compression without expired air resuscitation), devices and techniques to provide more effective external chest compression, devices for minimally invasive internal cardiac massage and improved technology for electrical therapy (biphasic cardioversion). Recent work suggests controlled hypothermia, using cold IV fluids, may be beneficial post-arrest in some patients. Broader public education, improved telecommunications and increased availability of defibrillators have also had considerable impact.

The daunting logistic task of teaching and maintaining competency in cardiopulmonary resuscitation, not only for healthcare professionals but for the general public, has meant that any changes in practice have

Table 1.1 Common causes of cardiac arrest

Adults (VF, VT, PEA)	Children (bradycardia, asystole)
Cardiac arrhythmia ± AMI	SIDS
Organ failure secondary to severe acute or acute-on-chronic illness	Severe medical illness
	Trauma/near-drowning
Trauma	Poisoning
Poisoning/overdose	Airway obstruction/respiratory failure
Pulmonary embolism	Primary cardiac causes (rare)

appropriately been adopted slowly and cautiously. Current recommendations call for an immediate assessment of the situation, including safety aspects for the patient and for rescuers, followed by a call for help, BLS and ALS as soon as possible.

BASIC LIFE SUPPORT (BLS)

The general principles of BLS are the same in neonates, children and adults, but their application differs because of the physiological and pathophysiological differences between these groups.

First assess safety and call for help, then initiate BLS. If there is life-threatening external bleeding, give immediate priority to controlling blood loss using direct pressure, elevation and, in cases of amputation, tourniquets.

Protect from the environment (including maintaining body temperature), perform constant reassessment, handle gently and reassure. Be aware that spinal injury may have occurred and take care to avoid neck movement whenever possible.

Complications of CPR include trauma to the ribs, sternum, lungs, liver, spleen or heart. Pneumothorax, haemothorax or fat embolism may all occur. Gastric distension (with air) and aspiration are also likely.

Simple (vagal) syncope
Neuropathology—seizure, stroke, meningitis/encephalitis, trauma
Hypoxia—airway, breathing or cellular
Hypovolaemia
Cardiac
Metabolic—hypoglycaemia, hyponatraemia, hyper/hypothermia
Toxins—drugs, alcohol, envenomation, electricity, anaphylaxis

Figure 1.1 A short, simple differential diagnosis of collapse/unconsciousness

Resuscitation of the newborn

Careful assessment and frequent observation (e.g. every 30 seconds) are required. Technique is as follows:

1. Clamp cord.
2. Dry and warm.
3. Assess:
   - Colour—initially blue but rapidly pink.
   - Tone—good tone and cries within minutes.
   - Respiratory rate—30 breaths per minute.
   - Heart rate—120–150 bpm (*Note:* palpation of peripheral pulses is unreliable. Use stethoscope or monitor.)
4. Position on back with head in neutral position.
5. Chin lift or jaw thrust.
6. Give five inflation breaths—prolonged (2 or 3 seconds) high pressure (30 cm H_2O).
7. Respiratory support—30–40 breaths per minute.
8. Chest compressions—thumbs of both hands can press on the sternum just below an imaginary line joining the nipples to reduce the anteroposterior diameter of the chest by about one third. The ratio of compressions to inflations in newborn resuscitation is 3:1.
9. Drugs—usually administered via an umbilical venous catheter (see Table 1.2).
10. Equipment—suction, Guedel airway, intubation equipment.

Table 1.2 Drugs used in paediatric resuscitation

Drug	Concentration	Dose	Volume
Adrenaline	1:10,000	10 μg/kg	0.1 mL/kg
Sodium bicarbonate	4.2%	1–2 mmol/kg	2–4 mL
Dextrose	10%	250 mg/kg	2.5 mL/kg

Resuscitation of children

Although asystole is a common initial rhythm in paediatric cardiac arrest, primary cardiac disease is uncommonly the cause. Infants (<1 year old) have a large head, big tongue and tonsils, a short neck, small chest with a soft sternum and ribs that are more horizontal than those of older children. Take care with landmarks and technique to account for these factors.

BLS procedure for children

Approach safely, call for help, then follow these steps.

A. AIRWAY. Clear and open airway

  DO NOT
  - do blind finger sweep if <1 year.
  - shake the child.
  - overly flex or extend the neck as this may worsen obstruction.
  DO
  - use a sucker and Guedel airway if available.

B. BREATHING. Check and support breathing
  - Look, listen and feel.
  - Give five rescue breaths immediately.
  - Mouth to mouth (or mouth to mouth and nose).
  - Blow only until chest rises. (Be careful not to overinflate the chest as this will promote regurgitation, and air in the stomach will also splint the diaphragm.)
  - Continue at 20 breaths per minute.

C. CIRCULATION. Check and support circulation
  - Check pulse and if absent begin chest compression. In an infant <1 year, the best pulse to feel is the brachial.
  - On firm surface, correct hand position (Table 1.3). Infant—two fingers, small child—heel of the hand, older child as for adult. Compress the chest by one-third of its depth.
  - Compression rate of 100 per minute, if more than one rescuer is present the pulse should be felt during compression to assess effectiveness.
  - Do one ventilation to five compressions (one or two rescuers).
  - Do 20 cycles then re-check pulse and breathing

  Continue until the patient recovers or until it can be clearly established that recovery is not possible. Prolonged CPR is more likely to be successful in children than in adults. If hypothermia is present, full resuscitation should continue with rewarming until the patient is normothermic.

Table 1.3 Technique for CPR in children

	Infant	Small child	Older child
Age	<1 year	1–8 years	>8 years
Position	1 finger breadth below inter-nipple line	1 finger breadth above xiphisternum	2 finger breadths above xiphisternum
Rate	100 per minute	100 per minute	100 per minute
Depth	1.5–2.5 cm	2.5–3.5 cm	3.0–4.5 cm
Use	2 fingers	Heel of one hand	Interlocked hands

If the child's airway is obstructed by a foreign body, dislodge by picking up the child, inverting over one arm and giving blows to the back with the flat of the hand between the shoulder blades. A smaller child can also be laid across the rescuer's lap face down and lateral chest thrusts used, compressing sharply, up to four times with a hand in each axilla.

Management for the older/larger child with complete obstruction is similar to adult management, placing the child in the lateral position and opening and clearing the airway. Back blows can be used and chest thrusts given with the child still in the lateral position and the rescuer pushing with both hands together into the same, uppermost chest wall/axilla. The Heimlich and other abdominal manoeuvres are no longer recommended. If obstruction is partial and the child is stable, transport to a facility with advanced airway skills and equipment if possible.

Resuscitation of adults

Cardiopulmonary arrest in an adult is more often due to cardiac disease, and management of arrhythmias and coronary artery occlusion is an urgent priority. The delivery of a DC shock as soon as possible after the onset of ventricular fibrillation (VF) or pulseless ventricular tachycardia (VT) improves the outcome.

In later pregnancy the arrested patient should be positioned supine but with something under the right buttock to provide pelvic tilt to relieve the major abdominal veins from uterine compression. Ventilation may also be more difficult because of uterine enlargement. Urgent caesarean section should be considered in cases of failed resuscitation.

BLS procedure for adults

Approach safely, call for help, then follow these steps.

A. AIRWAY. Clear and open airway
- Use finger sweep, suction and Guedel airway if available.
- Open the mouth, use chin lift, head tilt or jaw thrust.

B. BREATHING. Check and support breathing
- Look, listen and feel.
- Give five rescue breaths immediately, watching the chest rise with each.
- Remember to seal the nose.
- Tidal volume 800–1000 mL, observing chest movement.
- Continue at 20 breaths per minute.

C. CIRCULATION. Check and support circulation
- Check the carotids and if no pulse begin chest compression.
- Use a firm surface, correct hand position (lower half of sternum).
- Compression rate 100 per minute.
- Do five chest compressions then one ventilation (two rescuers) or 15 chest compressions then two breaths (one rescuer).
- Do 20 cycles then recheck pulse and breathing.

Continue until the patient recovers or until it can be clearly established that recovery is not possible. If the airway is completely obstructed by a foreign body, back blows or lateral chest thrust with the patient in the lateral position is recommended.

ADVANCED LIFE SUPPORT (ALS)

Advanced life support includes intubation and ventilation, and electrical and pharmacological therapy. When a defibrillator is available the highest priority, even before giving BLS, is to establish the underlying rhythm and give DC shocks, if indicated. If the rhythm cannot be determined but there is no cardiac output, a 'blind' shock of 200 joules should be given (150 joules for biphasic defibrillators).

Open (internal) cardiac massage is rarely indicated, but it may be beneficial for patients with tamponade or an anatomical abnormality who arrest in the operating room while the chest is open. It should also be considered for patients who have penetrating chest trauma and lose vital signs after arriving at the emergency department.

Advanced life support for children is outlined in Figure 1.2 and for adults in Figure 1.3.

Note: There should be minimal interruption to CPR between steps. Calcium chloride may be used in some settings: e.g. hyperkalaemia. Seek and treat reversible causes.

Defibrillation

Place one paddle/gelpad in the right second intercostal area parasternally and the other in the left midaxilliary line at the sixth intercostal space. Use firm pressure and suspend CPR as well as all other physical contact with the patient. Avoid ECG electrodes, medications, pacemakers or other devices. Avoid metal fixtures, flammable substances and high-flow oxygen near the chest or paddles.

Drug delivery

Ideally drugs should be given IV into a large (not lower) limb. Adrenaline, lignocaine and atropine can be given via the endotracheal tube (ETT) (give twice the IV dose and dilute to 10 mL, giving two large ventilations to disperse the drug). In paediatric cardiac arrest all drugs and fluids can be given via the intraosseous route if required.

ARRHYTHMIAS
Treatment of bradycardia

1. BLS and ALS as indicated.
2. Treat underlying cause and any secondary physiological disturbance, particularly hypothermia, coronary artery occlusion, hypoxia, acidosis and electrolyte disorders.

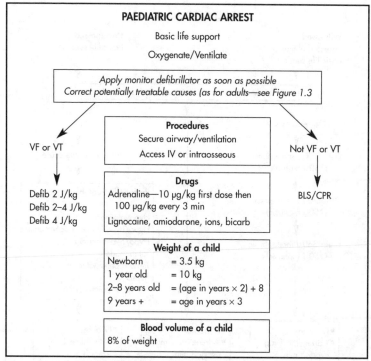

PAEDIATRIC CARDIAC ARREST

Basic life support

Oxygenate/Ventilate

Apply monitor defibrillator as soon as possible
Correct potentially treatable causes (as for adults—see Figure 1.3

VF or VT

Not VF or VT

Procedures
Secure airway/ventilation
Access IV or intraosseous

Defib 2 J/kg
Defib 2–4 J/kg
Defib 4 J/kg

Drugs
Adrenaline—10 μg/kg first dose then
    100 μg/kg every 3 min
Lignocaine, amiodarone, ions, bicarb

BLS/CPR

Weight of a child	
Newborn	= 3.5 kg
1 year old	= 10 kg
2–8 years old	= (age in years × 2) + 8
9 years +	= age in years × 3

Blood volume of a child
8% of weight

Figure 1.2   Procedure for paediatric cardiac arrest

3. Position supine legs elevated, if possible. *Note*: the presence of other factors such as pulmonary oedema (need to sit upright) may influence this. Supplement with oxygen and monitor.
4. Drugs and pacing (see arrhythmias, Chapter 12).
   • Cease ± reverse negative chronotropes/inotropes/dromotropes
   • Also treat cardiac failure, oliguria, hypotension

Treatment of tachycardia

Note that DC shock, when indicated (for example, in the presence of failing blood pressure), must be given as soon as possible. This may sometimes take precedence over all other therapies, including airway management.

1. BLS and ALS as indicated.
2. Treat cause and any secondary physiological disturbance, particularly hypoxia, hyperthermia, volume depletion, acidosis and electrolyte disorders.

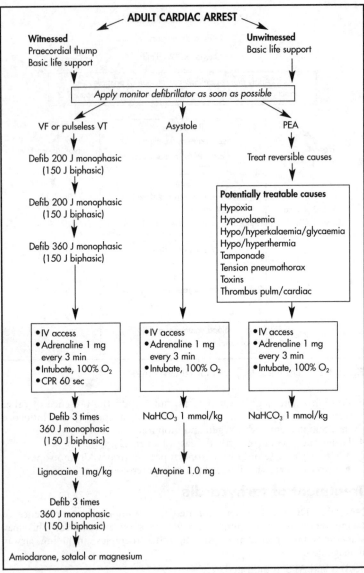

Figure 1.3　Procedure for adult cardiac arrest. There should be minimal interruption to CPR between steps. Calcium chloride may be used in some settings: e.g. hyperkalaemia. Seek and treat reversible causes.

3. Posture and positioning including oxygen, monitoring, IV access.
4. Drugs and defibrillation (see arrhythmias, Chapter 12).
   - Cease ± reverse positive chronotropes/inotropes/dromotropes
   - Also treat cardiac failure, oliguria, hypotension

EDITOR'S COMMENT

The vital skill of cardiopulmonary resuscitation is undergoing rapid change as the search for better outcomes continues. The key to good results is a prompt and orderly approach. The immediate call for help is paramount. Experience has proved that the sooner the simple manoeuvres of airway opening and rapid defibrillation are done, the more lives can been saved.

RECOMMENDED READING

Australian Resuscitation Council Guidelines for Cardiopulmonary Resuscitation website. Available: http://www.resus.org.au.
Cummins RO. Advanced cardiac life support. American Heart Association; 1997–1999.
European Resuscitation Council website. Available: http://www.erc.edu/uniweb/publicat/guidelines.html.

2 | Securing the airway and ventilation

Paul L Gaudry and Judy Alford

SECURING THE AIRWAY (Paul Gaudry)

Assessment and stabilisation of the airway take priority over other aspects of resuscitation in patients with life-threatening illness or injury.

Differences in airway anatomy of children and adults

The anatomy of the airways of infants and young children differs significantly from that of older children and adults, and this affects airway management.

1. Larger and more mobile head, which tends to flex the neck in the supine position.
2. Larger tongue, more prominent oropharyngeal tonsils and larger epiglottis.

3. Higher and more anterior larynx in infant (cervical vertebrae 3–4) than in child and adult (cervical vertebrae 5–6).
4. Narrowest at cricoid cartilage rather than at vocal cords.
5. Smaller diameter and shorter length of trachea.
6. Small amounts of mucosal swelling have major effects on airway resistance.

Causes of airway obstruction and respiratory failure

1. Decreased level of consciousness (cerebrovascular accident, seizure, infection, poisoning, head injury, near-drowning).
2. Trauma (maxillofacial fractures, blunt and penetrating neck injuries, laryngotracheal and bronchial rupture, chest injury, spinal cord injury).
3. Burns (face and neck burns, inhalational burns).
4. Foreign bodies (supraglottic, trachea, bronchus, oesophagus).
5. Infection (peritonsillar abscess, retropharyngeal abscess, epiglottitis, croup, pneumonia).
6. Inflammation (angioneurotic oedema, caustic ingestion, asthma, aspiration pneumonitis, parenchymal lung disease).
7. Shock (haemorrhagic, septic, anaphylactic, spinal).
8. Tumours (pharynx, larynx, trachea, bronchus).
9. Generalised weakness (neuropathies, myopathies).
10. Congenital anomalies in children (vascular ring).

Assessment and anticipation of airway obstruction

Establish whether the airway is patent and protected, threatened, or partially or completely obstructed. A patent airway is an absolute first priority. Protection from aspiration is only a relative priority and does not take priority over initial assessment and treatment of the patient's breathing and circulation.

1. Observe and listen for air movement and the rate and depth of respirations (at the mouth and nose, movement of chest wall, presence of tracheal tug).
2. Listen for noisy or abnormal sounds (gurgling, snoring, choking, coughing, stridor, wheeze).
3. Assess sound and quality of the voice (weak, painful, hoarse).
4. Determine the level of consciousness (Glasgow Coma Score).
5. Inspect mouth for foreign body.
6. Test the tone of the jaw, mouth and oropharyngeal muscles.
7. Test the gag reflex.
8. Feel the maxillofacial and neck regions (swelling, deformity, subcutaneous emphysema).

Factors affecting airway management

1. **Shape of face.** A poor seal between face and mask impedes bag-valve-mask ventilation. Causes of a poor seal are a beard, edentia, emaciation, obesity, facial trauma and burns.

2. **Difficult airway anatomy.** Impedes direct laryngoscopy and endotracheal intubation. Evaluate the anatomy before both elective and emergency endotracheal intubation. Focus on protruding maxilla relative to mandible (macrognathia), high arched palate, poor dentition, large tongue (macroglossia), short neck, limited mouth opening (intercisor gap). Test for neck mobility if cervical spine injury is not an issue. A sternomental distance less than 12.5 cm in an adult is the best predictor of 'difficult' intubation. Remember the differences in airway anatomy between children and adults. Anticipate 'difficult' intubation in certain congenital syndromes such as Down syndrome and Pierre Robin syndrome.

3. **Upper airway obstruction.** Initially the airway may only be threatened, but the pathological process may be progressive, as with burns and infection or movement of a foreign body. Priority must be given to securing the airway, as delay may precipitate complete obstruction. Intravenous sedation may also precipitate complete obstruction and should be avoided. If anaesthesia is required, inhalational induction may be preferred and relaxants avoided until bag-valve-mask ventilation is confirmed.

4. **Cervical spine injury.** Head and neck immobilisation must be maintained in the victim of blunt trauma until injury to the cervical spine is definitely excluded. If endotracheal intubation is indicated, it must be achieved without any flexion, extension or distraction of the neck. Intubation should be performed while an assistant maintains in-line immobilisation, without traction, of the head and neck.

5. **Full stomach.** All seriously ill or injured patients requiring intubation must be presumed to have a full stomach. Apply cricoid pressure during intubation to prevent regurgitation and aspiration.

6. **Limited haemodynamic reserves.** A patient with any form of shock is subject to haemodynamic deterioration during intubation, from the drugs used to facilitate intubation or from hypoxaemia before or during intubation. Preintubation oxygenation volume resuscitation and sometimes inotrope support are needed. The drugs used, and especially the drug dosage, must be individualised.

7. **Head injury.** Autoregulation of cerebral blood flow is impaired in head injury. The therapeutic aim before, during and after intubation is to maximise the chance to maintain arterial blood pressure and minimise the rise in intracranial pressure.

Manoeuvres to open or maintain the airway

1. **The coma position.** Turn the patient on the side. This allows the tongue to fall forwards and to one side to drain fluid from the mouth and reduce the risk of aspiration. When necessary, suction and laryngoscopy can be performed with the patient in the left lateral Trendelenburg position.
2. **Head tilt.** Extend the head at the atlanto-occipital joint by placing one hand on the forehead. This is usually combined with either chin lift or jaw thrust.
3. **Chin lift.** Lift the jaw forward and support it with the mouth slightly open.
4. **Jaw thrust.** Grasp the angles of the jaw and lift forward. Maximum jaw thrust may minimise the amount of head tilt needed to secure the airway when cervical spine injury is anticipated.
5. **Neck lift.** Lift the neck into the 'sniffing position'. This is less effective than the head tilt/chin lift or head tilt/jaw thrust manoeuvres. It is contraindicated when cervical spine injury is a possibility.

Manoeuvres to relieve foreign body obstruction

If the patient is capable of air movement, spontaneous coughing and breathing should be encouraged. The patient with poor or no air movement requires immediate help.

1. **Back blows.** Deliver four forcible blows between the scapulae with the heel of the hand. This may relieve partial or complete obstruction.
2. **Chest thrust.** Deliver four chest compressions with the hands over the sternum with the patient lying or sitting.
3. **Finger sweep.** To relieve obstruction in the oropharynx. Not recommended in infants.
4. **Heimlich manoeuvre.** Deliver thrusts with the fist over upper abdomen or lower chest with the patient standing, sitting or lying prone. Not recommended in infants.
5. **Repeated sequence.** Back blows, chest thrust, finger sweep, Heimlich manoeuvre and mouth-to-mouth ventilation is recommended.
6. **Infants under 1 year of age.** The recommended sequence is back blows, chest thrust and mouth-to-mouth ventilation.

Oropharyngeal and nasopharyngeal airways

1. **Oropharyngeal airway (Guedel airway).** Must be placed over the tongue, so that the tongue is lifted off the hypopharynx. Insert using a tongue depressor, or insert concave side up and then rotate 180°. Only tolerated if gag reflex is impaired. Can be used as a bite block in the intubated patient.
2. **Nasopharyngeal airway.** Lubricate well and insert through medial and inferior aspect of nasal cavity. Can be inserted in patients with tightly

clenched teeth. Tolerated even if the patient has an active gag reflex. Tip needs to lie behind tongue and low in hypopharynx but above the larynx.

Types of ventilation

Mouth-to-mask ventilation

1. Mask should incorporate a one-way valve. It is preferable to mouth-to-mouth ventilation.
2. Patients can be adequately ventilated until definitive assisted ventilation techniques are obtained.

Bag–valve–mask ventilation

1. Use 2 L bag for adults and children over 5 years of age, 500 mL bag for younger children and infants, 250 mL bag for premature infants.
2. Jackson Rees circuit is suitable for use only by an experienced resuscitator.
3. Mask–face seal is maintained with even pressure using thumb and index finger on the mask and the other fingers applying chin lift or jaw thrust, depending on the size of the patient. A second resuscitator may be needed to assist with jaw thrust.

Endotracheal intubation

Endotracheal intubation is the most effective and reliable means of securing an airway. It provides airway patency, prevents aspiration, assures oxygenation, and permits high ventilatory pressures and the use of positive end-expiratory pressure. It readily allows suctioning and can be used for administration of drugs if there is no intravenous access.

1. Approximate tube size (internal diameter) in adults is 7.5–8.0 mm in females and 8.0–8.5 mm in males. In pre-term infants use 2.5 mm, 3.0 mm in term infants, 3.5 mm in 3- to 9-month-olds, 4.0 mm for 9- to 24-month-olds. Tube size for patients over the age of 2 years is calculated from the formula:

$$\text{diameter (mm)} = \frac{\text{age}}{4} + 4$$

2. Uncuffed tubes are used in patients under the age of 8–10 years, allowing for an audible leak to prevent excessive pressure on the subglottis. Large-volume, low-pressure cuffs are used in older children and adults.
3. Orotracheal intubation is faster and easier than nasotracheal intubation.
4. In children, once orotracheal intubation is accomplished and the patient is stable, repeat direct laryngoscopy and nasotracheal intubation is often undertaken. This is because fixation and suctioning of a nasal tube is easier.

Technique of orotracheal intubation

1. Equipment should be prechecked (airways, tubes, introducers, forceps, bag-valve-mask, laryngoscopes).
2. Oxygen, suction and monitoring equipment must be available.
3. Skilled assistance is invaluable (with knowledge of the equipment used, to provide in-line manual immobilisation of the head and neck and to apply cricoid pressure).
4. The 'sniffing' position allows optimal visualisation of the vocal cords.
5. Be calm and orderly.
6. Monitor oxygen saturation, electrocardiogram and blood pressure during the procedure.
7. 'Stiffen' the tube to aid manipulation of the tube tip, by placing a lubricated 'introducer' inside the tube.
8. Aid visualisation of the larynx by the application of backward, upward, rightward pressure (BURP) to the thyroid cartilage.
9. Maintain visualisation of the tube passing through the vocal cords until the proximal end of the cuff is 2 cm beyond the cords.
10. Observation and auscultation should be performed to verify bilateral lung expansion.
11. Secure the tube in position, then insert an intragastric tube.
12. Capnography is ideal to confirm tube placement in the trachea.
13. Chest X-ray will ascertain the position of the tube tip in relation to the carina.

Rapid sequence induction (RSI)

RSI is used to induce unconsciousness and muscular paralysis to provide optimal intubating conditions, to avoid aspiration from a probable full stomach and to protect against reflex bradycardia and raised intracranial pressure resulting from manipulation of the airway. It is contraindicated if 'difficult' intubation is predicted and successful bag-valve-mask ventilation is considered unlikely. This will depend on the patient, the equipment and assistance available, and the skill of the operator.

1. **Preoxygenation.** Administration of 100% oxygen, using a well-fitting bag-mask for two minutes, will result in 95–98% nitrogen washout. This will protect against hypoxia during apnoea for up to 8 minutes. Manual ventilation is preferably avoided until intubation is accomplished.
2. **Simultaneous in-line manual immobilisation of the head and neck.** Used in the blunt trauma victim when cervical spine injury is a possibility.
3. **Cricoid pressure.** As soon as consciousness is lost, cricoid pressure is applied with the thumb and index finger to compress the oesophagus between the cricoid cartilage and the cervical spine. Compression is maintained until the tube cuff is inflated. This technique helps to prevent regurgitation and aspiration, but is contraindicated if the patient vomits. It should not be confused with BURP to bring the vocal cords into view.

4. **Secure intravenous infusion site**, for fluid and drug administration.
5. **Atropine** (10–20 mg/kg), as pretreatment to prevent bradycardia, which is more likely in children under 8 years of age and after repeated doses of suxamethonium.
6. **Induction.** Thiopentone 2.5% (3–5 mg/kg) induces unconsciousness within seconds of a single intravenous dose; its duration is a few minutes. Use a smaller dose (1–2 mg/kg) if depressed level of consciousness is already present. Its main side effects are cardiovascular and respiratory depression. Hypotension is managed with intravenous fluids. The dose must be reduced if there is already hypovolaemia or hypoxaemia. Propofol (2.0–2.5 mg/kg) also induces unconsciousness: a single induction dose lasts 5–10 minutes; avoid in children under 3 years. Alternatives are midazolam (0.1–0.2 mg/kg) combined with morphine (0.1–0.2 mg/kg) or fentanyl (2–4 mg/kg). Preinduction treatment of depressed cardiac output (from hypovolaemia, hypoxaemia, septic or cardiogenic shock) and titrating the drug dose against response are important, regardless of the agent. Lignocaine 1.5 mg/kg may be used as pretreatment in patients at risk of elevation of intracranial pressure.
7. **Suxamethonium** (1–2 mg/kg, 2–3 mg/kg in infants) induces neuromuscular depolarisation (fasciculations) followed by relaxation. Relaxation occurs within 60 seconds and generally lasts 3–10 minutes. Hypertension and tachycardia may occur as a result of stimulation of autonomic ganglia, or there may be bradycardia and salivation due to muscarinic effects. Other side effects include potassium flux from muscle cells, myoglobinaemia, muscle pain, a rise in intragastric, intraocular and intracranial pressure, and triggering of malignant hyperthermia. Prolonged relaxation occurs if there is pseudocholinesterase deficiency. An alternative is an 'intubating dose' of vecuronium (0.2–0.3 mg/kg), which produces relaxation by non-depolarising neuromuscular block, or rocuranium (1mg/kg). Onset is within 2–5 minutes and duration is 10–20 minutes.
8. **Propofol infusion** (1.0–3.0 mg/kg/h) is used to provide sedation to facilitate control of oxygenation and ventilation in adults. Alternatives are sedation and analgesia (midazolam and morphine). Add muscle relaxant if absolute control of ventilation is required. Under no circumstances give relaxants without sedation and analgesia. Usually vecuronium (0.1–0.15 mg/kg) or pancuronium (0.1–0.15 mg/kg) are used for maintenance relaxation. Vecuronium has a shorter duration of action, does not cause histamine release and produces less tachycardia and hypertension than pancuronium.
9. **Monitoring** is essential during and following the procedure—electrocardiogram, blood pressure, oxygen saturation, capnography.

Suctioning

1. Suctioning is an adjunct to manoeuvres to open or maintain the airway. It is used to remove tracheobronchial secretions via an endotracheal tube.

Table 2.1 Drugs in airway management

Drug	Dose	Important effects
Induction agents		
Thiopentone	3–5 mg/kg Less (0.5–1 mg/kg) in elderly or unstable	Hypotension esp. in hypovolaemia Respiratory depression Reduces cerebral metabolism, ICP Increased laryngeal sensitivity
Propofol	1–2.5 mg/kg	Decreases BP esp. in hypovolaemia Respiratory depression Reduces cerebral metabolism
Ketamine	1–2 mg/kg IV 3–5 mg/kg IM	Raises BP Raises HR Airway reflexes maintained Respiration not depressed Bronchodilation Raises ICP & IOP Hallucinations more common in adults
Fentanyl	2–3 μg/kg	Dose-related respiratory depression Analgesia Large doses may cause chest wall rigidity Relative cardiovascular stability
Midazolam	0.1–0.4 mg/kg	Some decrease in BP Respiratory depression
Muscle relaxants		
Suxamethonium	1 mg/kg	Drug of choice for RSI Raises K by 0.5 mEq/L, more in burns (>48 hours old), paralysis & denervation (>3 days old), crush injury Raises IOP (avoid in open eye injury) Triggers malignant hyperthermia Prolonged apnoea (rare, inherited)
Rocuronium	1 mg/kg for RSI 0.6 mg/kg for non-RSI 0.15 mg/kg prn	Use for RSI when suxamethonium contraindicated Use for maintaining paralysis
Vecuronium	0.1 mg/kg	Use for maintaining paralysis Not suitable for RSI

2. Yankauer sucker is used to remove secretions, blood, vomitus or foreign body from mouth and pharynx. In the unintubated patient, turn the patient on the side during suctioning.
3. Y-suction catheter with a soft tip is used for nasopharyngeal and tracheobronchial secretions. Catheter diameter should not be more than half the diameter of the endotracheal tube.
4. Preoxygenate and bag-valve-tube ventilate the patient before and after suctioning to prevent hypoxaemia and pulmonary collapse.

Oxygenation and ventilation

1. Ventilator settings require decisions about minute ventilation, respiratory rate, inspired oxygen concentration, peak airway pressure and the use of positive end-expiratory pressure. (See page 20.)
2. Monitor peak airway pressure as well as oxygen saturation, capnography and blood gases. Aim for oxygen saturation above 95% and mild hypocapnia.
3. A disconnection alarm must be used during mechanical ventilation.

Complications of intubation

1. **During intubation:** trauma to any structure from lips to the trachea; inability to oxygenate, ventilate or intubate; exacerbation of spinal cord injury; aspiration; haemodynamic collapse.
2. **While tube is in place:** misplacement; blockage; problems related to the ventilator.
3. **After extubation:** laryngospasm; aspiration; complications of trauma.

Extubation

1. The patient must be fully awake and have a gag reflex before extubation.
2. Non-depolarising neuromuscular blockade can be reversed with neostigmine (an anticholinesterase) and atropine (prophylactic antimuscarinic). Antagonists to midazolam and morphine are only rarely required.
3. Preoxygenation, suctioning of pharynx, trachea and intragastric tube should precede extubation, which is performed at the peak of inspiration.
4. Ensure oxygenation after extubation with a bag-valve-mask or a non-rebreathing mask.

Alternative airway techniques

1. **Nasotracheal intubation.** Can be performed without direct laryngoscopy in the non-apnoeic patient (the 'blind' technique). It is an appropriate alternative to orotracheal intubation in confirmed unstable cervical spine injury or spinal cord injury, in severely dyspnoeic awake patients who can be intubated in the sitting position, and in patients unable to fully open their mouth. It is contraindicated in patients with maxillofacial and anterior cranial fractures, and with conditions such as nasal polyps, upper airway foreign bodies and retropharyngeal abscesses.
2. **Laryngeal mask airway.** Consists of airway with elliptical cuffed 'mask' on distal end that rests over the larynx when inserted. Low-pressure ventilation may be performed, but it does not reliably prevent aspiration. Is quicker and an easier technique to learn than endotracheal intubation. Has an established role to provide an airway in the fasted patient during anaesthesia. Is a useful temporising technique if intubation skills are not available. When direct laryngoscopy and intubation fails it may serve to provide a functional airway until definitive intubation by cannulation of the trachea through the mask is performed. Intubation is possible through newer masks.

3. **Oesophageal-tracheal airway ('combitube').** Consists of twin-lumen tube with one lumen inserted into the oesophagus and the other lying above the trachea. A pharyngeal balloon provides a seal to enable ventilation. A distal balloon seals against gastric inflation and aspiration. An alternative to laryngeal mask airway if intubation skills are not available.

4. **Airway bougie.** An extension of the use of an 'introducer', this is used for a 'difficult' intubation. A long semi-rigid bougie is inserted between the vocal cords and the endotracheal tube is then passed over the bougie into the trachea. The bougie is then removed.

5. **Transillumination intubation.** Useful when a 'difficult' intubation is predicted. May be combined with rapid sequence induction. Distal end of tube is bent and a rigid lighted stylet is used to guide tube into larynx and signify correct placement. The rigid trocar is removed for nasotracheal intubation. Requires minimal training to use.

6. **Fibre-optic intubating laryngoscope.** This is an alternative to transillumination intubation if rapid sequence induction is contraindicated. Intubation is performed under local anaesthesia, preferably via the nasotracheal route. The laryngoscope is directed into the larynx and then acts as a guidewire for the tube. Requires a significant amount of training and is not in widespread use.

7. **Translaryngeal oxygenation.** Indicated when non-surgical airway management has failed, is contraindicated or is not available (total upper airway obstruction). Preferred to cricothyroidotomy in child under 8 years of age. Temporising oxygenating procedure, does not prevent aspiration, may lead to hypercarbia and is not effective if a foreign body is present below the cricoid cartilage.

8. **Cricothyroidotomy.** Alternative to translaryngeal oxygenation. May be used after temporising with translaryngeal oxygenation. Preferred to tracheostomy, which should be reserved for the operating room. A percutaneous approach (Seldinger technique) is easiest and fastest. Using a surgical approach, first insert a small endotracheal tube or tracheostomy tube. When the patient is stable, convert to tracheostomy or orotracheal tube.

Guidelines for 'difficult' intubation

1. If 'difficult' intubation is predicted but is not urgent, seek assistance from an experienced operator.
2. Assemble the available 'difficult' airway equipment.
3. Assess whether successful bag-valve-mask ventilation is likely.
4. Use an airway bougie (or transillumination intubation if available) if 'difficult' intubation is predicted.
5. Nasotracheal intubation, awake intubation or use of the fibre-optic intubating largyngoscope are options if successful bag-valve-mask ventilation is considered unlikely.
6. Avoid use of muscle relaxants if successful bag-mask-valve ventilation is considered unlikely.

7. If the initial attempt at orotracheal intubation fails and the patient has been paralysed, institute bag-valve-mask oxygenation and ventilation, then use BURP or an airway bougie and re-attempt intubation.

8. A 'difficult' intubation occurs if orotracheal intubation cannot be achieved after two attempts under direct laryngoscopy. Resume bag-valve-mask oxygenation and ventilation. Then re-attempt intubation using BURP or an airway bougie, or consider using a laryngeal mask airway, an oesophageal-tracheal airway or transillumination intubation.

9. If attempts at bag-valve-mask oxygenation and ventilation fail, escalate the use of a laryngeal mask airway or oesophageal-tracheal airway to reoxygenate. Consider passing airway bougie or endotracheal tube though the laryngeal mask.

10. Translaryngeal oxygenation or cricothyroidotomy are indicated when non-surgical airway management fails.

VENTILATORS (Judy Alford)

Ventilators are used in the emergency department to assist or control the respiration of patients. Patients requiring invasive ventilation need an artificial airway, most commonly an endotracheal tube. The level of ventilatory support needed by patients varies widely. Some have essentially normal lungs (e.g. patients with sedative overdose), while others have severe respiratory failure.

Indications for ventilation fall into three broad categories:

1. **Respiratory failure**
   - Airway obstruction.
   - Neuromuscular weakness: spinal cord injury, myasthenia gravis, organophosphate poisoning, exhaustion.
   - Chest wall disorders: deformity, flail chest, morbid obesity.
   - Pleural disease: massive effusions, pneumothorax or haemothorax.
   - Parenchymal lung disease: infection, adult respiratory stress syndrome (ARDS), pulmonary oedema, fibrosis, asthma, chronic airflow limitation (CAL).

2. **Central nervous system (CNS) disease**
   - Poisoning.
   - Trauma.
   - Cerebrovascular accident (CVA).
   - Infections.

3. **Circulatory failure**
   - Hypovolaemia.
   - Sepsis.
   - Cardiogenic shock.

Ventilators used in the emergency department are usually small and portable. The number of ventilatory modes available varies, but is usually less than is available on more complex machines in the intensive care unit (ICU). Nonetheless most patients can be managed in the short term.

Choosing initial settings for ventilation

Initially ventilator settings are estimated and then adjusted according to the patient's clinical progress and serial blood gas measurements.

Is the patient breathing spontaneously?

Spontaneously breathing patients are ventilated using a mode that assists each inspiratory effort by providing extra pressure or volume. Examples are continuous positive airways pressure (CPAP) and pressure support. Some ventilators and their circuits increase the work of breathing significantly and may not support spontaneous breathing. In these cases, the patient may need to be sedated and fully ventilated.

The patient who is not breathing adequately needs a mode that does all the work for them. Intermittent positive pressure ventilation (IPPV) or intermittent mandatory ventilation (IMV) provides a breath at a preset rate regardless of the patient's respiratory effort. Some ventilators can deliver a breath synchronised to an inspiratory effort. This is known as synchronised intermittent mandatory ventilation (SIMV).

How much oxygen does the patient need?

In all cases, start ventilation with 100% oxygen and titrate downwards according to the patient's arterial blood gases (ABGs) results. Some ventilators have limited options in selecting an inspired oxygen level. In patients who are inadequately oxygenated, positive end-expiratory pressure (PEEP) can increase the arterial oxygen tension for a given level of inspired oxygen.

How much gas should the patient receive?

The minute volume is the amount of gas moved every minute:

$$\text{Minute volume} = \text{respiratory rate} \times \text{tidal volume.}$$

The arterial tension of carbon dioxide is sensitive to changes in minute volume. Increasing the minute volume reduces the partial pressure of CO_2 ($PaCO_2$), and decreasing the minute volume raises $PaCO_2$. In patients with raised intracranial pressure, it may be necessary to deliberately hyperventilate to maintain a modest decrease in $PaCO_2$. In some patients with lung injury, trying to deliver a 'normal' minute volume may pose a risk of barotrauma. In these cases, the $PaCO_2$ may be allowed to rise quite significantly, an approach called permissive hypercapnia.

The ventilators in common use apply positive pressure to the lungs to enable gas movement. The amount of gas moved per breath depends on the ventilator settings and the lung compliance.

Ventilators can be set to deliver a given tidal volume at each breath. This mode is called volume control and is available on even the most basic machines. It may be possible to limit the delivery of the set volume if the airway pressures exceed a limit chosen by the operator (pressure regulated volume control (PRVC) mode).

Pressure control is a mode commonly used in the ICU but not always available on smaller ventilators. A constant airway pressure is provided during inspiration, with the tidal volume varying. This approach is often used where barotrauma is a concern.

Lung compliance is the change in lung volume for a given change in transpulmonary pressure. Diseased lungs often have abnormal compliance (e.g. in pulmonary oedema the lung is less compliant or 'stiffer'). Trying to deliver a 'normal' tidal volume to a poorly compliant lung can cause high airway pressures, increasing the risk of pneumothorax. Overdistension can worsen lung damage. The approach to ventilating is usually one of providing limited tidal volumes (6–8 mL/kg, sometimes less) with PEEP. This can be done using either volume or pressure control.

The choice of initial tidal volume depends on the clinical situation. In patients with respiratory failure or shock, a volume of 6–8 mL/kg is safest. Patients with normal lungs may tolerate tidal volumes of 10 mL/kg. Inspiratory pressures should not exceed 30 cm water.

Positive end-expiratory pressure (PEEP)

PEEP leaves a constant pressure on the lungs at the end of expiration, preventing the collapse of alveoli. Constant opening and closing of alveoli can damage them. Using PEEP may prevent further lung injury as well as maintaining functional residual capacity. As noted earlier, PEEP has a positive effect on oxygenation. However PEEP has a negative effect on cardiac output, because high intrathoracic pressures impede venous return. High levels of PEEP may not be tolerated in haemodynamically unstable patients. Another factor to be considered is 'auto-PEEP'. This is the pressure difference between the alveoli and the proximal airway at end-expiration, which can be raised in conditions with air-trapping, such as severe asthma. 'Auto-PEEP' can contribute to haemodynamic instability in some patients. Prolonging expiration may help to reduce air-trapping in affected patients.

Choosing a level of PEEP

PEEP of 5 cm water is tolerated by most patients. In patients with severe lung disease, increases in PEEP up to about 12 cm of water may be needed. PEEP may not be tolerated in patients with haemodynamic instability. Another group of patients who may not tolerate PEEP are those with raised intracranial pressure. In some cases the reduction in cerebral venous return may be enough to exacerbate the increase in intracranial pressure.

Special situations

Asthma

Use low respiratory rates with a prolonged expiratory phase to limit gas-trapping. Auto-PEEP may be significant, so additional PEEP may lead to hypotension. Avoid large tidal volumes. Permissive hypercapnia may be needed.

Raised intracranial pressure

Avoid hypercapnia. Maintain a $PaCO_2$ between 30 and 35, using end-tidal monitoring and arterial blood gases (ABGs). High levels of PEEP should be avoided.

Adult respiratory distress syndrome (ARDS)

ARDS is a difficult problem. The ideal ventilatory strategy is controversial. In the emergency department the key points are (a) to avoid barotrauma by using small tidal volumes and avoiding high airway pressures; (b) to use PEEP as tolerated and tolerate a high $PaCO_2$. Paralysis may be necessary. Frequent adjustments to tidal volume and respiratory rate may be needed.

Troubleshooting

- Ask for advice early.
- Never assume the monitor is the thing not working.
- If there is difficulty ventilating the patient, immediately remove the patient from the circuit and commence bag ventilation with 100% oxygen. Check the endotracheal tube (ETT) for kinking, displacement (in or out), obstruction and leaking. Examine the patient for equal and adequate breath sounds. Check the trachea is midline. If breath sounds are diminished, suction for mucous plugs and consider treating for a pneumothorax. Treat bronchospasm or pulmonary oedema if present. Get a chest X-ray. Consider bronchoscopy.
- If all of the above are normal, the problem may be with the machine. The ventilator may be disconnected (from the circuit, the gas supply or the power supply). There may be leaks in the tubing or valves, or tubing may be obstructed. Consider changing the circuit.

Non-invasive ventilation

Non-invasive ventilation using positive pressure via a face or nasal mask has become widely used in emergency departments. Most commonly a bi-level positive airway pressure (BiPAP) machine is used, although conventional pressure cycled ventilators can also be used.

The machine delivers a constant low level of positive pressure, which is increased upon sensing the patient's inspiratory effort. This increased inspiratory pressure is equivalent to pressure support ventilation, but when setting the machine the inspiratory positive airway pressure (IPAP) should be set at a level equal to the sum of PEEP and pressure support (e.g. an IPAP of 15 and an expiratory positive airway pressure (EPAP) of 5 is equivalent to pressure support of 10 and PEEP of 5).

Indications

1. Acute respiratory failure due to pulmonary oedema, CAL, asthma, pneumonia.
2. Chronic respiratory failure due to neuromuscular conditions.
3. Obstructive sleep apnoea.

Contraindications

1. Apnoea or impending cardiorespiratory arrest.
2. Haemodynamic instability.
3. Risk of aspiration.
4. Decreased level of consciousness.
5. Inability to cooperate with mask.

Problems with BiPAP

Mask may not be tolerated for the following reasons:

1. Skin irritation and pressure necrosis.
2. Conjunctival irritation or injury.
3. Aspiration.
4. Gastric over distension.
5. Hypotension due to raised intrathoracic pressure.
6. Progressive respiratory failure despite BiPAP, which is an indication for intubation.

PROCEDURAL SEDATION (Judy Alford)

Procedural sedation (also known as conscious sedation) refers to administration of sedative drugs to facilitate performance of a distressing or painful procedure. The level of sedation required varies with the procedure and the individual patient. The level of sedation falls short of general anaesthesia. The patient should retain the ability to respond to stimulus and airway reflexes should be maintained.

Indications

Procedures involving significant pain and/or anxiety are tolerated to varying degrees by individual patients. For example, a child may require sedation for wound suturing where an adult may not.

Nearly all patients

Procedures requiring sedation in nearly all patients include:

1. Reduction of dislocations of large joints.
2. Reduction & splinting of long bone fractures.
3. Cardioversion.

Some patients

Procedures requiring sedation in some patients include:

1. Lumbar puncture.
2. Central line insertion.
3. Lumbar puncture.
4. Wound suturing.
5. Foreign body removal.
6. Burn dressing.
7. Chest drain insertion.

Requirements

Procedural sedation should be undertaken in an area with working suction and oxygen. Pulse oximetry should be used. Continuous ECG and blood pressure monitoring may be used in selected patients (e.g. older or with cardiac history). Ready access to resuscitation equipment and emergency drugs is essential. At least one person should be present who has skills to manage any complications, including airway obstruction and cardiac arrest.

Fasting status does not necessarily preclude the use of sedation, but does influence the depth of sedation induced.

Drugs

The ideal drug for procedural sedation has rapid onset and offset, has no significant side effects, preserves airway reflexes and is easily titrated. Some commonly used agents are found in Table 2.2.

Aftercare

Patients should be monitored until they have emerged from sedation. It is not uncommon for patients to become more deeply sedated once painful stimulus has ceased.

Table 2.2 Drugs used in conscious sedation

Drug	Dose	Duration
Midazolam	0.02–0.1 mg/kg IV 0.05 mg/kg PO (onset about 20 minutes)	30 minutes IV, 45–60 minutes PO
Fentanyl	2–3 μg/kg IV	20–30 minutes
Propofol	0.2 mg/kg IV	10 minutes
Ketamine	1–2 mg/kg IV 3–5 mg/kg IM	15 minutes IV 30 minutes IM
Nitrous oxide	Given as 30–50% mix in oxygen Causes expansion of gas-filled structures (e.g. pneumothorax)	5 minutes

Patients should not be discharged from the emergency department until they have returned to their baseline mental state, are ambulant and have safe transport and supervision. Patients with poor social circumstances may require a longer period of observation.

EDITOR'S COMMENT

In the management of an urgent airway problem, always have a back-up plan in case the current manoeuvre is unsuccessful.

RECOMMENDED READING

Bongard FS, Sue DY. Current critical care diagnosis and treatment. 2nd edn. McGraw-Hill: Lange; 2002.
Emergency Life Support Manual. Emergency Life Support (ELS) Course Inc.
Finucane BT, Santora AH. Principles of airway management. 2nd edn. St Louis: Mosby; 1996.
Marx JA et al, eds. Rosen's emergency medicine: concepts and clinical practice. 5th edn. St Louis: Mosby; 2001.
Roberts JR, Hedges JR. Clinical procedures in emergency medicine. 3rd edn. Philadelphia: WB Saunders; 1997.
Tintinalli JE, Kelen GD, Stapczynski JS. Emergency medicine: a comprehensive study guide. American College of Emergency Physicians. 6th edn. New York: McGraw-Hill; 2003.

3 | Resuscitation procedures

Drew Richardson

This chapter gives a brief overview of major procedures that may be carried out in the emergency department. It is meant to be used as a reminder for a doctor who has already been trained in these techniques, and not as a training manual. The common procedures should be practised under supervision, and the uncommon procedures should be formally taught before they are attempted solo.

For all procedures, the following is essential.

1. Appropriate sterile technique and standard precautions. Minimally invasive procedures such as peripheral intravenous access require only gloves and a clean technique, but for more invasive procedures formal sterile technique with a sterile field, appropriate drapes, gown, gloves, mask and eye protection are mandatory. Less formal technique may be

acceptable only when the procedure is required within seconds (e.g. cricothyroidotomy or emergency department thoracotomy) and full protection for the staff must still be observed.

2. Obtain the patient's informed consent whenever possible. The level of explanation obviously varies with the invasiveness of the procedure and the urgency of the patient's condition, but all conscious patients should give their consent (even if only implied).

3. Ensure the patient's comfort and the safety of all parties by using appropriate analgesia and, if necessary, sedation. Do not attempt difficult procedures on patients who are unable or unwilling to lie still.

4. Ensure continuing care and resuscitation of the patient, particularly during long procedures, using other staff and patient monitoring throughout.

INTRAVASCULAR ACCESS TECHNIQUES

There are four basic intravascular access techniques:

1. Indwelling metal needle, now used only rarely and in peripheral sites, e.g. 'a butterfly'.

2. Catheter over needle technique, such as common intravenous cannula.

3. Catheter through needle technique, now used less often. A large-bore needle is inserted into the relevant vessel, and a smaller catheter advanced up the needle, usually into a central vein. The metal needle is then withdrawn and rendered safe in a plastic guard. This technique carries the disadvantage of a small-bore catheter and the risks of catheter tip embolisation with poor technique and ongoing ooze due to the diameter difference.

4. Seldinger technique, now widely accepted for all large or long intravascular lines. The vessel is punctured with a long needle on a syringe, and a flexible guidewire passed down the needle (often through the syringe). The syringe and needle are removed, and appropriate dilators passed over the wire, and then removed. The catheter is passed over the wire into the vessel, and the wire then removed. With this technique it is important to:
   a. check and understand the equipment before starting (various sets are available);
   b. have cardiac monitoring in place if the wire is to be near the heart;
   c. secure the catheter properly (usually by stitching);
   d. above all, never let go of the wire.

Intravenous lines—peripheral

Indications

1. Administration of fluid—resuscitative and/or maintenance.
2. Administration of drugs.
3. Obtaining blood (rare).

Contraindications

1. Overlying skin damage (e.g. burns) or infection.
2. Venous damage proximal to the insertion site.
3. Arteriovenous (AV) fistula in the limb.

Technique

1. Apply a venous tourniquet.
2. Identify a suitable vessel, ideally as peripheral as possible. Start looking on the back of the hands. Use cubital fossa veins only when large-volume resuscitation is required or other sites have proven unsuitable.
3. Prepare the area with a disinfectant-soaked swab, swabbing in a distal direction.
4. Stretch the skin slightly over the vein.
5. Insert the needle, bevel upwards, until a flushback is obtained.
6. Advance the catheter over the needle.
7. Remove needle, attach intravenous line or bung, and secure catheter.
8. Check position and patency by infusion or injection to clear blood from the catheter.

Complications

1. Haematoma.
2. Subcutaneous extravasation of fluid.
3. Damage to nearby structures.
4. Interarterial cannulation.

Intravenous lines—paediatric

The choice of a site for intravenous infusion in the neonate or young child should include consideration of the femoral vein in the groin and the scalp veins.

Of these, the femoral vein is probably the best to use in the critically ill child. Although no tourniquet can be applied, the vein is reliably located medial to the femoral artery pulse, just below the inguinal ligament.

The scalp veins can be rendered more visible by use of a rubber band tourniquet around the head and are entered in the usual fashion. Always inject saline and check for blanching to exclude arterial puncture. Careful strapping and use of a protector (e.g. plastic cup) are essential to avoid displacement of the scalp vein catheter.

Intraosseous infusion—paediatric

Intraosseous infusion is a rapid technique for reliably obtaining vascular access in sick, small children. Blood can usefully be drawn for biochemistry (not haematology) and large volumes of fluid or drug infused. It is highly recommended that this technique be practised on animal bones before it is attempted on a patient.

Indications

1. Critically ill child in urgent need of drug or fluid administration.
2. No other vascular access readily available.

Contraindications

1. Infection at puncture site.
2. Fracture of the bone.
3. Osteogenesis imperfecta.
4. Recent nearby intraosseous puncture (relative contraindication that is likely to lead to extravasation).

Technique

1. Identify infusion site: preferably upper medial surface of the tibia, 1–2 cm distal to the tibial tuberosity, but the lower tibia (at the junction of the medial malleolus and the shaft) may be suitable.
2. Prepare the area with an iodine swab.
3. Insert intraosseous needle (16–18-gauge special needle with stylet) into the bone at 45°, aiming distally. This will require a rotary 'grinding' motion until a 'crunch' is felt as the cortex is penetrated.
4. Remove stylet and attempt to aspirate marrow contents. Success clearly indicates correct placement, but failure sometimes occurs despite placement.
5. Begin infusion or injection of fluids and drugs. Flow should be relatively free.
6. Secure and protect the infusion site.

Complications

1. Extravasation of fluid.
2. Needle blockage.
3. Infection (rare, reduced by good technique and removal as soon as practicable).

Intravenous lines—central

Indications

1. Central venous pressure monitoring.
2. Infusion of concentrated/irritant solutions (e.g. inotropes, parenteral nutrition).
3. Insertion of specialised equipment (e.g. plasma exchange catheter, Swan-Ganz catheter, transvenous pacemaker).
4. Emergency venous access when peripheral access is impossible.

Contraindications

1. Distorted local anatomy.
2. Known or suspected vessel damage (current trauma, previous radiation therapy, previous surgery).
3. Coagulopathy or vasculitis.

4. Inability to provide cardiac monitoring.
5. Pneumothorax is a contraindication to central venous access on the opposite side (risk of bilateral pneumothoraces).

Technique—general

All of the techniques below carry different risks and benefits. All require ongoing cardiac monitoring but the choice of technique should depend on the experience of the operator and the technique favoured in the particular hospital. Remember that the ICU may have to care for 'your' catheter for days or weeks so, if a choice is available, use the method preferred by the inpatient team.

1. Use local anaesthesia liberally, following down the intended track.
2. Have cardiac monitoring in place, and always withdraw the catheter/ wire slightly when arrhythmias (usually ventricular ectopics) occur.
3. After catheter placement, always aspirate each part and then inject adequate saline to clear the line.
4. Secure catheter by stitching and apply dressing.

Complications

1. Arterial puncture. When detected, remove the needle or catheter and apply pressure over the site for a full 10 minutes, followed by arterial observation of the limb.
2. Pneumothorax. Always obtain chest X-ray (CXR).
3. Malposition of catheter tip. Always check X-ray.
   a. Wrong vein—passing into jugular vein to subclavian vein instead of superior vena cava (SVC). This is difficult to reposition without an image intensifier and may require repuncture.
   b. Excessive length—in right atrium or ventricle rather than SVC. The CXR should show that the tip is not below the carina. If it is too low, the catheter can be easily withdrawn.
4. Damage to mediastinal contents. Haemothorax, hydrothorax, arteriovenous fistula, and perforation of any structure in the chest (even an endotracheal cuff has been reported) may occur.
5. Infection.
6. Embolism—of air, wire or catheter parts.
7. Knotting/kinking of catheter.

Subclavian cannulation

Infraclavicular technique

1. Position the patient supine in 15° Trendelenburg with the arm adducted.
2. Enter at the junction of the middle and medial thirds of the clavicle.
3. Aim along the inferior surface of the clavicle towards the suprasternal notch, with a needle bevel facing inferomedially.
4. Advance 1–2 mm after first flush of blood to obtain reliable flow back into the syringe.

Complications

1. Pneumothorax.
2. Arterial puncture.
3. Others as described above.

Supraclavicular technique

1. Position the patient supine in 15° Trendelenburg.
2. Enter the neck just lateral to the lateral border of the clavicular head of sternocleidomastoid and just above the clavicle.
3. Aim approximately at the contralateral nipple with the bevel of the needle towards the patient's toes.
4. Advance 1–2 mm after first flush of blood to obtain reliable flow back into the syringe.

Complications

Although the full range of complications as above is described, they occur significantly less often with the supraclavicular approach.

Internal jugular vein catheterisation

Technique

1. Position head down at 10° and turned slightly away from side of entry.
2. Enter just above the point of the triangle formed by the two heads of sternocleidomastoid and 1 cm lateral to the internal carotid pulsation.
3. Aim parallel to the carotid artery ('straight down the neck').

Complications

1. Arterial puncture.
2. More easily displaced by movement than subclavian lines.
3. Others as above (rare).

CHEST DRAINAGE PROCEDURES

Needle thoracostomy

Needle thoracostomy is performed either with a soft flexible catheter 'over a needle' such as an intravenous cannula, or a specialised drainage set such as 'pneumocath' or 'pleurocath' (catheter through needle). The location depends on the setting and urgency. For a tension pneumothorax, the procedure is performed rapidly and without anaesthetic over the anterior chest wall. For therapeutic drainage of an effusion, it is performed posteriorly, and for aspiration of a simple pneumothorax, laterally or posteriorly.

Indications

1. Tension pneumothorax—drain direct to air.
2. Simple pneumothorax (spontaneous) up to 75% collapse.
3. Pleural effusion—drainage or sampling.

Contraindications

1. Traumatic pneumothorax—(unless tension is present) since tube thoracostomy indicated.
2. Haemothorax.
3. Bleeding dyscrasias (relative).

Technique

1. Check equipment. For drainage of fluid or simple pneumothorax, a large syringe and three-way tap are required in addition to the soft catheter. A syringe is normally attached if an IV cannula is being used.
2. Position the patient:
   a. Lying flat for anterior puncture of tension pneumothorax—2nd interspace, midclavicular line.
   b. Head of bed elevated for lateral puncture of simple pneumothorax—4th–5th interspace, midaxillary line.
   c. Leaning forwards over a pillow for posterior puncture of pleural effusion—8th–10th interspace, midscapular line.
3. Inject local anaesthetic if needed.
4. Insert the needle just over the lower rib of the interspace (in order to avoid the neurovascular bundle that lies beneath the rib above).
5. Aspiration of air/fluid through a cannula or a 'pop' into the pleural space indicates correct placement—advance the catheter and remove the needle.
6. For a tension pneumothorax, leave open and undertake subsequent tube thoracostomy.
7. For other drainage, connect a three-way tap and syringe to the catheter.
8. Aspirate air or fluid, emptying the syringe and sealing the catheter by means of the tap.
9. Remove catheter when aspiration is finished or when the tube thoracostomy is in place.
10. Always obtain repeat chest X-ray.

Complications

1. Damage to local structures—neurovascular bundle, internal thoracic artery (anterior approach).
2. Inadequate drainage due to small size of catheter, adhesions or blockage.
3. Underlying lung damage—a pneumothorax will be created if one is not already present.
4. Infection at the site.

Intercostal catheter—tube thoracostomy

Indications

1. Tension pneumothorax—only after needle thoracostomy.
2. Traumatic pneumothorax.

3. Simple pneumothorax that has not responded to needle drainage or is causing significant respiratory compromise.
4. Haemothorax.
5. Haemopneumothorax.
6. 'Prophylactic' use in the chest trauma patient who is to receive positive pressure ventilation or aeromedical transport. This indication depends on available skills and circumstance.

Contraindications (all relative)

1. Multiple adhesions.
2. Need for immediate thoracotomy.
3. Bleeding dyscrasias.

Technique

1. Provide appropriate sedation/analgesia. The majority of conscious patients will tolerate narcotics well and should receive them.
2. Position the patient:
   a. Elevate head of bed 45° if possible.
   b. Raise the arm on the relevant side over the head and place the fingers behind the head.
   c. Tilt the patient slightly away.
3. Select and mark the site, the fourth or fifth interspace and the midaxillary line, i.e. at the level of the nipple just behind the muscle bulk of the anterior chest wall muscles.
4. Select appropriate tube size, in general the largest reasonable tube (32 Fr to 36 Fr) should be used in adults with haemothorax, but much smaller tubes are appropriate if only air is to be drained.
5. Prepare drainage system—normally disposable plastic sets with an in-built water trap, but bag drainage with some form of flutter valve is often used in the field.
6. Prepare the area and inject local anaesthetic down to the pleura over the line of the rib below.
7. Incise skin 3–4 cm along the line of the rib below.
8. Bluntly dissect through the subcutaneous tissue and muscle layers to the pleura, passing just above the rib to avoid the neuromuscular bundle. A hiss will normally be heard when the pleural space is entered.
9. Enlarge the tract with a finger and insert finger into chest cavity to ensure full penetration and check for adhesions.
10. Insert tube without stylet in one of three ways:
    a. Hold tube and advance through hole manually.
    b. Grasp tip of tube in curved forceps and advance through hole.
    c. Use specially designed forceps (Pollard forceps) to open a path through which the tube is passed.
    Advance the tube upwards for a pneumothorax or downwards and backwards for a haemothorax to at least 3 cm beyond the last lateral hole.

11. Immediately connect the tube to the drainage system. If there is to be any delay, the tube should be clamped for a spontaneously breathing patient, but must not be clamped for a patient who is ventilated. 'Fogging' of the tube normally confirms its location inside the chest cavity.
12. Check that the underwater drain is bubbling or swinging—ask the patient to cough to confirm position. If it is not swinging, rotate the tube or remove and re-insert.
13. Close the skin wound with sutures and stitch the tube in place. Dress the wound and anchor the dressing to the tube.
14. X-ray to check position of tube and re-expansion of pneumothorax or drainage of haemothorax.

Complications

1. Blockage or failure to drain due to blood clots, position against chest wall, multiple adhesions or kinks.
2. Puncture of solid organs. Should not occur if stylet is not used and technique is followed, even in the presence of diaphragmatic hernia.
3. Reverse flow. Keep drainage bottle below patient.
4. Re-expansion pulmonary oedema.
5. Local injury or infection.
6. Persistent bubbling or failure of re-expansion due to leakage in circuit, intercostal catheter (ICC) drainage hole outside pleural cavity, or (rare) oesophageal rupture/broncopleural fistula.

Pericardiocentesis

Pericardiocentesis is an emergency procedure for the presumed diagnosis of pericardial tamponade, a diagnosis normally made clinically, on the basis of high central venous pressure, hypotension, tachycardia and muffled heart sounds. This is relatively common after penetrating chest trauma, relatively uncommon after blunt chest trauma, and is seen in left ventricular free wall rupture after myocardial infarction. Survival is poor unless the patient is reasonably fit and there is access to cardiothoracic surgery facilities. Diagnosis may also be made by echocardiography, which is gradually becoming available in the emergency setting.

Indications

1. Diagnostic—if the patient is stable, this is not indicated in the emergency department.
2. Pericardial tamponade or suspicion in deteriorating patient.
3. Electromechanical dissociation in cardiac arrest when other causes are excluded. This indication has a low success rate as tamponade is a rare cause of cardiac arrest unless there is a sizeable hole in the ventricular wall.

Contraindications

1. Immediate need for thoracotomy, particularly in cases of trauma.
2. Stable patient—seek echocardiographic evidence before proceeding.
3. Prolonged cardiac arrest when good outcome is not possible.

Technique

1. Position—head up at 45°.
2. Pass a nasogastric tube if abdominal distension present.
3. Prepare equipment—syringe, three-way tap and large needle. Ideally an insulated 10 cm needle, purpose-designed for such taps, or a pericardial catheter ('catheter over a needle') should be used. However, when the diagnosis is clear or when the patient is in cardiac arrest, then a large needle or large-bore IV catheter may be used. The metal hub of the needle should be attached to a V lead of the ECG monitor, and monitoring must be ongoing through the procedure.
4. Approach—insert needle between xiphoid process and left costal margin at 30–45° advancing towards the left shoulder.
5. The pericardium is normally entered 6–8 cm below the skin, and any fluid will be aspirated. If the needle touches the epicardium, an injury current with high ST segment should be seen on the ECG. In this case, withdraw the needle a few millimetres.
6. Aspirate with a syringe, using the three-way tap to disperse the contents if necessary. If a catheter has been inserted, withdraw the needle and re-connect the catheter to the tap.
7. Withdraw whatever fluid can be obtained, but if blood continues to flow freely, suspect ventricular penetration. Pericardial fluid may have a lower haematocrit than blood and may not clot, but neither of these tests is absolutely reliable or helpful within the first few minutes of aspiration.
8. If a response is obtained, leave the catheter in place and be prepared to re-aspirate prior to a thoracotomy.
9. Perform chest X-ray after the procedure to check for a pneumothorax.

Complications

1. Myocardial damage—ventricular puncture or coronary artery laceration.
2. Arrhythmias—ventricular ectopics, ventricular fibrillation (VF), cardiac arrest.
3. Pneumothorax or lung laceration.
4. Air embolism if accidental injection of air occurs.
5. Local infection.

URINARY CATHETERISATION

Indications

1. Urinary retention.
2. Monitoring of urinary output.
3. Drainage of neurogenic bladder.

4. Diagnostic urinary specimen.
5. Preoperative procedure for pelvic surgery.
6. Management of the unconscious patient.

Contraindications

1. Clinical suspicion of urethral injury—if there is a perineal haematoma and blood at the meatus, then an ascending urethrogram should be performed to identify urethral damage and/or a suprapubic catheter used as an alternative.
2. Urinary tract infection (UTI)—relative contraindication as introducing a foreign body to an infected area is undesirable.

Technique—males

1. Position—supine.
2. Prepare penis using no-touch technique, retracting the foreskin in and swabbing the glans and surrounding areas. Drape with a fenestrated sheet and repeat swab.
3. Instil lignocaine gel into urethral opening while holding the penis in the 'dirty' hand. From this point on, the hand holding the penis should be considered 'dirty' and only the other hand should touch the tray and catheter equipment.
4. After a delay for the gel to take effect, hold the catheter in forceps and insert into the bladder to a distance of 20–25 cm.
5. Inflate the catheter balloon using 5–10 mL sterile saline.
6. Check for free flow of urine and collect a specimen if necessary.
7. Connect an appropriate drainage bag.

Technique—females

1. Position—supine with heels drawn up and thighs abducted.
2. Prepare external genitalia by swabbing and drape with a fenestrated sheet. Separate labia with gauze squares and identify urinary meatus and re-swab.
3. Apply sterile lubricant liberally to the catheter.
4. Insert catheter into bladder using forceps, to a distance of 10–12 cm.
5. If catheter is to be left indwelling, inflate balloon with 5–10 mL sterile saline.
6. Collect any specimens necessary and connect appropriate drainage bag.

Complications—both sexes

1. Failure to catheterise:
   a. Inability to identify urethra (females). The urinary orifice is frequently displaced by gynaecological surgery or obscured by oedematous tissue. A more thorough examination, repositioning and better light are appropriate.

b. Strictures of the urethra. Excessive force should not be used, but a smaller catheter may be tried.

c. Prostatic obstruction—this is commonly the indication for catheterisation. Once again, a small catheter, and possibly an introducer, should be tried.

2. Trauma—creation of false passage, partial or complete urethral tear, long-term risk of stricture.
3. Infection—urethritis, epididymitis, pyelonephritis.
4. Haemorrhagic cystitis—rare complication of rapid decompression of a chronically distended bladder.
5. Paraphimosis in males—always replace a retracted foreskin.

Removal of trapped urinary catheter

Emergency medicine doctors may be called upon to remove a urinary catheter that is either blocked and unable to be removed or simply 'stuck' at a time of routine removal. The usual cause is a 'flap valve' in the balloon tubing, which prevents balloon deflation.

Various techniques are described. Cutting the catheter is rarely effective, since the blockage is usually proximal. If the patient's bladder is not excessively distended and the catheter balloon definitely lies within the bladder, the balloon may be overinflated with sterile water or saline until it bursts. If there is doubt about the position of the balloon, ultrasound should be used to identify it, since it must not be overinflated in the urinary tract. The balloon within the bladder can also be punctured using a suprapubic needle.

SUPRAPUBIC CYSTOSTOMY

Indications

1. As for urinary catheter, but catheter cannot be passed due to a suspected or definite urethral trauma.
2. Failed catheterisation, usually strictures or prosthetic disease.
3. Other reasons, such as blockage of an existing catheter.

Contraindications

1. Previous lower abdominal surgery/scarring/radiation.
2. Inability to palpate the bladder.
3. Bleeding diathesis.
4. Urinary tract infection.

Technique

1. Check equipment—a number of suprapubic catheter sets are available, mostly relying on a variant of the 'catheter over the needle' technique.
2. Position patient supine.

3. Inject local anaesthetic starting 2–3 cm above the symphysis pubis and heading down the expected track at approximately 20° towards the pelvis. When urine is drawn back into the anaesthetic syringe, the bladder has been reached.
4. Incise the skin with an appropriate scalpel blade.
5. Puncture the bladder down the same track used for the anaesthetic.
6. Follow appropriate technique to secure the catheter in the bladder. This varies between suprapubic catheter sets.
7. Collect any necessary specimens and connect the catheter to an appropriate drainage bag.
8. Apply adhesive and/or sutures as appropriate to maintain the catheter in place.

Complications

1. Failure to catheterise the bladder. If there is any doubt, ultrasound-guided catheterisation is essential.
2. Bowel perforation.
3. Extravasation of urine—intraperitoneal or extraperitoneal.
4. Local bleeding—intraperitoneal, extraperitoneal, or into bladder.
5. Infection.
6. Obstruction.

PERITONEAL LAVAGE

Indication

Cardiovascular instability in a patient with potential abdominal injury in whom other investigative measures, such as computerised tomography (CT) scan, are inappropriate or unavailable.

Note: Peritoneal lavage is now rarely used in emergency medicine. Although it is an effective screening technique, and is very sensitive for the presence of intraperitoneal blood, it lacks specificity, and its use as the primary investigation for abdominal trauma will result in relatively more negative laparotomies. Specific investigations such as CT scan are more appropriate.

Contraindications

1. Any indication for urgent laparotomy.
2. Significant scarring from previous abdominal or pelvic operations.
3. Pregnancy.
4. Morbid obesity.
5. Severe fractured pelvis. This is a relative contraindication because sufficient blood to cause a positive test often leaks into the peritoneum without any other intraabdominal injury.

6. Facilities for laparotomy unavailable. It is of no benefit to perform a peritoneal lavage and then have to transport the patient to another centre. The lavage fluid will simply further confuse the clinical picture.

Technique

1. Position—supine, preferably on tilting table.
2. Ensure urinary catheter and nasogastric tube are in situ and draining.
3. Prepare the abdomen (including shaving midline below umbilicus).
4. Anaesthetise with lignocaine and adrenaline in the midline below the umbilicus.
5. Incise the skin vertically for 3 cm. Continue the incision down to the linear alba and secure haemostasis.
6. Use an assistant or self-retaining retractor to hold the wound open.
7. Incise the fascia and peritoneum, grasping fascial edges with clamps to provide countertraction. The incision in the peritoneum needs to be only 5 mm long.
8. Insert the catheter into the peritoneum and advance downwards towards the pelvis.
9. Aspirate the catheter with a syringe.
10. If syringe aspiration negative, instil 10 mL/kg warmed saline.
11. Agitate the abdomen and briefly tilt the patient's head down if possible.
12. Lower the IV bag to the floor to siphon fluid out.
13. Send fluid for testing. A positive test is indicated by aspiration of more than 10 mL gross blood or obvious enteric contents initially, or by analysis of the fluid showing greater than 100,000 red blood cells per cubic millimetre, greater than 500 white blood cells per cubic millimetre or presence of bacteria/vegetable fibres. As a practical guide, if newsprint cannot be read through the IV set, then the test is regarded as positive.
14. Remove the catheter and close the wound unless the patient is to have immediate laparotomy.

Complications

1. Local bleeding and infection.
2. Perforation of intraperitoneal or retroperitoneal contents, including bowel, mesentery, vessels, bladder, uterus.
3. Peritonitis (usually due to bowel perforation).

ENDOTRACHEAL INTUBATION

Endotracheal intubation is an important part of airway management. The full range of airway management procedures is described in Chapter 2.

NON-INVASIVE VENTILATORY SUPPORT

Non-invasive techniques reduce the need for endotracheal intubation in some patients with respiratory failure. There are many different types, so knowing how to use the equipment available is critical. The procedure is usually simple and the benefit comes from ongoing treatment and monitoring.

Indications

1. Cardiogenic pulmonary oedema (continuous positive airway pressure, CPAP).
2. Exacerbation of chronic airways limitation (biphasic support, BiPAP).
3. Other causes of respiratory failure that are unresponsive to therapy and with no contraindication.

Contraindications

1. Absolute indication for intubation (e.g. risk of airway obstruction).
2. Inability to fit mask securely (e.g. abnormal anatomy).
3. Uncooperative patient.
4. Claustrophobia.

Technique

1. Ensure resuscitation and oxygenation continue while equipment is fully set up and tested.
2. Set appropriate starting levels of support and oxygenation. This is usually by protocol, with CPAP commonly beginning at around 5 cm water and oxygen concentration starting high (>50%) in pulmonary oedema but lower (30–40%) in chronic lung disease.
3. Rapidly apply the mask and remove previous oxygen therapy, ensuring snug fit of mask.
4. Continue monitoring and adjust parameters to patient's response.

Complications

1. Hypotension due to decreased venous return.
2. Pulmonary barotrauma such as pneumothorax (same as other forms of ventilation).
3. Excessive oxygenation—requires monitoring to prevent hypercarbia in chronic lung disease.

CRICOTHYROIDOTOMY

Indications

1. Supralaryngeal airway obstruction when tracheal intubation not possible (e.g. epiglottitis, burns, facial trauma).
2. Ventilatory support required (e.g. apnoea) and tracheal intubation failed.

Technique

1. Position the patient supine with the neck extended if possible.
2. Identify the cricothyroid membrane as a horizontal depression in the midline anteriorly between the notch of the thyroid cartilage and the cricoid cartilage. Prepare the area.
3. Make a 1.5 cm incision across the lower half of the cricothyroid membrane, then incise the membrane. This is best done with a guarded scalpel blade, usually supplied in cricothyroidotomy kits. However, it can be accomplished with any scalpel.
4. Open the cricothyroidotomy by dilating with artery forceps or gently twisting the scalpel blade.
5. Insert the tube (either a 6 mm cuffed endotracheal tube for an adult, or a 4.5 mm uncuffed cricothyroidotomy tube) in a downward direction.
6. Remove trocar, secure tube and ventilate the patient.
7. Check ventilation in the same way as for endotracheal intubation.

Complications

1. Local bleeding—external or into the airway.
2. Creation of a false passage.
3. Damage to larynx, trachea, oesophagus.
4. Local infection.

LUMBAR PUNCTURE
Indications

1. Clinical suspicion of central nervous system (CNS) infection, particularly meningitis.
2. Clinical suspicion of subarachnoid haemorrhage when CT scan unavailable or CT scan negative.
3. Sample of cerebrospinal fluid (CSF) required for non-emergent evaluation (e.g. Guillain-Barré syndrome).
4. Therapeutic—drainage of CSF or installation of chemotherapy.

Contraindications

1. Clinical or CT evidence of raised intracranial pressure or localising signs.
2. Infected site of puncture.
3. Bleeding diathesis.

Technique

1. Position the patient in the lateral recumbent position with knees drawn up. Mark the L4 spinous process which is palpable in a line connecting the posterior-superior iliac crests.
2. Prepare and drape the area.

3. Infiltrate local anaesthetic in L3/L4 or L4/L5. Gently insert a spinal needle in the midline. A non-cutting needle with side port is preferred, in which case the skin may need to be punctured first with a sheath. If a cutting needle is used, position the bevel horizontal. After penetrating the skin, aim approximately for the patient's umbilicus.
4. Advance, feeling for the loss of resistance as the needle penetrates the ligamentum flavum.
5. Remove the stylet to check for CSF flow. If the subarachnoid space has not been reached, carefully re-insert the stylet and continue.
6. When CSF is obtained, connect a manometer to measure CSF pressure and then collect a sample, normally into three sterile bottles.
7. Remove the needle and dress the site.

Note: The CSF pressure is of little diagnostic significance in the emergency department setting. If lumbar puncture is unsuccessful in the lateral recumbent position, it is appropriate to sit the patient up, leaning forward over a pillow. This position makes the procedure easier and is routinely used to administer spinal anaesthetics, although it does not allow manometry.

Complications

1. CSF infection—rare but potentially fatal.
2. Spinal cord or corda equina damage—should not occur if performed at the correct level.
3. Uncal herniation is described after lumbar puncture in cases with raised intercranial pressure.
5. Post – lumbar puncture headache.

EMERGENCY DEPARTMENT THORACOTOMY

Emergency department thoracotomy should be considered only if the operator is experienced, there is some hope of meaningful survival based on the patient's presentation, and facilities exist for rapid removal of the patient to a thoracic operating facility.

Indications

1. Penetrating chest trauma with all of the following:
   a. Signs of life present during pre-hospital phase.
   b. Any pneumothorax drained.
   c. Pericardiocentesis undertaken.
   d. Fluid load given.
   e. Continued poor response—in cardiac arrest or cardiac arrest clinically imminent.
2. Blunt trauma—only when signs of life have been present in the emergency department, no other lethal injuries (e.g. severe head injury) are present, no response to standard resuscitation, and electrical cardiac activity is still present.

Note: Even in these circumstances, the response rate to emergency department thoracotomy in blunt form is exceedingly low. The aim of emergency department thoracotomy is to drain pericardial tamponade, repair cardiac lacerations, or cross-clamp the aorta. Internal cardiac massage or internal defibrillation may be performed but do not constitute indications for thoracotomy alone.

Contraindications

1. Inadequately skilled personnel.
2. Thoracic operating theatre not available.
3. 'Medical' cardiac arrest.

Technique

1. Patient normally supine, intubated, undergoing CPR.
2. Prepare the left side of the chest.
3. Incise along the top of the left 5th rib down to the chest wall muscles. Begin 2 cm lateral to the sternum and extend beyond the posterior axillary line.
4. Dissect through the intercostal muscles into the pleura with Mayo scissors, stopping ventilation so that the lung collapses momentarily. Divide the intercostal muscles with a sweep of the Mayo scissors along the top of the 5th rib.
5. Insert rib spreaders with a handle and ratchet bar downwards and retract the ribs.
6. If pericardiotomy is required (history consistent with pericardial tamponade, pericardium swollen and tense), perform it with scissors starting at the diaphragm and moving upwards, 1 cm anterior to the phrenic nerve. Use fingers to gently sweep clots of blood from the pericardium.
7. If direct cardiac compression is required, use two hands anterior and posterior to the heart to gently compress.
8. If aortic cross-clamping is required, this is difficult to perform with a vascular clamp since the aorta must be separated from the oesophagus. It is easier to apply pressure through the pleura to compress the aorta against the thoracic spine.
9. Repair of lacerations in the myocardium is particularly difficult in the emergency setting, but may be attempted if necessary.
10. Proceed immediately to the operating theatre for further definitive treatment.

EDITOR'S COMMENT

Most problems arise when procedures are ill-prepared and done in haste.

RECOMMENDED READING

Roberts JR, Hedges JR. Clinical procedures in emergency medicine. 3rd edn. Philadelphia: WB Saunders; 1997.

Marx JA et al. Rosen's emergency medicine, concepts and clinical practice. 5th edn. St Louis: Mosby; 2001.

Tintinalli JE, Kelen GD, Stapczynski JS. Emergency medicine. A comprehensive study guide. 6th edn. New York: McGraw-Hill; 2003.

4 | Ultrasound in emergency medicine

Andrew Finckh and Gordian W O Fulde

Emergency department ultrasound is an area of rapidly expanding importance in the practice of emergency medicine. It is a safe and reliable technology that is relatively inexpensive and easily learned. Accompanying the developing acceptance and widening applications of emergency department ultrasound is an improvement in ultrasound technology, with more powerful and portable machines and an increasing focus on development of adjuncts for the performance of emergency department specific procedures.

The Australasian College for Emergency Medicine (ACEM) supports the use of ultrasound in the emergency department and indeed advocates the availability of timely ultrasound examinations around the clock. While emergency department ultrasound continues to expand and is an application limited only by the expertise of the clinician, the ACEM promotes the ability of the emergency physician and trainee to perform focused emergency department ultrasound examinations on trauma patients (focused assessment with sonography in trauma, or FAST) and on patients with suspected abdominal aortic aneurysm. The advantages of ultrasound examinations in these clinical cases have been clearly established.

BASIC PHYSICAL PRINCIPLES

'Ultrasound' is a sound whose frequency is above the range of human hearing.

The frequency of audible human range is 20–20,000 hertz (Hz), while that of diagnostic ultrasound is 1–20 megahertz (MHz), 3–12 MHz being the most common range.

Propagation of sound is the transfer of energy, not matter, from one place to another within a medium. Some of that energy is imparted to the medium.

Frequency and wavelength

Frequency and wavelength are inversely related. The higher the frequency, the shorter the wavelength. The shorter the wavelength, the less the tissue penetration but the greater the resolution and, therefore, the clearer the image.

Piezoelectric effect

Artificially grown crystals are commonly used for modern transducers. These are treated with high temperatures and strong electric fields to produce the piezoelectric properties necessary to generate sound waves. These properties mean that when a crystal in the ultrasound transducer has an applied voltage, the crystal is deformed and produces a pressure, i.e. the transducer sends an ultrasound. Conversely an applied pressure received by the transducer deforms the crystal to produce a voltage. This voltage is then analysed by the system. In essence, the piezoelectric crystal acts as both speaker and microphone.

Most transducers use many small crystal elements for the formation of each pulse.

Image resolution

Resolution is the ability to distinguish between echoes. It is clearly an important characteristic of an ultrasound machine. There are three kinds of image resolution.

1. **Contrast resolution** is the ability of an ultrasound system to differentiate between tissues with varying characteristics, e.g. between liver and spleen.
2. **Temporal resolution** is the ability of an ultrasound system to show changes in the underlying anatomy over time. This is particularly important in echocardiography.
3. **Spatial resolution** is the ability of an ultrasound system to detect and display structures that are close together. Spatial resolution can be axial or lateral:
   a. **Axial resolution** is the ability to display small targets along the path of the beam as separate entities. The most important determinant of this is the length of the pulse used to form the beam. The shorter the pulse length, the better the axial resolution. Simply put, the higher-frequency probes have better axial resolution but lower penetration.
   b. **Lateral resolution** is the ability to distinguish between two separate targets perpendicular to the beam. The wider the beam, the poorer the lateral resolution. Correct positioning of the focal zones is critical to gaining the best lateral resolution for a given transducer.

Interaction of sound with tissue

Attenuation is the term used to describe the factors affecting the echoes returning to the transducer.

The four main processes in attenuation are:

1. **Reflection.** This occurs at interfaces between soft tissues of differing acoustic impedance. Impedance is the resistance to propagation of sound. The percentage of the sound reflected is dependent on the magnitude of the impedance mismatch and the angle of approach to the interface. For example:

Soft tissue to air interface	99% reflected
Soft tissue to bone interface	40% reflected
Liver to kidney interface	2% reflected

2. **Refraction.** This is the deviation in the path of the beam that occurs when the beam passes through interfaces between tissues of differing speeds of sound when the angle of incidence is not 90°.
3. **Absorption.** This is the transfer of some of the energy of the beam to the material through which sound is travelling. It explains why high-frequency transducers cannot be used for examining deep structures within the body.
4. **Scattering.** This is the reflection of sound off objects that are irregular or smaller than the ultrasound beam. It occurs at interfaces within the sound beam path. The scatter pattern relies on the size of the interface relative to the wavelength of the sound.

Artefacts

Ultrasound systems operate on the basis of certain assumptions relating to the interaction of the sound beam with soft tissue interfaces. Some artefacts help ultrasound diagnosis. The common types of artefacts include:

1. **Acoustic shadowing.** This occurs when beam energy attenuation at a given interface is high, such as when an object with high density blocks signal transmission.
2. **Acoustic enhancement.** This occurs when there is an area of increased brightness relative to echoes from adjacent tissues.
3. **Edge shadowing.** This results from a combination of reflection and refraction occurring at the edge of rounded structures. It can be falsely interpreted as acoustic shadowing.
4. **Reverberation artefact.** This results from repeated reflections of sound between two interfaces. It is usually generated by high-level mismatch interfaces when the echo amplitude is very high.
5. **Beam width effect.** This occurs because the ultrasound beam is not a single line, although the system assumes that it is.
6. **Velocity artefact.** This occurs because various tissues have different velocities from the constant velocity assumed by the system. This results in incorrect placement of an object.

7. **Mirror image.** This is where a single image is displayed twice as a result of reflection off an interface.

Types of transducers

Linear and curved array transducers are most commonly used in general ultrasound.

1. A linear array transducer is constructed with multiple small crystal elements arranged in a straight line across the face of the probe. The beam generated by this transducer travels at 90° to the transducer face.

2. A curved array transducer is also constructed with multiple small crystal elements, except that the face of the transducer is convex. This results in a wider field of view at the bottom of the image and narrower image in the near field of view.

CHOICE OF EQUIPMENT

The ultrasound requirements of individual emergency departments vary depending on how the device will be used. For example, the emergency department that intends to limit studies to FAST and abdominal aorta scans will have different requirements from the emergency department that

Table 4.1 Choice of equipment

Type	Essential	Optional	Specialised
Ultrasound system	Variable send and receive focusing Support for flat linear and curved linear transducers Measurement calipers Internal memory	Small footprint intercostal probe Data disc Cineloop facility	Colour/amplitude mapping M-mode Obstetric biometry software package Sector size control Pulsed Doppler control Continuous wave Doppler control Transoesophageal echo facility
Transducers	Multifrequency (2.5–5.0 MHz) curved array Multifrequency (7–10 MHz) linear array (for foreign body and central line access)		Transvaginal probe Cardiac probe Transoesophageal probe
Peripherals	Video recorder hard copy device		

wishes to perform ultrasounds to assess a first trimester pregnancy, locate a foreign body, assess testicular blood flow or obtain central venous access. Not only should the current ultrasound needs of the emergency department be determined but the future needs also. Staff who become competent in the basic applications of ultrasound may wish to extend their skills with time.

Once the present and future ultrasound needs and the budgetary limitations of the emergency department have been determined, the items shown in Table 4.1 should be considered.

Like most emergency department equipment, ultrasound equipment should be assessed for:

1. Machine portability and stability.
2. Machine size. A larger machine may offer more features but be impractical in a resuscitation situation and difficult to store when not in use.
3. Ability to upgrade machine without replacing expensive items.
4. Servicing of machine, including transducers and peripherals.

An increasing number of manufacturers are now providing machines suitable for emergency department ultrasound. Trial of these machines before purchase is an effective way of determining suitability in individual emergency departments.

COMMON APPLICATIONS IN THE EMERGENCY DEPARTMENT

Focused assessment with sonography in trauma (FAST)

In recent years the FAST scan has emerged as a useful diagnostic test in the evaluation of the patient with blunt abdominal trauma (see Figure 4.1). The aim of FAST is to detect fluid as represented by anechoic (black) areas, particularly haemopericardium, haemoperitoneum and haemothorax. Ideally the FAST examination is performed in 5 minutes or less. The advantages and disadvantages of FAST are shown in Table 4.2.

A review of 11 studies has shown FAST to be a highly specific tool, with specificity of 98%. The sensitivity in these studies was 89%. In many trauma

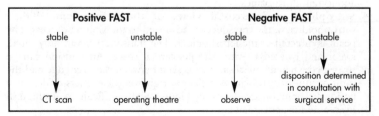

Figure 4.1   Blunt trauma algorithm

Table 4.2 Advantages and disadvantages or limitations of FAST

Advantages	Disadvantages
Safe for operator and patient	Positive examination requires presence of free intraperitoneal fluid (minimum of 600 mL)
Rapid	
Acceptable in the pregnant patient	Not reliable for excluding hollow visceral injury
Non-invasive	Not reliable for grading solid organ injuries
Easily performed and learned	Not reliable for excluding retroperitoneal haemorrhage
Can be performed concurrently with resuscitation	
Can be performed in a resuscitation area (i.e. monitored environment)	Patient anatomy or pathology may make examination technically difficult (obesity or subcutaneous emphysema)
Repeatable (of particular value in the monitoring of non-operative solid organ injuries)	
More cost effective when compared to DPL or CT	
Adult and paediatric application	

centres it has mostly eliminated the initial use of diagnostic peritoneal lavage.

FAST involves a minimum of four views.

1. **The hepatorenal interface (Morison's pouch) and the right diaphragm.** In this view, the transducer is placed at the right midaxillary line between the 11th and 12th ribs. The liver, kidney and diaphragm are viewed. Particular attention is paid to the hepatorenal interface.
2. **The splenorenal interface and left diaphragm.** In this view, the transducer is placed at the right posteroaxillary line (right side) between the 11th and 12th ribs. The spleen, kidney and diaphragm are viewed. The kidney usually lies more cephalad than on the right.
3. **The pouch of Douglas (retrovesical or retrouterine).** Ideally the bladder is full. The transducer is placed approximately 1 cm superior to the pubic symphysis. The examination is performed in both transverse and longitudinal planes.
4. **Subxiphoid or intercostal views of the pericardium.** With a subxiphoid view, the transducer is advanced to the xiphoid process. The beam is directed at the left shoulder. The transducer is variously tilted, swept and rotated to view the pericardial space. An effusion can be suspected when an anechoic area is seen between the liver edge and the right atrium or ventricle. A collapsed right ventricle offers evidence of pericardial tamponade. Clotting blood can be difficult to distinguish from anterior pericardial fat.

Other views include the bilateral paracolic gutters.

The applications of FAST are expanding and include penetrating thoracoabdominal trauma and unexplained hypotension in the trauma patient. The use of ultrasound-guided pericardiocentesis offers a safer therapeutic alternative in the presence of pericardial tamponade than traditional 'blind' methods.

Abdominal aortic scan

This is a continuous ultrasound scan of the aorta in both transverse and sagittal (transverse) planes from the diaphragm to the aortic bifurcation. The study includes measurement of the maximum aortic diameter in both planes.

If an aneurysm is present several additional items need to be assessed, including:

1. Proximal edge, especially relationship of aneurysm to origin of renal arteries.
2. Distal extent, especially relationship to origin of common iliac arteries.
3. Presence of thrombus.
4. Presence of dissection.
5. True aneurysmal diameter (outside to outside edge).
6. Residual lumen diameter.
7. Presence of haematoma surrounding the rupture.
8. Presence of free intraperitoneal fluid.

The presence of an abdominal aortic aneurysm (AAA) on ultrasound in the unstable patient confirms the need for laparotomy.

Indications for ultrasound to detect AAA include presence of syncope, shock, hypotension, abdominal pain, abdominal mass, and flank pain or back pain, especially in the older patient.

OTHER EVOLVING APPLICATIONS

1. Pregnancy:
   a. First trimester pelvic ultrasound to establish the location of the pregnancy and fetal heart rate in the symptomatic pregnant patient or the asymptomatic patient with risk factors for ectopic pregnancy.
   b. Second and third trimester pelvic ultrasound for detection of fetal cardiac movement, location of placenta and the evaluation of the pregnant trauma patient
2. Echocardiography, primarily entailing the assessment of presence of cardiac activity and pericardial effusion.
3. Biliary ultrasound—cholecystitis and cholelithiasis are best imaged with ultrasound.
4. Renal ultrasound—ultrasound images the kidneys well and can be a sensitive bedside test for hydronephrosis.
5. Assessment of above-calf deep venous thrombosis.
6. Procedural uses (see Table 4.3).

Table 4.3 Procedural applications for emergency department ultrasound

Application	Strengths and uses	Limitations
Intravenous lines	Body habitus Anticoagulation Lack of anatomic or palpable landmarks	Vessels may be difficult to visualise without Doppler technology
Bladder size and aspiration	Avoids dry taps Avoids urethral catheterisation	

Abscess location
  and aspiration
	Soft tissue infection without
	  clear fluctuation
		Other sonolucent structures

Thoracocentesis and
  paracentesis
Pericardiocentesis
	Localisation of fluid and
	  avoidance of viscera	

Foreign body localisation	Excellent visualisation in fluid
	  and uniform surrounding
	  tissue	

Lumbar puncture		
Arthrocentesis		

Ultrasound may localise the percutaneous insertion/incision site before the procedure or may provide real-time guidance of the procedure with needle, catheter or other device.

DOCUMENTATION

The results of emergency department ultrasound examinations used to facilitate patient care decisions should be documented in the patient's clinical record.

The following are basic items that should be documented:

1. Type of examination (e.g. FAST).
2. Reason for examination (e.g. blunt abdominal injury).
3. Views obtained. If a printer is attached, hard copies should be obtained and included in the clinical record.
4. Adequacy of views obtained. If inadequate, state reasons.
5. Findings—normal, abnormal or indeterminate.

Findings incidental to the examination should also be documented and the patient informed of them.

A patient undergoing an emergency department ultrasound should be informed that the examination is a focused one directed at determining the presence of specific pathologies or answering a specific clinical question. Radiologists still provide expertise in comprehensive examinations.

INITIAL TRAINING

The format of courses instructing individuals in emergency department ultrasound depends on the number of primary applications being taught. A single day course has proved to be adequate for those learning basic physics, knobology and how to perform FAST and abdominal aorta assessment. Sessions involve scanning live models that may include known pathology.

QUALITY REVIEW AND IMPROVEMENT

Quality review and improvement are important tools for monitoring ongoing performance of emergency physicians undertaking emergency department ultrasounds. The mechanisms for this review may include:

1. Static image review.
2. Videotape review.
3. Digital image review.
4. Clinical outcomes.

CREDENTIALLING PROCESS AND MAINTENANCE OF STANDARDS

The Australasian College for Emergency Medicine (ACEM) has determined the credentialling process that outlines the minimum standards deemed sufficient to maintain a level of competency in emergency department ultrasounds. Once a level of proficiency is attained, ongoing maintenance of standard is essential. ACEM has outlined what is deemed to be a sufficient number and standard of ongoing emergency department ultrasounds to maintain an acceptable quality of examinations. Individual institutions can adopt or adapt these standards according to local needs. An integral component of the credentialling process is a clear statement of the clinical question to be answered, such as:

1. Haemoperitoneum—yes/no.
2. Haemopericardium—yes/no.
3. AAA—yes/no.

A process of measuring and documenting performance, accuracy and image quality is an essential part of continuous quality improvement, e.g. maintaining log books and keeping hard copy images, and regular review with radiology staff.

EDITOR'S COMMENT

Ultrasound will not remain optional for major emergency departments for long.

RECOMMENDED READING

ACEM Policy Document. Credentialling for ED ultrasonography. Online.
    Available: http://www.acem.org.au; July 2000.
ACEM Policy Document. Use of bedside ultrasound by emergency physicians.
    Online. Available: http://www.acem.org.au; July 1999.
ACEP Policy Statement. Use of ultrasound imaging by emergency physicians.
    Online. Available: http://www.acep.org; June 2001.
Australian Institute of Ultrasound. Ultrasound in emergency medicine handbook.
    Mermaid Beach, Queensland: Australian Institute of Ultrasound; 2001.
Eastern Association for Surgery of Trauma (EAST) Practice Management
    Guidelines Work Group. Evaluation of blunt abdominal trauma. Online.
    Available: http://www.east.org; 2001.

5	Physiological monitoring in the emergency department

Mark Gillett

Physiological vital signs are just that—'vital'. Numerous adverse events in emergency departments can be traced back to the failure to elicit initial vital signs and to follow their trends over time, or to misinterpretation or disregard of their significance.

An abnormal pulse rate in an adult is outside the range of 50–100 beats per minute (bpm). Normal values for children are noted in Table 5.1. There is always a reason for an abnormal pulse rate and some causes are life threatening, e.g. pulmonary embolus, occult haemorrhage or complete heart block. A patient with unexplained brady- or tachycardia should never be discharged, even if all other facets of the history, examination and investigations are normal. Observation in the emergency department and discussion with senior colleagues is necessary to elicit a diagnosis.

Respiratory rate is the most often overlooked and poorly taken clinical vital sign. The normal range varies with age (see Table 5.1). Slow ventilation <10/min is always abnormal and may rapidly lead to apnoea. Tachypnoea has multiple causes and should not be assumed to be anxiety unless other causes such as pulmonary embolus and overdose have been considered and excluded. Always take the respiratory rate yourself, as it is remarkable how often the rate of 16 breaths per minute is recorded on observation charts when the true rate is very different.

Table 5.1 Normal vital signs by age

Age (years)	Respiratory rate (breaths per minute)	Heart rate (bpm)	Systolic blood pressure (mmHg)
<1	30–40	110–160	70–90
2–5	25–30	95–140	80–100
6–12	20–25	80–120	90–110
>12	15–20	60–100	100–120

Blood pressure (BP) is the most difficult clinical vital sign to record. The taking of a manual blood pressure is now often superseded by the use of electronic non-invasive blood pressure (NIBP) machines. All NIBP devices should be regarded as random number generators and a manual BP performed on all emergency department patients is regarded as a baseline.

Temperature elevations are rarely overlooked but beware of the hypothermic patient (T ≤35°C) whose temperature may reflect sepsis, especially in groups such as infants, the elderly and others with any kind of immune suppression.

ELECTRONIC MONITORING

Until 15 years ago, any form of electronic monitoring other than continuous electrocardiographic (ECG) tracings was rare. Today any patient undergoing a procedure in the emergency department, or with an acute illness or injury, routinely undergoes electronic monitoring.

The reasons underlying this explosion in technology include:

1. The availability of compact, reliable and affordable monitoring devices.
2. A push towards improved quality of patient care.
3. Fear of litigation.
4. Universal acceptance that all patients with comparable health conditions should receive identical care, regardless of the hospital department in which they are treated.
5. ACHS/College guidelines.

Because of this, we have seen pulse oximetry and, more recently, capnography evolve from luxuries to necessities. Despite this, some physicians argue that there is little proof that monitoring devices enhance outcome. Good studies verifying decreased morbidity and mortality are lacking for many aspects of the use of these devices.

In no circumstances should electronic monitoring replace direct observation of the patient. The devices are prone to both mechanical faults and observer misinterpretation. The extent of monitoring employed should reflect the individual patient's condition.

Future trends include the use of modular systems, facility-wide approaches, and the marriage of physiological monitoring and information systems.

CONTINUOUS ECG MONITORING

The simplest and least invasive form of cardiac monitoring—continuous ECG monitoring—was introduced to emergency departments in the 1960s, following its successful application to the then new coronary care units. It was significantly responsible for the decrease in mortality from early arrhythmias after acute myocardial infarction (AMI). Its indications have widened considerably since then.

In this technique, electrical signals generated by the heart are detected by skin electrodes, conveyed to a high-gain amplifier and displayed on an oscilloscope. These devices may be stand-alone or part of multichannel systems. They can be fixed or portable. Most units employ a three-electrode system with a choice of leads I, II or III. Lead II is most commonly used in order to optimise P wave definition. Praecordial leads are occasionally used, as they may allow identification of ischaemic changes. They should not replace the 12-lead electrocardiogram for definitive diagnostic purposes.

Added features include freeze, print-out, memory, ST segment analysis, central monitoring, alarms and filter capabilities.

NON-INVASIVE BLOOD PRESSURE (NIBP) MONITORING

In 1896, Riva-Rocci first described the use of an inflatable cuff to determine systolic blood pressure by palpation. Two current mechanical ways of measuring blood pressure make use of the Doppler and oscillometric principles.

Oscillometry

Oscillometry is the most commonly used of these technologies (e.g. Dinamap™). It is based on the observation that, as blood flows through an artery, the vessel wall oscillates. The oscillations are transmitted to the overlying cuff and are sensed by pressure transducers. These changes are relayed to a microprocessor in the main unit, which calculates and displays systolic, diastolic and mean blood pressures as well as heart rate.

Ideal units feature high and low alarms for all modalities, record, print, trend and automatic/manual cycling facilities.

Potential problems

1. Systolic blood pressure is the most accurate measurement, followed by the mean pressure. Diastolic measurements are fully derived values and hence are very inaccurate.
2. Systolic values are generally overestimated at low blood pressures and underestimated at high blood pressures.
3. Accuracy is poor in atrial fibrillation and other irregular rhythms, as these units rely on a regular cardiac rhythm.

4. Cuff width is critical—too wide underestimates and too narrow overestimates systolic blood pressure.
5. Cuff movement caused by the patient or staff invalidates measurements.

Caveats

1. Useful in following trends in essentially normotensive patients.
2. Always validate initial NIBP values against a manual measurement. If there is any discrepancy, don't believe the machine!

MONITORING TEMPERATURE

Temperature is one of the most difficult physical signs to record. Gold standard techniques are invasive while non-invasive techniques are prone to inaccuracies. In addition, even the basic question of what is an abnormal temperature range is still controversial, especially in infants.

Devices

Technologies available include thermophototropic devices, thermocouples, thermisters, mercury/glass thermometers and infrared emission detectors (IREDs). The latter three are the most commonly used in the emergency department.

1. **Thermophototropic skin strips** are unreliable, as they readily reflect the environmental temperature.
2. **Thermisters** are very accurate and allow continuous measurements. They can be used by the rectal, oral and oesophageal routes. They suffer from being invasive, expensive and requiring regular calibration.
3. **Mercury thermometers** are cheap, widely available and lend themselves to oral, axillary and rectal readings. Problems include the risk of mucosal damage due to glass breakage, a low limit of only 35°C and a long equilibration time.
4. **IREDs** give rapid, relatively non-invasive measurements. They are limited to the tympanic route, expensive, unreliable in infants and rely significantly on operator technique.

Sites of measurement

Temperature may be measured at multiple body sites, which are (in order of decreasing reliability) oesophageal, tympanic, rectal, oral, axillary and skin. Each site has its own practical advantages and disadvantages:

1. Oesophageal measurements reflect core temperature well, but an invasive thermister probe is needed. They are rarely used in emergency departments.
2. Tympanic measurements reflect core temperature moderately well and are unaffected by local aural inflammatory conditions or the presence of cerumen. There is a potential for mucosal abrasion and/or tympanic membrane rupture.

3. The rectal route reflects core temperature well but faecal insulation may invalidate readings. Problems include a lag time in reflecting core temperature changes and a risk of rectal trauma, profound vagal stimulation and staff infection.
4. The axillary and oral routes can be more than 1°C lower than core temperature. They require significant equilibration time and are susceptible to inaccuracy due to environmental and positional influences.

CAPNOGRAPHY

Capnography refers to the measurement and display of carbon dioxide partial pressure (PCO_2) levels in expired gases. End-tidal CO_2 ($P_{ET}CO_2$) roughly equals alveolar PCO_2 ($PaCO_2$) and therefore arterial PCO_2 ($PaCO_2$). The $PaCO_2/P_{ET}CO_2$ gradient is usually 2–4 mmHg: e.g. $P_{ET}CO_2$ of 36 mmHg equals $PaCO_2$ of 40 mmHg. This relationship is invalid in the presence of a significant pulmonary diffusion defect.

Most devices rely on infrared absorption techniques. Two main types exist, sidestream and mainstream samplers.

1. **Sidestream samplers** draw a continuous gas sample into a measuring cell for analysis. Their advantages include their light weight, adaptors which decrease the risk of endotracheal tube (ETT)/circuit kinking or displacement, and their lower cost. A delay of several seconds in analysis is their disadvantage.
2. **Mainstream samplers** directly straddle the ventilatory circuit between the ETT and the circuit tubing. They give instantaneous readings, but are bulky and may add clinically significant dead space in neonates.

Full capnography comprises real-time analogue or digital display of the CO_2 waveform throughout the respiratory cycle, plus alarms for apnoea and low/high CO_2 measurements. The capnographic waveform itself can give added information, e.g. airway obstruction.

Increased $P_{ET}CO_2$ values are seen with alveolar hypoventilation, malignant hyperthermia, tourniquet release and bicarbonate administration. Low values are associated with hyperventilation, ventilatory circuit leaks/obstruction and low cardiac output states. Capnography's main uses in the emergency department are in the verification of ETT placement and as an aid in determining ventilator parameters in patients undergoing controlled ventilation. In the latter situation, a set of arterial blood gases should be performed to validate the $P_{ET}CO_2$ measurement before the capnography is viewed as reliable. The Australian and New Zealand College of Anaesthetists currently recommends that these devices be used in all intubated and/or ventilated patients from the moment of intubation until extubation.

Colorimetric $P_{ET}CO_2$ devices (mushroom devices) are unreliable owing to subjective colour interpretation and variable reagent lifespan.

PULSE OXIMETRY

Described by some authors as the 'fifth vital sign', pulse oximetry has become a universal monitoring standard in the modern emergency department. Pulse oximeters provide an immediate determination of arterial oxygenation by estimating the colour of arterial blood between a light source and a photodetector. The differential spectral absorption of oxyhaemoglobin (HbO_2) and deoxyhaemoglobin (Hb) at two wavelengths of light, 660 nm (red) and 940 nm (infrared), allows an estimation of the percentage saturation of haemoglobin with oxygen (SaO_2).

Oxygen-haemoglobin dissociation curve

The PaO_2 can be calculated from the SaO_2 by reference to the oxygen-haemoglobin dissociation curve (Figure 5.1). The curve is shifted to the right by increasing PCO_2, increasing temperature and falling pH. Two figures worth committing to memory are:
1. An apparently good SaO_2 of 90% correlates with a PaO_2 of only 60 mmHg.
2. A 50% SaO_2 translates to a very low PaO_2 of 27 mmHg.

Advantages of pulse oximeters

Pulse oximeters are easy to apply, non-invasive and require no regular calibration. They are accurate within the SaO_2 range of 80–100%. The probes are usually placed on fingers or toes, but may be placed more centrally if not reading peripherally. They provide continuous audio and visual displays. All pulse oximeters indicate their sensing of a pulse by

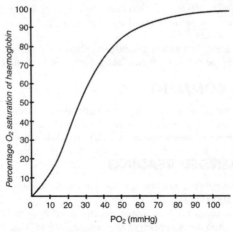

Figure 5.1 Oxygen-haemoglobin dissociation curve

emitting a beep. Most machines make the pitch of this beep proportional to the SaO_2. As the SaO_2 falls, the beep becomes a 'sicker' sound. Ideally all such devices should have alarms for low SaO_2 and low/high pulse rates. Very compact pocket designs are now becoming available.

Disadvantages of pulse oximeters

A number of situations make pulse oximetry unreliable or unusable. These include:

1. Poor peripheral circulation, e.g. shock, cold. Absence of a waveform prevents meaningful results.
2. Patient or probe movement. Most machines indicate malfunction unless movement is rhythmic at around heart rate. In this latter case it may record a false SaO_2.
3. Saturations of less than 80%. These are unreliable as machines are only calibrated between levels of 80% and 100%. Lower levels are extrapolations, which are prone to error.
4. Dyshaemoglobinaemias. Carboxyhaemoglobin (COHb) has similar spectral absorption to HbO_2. Thus haemoglobin saturated with carbon monoxide (CO) is read as HbO_2 giving a falsely high SaO_2. Methaemoglobin has similar absorption at 660 nm and 940 nm, thus giving a value of 85% regardless of the true SaO_2.
5. IV dyes (e.g. methylene blue), bilirubin and nail polish may all interfere with light absorption, causing a lower SaO_2 than is truly present.
6. Electromagnetic interference (e.g. diathermy and cellular phones) causes unreliable measurements.
7. Bright or pulsatile light, especially at physiological frequencies, floods the sensing diode and confounds the results.
8. Shifts in the O_2-Hb dissociation curve (see above) due to pH, PCO_2 and temperature. These alter the PaO_2 for a given SaO_2. However, such changes are rarely clinically significant.
9. Sudden changes in oxygen saturation. These may not be sensed by the device for up to 60 seconds, leading to possible hypoxic organ damage.

EDITOR'S COMMENT

In the majority of patients who 'suddenly' deteriorate, quite abnormal observations are taken and recorded some time before they crash. This provides the basis of intervention by METs (mobile emergency teams).

RECOMMENDED READING

Soubani AO. Noninvasive monitoring of oxygen and carbon dioxide. Am J Emerg Med 2001; 19:141–146.

Lewinter JR, Terndrup TE. Vital sign measurement. In: Roberts JR, Hedges JR, eds. Clinical procedures in emergency medicine. 3rd edn. Philadelphia: WB Saunders; 1997.

6 The patient with chest pain, dyspnoea or haemoptysis

Patricia A Saccasan-Whelan and Anthony J Whelan

Cardiorespiratory disorders are common and are major reasons for patients to present to the emergency department. Accurate and timely diagnosis, treatment and disposition are important to minimise morbidity and mortality. At the same time, the clinician must be aware of the costs associated with inappropriate admission and investigation.

CHEST PAIN

Many patients come to the emergency department with a principal complaint of chest pain. While there are many causes of chest pain, there are a few life-threatening disorders that must be considered in any patient with this as the chief complaint (Table 6.1). Much of the literature is devoted to the diagnosis and management of unstable coronary syndromes, which is appropriate given the prevalence of ischaemic heart disease. In the United States a 'missed diagnosis' of myocardial infarction is the commonest (and most expensive) cause of malpractice proceedings against emergency physicians. Nevertheless, the other important causes must be recalled, particularly in the atypical patient.

Myocardial ischaemia

History

A 'textbook' history suggestive of myocardial ischaemia is highly suggestive of that diagnosis, particularly in middle-aged male patients.

Table 6.1 Causes of chest pain	
Potentially life-threatening	**Not life-threatening**
Acute myocardial infarction	Musculoskeletal pain
Unstable angina	Oesophageal pain
Pulmonary embolism	Pericarditis
Aortic dissection	Pleurisy, pneumonia
Tension pneumothorax	Mitral valve prolapse
Ruptured oesophagus	Herpes zoster

Classical ischaemic pain should be easy to recognise: central, heavy or oppressive chest discomfort, often with radiation to the arms or neck or jaw. Patients prefer to lie still, and there is no relationship to posture, food or the respiratory cycle. The pain may be very distressing but the severity of the discomfort is no guide to the extent of the pathology. Autonomic accompaniments such as nausea and sweating are highly suggestive of myocardial ischaemia, but are non-specific. Heaviness of the arms accompanying chest pain is also very suspicious. A previous history of angina is inconstant, but any preceding symptom exacerbated by exercise should be thoroughly examined. The pain of angina is usually of less than 20 minutes' duration, and may be relieved by nitrates.

Unstable angina and myocardial infarction comprise the acute coronary syndromes. The description of the pain is similar, but the time course and response to nitrates help to distinguish these entities. Recognition of these syndromes is crucial in the evaluation of the patient with chest pain (Table 6.2).

However, atypical presentations are common, particularly in women and those outside the usual age range for ischaemic heart disease. Pain may be felt primarily in the epigastrium, neck or arm without any discomfort in the chest. Some patients deny that they have pain but agree to tightness or heaviness. A high index of suspicion for myocardial ischaemia should be maintained in any patient complaining of chest discomfort of recent origin.

Risk factors

The risk factors for atherosclerosis should be sought, but the presence or absence of risk factors does not rule the diagnosis of myocardial ischaemia in or out. Increasing age and a history of previously proven ischaemic events are the most important risk factors influencing the likelihood of ischaemic heart disease.

Hypertension is the primary risk factor for aortic dissection but a positive family history could suggest a genetic disorder such as Marfan's syndrome.

The risk factors for deep venous thrombosis (hypercoagulability, stasis or damage to the vein wall) should be looked for in the patient presenting with possible pulmonary embolism.

Table 6.2 Unstable angina—Braunwald classification[6]

Class	Description	Risk of AMI/death in next year
I	New onset of exertional angina; angina with less effort; no rest pain	7%
II	Angina at rest within the last month but no pain in last 48 hours	10%
III	Angina at rest in the last 48 hours	11%

Other potentially life-threatening causes of chest pain

Aortic dissection

Aortic dissection is a rare but important disorder that must be promptly recognised in patients presenting with severe chest pain. The pain of aortic dissection is usually of abrupt onset and is maximal from the outset, as opposed to the pain of a myocardial infarction which builds up to crescendo. Dissection pain often radiates to the back, which is unusual in myocardial infarction. The pain is often severe and may require large doses of narcotics for relief. The appearance of a patient with severe pain and a non-specific ECG who appears shocked yet has a high blood pressure is a strong clue to this disorder.

Pneumothorax

Pleuritic chest pain is pain which varies with the respiratory cycle, usually worse with inspiration. Pleuritic chest pain associated with dyspnoea may indicate pneumothorax, due to air in the pleural space. Primary spontaneous pneumothorax is frequently associated with a tall thin body habitus in younger male patients. Secondary spontaneous pneumothorax complicates chronic lung disease, especially chronic obstructive pulmonary disease (COPD) and cystic fibrosis.

Pulmonary embolism

Pulmonary embolism may produce two chest pain syndromes: pleuritic chest pain secondary to pulmonary infarction, or central chest discomfort (suggestive of myocardial ischaemia) associated with dyspnoea and haemodynamic collapse, in massive pulmonary embolism. A predisposing cause can be found in 90% of cases. Nearly all cases of pulmonary embolism are secondary to deep vein thrombosis (DVT). However, clinical examination is relatively insensitive in the detection of DVT.

Ruptured oesophagus

Severe anterior chest pain following vomiting is characteristic of oesophageal perforation (Boerhaave's syndrome). While vomiting may accompany acute myocardial infarction (AMI), it usually follows rather than precedes the onset of chest pain. Oesophageal perforation may also follow instrumentation, especially oesophageal dilatation.

Other causes of chest pain

Pericarditis

Pain is usually felt in the anterior chest and may be severe. Often the pain varies according to posture and the respiratory cycle. A pericardial rub is diagnostic but inconstant.

Reflux

The pain of reflux is usually described as burning, with a 'rising' sensation coming up into the throat. Often there are associated oesophageal symptoms such as odynophagia, dysphagia, belching and waterbrash. Antacids give relief.

Oesophageal spasm

The pain of oesophageal spasm is more severe and may be indistinguishable from myocardial ischaemia. There may even be relief with nitrates.

Chest wall pain

Chest wall pain is the commonest type of chest pain in non-hospitalised patients. Pain is generally well-localised, jabbing or stabbing, and lasts either for a fraction of a second or for hours or days at a time. While a number of syndromes are described, precise diagnosis may not be possible. Pain that comes from 'outside' into the chest like a knife or with a stabbing sensation is unlikely to be due to myocardial ischaemia.

Anxiety

Chest pain may be associated with anxiety states, and is an important component of the hyperventilation syndrome.

Abdominal disease

Upper abdominal disorders such as cholecystitis, peptic ulcer disease and pancreatitis may all be associated with chest pain out of proportion to the abdominal signs. Some of these syndromes may be associated with ECG abnormalities.

Physical examination

A rapid assessment of the patient's general condition is the first step. In general, patients with chest pain should be triaged to a monitored bed for rapid assessment and management. The acutely ill patient with hypotension, or with other important abnormalities of vital signs, must be recognised quickly, IV access obtained and oxygen commenced. In addition look for:

1. Impaired level of consciousness, presence of respiratory distress, diaphoresis, pallor and peripheral hypoperfusion.
2. Signs of cardiac failure. Oedema is relatively non-specific, but a raised jugular venous pressure (JVP) or a third heart sound are very suggestive of cardiac failure.
3. Peripheral pulses. Peripheral vascular disease is strongly associated with coronary artery disease. Compare pulses in both arms and consider blood pressure in both arms if there is a clinical suspicion of aortic dissection.
4. The precordium. Cardiomegaly is an important sign. A fourth heart sound, however, is non-specific particularly in elderly or hypertensive

patients. Murmurs are frequently not contributory but severe aortic stenosis, mitral valve prolapse and hypertrophic cardiomyopathy may be associated with chest pain. A mitral regurgitant murmur that coincides with the patient's pain and disappears with relief of pain is highly significant for high-risk ischaemia. In general, chest wall tenderness in unreliable: it is a common finding and does not necessarily imply a benign cause for the patient's chest pain. A pericardial rub is an important sign but may be transient or positional.

5. The chest. Symmetry of breath sounds and deviation of the trachea should be sought. Look also for crackles, rubs and features of consolidation or pleural effusion.

6. Abdominal tenderness may indicate a non-cardiac cause for the patient's symptoms.

7. Limbs. Look for oedema, pulses and clinical signs of DVT.

Investigations

ECG

All patients complaining of chest pain should have an ECG, and old ECGs should be obtained for comparison. If the initial ECG is unhelpful and symptoms continue, a repeat ECG in 20–30 minutes may be more informative. The ECG helps to triage patients into high, intermediate and low risk for unstable coronary syndromes (see Table 7.1, p 71). ECG patterns are discussed in more detail in other chapters.

Cardiac enzymes

The development of rapid troponin assays has greatly assisted in the assessment of risk in acute coronary syndromes. Cardiac troponins are elements of the contractile apparatus of the muscle, and the two cardiac troponins (I and T) are immunologically distinct from those derived from skeletal muscle. Troponins are thus much more specific than creatine kinase (CK) and older cardiac markers. Troponins are also considerably more sensitive than CK and small increases occur in many acute coronary syndrome patients without a rise in CK.

A rise in troponin is a major risk factor for adverse events in this setting. A rise in the level of troponin I to greater than five times the upper limit of normal indicates a risk of adverse events (death or reinfarction) three to six times higher in the next 30 days than for patients with normal troponins.[1] Two normal troponin values (on admission to the emergency department and 6 hours later) may allow discharge home with safety in patients presenting with chest pain and non-diagnostic ECGs.[2]

Other tests

Bedside transthoracic echocardiography can allow detection of wall motion abnormalities which indicate areas of ischaemia or infarction. Echocardiography may also detect pericardial effusions, aortic dilation or evidence of aortic dissection. The usefulness of transthoracic echocardiography is dependent on the skill and experience of the operator, and access to this technique is not as widespread as in the United States. A chest X-ray is a simple and important part of the work-up of the patient with chest pain. Pulmonary pathology and evidence of left ventricular failure are valuable findings.

Chest pain units

Some emergency departments offer dedicated services to rapidly assess patients with chest pain.[3] High-risk patients are identified and appropriate treatment such as reperfusion therapies instituted. Lower-risk patients are monitored, receive serial troponin and ECG testing, and may also have a provocative test such as a treadmill stress test or a nuclear myocardial perfusion scan. Chest pain units have been shown to allow rapid, safe discharge of low-risk patients, and to reduce inappropriate admissions and costs.[4]

Disposition

Figure 6.1 summarises the processes to be followed in the management of chest pain. Decisions regarding patient care and admission are based on diagnosis and assessment of risk based on clinical assessment, ECG findings and tests. If clinical suspicion remains high despite the emergency department work-up, admission may be the safest option.

DYSPNOEA

Dyspnoea is the unpleasant awareness of the work of breathing. Dyspnoea may or may not be associated with hypoxaemia, and tachypnoea (rapid breathing) is a common but not inevitable accompaniment to dyspnoea. Accurate assessment of the dyspnoeic patient depends on history, physical examination and appropriate tests, especially chest X-ray. Physical signs in the severely distressed, breathless patient may be difficult to interpret. Many patients with acute cardiogenic pulmonary oedema have prominent wheezing, but wheezing is also a cardinal physical sign in airflow obstruction.

History

Important points in the history include:

1. Previous cardiorespiratory disease.
2. Previous best exercise tolerance.
3. Paroxysmal nocturnal dyspnoea—although this may be seen in both asthma and left ventricular failure (LVF).
4. Orthopnoea—this is more specific for LVF.
5. Time course and onset of dyspnoea.
6. Chest pain (pleuritic, anginal).

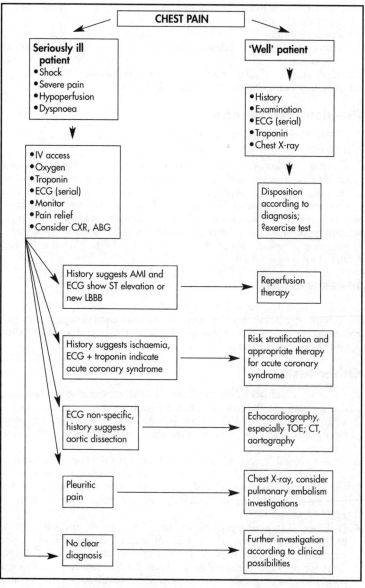

Figure 6.1 Algorithm for the management of the patient presenting with chest pain

7. Peripheral oedema.
8. Smoking history.
9. Presence of atopy.
10. History to suggest infection—fever, sweats, purulent sputum, coryzal symptoms.
11. Medications, including response to bronchodilators.
12. Risk factors for deep venous thrombosis (DVT).

Physical examination

An immediate assessment is necessary to differentiate the critically ill patient from the less sick. Look for:

1. General appearance. Level of consciousness—is immediate respiratory support necessary? Other features include cyanosis, respiratory distress, stridor (suggesting upper airway obstruction), vital signs including oximetry, and a general assessment of the efficacy of ventilatory effort.
2. Cardiorespiratory assessment. Chest wall configuration and symmetry of movement, tracheal position, presence of subcutaneous emphysema, evidence of cardiac failure, focal signs in the chest, murmurs, oedema and clinical signs of DVT.

Investigations

Examination of the chest X-ray is crucial in the assessment of the patient with dyspnoea. Recall the limitations of portable chest X-rays, particularly regarding heart size. Figure 6.2 is a guide to the interpretation of chest X-rays in breathless patients.

Other tests

1. Spirometry and peak expiratory flow. In the patient able to cooperate, these simple procedures are excellent tools to diagnose and quantify airflow obstruction. The flow–volume loop, available on many electronic spirometers, may demonstrate typical findings in upper airway obstruction.
2. Arterial blood gases (ABGs) are indicated in all dyspnoeic patients. Measurement of the alveolar–arterial gradient is a valuable tool in the assessment of hypoxaemia. Blood gas patterns are non-specific but indicate the severity of the disease process and guide oxygen therapy.
3. ECG.
4. D-dimer. Later generations of this test, which measures fibrin breakdown products, are useful in excluding significant recent pulmonary embolism. A positive test is non-specific.
5. Tests for pulmonary embolism. Computerised tomography (CT) spiral pulmonary angiography now rivals nuclear ventilation-perfusion lung scans in the diagnosis of pulmonary embolism. In patients with haemodynamic derangement (hypotension, acute cor pulmonale,

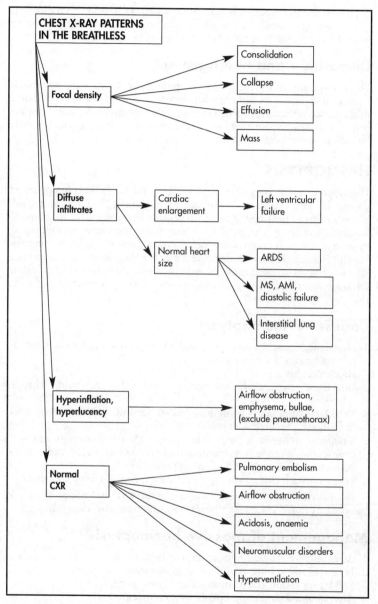

Figure 6.2 Guidelines for the interpretation of chest X-rays in breathless patients

abnormal ECG suggesting right heart strain), a CT study is very likely to be diagnostic. Similarly, coexisting lung problems reduce the specificity of the ventilation-perfusion lung scan for pulmonary embolism.

Disposition and management

Disposition and management depend on the cause. Oxygen therapy should be started early and monitored with oximetry. Carbon dioxide retention is of less concern than hypoxaemia in the acutely ill patient. A clear sensorium is strong evidence against serious acute carbon dioxide retention, but serial blood gases may be necessary.

HAEMOPTYSIS

Haemoptysis is the coughing of blood from the lungs. It is important to distinguish between haemoptysis and haematemesis, and also to exclude blood loss from the upper airway, particularly the nose. Most haemoptysis is minor, indicating the need for a search for the cause rather than an immediate threat. Large-volume haemoptysis, however, is frightening and life-threatening. It may be difficult for either the patient or the medical staff to estimate the volume of blood loss. Loss of greater than 600 mL in 24 hours constitutes massive haemoptysis, carrying a mortality of more than 50% in some series.[5]

Causes of haemoptysis

1. Neoplasia. Bronchial carcinoma and adenoma often cause haemoptysis, but only rarely is this massive.
2. Bronchiectasis.
3. Infections, particularly tuberculosis and other cavitating chronic infections.
4. Vascular. Pulmonary infarction, mitral stenosis, arteriovenous malformations, ruptured aneurysm.
5. Vasculitis. Systemic lupus erythematosus (SLE), Goodpasture's syndrome and Wegener's granulomatosis may be associated with diffuse pulmonary haemorrhage and haemoptysis.
6. Other causes include anticoagulant therapy, coagulopathy and trauma.

In Australia the commoner causes of massive haemoptysis include bleeding from old cavitatory disease, bronchiectasis and vasculitis.

Management of massive haemoptysis

1. Assess airway—urgent intubation may be necessary.
2. IV access and volume replacement as necessary.
3. Full blood count, coagulation screen, crossmatch.
4. Arterial blood gases, appropriate oxygen therapy.
5. Urgent chest X-ray.

6. If the affected side is known, nurse with the diseased side down, to protect the unaffected lung.
7. Urgent consultation with a cardiothoracic surgical unit.
8. CT scan.
9. Bronchoscopy. Rigid bronchoscopy may be preferred, at least initially, because of better suctioning ability and maintenance of airway patency.

Definitive management depends on the cause. Options include bronchoscopic techniques to identify and occlude the bleeding airway, angiography and embolisation of feeding arteries, and thoracotomy with resection.

Lesser degrees of haemoptysis

Management depends on the cause, based on history, risk for malignancy and chest X-ray. If admission is not indicated, quick follow-up, perhaps for bronchoscopy, is necessary.

REFERENCES

1. Antman EA. Decision making with cardiac troponin tests. N Engl J Med 2002; 346:2079–2082.
2. Hamm CW, Goldmann BU, Heeschen C et al. Emergency room triage of patients with acute chest pain by means of rapid testing for cardiac troponin T or troponin I. N Engl J Med 1997; 33:1648–1653.
3. Unstable Angina Writing Group. Management of unstable angina, 2000. Med J Aust Oct 2000; 173:S66–S88.
4. Lewis WR, Amsterdam EA. Chest pain emergency units. Curr Opin Cardiol 1999; 14:321–328.
5. Jean-Baptiste E. Clinical assessment and management of massive haemoptysis. Crit Care Med 2000; 28:1642–1647.
6. Cannon CP, Braunwald E. Unstable angina. In: Braunwald E, Zipes PZ, Libby P, eds. Heart disease—a textbook of cardiovascular medicine. 6th edn. Philadelphia: WB Saunders; 2001:1233.

Coronary syndromes and myocardial infarction

Paul Preisz

Rapid recognition of acute coronary artery occlusion is critical because timely treatment may prevent life-threatening early complications such as arrhythmias or save the patient's life, or quality of life. Active intervention may lead to revascularisation before irreversible myocardial damage has occurred.

As treatment is time-critical, systems for the early identification of patients at risk, as well as audit systems and quality control programmes, are required to ensure that delays are minimised. Public education and awareness as well as coordination with general practitioners and ambulance services may also shorten the period between the onset of ischaemia and definitive care.

All patients who present with chest pain or other symptoms that may be due to myocardial ischaemia should be triaged as high acuity patients and should be assessed in a monitored area with supplemental oxygen and an intravenous cannula in situ from the outset. History, examination, investigation and management should proceed rapidly and concurrently, and senior staff should be contacted as soon as possible. The ECG should be done on arrival and patients with new ST elevation or new left bundle branch block should be considered for reperfusion therapy.

Significantly, a variety of interventions have now been shown to be beneficial in some groups but not in others, and this has meant that the stratification of cardiac patients based on the likely pathophysiology at the time of presentation has assumed considerable importance. History, physical examination, the ECG, troponin measurement and other tests all play a role.

Monitoring and repeated assessment over time greatly improves the accuracy of diagnosis, and appropriate early intervention allows better subsequent outcomes. This has led emergency departments to play a much greater role in both the initial and subsequent care of these patients.

PATHOLOGY

Plaque in coronary arteries contains lipid, connective tissue, inflammatory cells, mediators and enzymes. Plaques may erode or rupture and subsequent platelet aggregation, thrombus formation and vessel spasm will result in decreased blood flow.

The severity and duration of obstruction, the available collateral flow and the nature of the thrombus formed will determine the resultant coronary syndrome. **Platelet thrombi** are white and more often associated with unstable angina and non-ST-elevation infarcts, whereas **red thrombi** contain red blood cells and are more often associated with ST-elevation infarct.

DIAGNOSIS

It is important to maintain a high index of suspicion, as presentation with myocardial ischaemia may be typical or atypical. Diagnosis of coronary artery occlusion should be made early in the course of the illness, if possible before infarction is established.

Acute coronary syndromes have recently been redefined as:

- low-risk unstable angina, high-risk unstable angina
- non-ST-elevation myocardial infarction
- ST-elevation myocardial infarction

The diagnosis of coronary artery occlusion may not be immediately apparent and a high index of suspicion is required, even if risk factors are not present. Women and elderly patients are prone to late or missed diagnosis. It may well be necessary to admit and observe a patient, and perform serial ECGs and cardiac enzymes, followed by further evaluation, before the diagnosis can be confidently excluded (Table 7.1).

Table 7.1 Coronary syndromes

Syndrome	ECG	Markers	Myocardial damage	Morbidity/ mortality
ANGINA				
Low-risk unstable angina	No new changes	Troponin normal CK normal	No	Low
High-risk unstable angina	ST depression or transient ST elevation No Q waves	Troponin elevated CK normal	Minimal damage	++
INFARCTION				
Non-ST elevation AMI (non-STEMI)	ST depression or transient ST elevation No Q waves	Troponin elevated CK elevated	Infarction	+++
ST elevation AMI (STEMI)	ST elevation May have Q waves	Troponin elevated CK elevated	More extensive infarction	+++++

Adapted from The National Heart Foundation guidelines for management of unstable angina, 2000. MJA 16 Oct 2000; 173 (supplement).

Highest-risk groups for ischaemic heart disease (IHD)

1. Those with established diagnosis of coronary artery disease, positive angiogram or other diagnostic tests, previous revascularisation, previous AMI.
2. Age is the most important predictor. Chest pain in a patient over 40 years of age presenting to the emergency department has a relatively high probability of being cardiac in origin.
3. Cardiac risk factors are relatively more useful in predicting the likely presence of ischaemic heart disease in patients under 40 years of age. Family history of IHD at an early age (may also have a family history of other risk factors), hypertension, smoking, diabetes and cholesterol abnormality (high total cholesterol, high LDL, low HDL).
4. Other factors such as inactivity, obesity and excessive alcohol consumption play a role by contributing to cardiac risk factors.
5. Drug usage, particularly cocaine and amphetamines, should be taken into consideration with some patients.

CLINICAL PRESENTATION
Cardiac chest pain

1. Chest pain may have 'typical' features such as central retrosternal location, crushing heavy or tight quality, radiation to the jaw and arm, nausea, sweating and pallor. Prolonged pain and pain during or after exertion suggests a cardiac cause.
2. Pain may be atypical, or infarction with little or no pain may occur, particularly if the patient is elderly or diabetic. Sharp pain or even chest wall tenderness may be present.

Dyspnoea

Pulmonary oedema may be present and may dominate the clinical picture.

Presyncope or syncope

Coronary artery occlusion may present as cardiac arrest due to a complicating arrhythmia or it may be precipitated by an arrhythmia.

Other

Patients may also present with symptoms or signs due to rhythm disturbance and/or low cardiac output such as palpitations, weakness, dizziness, confusion, breathlessness or collapse. In older patients tiredness, weakness or confusion may be the presenting problem.

Abnormal physical findings

1. The following may or may not be present: tachycardia, bradycardia, arrhythmias, added heart sounds, new murmurs, left or right heart failure.
2. Hypotension suggests extensive infarction, arrhythmias, pre-existing disease, medications (such as nitrates, beta-blockers) or sometimes, when seen in inferior infarction, right ventricular involvement.
3. In more extensive infarction (>40% of left ventricle) cardiogenic shock may occur. Mitral valve dysfunction, free-wall or septal rupture may lead to hypotension and cardiac failure.

INVESTIGATIONS

Electrocardiogram (ECG)

A 12-lead ECG should be performed urgently on all patients with any chest pain, dyspnoea, syncope or other suggestive symptoms. A significant proportion of patients with AMI may initially have a normal or non-diagnostic ECG. Comparison with a previous ECG is often helpful.

ECG abnormalities

1. Bradycardia (often with inferior AMI).
2. Tachycardia, often related to sympathetic response, pain and fear.
3. Arrythmias, increased ectopy.
4. ST segment changes, such as horizontal ST segment elevation, may occur within minutes and suggest infarction.
5. ST depression, peaked T waves or deep symmetrical T wave inversion are also suggestive of injury or ischaemia.
6. Pathological Q waves appear within hours and are associated with transmural infarction.

The distribution of the ECG abnormalities indicates the anatomical territory involved (Table 7.2).

Table 7.2 Distribution of ECG abnormalities seen with acute coronary syndrome

ECG lead	Area	Artery
1, aVL, V4-6	Lateral	Circumflex
II, III, aVF	Inferior	Circumflex, right coronary
V1 (large R & ST?)	Posterior	Right coronary
V2-4	Anterior	Left anterior descending

Chest X-ray (CXR)

A portable CXR should be performed as soon as possible. The patient should continue to be closely monitored and urgent therapy, when required, should not be delayed.

Congenital, valvular and hypertensive heart disease, as well as ischaemic heart disease and cardiac failure, may show X-ray changes. Less commonly, thoracic aortic dissection may present with chest pain, collapse or heart failure with or without ECG abnormalities. CXR findings such as a widened mediastinum may be present; however, if the clinical pattern is suggestive, transoesophageal echocardiography or other definitive investigation to exclude dissection is urgently required, even if the CXR is normal.

Blood tests

Urgent blood tests, including a full blood count, urea, creatinine, electrolytes and cardiac enzymes, should be performed. In particular, the serum potassium level should be obtained and supplementation given if hypokalaemia is present, as arrhythmias may otherwise occur. Blood should also be sent for serum cholesterol and triglycerides. Thyroid function and liver function tests and serum drug levels will also be indicated in some patients.

Cardiac enzymes

Cardiac enzymes are useful but must be interpreted with care. Normal cardiac enzymes do not in themselves exclude cardiac disease.

Troponin

Elevated troponin T and I measurements indicate myocardial damage and are predictors of increased risk of cardiac mortality. It may take several hours for troponin levels to rise and a series of tests may be required, with an initial measurement at presentation and subsequent testing at 6 or more hours from the time of onset of the pain. Troponin may also be elevated in patients with heart failure, tachycardia, myocarditis, pericarditis or other non-ischaemic cardiac injury.

Creatine kinase (CK)

Creatine kinase rises within 8 to 12 hours and is generally normal by 72 hours. The fraction derived principally from cardiac muscle is known as creatine kinase isoenzyme (CKMB). If the total CK is elevated but the CKMB is normal, this suggests a non-cardiac source such as skeletal muscle. When the CK is elevated, the ratio or index of CKMB to total CK is predictive of acute myocardial injury when it exceeds 4%. Note that patients in the high-risk unstable angina group (minor myocardial damage) may present with a normal CK but elevated troponin. CK may also be useful in patients who have had a cardiac event with resultant elevated troponin (which will stay elevated for up to a week) followed by a further event some days later (the rise in CK from the initial event should have abated and a subsequent rise in CK marks a new event).

Other markers

Other markers may be validated in the future as changes occurring in coronary artery plaque are associated with inflammation and elevated markers such as C reactive protein (CRP) may prove helpful. CRP and other markers such as brain naturetic peptide (BNP) are now under investigation as predictors of longer-term risk as well as of acute events.

Stress ECG, echocardiography, perfusion and scintillation scans have a role in the emergency department assessment of patients stratified as low risk who have normal serial ECGs and troponins. Coronary angiography will be discussed in detail, as it has both diagnostic and therapeutic applications in the acute setting.

MANAGEMENT

Initial management of myocardial infarction

Emergency treatment begins as soon as the diagnosis is suspected and continues concurrently with assessment. Initially, steps are taken to ensure safety:

1. Ensure adequate airway and ventilation.
2. Administer oxygen via a face mask or nasal prongs.
3. Ensure adequate circulation.
4. Monitor ECG in a resuscitation cubicle.
5. Provide intravenous access.

The rate, rhythm, preload and afterload should be optimised to maintain adequate cardiac output without excessive oxygen demand. Any abnormalities that adversely affect this balance, or that may increase the chance of complications, should be addressed urgently.

Arrhythmias

Generally, arrhythmias are common and require treatment if causing heart failure or haemodynamic compromise, if associated with excessive myocardial oxygen consumption or if likely to lead on to other more dangerous arrhythmias. General guidelines are as follows (see also Chapter 12):

1. Direct current (DC) shock, if required (ventricular fibrillation—VF; ventricular tachycardia—VT, with compromise), takes precedence and should be performed urgently before other therapy or manoeuvres.
2. Position appropriately—for pulmonary oedema, position upright; for hypotension, position supine ± elevate legs.

3. Give supplemental oxygen.
4. Treat underlying causes and secondary physiological disturbances—e.g. coronary artery occlusion, hypoxia (e.g. with left ventricular failure, or LVF), electrolyte abnormality (e.g. ↓K+), acidosis, drug toxicity, anaemia.

Bradyarrhythmias in the setting of inferior infarction may be transient and are often due to increased vagal tone or to AV nodal ischaemia. When present in patients with anterior infarction, conducting tissue involvement is more common and specific treatment is more often required.

Tachyarrhythmias may be associated with excessive myocardial oxygen consumption, and inadequate cardiac function and treatment should usually be considered. Pain and fear as underlying factors should be taken into account in patients with sinus tachycardia.

Heart failure

Pulmonary oedema, if present, should be treated at the outset. Hypotension with inadequate peripheral perfusion and/or oliguria should be managed by optimising heart rate and rhythm and by the careful use of fluids, and inotropes. When shock is present, surgical causes such as ventricular rupture and mitral valve dysfunction should be excluded. Medical causes apart from myocardial muscle damage, such as drug allergy or toxicity, should also be considered. Re-establishing coronary artery patency in patients with cardiogenic shock is critical, and urgent angiography is indicated if available. Diuretics and continuous positive airways pressure (CPAP) or bi-level positive airways pressure (BiPAP) may be required if pulmonary oedema is present.

Angiotensin-converting enzyme (ACE) inhibitors are beneficial in patients with acute myocardial infarction (AMI), particularly in those with heart failure, and should be introduced at an early stage unless contra-indicated (e.g hypotension, allergy). Their role in the absence of left ventricular impairment or hypertension has not been so clearly defined.

Pain relief

The initial management of cardiac pain is often with nitrates, particularly sublingual sprays or tablets, which have a rapid onset of action. They should be administered at the outset and the dose repeated as often as required. Their use is limited only by side effects such as headache and hypotension.

Intravenous nitrate infusions have the advantage of being readily titratable to individual patient requirements. If the volume of fluid is a critical factor a more concentrated (double-loaded) intravenous solution can be used. Nitrates also significantly reduce preload, which is beneficial in some patients with left ventricular failure.

Morphine is useful as an analgesic and an anxiolytic and may also reduce preload (and afterload). Doses of 2.5–5.0 mg IV are given as required and an antiemetic such as metoclopramide 10 mg IV should be given concurrently. Hypotension, clouding of consciousness and respiratory depression limit the amount of morphine used.

Restoring coronary artery patency

Restoring coronary artery patency is an urgent priority.

Unless there is a history of major aspirin allergy, all patients should initially receive aspirin 150–300 mg orally.

The selection of an appropriate reperfusion strategy depends on the clinical setting. If it is not possible to reach hospital within 90 minutes from the time of coronary artery occlusion, out-of-hospital thrombolysis should be considered. If it is not possible to perform angioplasty within 60 minutes, thrombolysis should be undertaken as soon as possible in the emergency department. It is likely that urgent coronary angiography with angioplasty may yield the best results if it is immediately available in an experienced unit. Extended travelling times and delays must be avoided. The potential benefits of thrombolysis followed by coronary angioplasty are currently being assessed. Angioplasty is now increasingly available, often with stenting and adjunctive antiplatelet therapy (e.g. GP IIb/IIIa inhibitors such as abciximab) on a 24-hour basis. The role of drug-eluding stents is now being considered.

Choosing a thrombolytic agent

Several thrombolytic agents are currently in common use and all are effective, although risks, benefits and costs of the available agents vary. Newer drugs such as tenecteplase have the advantage of simplified dosing and bolus administration.

Contraindications

Exclusion criteria for thrombolytic therapy are as follows:

1. Known bleeding diathesis or significant risk of life-threatening haemorrhage—e.g. actively bleeding peptic ulcer, puncture of non-compressible vessel.
2. Stroke within the preceding year, intracranial or intraspinal surgery within the preceding 2 months, intracranial or intraspinal aneurysm, arteriovenous malformation or neoplasm.
3. Prolonged and traumatic cardiopulmonary resuscitation (CPR) within the preceding 2 weeks. Limited CPR and DC shock are not contraindications.
4. Persistent hypertension with diastolic blood pressure of 110 mmHg or more which cannot be controlled.

Contraindications should exclude thrombolysis only where the risks associated with therapy outweigh the potential benefits. The risk of haemorrhagic stroke is higher in hypertensive and elderly patients. Re-establishing patency improves the outlook to such an extent that contraindications tend to be relative rather than absolute. Any major medical illness may be a relative contraindication, but advanced age alone is not.

Adverse reactions and complications of thrombolysis

1. **Hypotension and bradycardia.** Agents such as streptokinase and less commonly tissue plasminogen activator (TPA) can be associated with hypotension and bradycardia during administration. Treatment consists of stopping the infusion, placing the patient supine, administering fluids if possible and withdrawing other agents, such as nitrates, which may also lower blood pressure. When the blood pressure recovers (i.e. >100 mmHg systolic), the infusion is restarted.
2. **Arrhythmias** may occur when coronary artery patency is restored and should be treated as required. Allergic reactions may occur with streptokinase and should be managed in the usual way.
3. **External bleeding** should be controlled with pressure and the patient should be carefully observed for signs of internal bleeding, e.g. gastrointestinal bleeding or stroke. Should haemorrhage become life-threatening, the thrombolytic agent should be ceased and intravenous heparin should be reversed with 1 mg protamine for every 100 units heparin given as a bolus, or for every 100 units heparin given by infusion during the preceding 4 hours. Blood transfusion may be indicated and platelets are often required if several units of blood have been given. Either cryoprecipitate or fresh frozen plasma should also be provided and use of other agents such as tranexamic acid or aminocaproic acid considered.

Beta blockade

Beta blockade reduces both immediate and late mortality and should be undertaken unless contraindicated. If patients are already taking these medications, they should be continued while in hospital. Where therapy is to be initiated, an intravenous dose may be given first, e.g. metoprolol 2.5–5 mg IV (can be repeated if required) until the heart rate is less than 70 bpm. Oral therapy should then follow 25–100 mg twice daily.

Contraindications to beta-blockers are:

1. Bradycardia or heart block.
2. Hypotension.
3. Left ventricular failure.
4. Asthma or chronic airflow limitation.
5. Inadequate peripheral perfusion or peripheral vascular disease.
6. Drug interactions, e.g. calcium channel blockers.
7. Known allergy or unacceptable side effects.

Initial management of angina

Patients presenting with possible myocardial ischaemia but not initially with infarction should undergo risk stratification as this will determine their optimal management. This is a dynamic process and it is important to reassess each individual case, as clinical circumstances may change. Monitoring over 8–12 hours with frequent ECGs or continuous ST

Table 7.3 Therapy for unstable angina to be considered in the absence of contraindications

	Low-risk unstable angina	High-risk unstable angina
Aspirin	♥	♥
Nitrates	♥	♥
Beta-blockers	♥	♥
Treat elevated lipids*	♥	♥
ACE inhibitors**	♥	♥
Heparin LMW or IV UFH		♥
ADP blocker*** (clopidogrel)		♥
IIb IIIa inhibitors*** (abciximab, tirofiban)		♥
Consider PCA		♥

*Total cholesterol >4.0 mmol/L
**In the presence of hypertension, diabetes or congestive cardiac failure
***Not for patients who may require coronary artery bypass grafting (CABG) within 5 days
***For patients undergoing percutaneous coronary angioplasty (PCA)
LMW   Low molecular weight
UNH   Unfractionated heparin

segment monitoring and repeated troponin levels should be undertaken, looking for features of high-risk unstable angina, as follows:

1. Diabetes.
2. Associated syncope.
3. Heart failure, mitral regurgitation, gallop.
4. Low blood pressure or poor peripheral perfusion.
5. Prolonged (>10 min) rest or repetitive chest pain.
6. ECG changes or elevated troponin.

Patients who do not have high-risk features after observation and monitoring as above may be suitable for discharge and outpatient follow-up, e.g. stress test.

Therapy for unstable angina

See Table 7.3. Monitoring and oxygen therapy should be instituted. Consider and treat secondary causes of angina such as arrhythmias, anaemia, thyroid disease, cardiomyopathy and valvular heart disease.

RECOMMENDED READING

Australian Heart Foundation. Management of unstable angina, guidelines. Online. Available: http://www,heartfoundation.com.au; 2000.
Australian Heart Foundation. Reperfusion therapy for acute myocardial infarction. Online. Available: http://www.heartfoundation.com.au.
British Heart Foundation. Website. Available: http://www.bhf.org.uk.

Harrison TR, Braunwald E. Harrison's principles of internal medicine. 15th edn.
  New York: McGraw-Hill; 2001.
Fonarow GC. UCLA clinical practice guidelines. UCLA Clinical Guidelines
  Committee, UCLA Division of Cardiology; 2001. Online. Available:
  http://www.mea.ucla.edu.

8   Acute pulmonary oedema

Anthony F T Brown

Decompensated heart failure, or acute pulmonary oedema (APO), now
accounts for 1% of emergency department (ED) visits, with a 16% in-
hospital mortality for those admitted with frank pulmonary oedema.

Although the typical frail, elderly patient may dominate the physician's
perspective, APO in the ED can present in a diverse group of patients,
from those suffering from an underlying acute myocardial infarct to
chronic decompensated heart failure to non-cardiogenic causes, all of
which often have subtly different historical, examination and investigation
findings, and may require a wide variety of urgent treatments.

PATHOPHYSIOLOGY OF APO

Acute pulmonary oedema may be divided into cardiogenic and non-
cardiogenic causes.

Acute cardiogenic pulmonary oedema

Acute cardiogenic pulmonary oedema is the most severe manifestation of
congestive heart failure, and is associated with an increase in lung fluid
secondary to leakage from pulmonary capillaries into the alveoli and
interstitium of the lungs. Underlying this is a rise in left atrial pressure
related to left ventricular dysfunction.

The causative heart disease leading to left ventricular failure may be
predominantly systolic failure with impaired cardiac contractility, i.e. an
ejection fraction (EF) under 40%, diastolic failure with impaired
myocardial relaxation (but a normal or even supranormal EF), or a
combination of both.

APO may develop out of the blue, or be precipitated in patients with
existing heart disease as a result of an acute cause such as ischaemia, an
arrhythmia or medication change. Table 8.1 gives the causes of cardiogenic
pulmonary oedema.

Table 8.1 Causes of cardiogenic pulmonary oedema

Precipitating factors
- Inappropriate reduction of therapy or non-compliance
- Arrhythmia
  —tachycardia, including atrial fibrillation
  —bradycardia, conduction abnormality
- Pulmonary embolism
- Systemic infection including septic shock
- Cardiac infection—myocarditis, endocarditis
- High output state—anaemia, thyrotoxicosis, beri beri
- Cardiac depressant (beta-blocker) or salt-retaining (non-steroidal anti-inflammatory) drugs
- Volume overload
- Alcohol excess or withdrawal

Predominant systolic heart failure
- Myocardial ischaemia
- Hypertension
- Cardiomyopathy
- Myocarditis
- Valvular disease, ruptured valve leaflet

Predominant diastolic heart failure
- Hypertension
- Aortic stenosis (severe)
- Cardiomyopathy (HOCM or restrictive)
- Myocardial ischaemia

Non-cardiogenic pulmonary oedema

Non-cardiogenic pulmonary oedema may result from a wide variety of causes, such as:

1. Altered capillary permeability in adult respiratory distress syndrome (ARDS), septicaemia, pancreatitis, inhaled toxins, uraemia or near-drowning.
2. Increased pulmonary capillary pressure, including pulmonary venous thrombosis.
3. Decreased oncotic pressure such as hypoalbuminaemia.
4. Mixed or unknown mechanisms such as neurogenic pulmonary oedema, high-altitude pulmonary oedema (HAPE), heroin overdose, eclampsia and post-cardioversion.

Neurogenic pulmonary oedema

Neurogenic pulmonary oedema is a relatively rare cause of APO, developing within a few hours of an acute neurologic insult, and is usually associated with intracranial hypertension such as from a head injury, intracerebral haemorrhage or prolonged seizures.

CLINICAL FEATURES OF APO

History

Patients may be too distressed to give a history until after aggressive medical management, but may report chest pain, a change in medication or recent fever (see Table 8.1) as a precipitating cause, or remember previous episodes of 'fluid on the lung'.

Acute breathlessness is universal, and may occur on a background of cough, exertional dyspnoea, orthopnoea, paroxysmal nocturnal dyspnoea (PND) and dyspnoea at rest. Other non-specific features such as fatigue and nocturia may occur in compensated heart failure. Finally, confusion, coma and respiratory arrest may ensue.

Examination

Patients with APO are terrified, sweaty, unwilling to lie down, restless and may wheeze or froth pink sputum in extreme cases.

Tachypnoea, tachycardia, reduced oxygen saturation, hyper- or hypotension and cyanosis may all occur.

Basal crackles, a raised jugular venous pressure (JVP) from secondary right-heart failure and a third heart sound gallop are typical, whereas in non-cardiogenic pulmonary oedema patients may have a warm periphery, bounding pulse and absence of a gallop or jugular venous distension.

A new systolic murmur may indicate an acute mechanical complication such as papillary muscle rupture or an acquired ventricular septal defect (VSD) in the setting of an acute myocardial infarction.

INVESTIGATIONS FOR APO

Electrocardiogram (ECG)

This is essential to diagnose an acute myocardial infarction, arrhythmia or heart block and may determine the need for time-critical reperfusion therapy in the presence of chest pain (see Chapter 7). It may also indicate underlying heart disease with left ventricular hypertrophy, pre-existing coronary artery disease or even an electrolyte disturbance.

Chest X-ray (CXR)

CXR will confirm the presence of APO, and is particularly useful early to help differentiate APO from an exacerbation of chronic obstructive lung disease (COLD) or asthma.

1. Cardiomegaly, pulmonary venous congestion with upper lobe diversion, perihilar 'batswing' infiltrates, Kerley B engorged subpleural lymphatics, interstitial oedema and small pleural effusions are typical.

2. A normal heart size may occur in acute valvular rupture, diastolic dysfunction, myocarditis or non-cardiogenic causes of pulmonary oedema.

Laboratory tests

A full blood count, electrolyte and liver function test, cardiac enzymes including troponin, coagulation profile and thyroid function test should be sent, but add nothing to the immediate management.

Arterial blood gases

As with laboratory tests, arterial blood gases add nothing to the initial management and serve only to delay therapy. They may be useful to monitor hypercapnoea in the non-responding patient.

MANAGEMENT OF APO

1. Sit the patient upright, apply high-flow oxygen and commence non-invasive monitoring in a resuscitation area.
2. Commence nitrates to reduce preload.
   a. Give glyceryl trinitrate (GTN) 150–300 μg sublingually. This dose may be repeated. Remove the tablet or cease if hypotension (systolic blood pressure, SBP, below 100 mmHg) occurs.
   b. In resistant cases, particularly those associated with ischaemic chest pain, change to a glyceryl trinitrate infusion. Add 200 mg GTN to 500 mL 5% dextrose (i.e. 400 μg/mL in a glass bottle with low-absorption polyethylene infusion set). Commence at 1 mL/h and gradually increase to 20 mL/h or more, maintaining SBP above 100 mmHg.
3. Give frusemide 40 mg IV or twice their usual oral daily dose if already taking frusemide tablets. This may be repeated after 20 minutes, but avoid overdiuresis.
4. If there is marked dyspnoea and agitation, give small increments of morphine, starting at 0.5 mg IV in the elderly up to 2.5 mg in younger patients. Do not use morphine routinely, particularly if the patient is tired, may have COLD/asthma, or is becoming obtunded with a rising partial pressure of CO_2 ($PaCO_2$).
5. Commence mask continuous positive airways pressure (CPAP) in those who do not respond to the above standard pharmacologic therapy.
   a. Use a tight-fitting face mask, high-flow gas circuit and start with 5–10 cm H_2O. CPAP improves lung mechanics and enhances left ventricular performance, reducing the need for intubation.
   b. Do not use bi-level positive airways pressure (BiPAP) or non-invasive positive pressure ventilation (NPPV), as this appears to be negatively associated with increased rates of acute myocardial infarction (AMI) in cardiogenic pulmonary oedema.

DISPOSAL

1. Patients who present hypotensive, or deteriorate and/or do not tolerate vasodilation, have a poor prognosis, with up to 80% mortality.
   a. Call for senior help if you have not already done so! Manage the patient as for cardiogenic shock with intubation and mechanical ventilation, applying 5–10 cm H_2O positive end-expiratory pressure (PEEP).
   b. Support the circulation with inotropes such as dopamine 2–20 µg/kg/min and dobutamine 2–30 µg/kg/min. Adrenaline may be required for extreme hypotension, but the higher myocardial oxygen demand may ultimately be deleterious.
   c. Look for a treatable mechanical cause with a transthoracic echocardiogram, such as an acute valvular rupture or VSD, and organise cardiac surgical care if these are found.
   d. Admit the patient to intensive care. Consider an intraaortic balloon pump as a temporising measure while reperfusion therapy—such as acute angioplasty or coronary revascularisation—is performed in the setting of an ST-elevation myocardial infarction, or while valvular or VSD repair is organised (see above).
2. In the majority of patients who respond to standard therapy, arrange admission to a coronary care unit if there are ongoing cardiac issues such as pain, ischaemia, arrhythmias or electrolyte disturbances, and close monitoring or respiratory support is necessary. Otherwise, particularly in the elderly patient with brief decompensation of chronic heart failure, admit the patient to a non-monitored medical bed.
3. Non-cardiogenic pulmonary oedema is managed according to the underlying primary cause, with non-invasive or invasive respiratory support as necessary.

RECOMMENDED READING

Brisbane Cardiac Consortium. Clinical practice guidelines: hospital management of congestive cardiac failure. Clinical Support Systems Program; 2001. Online. Available: http:/www.health.qld.gov.au/BCC; July 2002.

Congestive heart failure. In: Ball CM, Phillips RS, eds. Evidence-based on call: acute medicine. Edinburgh: Churchill Livingstone; 2001:210–233.

Cotter G, Metzkor E, Kaluski E et al. Randomised trial of high-dose isosorbide dinitrate plus low-dose furosemide versus high-dose furosemide plus low-dose isosorbide dinitrate in severe pulmonary oedema. Lancet 1998; 351:389–393.

Kosowsky JM, Kobayashi L. Acute decompensated heart failure: diagnostic and therapeutic strategies for the new millennium. Emergency Medicine Practice: An Evidence-based Approach to Emergency Medicine 2002; 4(2):1–28.

Pang D, Keenan SP, Cook DJ et al. The effect of positive pressure airway support on mortality and the need for intubation in cardiogenic pulmonary oedema: a systematic review. Chest 1998; 114:1185–1192.

9 Pulmonary emboli and venous thromboses

George Jelinek and Martin Duffy

PULMONARY EMBOLI (George Jelinek)

Pulmonary embolism (PE) is a diagnosis to be made in the emergency department. If diagnosed and treated appropriately, the mortality is of the order of 8–10%, with most patients dying of comorbidity. If the diagnosis is not made initially, the mortality rises to about one-third of cases.[1]

The diagnosis is often difficult and approaches to diagnosis are currently in a state of flux. Classical signs and symptoms occur only occasionally. Clinical judgment enhances the ability of investigations to predict PE, and is now used in most PE investigation algorithms, in association with calculation of pre-test probability (PTP) of PE based on symptoms, signs and risk factors.[2]

The Prospective Investigation of Pulmonary Embolism Diagnosis (PIOPED) study found that, although an abnormal (low, intermediate or high probability) ventilation/perfusion lung scan was very sensitive (98%) for PE, it was not nearly as specific (10%) as previously thought, and only a minority of patients with PE had high-probability scans.[3] Ultrasonography of leg veins (to look for deep vein thrombosis—DVT) and pulmonary angiography should be used much more liberally when there is strong clinical suspicion of PE. Increasingly, D-dimer assay and CT pulmonary angiography (CTPA) are being used to refine diagnosis. D-dimer has gone in and out of favour, owing to differences in sensitivity of the various testing methods, but with rapid, modern ELISA D-dimers sensitivity is virtually 100% and the test can be reliably used to exclude PE, provided patient selection is good.

Clinical features[4]

Commonest symptoms

1. Chest pain	88%
• pleuritic	74%
• other	14%
2. Dyspnoea	84%
3. Apprehension	59%
4. Cough	53%
5. Haemoptysis	30%
6. Sweats	27%

Commonest signs

1. Tachypnoea (>16/min)	92%
2. Crackles/rales	58%
3. Loud P_2	53%
4. Tachycardia (>100/min)	44%
5. Fever (>37.8°C)	43%
6. Diaphoresis	36%
7. Gallop rhythm	34%
8. DVT clinically	32%
9. Peripheral oedema	24%
10. Pulmonary/tricuspid murmur	23%
11. Cyanosis	19%

Risk factors

1. Prolonged immobility 55%
2. Current venous disease 49%
3. Congestive cardiac failure/
   chronic airflow limitation (CAL) 38%
4. Others (systemic malignancy, trauma to pelvis/lower extremity, surgery, peripartum, oestrogen intake including contraceptives, age >50, obesity).

Note: only 6% of patients with PE have no recognised coexistent illness or risk factor.

Pre-test probability (PTP)[2]

Points are awarded as follows:

Signs of DVT	3
PE most likely cause	3
Active cancer	1.5
Recent immobilisation (bed rest of 3 days or more, leg plaster for 2 weeks or more, surgery within 3 weeks)	1.5
Tachycardia (pulse rate>100/min)	1
History of haemoptysis	1

PTP is considered high if over 6, intermediate for a score of 3–6, and low for a score of 2 or less.

Investigations

Chest X-ray (CXR)

CXR is usually abnormal, but no changes are specific. Only 7–22% are normal. The commonest findings are:
1. Raised hemidiaphragm with atelectasis 50%
2. Consolidation/infiltrates/effusion 30–50%
   Hampton's hump and Westermark's sign are uncommon.

ECG

ECG is usually abnormal. Only 13% are normal or unchanged. The commonest findings are:

1. Tachycardia (>100/min)   44%
2. ST–T wave changes   42%
3. Acute cor pulmonale ($S_1Q_3T_3$)   12%

Arterial blood gases (ABGs)

ABGs are usually hypoxic. Only 10–15% of patients have a PO_2 >80 mmHg, 5% have PO_2 >90 mmHg. Pulse oximetry, as in other respiratory emergencies, is invaluable.

D-dimer

A negative D-dimer, in conjunction with a low or intermediate PTP, effectively excludes PE. A D-dimer is, however, unreliable and should not be performed in the following circumstances: for inpatients, for patients with recent (within 2 weeks) invasive surgery or major trauma or with active cancer, or where the duration of symptoms is 7 days or more.

Special investigations

Radionuclide ventilation-perfusion lung scan

If normal or near-normal, the diagnosis is reasonably excluded (about 4% will have PE).[2]

- Low probability   PE in 16%
- Medium probability   PE in 33%
- High probability   PE in 88%

A history of PE decreases the accuracy of diagnosis based on a high-probability scan. If the CXR is abnormal, CTPA is preferred to ventilation-perfusion (V/Q) scanning.

CT pulmonary angiography (CTPA)

CTPA is useful in the setting of patients with markedly abnormal CXRs. It is more sensitive for central than peripheral PEs and has the advantage of detecting other pulmonary pathology if present. Magnetic resonance imaging (MRI) is available in a few centres.

Pulmonary angiography

Nearly 100% specific and sensitive, pulmonary angiography is the 'gold standard'. A negative study essentially excludes the diagnosis of PE. However, morbidity is 1–4% and mortality 0.1–0.4%.[1] It should be used more often when clinical suspicion is very high but other investigations are normal.

Diagnostic pathway

A reasonable approach is to base the use of invasive investigations on a combination of PTP and D-dimer assay. A PTP of 6 or less, together with a negative D-dimer, excludes PE. Otherwise, invasive testing should be undertaken. The choice of test depends on CXR findings. If the CXR is essentially normal, a V/Q scan should be performed; if the CXR is abnormal, a CTPA. Results of these tests should again be interpreted in light of the PTP. A low PTP in association with normal or low-probability V/Q scan or negative CTPA effectively excludes PE. A high-probability V/Q scan, in association with an intermediate or high PTP, makes the diagnosis of PE. For other combinations of PTP and V/Q results, leg ultrasonography and/or pulmonary angiography are needed to make a definitive diagnosis.

Management

Treatment may need to begin on suspicion, particularly if definitive investigations are unavailable out of hours. Conventional anticoagulation with heparin in currently recommended dose regimens (e.g. 5000 units IV stat followed by 800–1600 units/hour by continuous infusion) is standard therapy, although low molecular weight heparins now appear to be equally effective. For haemodynamically compromised patients, thrombolysis with tissue plasminogen activator (TPA) or streptokinase should be considered, although the evidence of their effectiveness is still limited.

VENOUS THROMBOEMBOLISM (Martin Duffy)

Venous thromboembolism is a common disease. The underlying abnormality, as described by Virchow many years ago, is a problem with one or more of the following:

- venous stasis
- injury to the vessel wall
- hypercoagulability

Although it can occur in any part of the venous system, clinically important sites are the deep veins of the lower limbs and the pelvic veins. Less commonly, the axillary/subclavian veins may be affected.

Patients presenting to the emergency department with possible venous thromboembolism often have myriad signs and symptoms, making diagnosis a challenging exercise. Importantly, we need to be accurate with this diagnosis. If we miss it, the patient may suffer significant morbidity or mortality, ranging from postphlebitic syndrome to pulmonary embolism and death. If we overdiagnose it, the patient may be exposed to the risks of unnecessary therapy, such as haemorrhage from anticoagulation.

The problem

A typical scenario in the emergency department is the patient who presents with a painful, swollen calf for assessment and management of possible underlying DVT.

In the past, experience had shown us that the clinical examination was unreliable in diagnosing or excluding DVT, hence the mere suggestion of the possibility virtually compelled the physician to perform some form of medical imaging as part of the diagnostic work-up.

Nowadays, this is no longer the case. The use of a set of standardised clinical criteria enables patients to be stratified into low, moderate or high pre-test probabilities of DVT. When this stratification is combined with the results of a D-dimer level many patients may not require any further investigation.

Diagnostic approach

The algorithm shown in Figure 9.1 summarises one approach to the investigation of the patient with a possible DVT, based on evidence at present available in the literature.

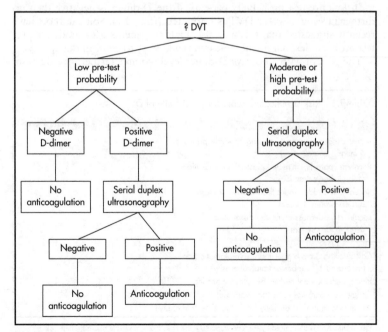

Figure 9.1   Algorithm for the investigation of suspected DVT

Step 1: Determine the patient's pre-test probability

Clinical 'impression' alone is not sufficient. Wells and colleagues[2] have developed and validated a set of clinical criteria incorporating signs, symptoms, risk factors and alternative diagnoses for stratifying a patient's pre-test probability of DVT (Table 9.1). Some authors have argued that the criteria specifically exclude patients with a history of DVT, and are therefore applicable to first-time presentations only, thus limiting their usefulness. However, further research suggests that the criteria appear to be useful in recurrent episodes as well. A notable exclusion is the pregnant patient.

The approximate rate of DVT in these categories in the original study was 5%, 33% and 85% respectively.

Step 2: Determine the D-dimer level

D-dimer is a degradation product from cross-linked fibrin. It rises acutely in the presence of venous thrombosis—and unfortunately it rises in many other conditions as well (malignancy, infection, trauma, haemorrhage and even recent major surgery). Numerous assays are available, so it is important that you know which one your laboratory uses—a highly sensitive assay is a must.

In low pre-test probability patients, if the D-dimer is negative then no further investigation for DVT is warranted (risk ~1%). Some authors have recently suggested that this may also apply to patients with moderate pre-test probabilities, but further research is necessary to confirm this approach.

The patient with a positive D-dimer level requires further investigation.

Table 9.1   Risk stratification score for probability of DVT

	If present, score:
Active cancer (treatment ongoing or within previous 6 months or palliative)	1
Paralysis, paresis, or recent plaster immobilisation of the lower extremities	1
Recently bedridden more than 3 days or major surgery within 4 weeks	1
Localised tenderness along the distribution of the deep venous system	1
Entire leg swollen	1
Calf swelling 3 cm bigger than asymptomatic side (measured 10 cm below tibial tuberosity)	1
Pitting oedema confined to the symptomatic leg	1
Collateral superficial veins (non-varicose)	1
Alternative diagnosis as likely or greater than that of DVT	−2

Risk stratification is determined by the total score: ≤0 = low risk, 1–2 = moderate risk, ≥3 = high risk.
In patients with symptoms in both legs, the more symptomatic leg is used.

Step 3: Further investigation

The next investigation in most Australasian settings is duplex ultrasonography of the affected lower limb. Sensitivities and specificities of 97% and 94% respectively are quoted in the literature. However, it is important to remember two points:

1. The test is operator-dependent.
2. The sensitivity for detecting isolated calf vein DVT is only 73%. Interestingly, 20–30% of calf vein DVTs may extend proximally. Hence, if the initial examination is negative, it is necessary to perform a repeat ultrasound examination in approximately 1 week's time (i.e. serial testing is a must).

If the ultrasound is positive at any stage for DVT, treat the patient. If the ultrasound is negative on serial testing, the likelihood of DVT is exceedingly small and treatment can be withheld.

Other imaging modalities include:

1. Impedance plethysmography—non-invasive, but not as accurate as ultrasound.
2. Venography—the 'old' gold standard', rarely used nowadays because it is invasive and has associated complications.
3. CT and MRI—accurate, but their place in the diagnostic algorithm has yet to be determined based on cost, incremental value etc.

Treatment

The treatment of DVT has changed significantly over recent years, with many patients now being treated as outpatients, largely as a result of the numerous advantages low molecular weight heparin has over unfractionated heparin—i.e. weight-based dosing that does not require any specific monitoring and simple subcutaneous administration once or twice daily.

Consider whole picture

It is important to remember to look at the whole picture when deciding on a treatment plan for each individual, including the following:

- Age.
- Comorbidities—including active bleeding/familial bleeding disorder/marked renal disease/severe liver disease.
- Proximal versus distal thrombus.
- Accompanying pulmonary embolism.
- Social supports.
- Ability to access further medical care if/when required.

Baseline investigations

Baseline investigations prior to commencing therapy may include:

- Full blood count.
- Electrolytes/urea/creatinine.

- Liver function tests.
- Coagulation profile.

Above-knee DVT

A suitable treatment plan for an above-knee DVT is as follows:

1. Non-drug therapy—mobilisation and thromboembolism (TED) stockings.
2. Analgesia as required.
3. Enoxaparin 1.5 mg/kg/day as a single dose (if >100 mg/day, divide the dose into two equal doses). Reduce the dose to 0.75–1 mg/kg/day if Hb <100 g/dL, thrombocytopenia, renal impairment, liver disease or elderly patient.
4. Start warfarin on day 2 or 3 (can be done by local medical officer).
5. Continue enoxaparin until the international normalised ratio (INR) is therapeutic (2–3) for at least 24 hours.
6. Anticoagulate for 3 months.

Below-knee DVT

A suitable treatment plan for a below-knee DVT is:

1. Non-drug therapy—mobilisation and TED stockings.
2. Analgesia as required.
3. Enoxaparin 1.5 mg/kg/day as a single dose (if >100 mg/day, divide the dose into two equal doses).
4. Treat for 7–10 days.
5. Repeat lower limb duplex ultrasound at 7–10 days.
6. If ultrasound the same or unchanged, stop anticoagulation.
7. If ultrasound shows progression, treat as for above-knee DVT.

Many new drug therapies for both prophylaxis and treatment of venous thromboembolism are currently undergoing development and testing. Most of these specifically target individual components of the coagulation system. Of considerable interest is the small direct thrombin inhibitor ximelagatran. It is an orally administered prodrug that is rapidly metabolised to its active metabolite melagatran. Trials to date suggest it requires no dose adjustment and no patient monitoring, and it appears to be as effective as present-day anticoagulants. The potential to simplify outpatient therapy is enormous.

The role of thrombolytics in the management of DVT remains unclear at this point in time. Studies show improvement in clot lysis, but usually at the expense of an increase in haemorrhagic complications. Restricted use in the patient with a massive DVT, after serious consideration of the risk–benefit ratio for the individual patient, seems to be the only scenario when thrombolytics may be considered at present.

Other treatments

1. **Vena caval filter.** The placement of a filter to prevent pulmonary embolism should be considered in any patient who has a contraindication

to anticoagulation, serious bleeding complications on anticoagulation, or disease progression despite adequate anticoagulation.

2. **Surgery**—reserved for massive DVTs that threaten limb or life.

Further investigations

Patients with comfirmed DVT, and no obvious reason for the development of such a problem, require further investigation. Apart from the possibility of an underlying hypercoagulable state, always keep in mind the possibility of an as yet undiagnosed malignancy.

Investigations ordered as part of a procoagulant screen include:

- Activated protein C resistance.
- ANA.
- Anticardiolipin antibody.
- Antithrombin III (note that the use of low molecular weight heparin interferes with antithrombin III testing).
- Factor V Leiden.
- Homocysteine.
- Lupus inhibitor.
- MTHFR gene mutation.
- Protein C and S.
- PT20210 gene.

Axillary/subclavian vein thrombosis

Axillary/subclavian vein thrombosis is a much less common clinical problem. The underlying cause is similar to those of other DVTs, although other factors that play a more prominent role include excessive/unusual exercise, intravenous catheters and intravenous drug use. Often there is an underlying predisposing narrowing, e.g. cervical rib. Although commonly thought to be of less concern in terms of embolisation, axillary/subclavian vein thrombosis has been known to occur in up to 30% of cases, and should therefore be treated as aggressively as lower limb DVT.

Pearls/pitfalls

- Venous thromboembolism is a common but difficult clinical problem.
- Use Wells' criteria to risk-stratify patients.
- A sensitive D-dimer assay is a MUST.
- Many patients are suitable for outpatient therapy.
- New oral drugs are on the horizon.

EDITOR'S COMMENT

Pulmonary embolism and venous thrombosis are classical and critical diagnoses that need to be excluded by investigation, as clinical signs are unreliable and the consequences can be very significant. A high clinical suspicion and no confirmatory test may still warrant admission/treatment.

REFERENCES

1. Dunmire SM. Pulmonary embolism. Emergency Medicine Clinics of North America 1989; 7:339–354.
2. Wells PS, Ginsberg JS, Anderson DR et al. Use of a clinical model for safe management of patients with suspected pulmonary embolism. Ann Intern Med 1998; 129:997–1005.
3. The PIOPED investigators. Value of the ventilation/perfusion scan in acute pulmonary embolism. Results of the prospective investigation of pulmonary embolism diagnosis (PIOPED). JAMA 1990; 263:2753–2759.
4. Urokinase-streptokinase embolism trial: phase II results. JAMA 1974; 229:1606–1613.

RECOMMENDED READING

Bates S, Kearon C, Crowther M et al. A diagnostic strategy involving a quantitative latex D-dimer assay reliably excludes deep venous thrombosis. Ann Intern Med 2003; 138(10):787–794.

Cornuz J, Ghali W, Hayoz D et al. Clinical prediction of deep venous thrombosis using two risk assessment methods in combination with rapid quantitative D-dimer testing. Am J Med 2002; 112(3):198–203.

Forster A, Wells P. The rationale and evidence for the treatment of lower-extremity deep venous thrombosis with thrombolytic agents. Current Opinion in Haematology 2002; 9(5):437–442.

Hyers T. Management of venous thromboembolism: past, present, and future. Arch Intern Med 2003; 163(7):759–768.

Kelly J, Hunt B. Role of D-dimers in diagnosis of venous thromboembolism. Lancet 2002; 359 (February 9):456–458.

Kraaijenhagen R, Piovella F, Bernardi E et al. Simplification of the diagnostic management of suspected deep vein thrombosis. Arch Intern Med 2002; 162 (April 22):907–911.

Wells P, Anderson D. Diagnosis of deep-vein thrombosis in the year 2000. Curr Opin Pulm Med 2000; 6(4):309–313.

10 Shock

Steve Dunjey

Shock is a clinical condition resulting from inadequate tissue perfusion. There are multiple causes but the final common pathway of inadequate perfusion means that insufficient metabolic substrates (primarily oxygen) are provided to sustain cellular homeostasis.

CAUSES AND EFFECTS

Causes of shock are loosely grouped as follows:

- Hypovolaemia (inadequate circulating volume).
- Cardiogenic (inadequate myocardial contractility).
- Distributive (adequate volume, which is maldistributed).
- Obstructive (impedance to venous return).

A complete list of the causes is given in Table 10.1. A patient in shock will manifest signs of:

- Inadequate tissue perfusion, with end organ dysfunction (confusion, agitation, acidosis, decreased urine output etc). (See Table 10.2.)
- Compensation. This includes tachycardia, peripheral vasoconstriction (sweaty, pale, cold peripheries with decreased capillary return), central vasoconstriction (narrowed pulse pressure) and decreased blood flow through nonvital structures, such as abdominal viscera (manifested by decreased urine output, decreased bowel sounds). Compensation can be so effective in young patients that the underlying shock state is manifest only by tachycardia, and more fully revealed by measuring postural

Table 10.1 Causes of shock

Type of shock	Causes	Signs
Hypovolaemia	Haemorrhage Vomiting/diarrhoea Dehydration Addison's	Obvious external blood Skin turgor Dry mucous membranes ↓ JVP
Cardiogenic	Myocardial infarction (esp. anterior, R ventricular) Myocardial contusion Acute valvular lesion Cardiomyopathies Arrhythmias	Extremes of pulse rate ↑ JVP ECG evidence of AMI, arrhythmia New murmurs
Distributive	Neurogenic/spinal Injury Anaphylaxis Sepsis	Flaccid paralysis, warm peripheries, relative bradycardia, priapism Urticaria, angiodema, wheeze Febrile, warm peripheries, evidence of focus
Obstructive	Pulmonary embolism Cardiac tamponade Tension pneumothroax	Evidence of DVT, pulmonary hypertension ↑ JVP Distant muffled heart sounds, pulsus paradoxus, electrical alternans Subcutaneous emphysema midline shift trachea, ↓ breath sounds

JVP Jugular venous pressure

Table 10.2 Adverse effects of shock

1. Kidney: oliguria and renal failure.
2. CNS: confusion, restlessness and decreased level of consciousness.
3. Lung: hypoxia and adult respiratory distress syndrome (ARDS).
4. Liver: elevation of hepatic transaminases and bilirubin.
5. Gastrointestinal tract (GIT): ischaemia, ileus, diarrhoea, stress ulceration and bacterial translocation into the systemic circulation.
6. Myocardium: may impair myocardial function in severe cases.
7. Other tissue damage: all tissues are probably impaired, but the processes involved are difficult to quantify

blood pressure drop (greater than 20 mmHg systolic). Younger patients are able to maintain an increased heart rate and cardiac output but may suddenly deteriorate when they are unable to compensate further. Elderly patients may be incapable of mounting a tachycardiac response to shock because of medications (especially beta-blockers) or underlying heart disease.

- The cause of the shock.

OVERVIEW OF MANAGEMENT

Shocked patients should be managed in a fully monitored area. The assessment and treatment of the shocked patient should occur in parallel. Initial treatment focuses on resuscitation, monitoring (to assess response to treatment) and seeking a specific cause (history, examination and investigations).

Airway and breathing

- Secure the airway.
- Enhance oxygenation. All patients will benefit from supplemental oxygen: initially provide the highest level of inspired O_2 available.
- Support ventilation if necessary.

Circulation

- Control accessible haemorrhage.
- Gain intravenous access with a minimum of two large-bore peripheral IV lines.
- Begin fluid replacement. The volume of fluid replacement required will depend to a great degree on the type of shock being treated. Hypovolaemic shock commonly requires large volumes of fluid replacement, whereas patients with cardiogenic shock may require very little. It is reasonable to begin with 300–500 mL boluses of fluid, and to review the response.

- If the patient demonstrates ongoing signs of shock despite adequate volume replacement, the use of inotropic/vasopressor support should be considered.

Monitoring

Monitoring may include—pulse rate, non-invasive blood pressure, urine output, temperature, central venous pressure (CVP), pulse oximetry, ECG. If the blood pressure remains low, invasive arterial monitoring may be appropriate. Other modalities may include capnography in intubated patients, and pulmonary artery wedge pressure (PAWP).

Investigations

Once the cause of shock has been determined, specific therapy should be considered and commenced if necessary. The steps described below are relevant and appropriate in all patients with shock.

HYPOVOLAEMIC SHOCK

Hypovolaemic shock involves the loss of intravascular volume. Among the most common causes in patients presenting to the emergency department are blood loss (external, internal) and dehydration. The aims of management are to limit further fluid loss and replenish circulating intravascular volume. External haemorrhage is best controlled with direct pressure. Currently the use of military antishock trousers (MAST) is controversial and appears limited to patients with major pelvic and lower limb injuries where the device stabilises fractures and produces pelvic compression, which limits further blood loss. Adequacy of fluid resuscitation can be judged by the response of measured cardiovascular parameters. Fluids used include crystalloids and colloids, although currently crystalloids appear to be used more often.

Management

1. Assess and treat airway, breathing and circulation (ABCs).
2. The initial fluid of choice is usually an isotonic crystalloid, which is probably best delivered as 300–500 mL IV aliquots rapidly infused (or 20 mL per kilogram aliquots for children).
3. Consider the use of blood products if blood loss is the primary cause of shock. If necessary (e.g. in established shock, with ongoing loss of blood) transfuse O-negative blood until either group-specific or fully crossmatched blood is available.
4. Large-bore peripheral lines are preferred. Central venous catheters (CVCs) can be time consuming, difficult to perform, and have the potential to cause injury. CVCs can be used if peripheral access proves impossible, or at a later stage when resuscitation is well established.

5. Surgically correctible sources of blood loss should be sought, and haemorrhage arrested. Some sources of haemorrhage (e.g. oesophageal varices) may be controlled medically (e.g. IV infusion octreotide).
6. The end point of fluid therapy is currently the subject of fierce debate. This is discussed more fully at the end of this chapter under the heading 'Controversies'.

CARDIOGENIC SHOCK

Cardiogenic shock results from cardiac dysfunction with decreased cardiac output. With increasing ventricular dysfunction, florid pulmonary oedema may develop. There are often prominent signs of right ventricular failure, such as jugular venous distension.

The most common initiating event for cardiogenic shock is acute ischaemic damage to the myocardium. Once more than 40% of the myocardium is affected, cardiogenic shock may result as a consequence of reduced ejection fraction and cardiac output. Ischaemia can also trigger cardiogenic shock by producing papillary muscle dysfunction septal defects or a free-wall rupture or right ventricular infarction. Other causes are listed in Table 10.1. Traditionally, tachy- and bradyarrhythmias are listed separately.

Cardiogenic shock is a highly lethal condition with a mortality rate in excess of 80% if a non-invasive, supportive approach is used. Preventing cardiogenic shock from developing is the most effective therapy, and every effort should be made to limit infarct size in patients with acute myocardial infarction (AMI) (including early coronary artery reperfusion, controlling hypertension and correcting tachy/bradyarrhythmias). It seems clear that percutaneous transluminal coronary angioplasty (PTCA) or emergency bypass are more effective than thrombolytic therapy.

Management

1. Assess and treat ABCs.
2. Maintaining an adequate blood pressure can be difficult, particularly because the volumes of fluid used in normal resuscitation can adversely affect myocardial oxygen consumption and exacerbate the problem. The patient's condition does not always allow time for institution of monitoring or for sophisticated monitoring (e.g. Swan-Ganz catheter) and may force the clinician to administer empiric therapy. If the patient is already in pulmonary oedema, a fluid bolus should be avoided, but for other patients it is acceptable to try incremental small boluses of crystalloid as a first step.
3. If there is no response to a fluid challenge, a vasopressor is required. Commonly used agents include dobutamine and dopamine.
4. Afterload reduction leads to improved cardiac function, but further reduction in blood pressure may compromise the function of other vital

organs. Afterload reduction is therefore something to institute with caution to prevent exacerbation of hypotension.

5. Specific therapy includes aspirin control of arrhythmias and reperfusion of the infarcted area.

6. Consider use of intraaortic balloon pump for patients who remain haemodynamically unstable.

DISTRIBUTIVE SHOCK

A number of pathological conditions cause distributive shock, the hallmarks of which are maldistribution of intravascular fluid through microvascular leak and/or vasodilation.

Septic shock

Septic shock results from a host response to infection with triggering of an immunologic cascade. While the microbiological products are harmful, the widespread and unregulated host response produces chemical mediators which harm the host as well as the infecting organism. Chemical mediators involved include the complement system, leukotrienes, prostaglandins, thromboxanes, histamine, bradykinins, tumour necrosis factor (TNF) and interleukin-1.

Septic shock occurs in approximately 50% of those with gram-negative bacteraemia, and in about 20% of those with *Staphylococcus aureus* bacteraemia. The gram-negative organisms most often implicated are *E. coli, Klebsiella, Pseudomonas, Enterobacter* and *Proteus* species.

Septic shock is marked clinically by signs of underlying infection (although this may not be obvious in the immunocompromised or those at extremes of age) and vasodilation (with warm peripheries despite hypotension). Eventually myocardial dysfunction adds to the instability caused by microvascular leak and vasodilation.

Management

1. Assess and treat ABCs.

2. Large volumes of fluid may be required.

3. In addition to fluids, inotropes are likely to be necessary, and should be chosen to address the twin problems of decreased systemic vascular resistance as well as decreased myocardial function. Noradrenaline is an appropriate agent.

4. Sophisticated, invasive monitoring is often required, including arterial monitoring, CVP and PAWP.

5. The source of sepsis should be aggressively and rapidly sought. It may be appropriate to administer empiric antibiotic therapy, unless a focus can be established. Other treatments may include surgical drainage, debridement or laparotomy.

Anaphylactic shock

Anaphylactic shock results from the release of chemical mediators from mast cells and basophils. These chemicals (including histamine, prostaglandins, kallikrein etc) cause vasodilation and capillary leakage, and subsequently hypotension. In addition, they can cause life-threatening compromise of the upper airway (angio-oedema) and ventilation (bronchospasm).

Clinically the syndrome is marked by a recent exposure to an allergen (normally within half an hour), the presence of urticarial angio-oedema (90% of patients), rhinitis, conjunctivitis, gastrointestinal cramping and bronchospasm.

Management

1. Assess and treat ABCs. Be ready to deal with rapid progressive loss of airway. Endotracheal intubation may be difficult or impossible in the face of massive angio-oedema, and a surgical airway may be necessary. Be prepared for resistant bronchospasm.
2. All patients will benefit from supplemental oxygen and IV fluids.
3. The specific agent of choice is adrenaline, which can be life-saving. It can be administered IM or IV, but if administered IV should be given in small (50–100 µg) titrated boluses as required.
4. Other agents frequently used include antihistamines and corticosteroids, but adrenaline is the agent of choice. Steroids may reduce the incidence of recurrence that occurs hours after the first presentation. Promethazine is a commonly used antihistamine (25–50 mg IV for adults), and an H_2 blocker like cimetidine can be used in resistant cases.
5. Bronchospasm can be treated on its merits.
6. Remove the offending agent, if possible.
7. Consider glucagon if the patient is on beta-blockers and is not responding to standard treatment.
8. Re-examine the patient frequently to assess progress.

Neurogenic shock

Neurogenic shock occurs when sympathetic tone is lost following spinal cord transection above the T6 level. Loss of sympathetic tone causes peripheral vasodilation and is classically associated with bradycardia.

Management

1. Assess and treat ABCs. If the level of injury is high enough (e.g. high cervical), there may be compromised ventilatory effort.
2. Engage in a thorough search for other causes of hypotension. Blood loss should be sought and confidently excluded before hypotension is attributed to neurogenic causes alone.
3. If neurogenic shock does need to be treated, it is relatively unresponsive to fluid resuscitation, and overhydration is to be discouraged. Patients

may require treatment with inotropic/vasopressor agents to effectively raise blood pressure.

OBSTRUCTIVE SHOCK

Obstructive shock is hypotension due to impeded venous return. Circulatory volume is normal, but blood is prevented from entering the heart.

Specific clinical signs are of impeded venous return (distended neck veins) and also of the cause.

Pericardial tamponade

Pericardial tamponade occurs when fluid accumulates in the pericardial space, eventually impairing cardiac filling. Classically, patients manifest Beck's triad (hypotension, elevated venous pressure and muffled heart sounds), and may have pulsus paradoxus greater than 10 mmHg. Clinical deterioration can be rapid. ECG may show electrical alternans, and the diagnosis can be established definitively with echocardiography.

1. Assess and treat ABCs.
2. All patients benefit from IV fluids and oxygen.
3. Specific therapy is emergent pericardiocentesis, which ideally should be done with echo and ECG guidance.
4. Other specific therapies depend on the cause, and may include cardiac surgery for penetrating injuries to the myocardium.

Tension pneumothorax

Obstructive shock results from a tension pneumothorax when raised intrathoracic pressure induces collapse of cardiac chambers and impairs cardiac function. Specific signs include respiratory distress, with shift of the trachea from the midline and a hyperresonant, quiet chest on the side of the pneumothorax. The diagnosis is clinical, and should not depend on a confirmatory chest X-ray.

Management

1. Assess and treat ABCs.
2. Specific therapy is to drain the pneumothorax, initially by needle thoracostomy, immediately followed by a formal intercostal catheter.
3. Sucking chest wounds can cause a tension pneumothorax and should be covered with a non-permeable dressing stuck down on three sides.
4. A pneumothorax that resists drainage and continues to bubble vigorously may represent an injury to a major airway. Cardiothoracic help should be sought.

Pulmonary embolism

Massive pulmonary embolism can cause obstructive shock (see Chapter 9).

CONTROVERSIES
Crystalloid versus colloid

It is fair to say that, at the time of publication, crystalloids are enjoying a resurgence. Most readers will be familiar with the arguments for and against, and should direct their attention to any of the excellent arguments written on the subject.

Volume of fluids

There is currently a great deal of discussion about the extent to which we should attempt to normalise blood pressure in hypotensive patients suffering from blood loss. It seems clear that hypotension is deleterious in the setting of major head injury, and every effort should be made to achieve normotension in such patients.

Recent evidence seems to suggest that for other conditions (e.g. penetrating torso injury, ectopic pregnancy, aortic aneurysm rupture) aiming for normal blood pressure through fluid therapy may be dis-advantageous, and certainly that supranormal blood pressure may encourage bleeding. For this second group subnormal blood pressure may be acceptable and even desirable, providing surgery can be arranged expeditiously.

Most clinicians have responded to these conflicting pieces of evidence by maintaining normal blood pressure values in any patient with a head injury, but limiting fluid in patients with penetrating injuries and certainly avoiding blood pressures which are supranormal.

Other controversies

Other controversies that episodically resurface include the use of steroid in sepsis and the use of MAST suits.

SUMMARY

There are multiple causes of shock, but the initial approach is always the same. Secure an airway, supplement ventilation if possible, provide oxygen and resuscitate with IV fluids (except for cardiogenic shock). Further fluid loss should be prevented, if hypovolaemia is the cause of shock. The specific cause should be sought and treated as appropriate.

EDITOR'S COMMENT

Inadequate fluid replacement, especially in younger shocked patients, is still a major cause of preventable morbidity.

RECOMMENDED READING

Annane D, Sebille V, Charpentier C, et al. Effect of treatment with low doses of hydrocortisone and fludrocortisone on mortality in patients with septic shock. JAMA 2002; 288(7):862–871.

Burris D, Rhee P, Kaufmann C, et al. Controlled resuscitation for uncontrolled haemorrhagic shock. J Trauma 1999; 46(2):216–222.

Dutton R, Mackenzie C, Scalea T. Hypotensive resuscitation during active haemorrhage: impact on in-hospital mortality. J Trauma 2002; 52(6):1141–1146.

McCunn M, Karlin A. Nonblood fluid resuscitation. Anaesthesiology Clinics of North America 1999; 17(1):107–121.

McGee S, Abernethy W, Simel D. Is this patient hypovolaemic? JAMA 1999; 281(11):1022–1029.

11 Emergency treatment of hypertension

Diane King

Hypertension is a common condition. The most common aetiology is unknown (essential hypertension). The other major causes are renal disease, glucocorticoid excess (endogenous or iatrogenic), coarctation of the aorta and phaeochromocytoma.

Hypertension in the emergency department is seen in a number of situations:

- An acute rise related to pain and anxiety—which should be treated symptomatically.
- An incidental finding—which requires appropriate investigation and follow-up.
- In a patient with a known history of hypertension on treatment.
- Long-term complications of hypertension—for example stroke, ischaemic heart disease, peripheral vascular disease and aortic dissection.
- Hypertension related to a catastrophic intracranial event.
- Hypertensive emergencies—which occur in the presence of end organ dysfunction related to a relatively acute increase in blood pressure.

MALIGNANT HYPERTENSION

Malignant hypertension is severe hypertension associated with acute and progressive end organ damage. If untreated it may result in acute renal failure, an intracerebral bleed, papilloedema, encephalopathy and cardiac involvement, including acute left ventricular failure or myocardial infarction. The diastolic blood pressure is usually above 130 mmHg.

The severity of the end organ damage and the speed of progression dictate the speed required to control the blood pressure and the agents used.

HYPERTENSIVE ENCEPHALOPATHY

Hypertensive encephalopathy occurs with an acute rise in blood pressure to the extent that cerebral autoregulation is lost and cerebral ischaemia secondary to vasospasm occurs. This occurs at a mean arterial pressure (MAP) of 150–200 mmHg. Patients present with headache, vomiting, drowsiness, papilloedema and possibly focal neurological deficits. Treatment must be instituted to rapidly reduce the MAP to about 120 mmHg. This is best achieved in an intensive care environment with an infusion of sodium nitroprusside. Alternative drug therapies include glyceryl trinitrate, labetalol or diazoxide.

PULMONARY OEDEMA

Hypertension frequently accompanies acute left ventricular failure, and may be causative. Myocardial ischaemia may also be present in this setting. The treatment includes oxygen, intravenous diuretic (frusemide) and an intravenous glyceryl trinitrate infusion. In severe cases continuous positive airway pressure or ventilation may be required. Glyceryl trinitrate is particularly useful in this setting as its venodilator effect lowers blood pressure, improves myocardial ischaemia and decreases total peripheral resistance, thereby improving myocardial function.

THORACIC AORTIC DISSECTION

Chronic hypertension is the underlying cause of thoracic aortic dissection in 90% of cases. The patient presents with severe, unremitting chest and back pain, may have differential arm blood pressure readings and/or neurological deficits. Chest X-ray may show a widened mediastinum. The blood pressure at the time of dissection is usually, although not always, elevated. Treatment may be medical or surgical or both, and depends on the site and extent of the dissection. Surgery is usually indicated in proximal dissections. Medical therapy consists of control of heart rate, force of contraction, and blood pressure. This is achieved by use of beta-blocking agents such as propranolol, metoprolol or esmolol, possibly with the addition of a sodium nitroprusside infusion, or a combined alpha- and beta-blocking agent such as labetalol.

CATASTROPHIC INTRACRANIAL EVENT

Hypertension may be seen in a patient with severe head trauma, acute ischaemic stroke, subarachnoid haemorrhage or intracranial haemorrhage. Control of blood pressure in this setting is best managed by supportive care, with sedation and analgesia rather than antihypertensives, as loss of cerebral perfusion pressure by too rapid a drop in blood pressure can be harmful. This must be balanced, however, by the risk in severe hypertension of intracerebral vasospasm or rebleeding.

PREECLAMPSIA AND ECLAMPSIA

Hypertension in pregnancy increases risk to both the mother and fetus. Because the blood pressure in pregnancy is normally lower than in the non-pregnant state, significant effects from hypertension occur at relatively lower blood pressures. Preeclampsia occurs when there is systolic blood pressure greater than 140 mmHg or diastolic pressure greater than 100 mmHg, and proteinuria. It occurs most commonly in primiparous women or older multiparous women. Preeclampsia is usually gradual in onset, occurring mostly after 32 weeks' gestation, and is manifest by hypertension, proteinuria and oedema. As severity increases, central nervous system involvement occurs, with visual disturbance, headache, confusion and then seizures. The presence of seizures defines eclampsia. Optic fundal examination is abnormal, and hyperreflexia and muscle clonus may be present. Renal function is impaired, and multiorgan impairment may be evident.

Preeclampsia requires urgent obstetric consultation, hospitalisation with bed rest and blood pressure control. Blood pressure control is with hydralazine, which in an emergency situation is given in intravenous boluses to achieve a diastolic blood pressure of less than 100 mmHg. Other agents that can be used are diazoxide or labetalol.

If eclampsia is present, blood pressure control is achieved in the same way, and occasionally sodium nitroprusside may be required, although this should be used only if other agents have failed, as there are fetal risks with its use. Seizure prevention and control is achieved with the use of intravenous magnesium sulphate in 4–6 mg boluses. Magnesium may be given up to the point of loss of reflexes. Urgent delivery of the fetus is the definitive therapy for severe preeclampsia and eclampsia.

DRUG THERAPY IN HYPERTENSIVE EMERGENCIES

Beta-blockers

Intravenous beta blockade may be achieved with metoprolol, which is injected in a dose of 5 mg slowly over 1–2 minutes. This is repeated up to a dose of 15 mg as required. This is most commonly used in aortic dissection. Oral therapy should also be commenced. Labetalol is a nonselective beta-blocking agent with alpha-blocking effects. Used intravenously, it is given in 20 mg aliquots infused over 2 minutes. It acts rapidly, taking effect in 5–10 minutes.

All beta-blocking agents are contraindicated in asthma, heart block, and left ventricular failure.

Glyceryl trinitrate

Intravenous glyceryl trinitrate is a rapidly acting agent with predominant venodilator effect and has coronary vasodilating properties. This makes it an ideal choice for myocardial hypertensive emergencies. It is given as an intravenous infusion requiring close blood pressure monitoring, and is titrated to effect. The usual preparation is 50 mg in 500 mL 5% dextrose solution. Because the drug migrates into plastics, it must be given from a glass solution bottle through a specific latex-free set.

Sodium nitroprusside

Sodium nitroprusside is the most potent antihypertensive agent, and requires continuous arterial pressure monitoring in an intensive care environment. It becomes inactive if exposed to light, and the whole infusion should be covered with aluminium foil. The dose is titrated to effect, and the infusion is prepared as 50 mg in 500 mL 5% dextrose, given through a microdrip.

Hydralazine

Hydralazine is used in obstetric hypertensive emergencies and is given intravenously initially as bolus doses over 1 minute. The initial dose is 5 mg, and repeat doses of 10 mg may be given every 20 minutes if required. Oral therapy can also be instituted.

Other antihypertensive agents

The common antihypertensive agents are used for less immediate blood pressure control and are given orally. The calcium channel blocker nifedipine may be given in a dose of 10–20 mg orally. It is a potent arteriodilating agent, with rapid onset of action. It has negligible effect on the myocardial conduction system, but does have negative inotropic effects and may cause an unpredictable blood pressure drop. It should therefore be used with caution in urgent situations.

Angiotensin-converting enzyme (ACE) inhibitors are best reserved as the agents of choice for long-term blood pressure control.

RECOMMENDED READING

Marx JA, Hockberger RS, Walls RM, et al. Rosen's emergency medicine: concepts and clinical practice. 5th edn. St Louis: Mosby; 2001.

Tintinalli JE, Kelen GD, Stapczynski JS. Emergency medicine: a comprehensive study guide. American College of Emergency Physicians. 6th edn. New York: McGraw-Hill; 2003.

12 Clinical electrocardiography

Allen Yuen

This chapter examines the clinical use of the ECG, one of the most important diagnostic tools in an emergency department. It must be stressed, however, that the ECG may appear normal, even in the presence of severe cardiac disease.

The reader should have knowledge of basic cardiac electrophysiology and anatomy, which will help in localising lesions from the ECG.

INDICATIONS

ECGs are indicated as follows:

1. Early, to assist in the diagnosis and treatment of potentially life-threatening disorders.
2. Routinely, as part of cardiac assessment.

They should be performed in all cases of chest pain, upper abdominal pain, dyspnoea, collapse, arrest, palpitations, syncope, dizziness, nontraumatic loss of consciousness and shock; also in any patient with a history of hypertension, fluid or electrolyte imbalance, drug overdose or other conditions that may affect the heart.

ECG INTERPRETATION

This is most usefully done in the context of the presenting symptoms and signs, which fall into three main groups:

1. Chest and upper abdominal pain, dyspnoea, shock.
2. Collapse, palpitations, syncope, dizziness, altered consciousness.
3. Electrolyte disturbances, drug overdose, environmental emergencies.

The ECG should be examined for rate, rhythm, P wave, PR interval, QRS morphology and axis, ST-T segment, T wave and Q-T interval.

With chest pain, particular attention is paid to the ST-T segment and Q waves. The underlying lesions may be determined by ECG pattern recognition. It is useful to have a previous ECG for comparison, so that the significance of any changes can be better understood.

1. Chest and upper abdominal pain, dyspnoea, shock

History and examination are the mainstays of assessment, with the ECG playing a complementary role. The main conditions requiring early diagnosis are acute myocardial infarction (AMI), unstable angina, aortic dissection and pulmonary embolism (PE).

Myocardial infarction

Note that the initial ECG may be normal in about half of patients with AMI. The earliest change is ST elevation, which may occur within 30 minutes of onset of pain, and is the basis upon which a decision regarding thrombolysis or angioplasty is made.

ST elevation

- ST elevation = or >1 mm in LI & aVL suggests a lateral AMI (Figure 12.1), usually due to occlusion of the circumflex artery .
- ST elevation = or >1 mm in LII, III & aVF suggests inferior AMI, usually due to occlusion of the right coronary artery. In some cases, the left coronary system may be the site, if the left coronary artery (LCA) is 'dominant'.
- ST elevation = or >2 mm in chest leads suggests anterior or anteroseptal (if only in V_{1-3}) AMI, which occurs with occlusion of the left main coronary or its branches.

If treated early with thrombolysis or angioplasty, the ST elevation can regress, and further myocardial damage prevented.

Normal 'high ST-take-off' in anterior chest leads can confuse the diagnosis when the chest pain is atypical, but when in doubt it is better to suspect an acute cardiac event than to clear the patient. Consult an emergency physician, cardiologist or registrar.

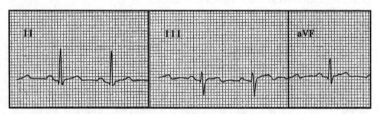

Figure 12.1 Inferior AMI, earliest changes: minimal ST elevation in II, III, aVF

ST depression

ST depression >2 mm in V_1 may indicate a posterior infarct, and this may be confirmed in ECG leads $V_{7,8,9}$. $V_{1,2}$ will also have a prominent R wave and tall T waves. Posterior infarcts are usually caused by occlusion of the right coronary artery (RCA).

The RCA also supplies the sinoatrial (SA) and arteriovenous (AV) nodes and the bundle of His. Occlusion of the RCA is associated with potentially serious bradyarrhythmias.

Table 12.1 Infarct localisation—the ECG pattern distribution will help to localise the site of infarction and the usual infarct-related artery

ECG pattern distribution	Site	Infarct-related artery
V_{2-5}	Anterior	Left main & branches
V_{1-3}	Anteroseptal	Left main & branches
V_{5-6} , I, aVL	Anterolateral	Left anterior descending
I, aVL	Lateral	Left anterior descending
II, III, aVF	Inferior	Right coronary or circumflex
$V_{7,8,9}$	Posterior	Right coronary or circumflex
Reciprocal changes $(R,\downarrow ST,\downarrow T)V_{1,2}$ RV_4	Right ventricular	Right coronary

Minor ST or Q wave changes in V_1 with signs of right ventricular failure, e.g. elevated jugular venous pressure (JVP), may point to a right ventricular infarct: right ventricular leads $RV_{3,4,5}$ may show characteristically slight ST elevation.

Q waves

Q waves >2 mm, >40 msec follow in those leads showing ST elevation, if the infarct evolves (Table 12.1). They may appear within the first hour or, more commonly, within 2–6 hours (Figure 12.2). Differentiate from septal Q waves in LI, LII, aVF or V_5, V_6, which are small (<2 mm) and narrow.

A nonpathological Q wave can occur in LIII; it is narrow, <2 mm and less than one-third the height of the QRS complex, and may disappear during deep inspiration. A small Q wave in LIII is significant if associated with one in LII.

Sometimes Q waves don't develop, but AMI can still be suspected if there are small R waves with 'lack of progression of R waves' across the anterior leads (normally the R wave increases in amplitude from V_2 to V_4). These infarcts are often associated with inverted T waves.

Non-Q AMI refers to subendocardial infarcts. Up to 40% of infarcts are not transmural, but they predispose to reinfarction.

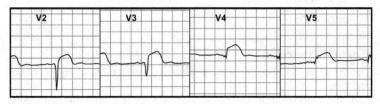

Figure 12.2 Anterior AMI, later changes: Q waves, prominent coved ST elevation V_{2-5}

R wave

A prominent R wave in V_1, and often in V_2, suggests a posterior infarct, as well as incomplete right bundle branch block (RBBB), right ventricular hypertrophy (RVH) or left accessory pathway.

T waves

Hyperacute peaked T waves in V leads may be the only sign of AMI; they may occur in hyperkalaemia or without a known cause.

Left bundle branch block (LBBB)

New LBBB with chest pain indicates AMI. The location may be diagnosed by inspecting the affected leads to see whether there is concordance of ST segments with QRS complexes (in non-AMI LBBB, the ST segments are discordant with the QRS, i.e. they point in opposite directions).

In LBBB, AMI is present if the following occur:

- The QRS is upright and the ST is elevated >5 mm.
- The QRS is depressed and the ST is also depressed.
- There are Q waves in LI and aVL, which indicate a lateral AMI.

Right bundle branch block (RBBB)

RBBB does not mask AMI, as ST elevation does not occur in non-AMI RBBB.

Unstable angina, acute coronary syndrome, acute ischaemia

The ECG may be normal, but acute ischaemia is confirmed by 2 mm or more ST depression in anterior or standard leads. This may be induced by exercise. If angina is prolonged greater than 20 minutes, then this can be regarded as preinfarctional.

Left ventricular hypertrophy

LAD

- S inV_2 + R inV_5 >35 mm.
- ST depression anterior chest leads (LV strain).

Pericarditis

- Extensive ST elevation, concave upwards.
- P-R depression.

Myocarditis

Nonspecific ST-T changes.

Aortic dissection

The ECG is nonspecific, with associated hypertensive changes in the majority.

If the dissection involves the coronary ostia, resultant myocardial ischaemia or infarction may be seen. The cardiac surgeon should be notified urgently.

Pulmonary embolus

Over 40% of cases show no significant change, therefore a normal ECG does not rule out a pulmonary embolus. ECG findings include:

- Sinus tachycardia.
- RBBB, usually partial.
- R axis deviation.
- $S_1Q_3T_3$ (acute cor pulmonale).
- ST elevation in aVR.
- Anterior T wave inversion V_{1-4} (Figure 12.3); differentiate from the normal T wave inversion found in some youths, athletes and negroid people in V_{1-3}.

Compromised patients may need urgent thrombolysis or embolectomy.

2. Collapse, palpitations, syncope, dizziness, altered consciousness

The ECG can help to determine a cardiac cause.

AMI, acute ischaemia, unstable angina or acute coronary syndrome

These can cause syncope or coma as a result of vasovagal reaction, cardiogenic shock, tamponade or any of the following arrhythmias.

Ventricular asystole

Absence of any electrical activity with a 'flat' ECG is asystole requiring cardiac massage, full cardiopulmonary resuscitation (CPR) and the use of adrenaline as in advanced life support (ALS) guidelines.

Ensure that leads are attached and recording amplitude is correct, as low-voltage ventricular fibrillation (VF) may be misinterpreted as asystole. Direct current reversion should be tried, if there is any doubt.

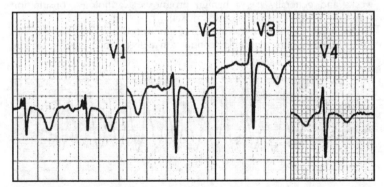

Figure 12.3 Acute pulmonary embolism: partial RBBB, inverted T waves V_{1-4}

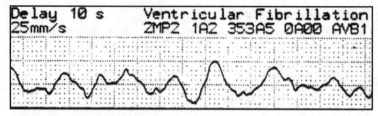

Figure 12.4   Ventricular fibrillation

Ventricular fibrillation

The grossly irregular and variable amplitude rhythm is unmistakeable (Figure 12.4). It requires immediate defibrillation and full CPR and ALS, with adrenaline and lignocaine or amiodarone as the mainstays of drug therapy.

Lack of response to treatment will lead to deterioration, agonal rhythm with a sine-wave pattern, asystole and death. Rarely, continued ALS may still rescue a patient with a preterminal rhythm.

Ventricular tachycardia (VT)

A wide-complex tachycardia represents VT (Figure 12.5) in over 90% of cases, approaching 100% in patients with prior AMI. If in doubt, treat as VT. Most VT occurs in the setting of structural heart disease, usually ischaemic.

If the patient is not haemodynamically compromised, chemical cardioversion should be attempted, with lignocaine, procainamide or amiodarone. Otherwise, prompt electrical cardioversion should be performed (once sedated or consciousness lost).

In the absence of structural heart disease, VT may last for seconds to weeks and generally has a benign prognosis. Cardiology consultation regarding medical management is advised.

Diagnostic difficulty occurs in cases of supraventricular tachycardia (SVT) with aberrancy/intraventricular conduction defect, which can mimic the

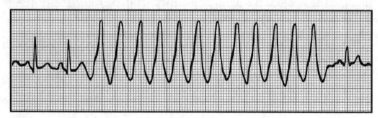

Figure 12.5   Ventricular tachycardia: onset from sinus rhythm

ECG appearances of VT. There should be typical LBBB or RBBB changes, otherwise it is not aberrancy and must be regarded as VT.

Torsades de pointes

Torsades de pointes is a polymorphic broad-complex VT with 'twisting of the axes', often several complexes alternating above and below the isoelectric line. The danger is that it may degenerate into VF, but it is more often self-limiting. Causes include drugs which prolong the Q-T interval, electrolyte disturbances and ischaemia; it may be congenital.

Treatment involves drug withdrawal, magnesium, correction of electrolytes or ischaemia, and pacing if bradycardic.

Heart block

High-degree heart block, particularly if associated with AMI, may deteriorate to complete heart block requiring urgent pacing. Incomplete occlusions can cause intermittent blocks.

First-degree AV bloc

The P-R interval is >0.2 seconds.

Second-degree, Mobitz Type I, Wenckebach

The P-R interval increases progressively until a 'dropped beat', with no QRS/ventricular response, occurs. The subsequent P-R interval is shorter than the P-R before the dropped beat.

Second-degree, Mobitz Type II

The P-R interval is constant, resulting in frequent dropped beats, often regular, e.g. 1 in 3. Deterioration results in a high rate of progression to complete heart block.

Third-degree, complete AV/heart block (CHB)

There is no P to QRS relationship; all of the atrial impulses are blocked at the AV node, so that regular P waves (rate >50) are seen with an independent, idioventricular QRS with a rate of around 30–40. If the QRS complex arises just below the AV node, the QRS may be narrow and normal in appearance (junctional AV block). More distal rhythms are relatively wide (>0.12 s). In general, the broader escape rhythms are more unstable and more likely to progress to ventricular standstill. Patients with CHB (complete heart block) may decompensate with poor cardiac output, hypotension or loss of consciousness (Stokes-Adams attack). Urgent treatment with atropine, isoprenaline and/or pacing are indicated. It seems atropine is more effective for narrow complex CHB, and may worsen the block in broad complex CHB.

Bundle branch block (BBB)

BBB generally indicates disease in the main conducting system, and syncope can result from an associated AMI with decompensation, progression to CHB and asystole.

LBBB (Figure 12.6), due to functional or anatomical block of the LBB and delayed depolarisation of the left ventricle, is seen as an rS in V_1 and a broad RR^1 in $V_{5,6}$ with a wide QRS (>0.12 s). It can be benign, but it is more commonly associated with ischaemic heart disease (IHD) and hypertension. It is important to note that evidence of AMI may still be seen on the ECG (see above, under 'Myocardial infarction').

RBBB (Figure 12.7), due to functional or anatomical block of the RBB and delayed depolarisation of the right ventricle, is seen as an RSR^1 pattern in $V_{1,2}$ with a wide QRS (>0.12 s) and is often benign, but can also be a sign of acute right heart strain, such as acute pulmonary embolism. AMI is not disguised by a RBBB.

LAFB (left anterior fascicular block, anterior hemiblock) is seen as left axis deviation ($Q_1R_1S_3$) and a normal duration QRS. In patients with chest pain, it signifies partial occlusion of the left anterior descending artery and occurs in about half of anterior infarctions. If the LAD occlusion is more extensive, RBBB will also be present.

LPFB (left posterior fascicular block, posterior hemiblock) is rare and seen as right axis deviation (S_1R_3) and a normal duration QRS. Since the posterior fascicle is broad, its occurrence indicates a widespread lesion such as an inferolateral infarct, cardiomyopathy or cor pulmonale. If associated

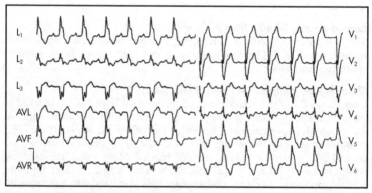

Figure 12.6 Left bundle branch block

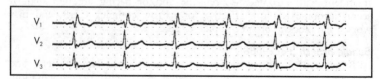

Figure 12.7 Right bundle branch block

with RBBB, this signifies extensive coronary artery disease with high risk of complete AV block.

Atrial fibrillation (AF)

In atrial fibrillation there are no P waves, and the rhythm is irregular (Figure 12.8). It is the most common supraventricular tachycardia and its incidence increases with age.

When caused by AMI or PE, with rapid irregular ventricular response (130–180), AF may result in poor cardiac output with palpitations and syncope. It usually coexists with hypertensive, dilated, valvular or rheumatic heart disease, although up to 25% patients have 'lone' AF with no structural heart disease.

Acute management involves rate control and reversion to sinus rhythm. Rate control is best achieved with drugs which prolong AV nodal conduction, such as IV beta-blockers (e.g. metoprolol) or calcium channel blockers (e.g. verapamil) or digoxin. Reversing the arrhythmia is best achieved with sotalol, amiodarone or DC cardioversion.

Digoxin has long been the mainstay of therapy, but while it slows the rate, it may prolong the arrhythmia. It must not be used in AF with preexcitation (Wolff-Parkinson-White syndrome—WPW), where it may cause serious tachyarrhythmias.

Flecainide is effective for reversion, but is contraindicated in IHD and congestive cardiac failure (CCF).

Curative radiofrequency ablation is used in selected cases.

If AF has been present for more than 1–2 days, anticoagulation must be considered, to prevent atrial thrombosis and embolus (cerebral, mesenteric, peripheral). Echocardiography will help detect atrial thrombus.

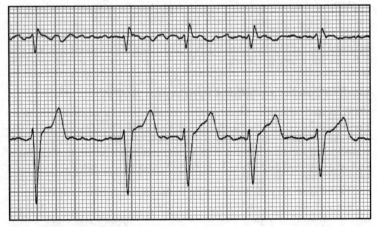

Figure 12.8 Atrial fibrillation

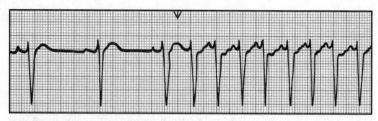

Figure 12.9 Paroxysmal supraventricular tachycardia

Atrial flutter

Generally, atrial flutter has an atrial rate of 300 with variable block (commonly 2:1 or 3:1).

It has the same causes as atrial fibrillation and may be treated similarly. Despite its regular rate, it may still result in atrial thrombus.

Paroxysmal supraventricular tachycardia (PSVT)

PSVT has a regular rate, usually 150–200 (range 100–280, see Figure 12.9). It is a junctional tachycardia where the AV node is an integral part of the arrhythmia circuit.

AV nodal re-entry tachycardia (AVNRT) is where the circuit is within the AV node itself, while AV re-entry tachycardia (AVRT) is where an additional (accessory) pathway is involved.

Vagal manoeuvres such as carotid sinus massage may terminate PSVT. Adenosine is relatively safe to use for chemical reversion. Verapamil may be used with care but it can cause intractable hypotension, CHB and asystole, especially if the patient is also on a beta-blocker or digoxin.

SVT with intraventricular conduction defect (aberrant conduction), such as when a concurrent bundle branch block or WPW syndrome causes a broad QRS complex, is difficult to differentiate from VT. Adenosine is safe for SVT with BBB, but in WPW it may cause hypotension and unstable VT. Radiofrequency ablation (RA) may be needed if adenosine is unsuccessful.

Wolff-Parkinson-White syndrome (WPW)

WPW is due to preexcitation of the ventricles by an accessory pathway, bypassing the AV node, resulting in a short P-R interval, and a slurred upstroke or 'delta wave' on the R wave, best seen in V_{2-6} (Figure 12.10). If associated with a dominant R in V_1 and inverted T waves in V_{1-4}, this is due to a left accessory path (Type A WPW), otherwise the accessory path is on the right (Type B WPW).

The ECG of Type A WPW can be mistaken for a posterior AMI.

Serious paroxysmal tachyarrhythmias can occur by retrograde re-entry mechanisms or by rapid conduction of superimposed AF/atrial flutter, such as when digoxin is used for treating AF when WPW is unrecognised.

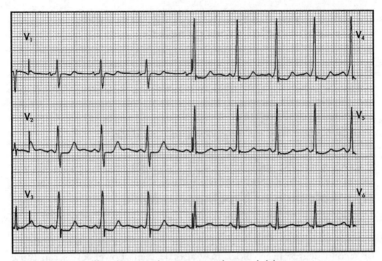

Figure 12.10 Wolff-Parkinson-White Type A with typical delta waves

Impulses may be rapidly conducted down the accessory path and cause a bizarre ECG with variable width QRS tachycardia, hypotension and eventual VF arrest.

Treat WPW tachyarrhythmias with IV procainamide if stable, or cardioversion if decompensated. Other drugs may be used, but there is risk of exacerbating aberrant conduction. RA or surgery may be needed.

Holter monitoring

Despite a history suggestive of an abnormal rhythm, none may be detected during emergency department assessment. The patient should be considered for admission for cardiac monitoring or Holter monitoring as an outpatient.

Holter monitoring involves attaching a patient to a portable personal ECG monitor, which records usually two ECG channels on tape or computer for 24 hours. A technician then scans the recordings by computer and identifies periods of arrhythmia, which are then presented to the cardiologist for review to see if episodes of palpitations, syncope, angina etc can be explained.

Sinus bradycardia <35 bpm, sinus pauses <3 s, Wenckebach, brief runs of AF, multiple atrial ectopics and isolated ventricular ectopic beats are all found in otherwise normal people and do not warrant treatment.

Sustained arrhythmias are more significant, particularly in symptomatic patients.

Holter monitoring is also useful in checking response to antiarrhythmics.

3. Electrolyte imbalance, drug overdose, environmental emergencies

Arrhythmias can arise as a result of any of the above conditions.

Potassium or magnesium imbalance

Potassium imbalance and magnesium imbalance cause similar effects and are important to recognise early, as each may progress to serious arrhythmias if uncorrected.

Hyperkalaemia or hypermagnesaemia

Hyperkalaemia or hypermagnesaemia may cause tall, peaked T waves, flat P waves, wide QRS and undefined ST-T changes. Higher levels will cause various tachyarrhythmias including VT and, eventually, asystole.

Hypokalaemia or hypomagnesaemia

Hypokalaemia or hypomagnesaemia may result in a prolonged Q-T, flattened T waves and small U waves; note that U waves may occur in healthy people in V_{2-4}, but the T waves are normal. ST depression and first- or second-degree heart block may also be seen. Lower levels can cause atrial and ventricular arrhythmias, notably torsades de pointes.

Calcium imbalance

Hypercalcaemia

Hypercalcaemia shortens the ST and the Q-T intervals, but widens the T wave. Bradycardias, BBB, second-degree heart block and CHB can deteriorate to asystole if levels are markedly elevated.

Hypocalcaemia

Hypocalcaemia lengthens the ST and therefore the Q-T interval, with risk of VT and torsades. A prolonged Q-Tc may be caused by any drug which causes hypocalcaemia, hypokalaemia and hypomagnesaemia.

Prolonged Q-Tc Interval

A Q-Tc (corrected for the rate) of over 0.44 s predisposes to VT and torsades, and should be corrected as soon as possible.

Drugs that cause this include the macrolide antibiotics, tricyclic antidepressants, antifungals, antihistamines, trimethoprim, cisapride and Class 1A & C antiarrhythmic agents.

Any serious tachycardia associated with prolonged Q-Tc should be treated by correcting the underlying cause and cardioversion or Class 1B antiarrhythmics such as amiodarone or phenytoin, and not the usual Class 1A drugs. Pacing may be needed.

Environmental emergencies

Hypothermia and electrocution are examples of emergencies that cause cardiac effects.

Hypothermia

With severe hypothermia, cardiac effects can be related to the temperature. The initial response is a sinus tachycardia with temperatures down to 32°, then bradycardia with temperatures down to about 30°. Osborn waves, which are deflections at the end of the QRS complex and in the same direction as the QRS, appear at around 30°, and increase in height as the temperature falls. Various arrhythmias occur down to 27°, when VF may occur and cause death. In some patients VF does not occur, and the temperature can fall as low as 22°, culminating in fatal asystole. Gradual rewarming and ALS should be instituted early to avoid this. See also Chapter 32.

Electrocution

Cardiac effects can vary from nil to ST changes, transient arrhythmias, BBB, heart block, myocardial necrosis and cardiac asystole. If the route from entry to exit points traverses the torso, cardiac damage is more likely.

A low current of 10–100 microamps (μA), resulting from stray currents or earthing faults in household equipment, can cause a microshock, which can result in VF arrest. If the skin resistance is lowered by moisture, a 0.24 milliamp (mA) current from a 240 V source can be increased to a current of 240 mA and cause a macroshock, with resultant VF.

Contact with high-tension power lines (>1000 A) or a lightning strike (>12000 A) can cause cardiorespiratory arrest from asystole (more commonly) or VF. Early advanced life support may save these patients, but the severity of their burns will determine their survival.

See also Chapter 31.

Axis (electrical pathway mapping)

Axis generally refers to the QRS axis and the direction of depolarisation in the ventricles as reflected in the frontal plane (the anterior chest wall). It is best illustrated by a clock face with each numerical division representing 30° (Figure 12.11).

The horizontal direction can be determined by inspecting LI, to see whether the QRS deflection is mainly up (positive impulse moving from right to left), or down (negative impulse from left to right).

The vertical direction is reflected in aVF (the vertical axis). If the QRS deflection is mainly up, the impulse is travelling towards the foot, and if the QRS is down, the impulse is towards the head.

Combining this information, the quadrant in which the QRS vector lies can be determined.

- QRS in LI up, in aVF up—vector in left lower quadrant (normal axis).
- QRS in LI up, in aVF down—vector in left upper quadrant (left axis deviation).
- QRS in LI down, in aVF up—vector in right lower quadrant (right axis deviation).

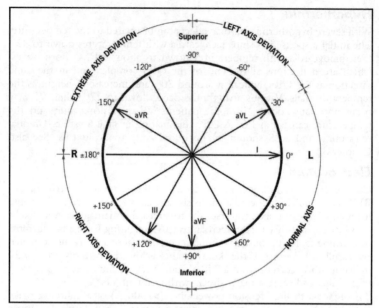

Figure 12.11 The QRS frontal plane cardiac axial reference system (Yuen Derek, after Fisch C, Electrocardiography (in Braunwald E, Heart disease, 5th edn) and Mirvis D, Goldberg A, Electrocardiography (in Braunwald E, Heart disease, 6th edn). Philadelphia: WB Saunders; 1997 and 2001)

- QRS in LI down, in aVF down—vector in right upper quadrant (indeterminate or extreme right axis deviation (RAD).

To determine the axis more accurately (within 30°), note which limb or standard lead has the most isoelectric QRS (equally up and down): the axis is at 90° to this in the predetermined quadrant (see Figure 12.11). The range of normal axis can extend from –30° to +90°, as patients who are obese can have a more horizontal heart (vector in left upper quadrant), while those who are asthenic have a more vertical heart (90° axis). Thus, if the QRS is isoelectric in lead aVR, and the above criteria point to the left upper quadrant (left axis deviation), then a perpendicular (90°) to the aVR axis gives an axis of –60° in the left upper quadrant. The QRS axis is then –60° in the frontal plane.

While the above is more accurate, a simple summary is:

- QRS in LI negative = RAD.
- QRS in LII negative = LAD.

Significance

Left axis deviation

Left axis deviation should raise the suspicion of anterior hemiblock (left anterior fascicular block—LAFB), often as a result of occlusive disease of the left anterior descending artery or cardiomyopathy.

Right axis deviation

Right axis deviation suggests posterior hemiblock (right posterior fascicular block—RPFB) and usually right (occasionally, left) coronary artery disease, right ventricular hypertrophy, acute cor pulmonale (as in massive pulmonary embolus) or cardiomyopathy.

Note: In general, the vector moves towards hypertrophy and away from infarction.

QRS axis

QRS axis can also be described in the horizontal plane, looking up. Using the chest leads, the QRS is normally isoelectric in V_3 or V_4. If the QRS is isoelectric over $V_{1\,or\,2}$, this is counterclockwise rotation, and if in $V_{5\,or\,6}$, it is clockwise rotation.

EDITOR'S COMMENT

The ECG, which is a very routine test, will give many clues and information if they are looked for.

RECOMMENDED READING

Bersten AD, Soni N, Oh TE, eds. Oh's intensive care manual. 5th edn. Edinburgh: Butterworth-Heinemann; 2003.

Dubin D. Rapid interpretation of EKGs. 6th edn. Cover Publishing; 2000.

Hampton JR. The ECG in practice. 3rd edn. Edinburgh: Churchill Livingstone; 2001.

Mirvis DM, Goldberger AL. Electrocardiography. In: Braunwald E. Heart disease: a textbook of cardiovascular medicine. 6th edn. Philadelphia: WB Saunders; 2001.

Wagner G. Marriott's practical electrocardiography. 10th edn. Philadelphia: Lippincott Williams & Wilkins; 2001.

Acknowledgment: The author would like to thank Dr Bruno Martin, FRACP, Cardiologist, Epworth Hospital, who kindly reviewed the manuscript of this chapter.

GENERAL PRINCIPLES

Acute shortness of breath may herald a life-threatening condition.

Your role in the emergency department includes appropriate triage, immediate resuscitation and stabilisation, initial broad diagnosis and specific therapy (these may be concurrent).

Life-threatening conditions presenting with breathlessness

1. Acute asthma.
2. Acute exacerbation of chronic airflow limitation.
3. Acute cardiogenic pulmonary oedema.
4. Pneumonia.
5. Pneumothorax.
6. Pulmonary embolism.
7. Acute lung injury: contusion, aspiration, inhalation.
8. Anaphylaxis with acute bronchospasm.

OXYGEN THERAPY

Initial high-flow oxygen therapy is essential for any acutely breathless patient. The uncommon complications of oxygen therapy develop slowly, whereas acute hypoxaemia is immediately life-threatening.

If the patient is acutely breathless, oxygen must never be withheld (even to carry out tests). Stabilisation always comes before investigation.

Methods for delivering oxygen

1. Hudson mask

This method delivers between 30% and 60% oxygen, depending on flow rate and the patient's ventilation. Flow rates below 4 L/min should not be used, as rebreathing may occur.

2. Venturi mask

This system delivers controlled oxygen therapy, between 24% and 60%. Ideal for tailoring oxygen therapy after initial stabilisation, such as in patients with chronic airflow limitation (CAL) and CO_2 retention.

3. Non-rebreathing reservoir mask

With a well-fitting mask and full reservoir bag, this may deliver close to 100% oxygen. Suitable for alert patients with hypoxaemia, while contemplating ventilation.

4. Continuous positive airway pressure (CPAP)

Circuit requires air-tight mask, variable gas mixture and cooperative patient. Delivers up to 100% oxygen. Particularly useful in acute pulmonary oedema.

5. Bi-level positive airways pressure (BiPAP)

Similar to CPAP, but delivers cycled pressure. Effective in patients with CAL.

6. Bag–valve–mask circuit

This may deliver 100% oxygen, but requires a supine patient and is labour intensive. Ideal for preoxygenation prior to intubation.

Monitoring oxygen therapy: oximetry and arterial blood gases

Pulse oximetry should be a standard part of monitoring any acutely unwell patient. Below 90% oxygen saturation, arterial oxygenation falls precipitously. Oximetry is a rapid method of determining the method and amount of oxygen supplementation.

Arterial blood gases (ABGs) give information about oxygenation, ventilation, chronicity and acid–base status. Oxygen must not be withdrawn for 'blood gases on room air' while the patient is still unwell—oxygenation is vital and tests can wait until after stabilisation. Blood gases done initially on oxygen can give important information about the patient.

ACUTE ASTHMA

Asthmatic patients generally have a known diagnosis and a history of previous episodes. They may deteriorate suddenly and may present late, so assessment of severity and adequate initial treatment are vital. Asthmatic patients still die in hospital.

Initial stabilisation

1. Triage to an acute bed.
2. Apply high-flow oxygen immediately.
3. Obtain IV access.
4. Monitor respiratory rate, blood pressure, heart rate and pulse oximetry. Measure peak flow or spirometry (if possible).

Assessment of severity

High-risk features

1. **History**—childhood onset, steroid dependence, previous intensive care unit (ICU) admissions or need for ventilation.
2. **Examination**—inability to speak in sentences, use of accessory muscles, poor air entry, forced expiratory volume (FEV) or peak expiratory flow rate (PEFR) <50% predicted.

Features of life-threatening attack

Silent chest, sweating, vomiting, panic, inability to speak, pulse oximetry <90%.

Immediate treatment

1. Apply nebulised salbutamol in the appropriate dose (5 mg = 1 mL solution for adults).
2. If **life-threatening** features, give continuous nebulised salbutamol, concurrently prepare adrenaline and intubation equipment and summon help (senior staff skilled in intubation and ventilation). Make sure you have two secure IV lines and give a fluid volume load of 500 mL IV.
3. If **pre-arrest**, give intravenous salbutamol and aliquots of 0.1 mg adrenaline intravenously. Do not sedate—panic is a sign of impending arrest. Intubate and ventilate as a last resort—use low tidal volume and respiratory rate to avoid barotrauma (permissive hypercarbia).
4. If **stable**:
   - Further history: onset and duration of attack, medication, precipitants, past history, high-risk features, allergies. Check old notes.
   - Further examination: respiratory rate, air entry, accessory muscle use.
   - Investigations: not routinely indicated initially unless poor response to treatment.

Further treatment

1. Continue nebulised salbutamol—continuous or intermittent, as indicated by response. May add ipratropium bromide. Continue oxygen.
2. Give hydrocortisone, 100–200 mg IV or equivalent.
3. Assess response to treatment both clinically and by objective measurement (PEFR or spirometry).
4. Observe for a number of hours to assess need for admission. Err on the side of caution, especially at night.
5. If patient is discharged, ensure follow-up and education.

ACUTE EXACERBATION OF CHRONIC AIRFLOW LIMITATION (CAL)

Exacerbations are commonly precipitated by infection (viral or bacterial). Patients may still smoke, and may be oxygen-dependent. While chronic

CO_2 retention may be a feature, hypoxaemia is the immediate threat to life, and supplementary oxygen is required immediately. The oxygen delivery can be fine-tuned as the patient's condition stabilises.

Initial stabilisation

1. Triage to an acute bed.
2. Give oxygen immediately.
3. Obtain IV access.
4. Monitor respiratory rate, ECG, BP, pulse oximetry. Measure spirometry if possible. Aim to maintain SaO_2 above 90% by oximetry.
5. Commence nebuliser therapy—salbutamol with or without ipratropium.
6. If in **acute distress** and not improving: apply BiPAP (commencing with 50% oxygen and titrating to pulse oximetry of 90–95%). CPAP is useful if pulmonary oedema coexists.
7. If stable:
   - History: onset and duration of attack, medications, precipitant, other illnesses, smoking, home oxygen, general clinical state. Check old notes.
   - Examination: colour, respiratory rate, air entry, crepitations, accessory muscle use, oedema.
   - Investigations: chest X-ray (CXR) to exclude infection, pneumothorax; ABGs (initially on oxygen); white cell count (WCC) if infection suspected.

Further treatment

1. Continue nebulised salbutamol with or without ipratropium bromide—continuously or intermittently as required.
2. Hydrocortisone 100–200 mg IV.
3. Antibiotics if evidence of infection.
4. If concurrent pulmonary oedema, add nitrates and diuretics.
5. Admit to hospital (unless very mild exacerbation).

ACUTE PULMONARY OEDEMA

These patients generally present acutely distressed, sitting up, sweaty, anxious, and with widespread crackles in their chests. Wheezes may sometimes be heard, which may mean coexisting chronic airflow limitation or bronchospasm secondary to oedema. The common precipitants include myocardial ischaemia (chest pain), arrhythmias (commonly atrial fibrillation) and changes in medication (reduction of diuretics or addition of non-steroidal anti-inflammatory drugs—NSAIDs).

Cardiogenic pulmonary oedema is relatively easy to treat if associated with hypertension, but very difficult if associated with low BP (cardiogenic shock).

See also Chapter 8.

PNEUMONIA

Pneumonia generally presents with a combination of chest pain, shortness of breath and fever, sometimes with purulent sputum. It is uncommon for pneumonia to present as acute respiratory distress unless the condition is advanced, rapidly progressive (e.g. the immunosuppressed patient with *Pneumocystis carinii*) or associated with poor respiratory reserve. The immediate threats to life include hypoxaemia and systemic sepsis.

Initial stabilisation

1. Triage to acute treatment area.
2. Apply high-flow oxygen immediately.
3. Obtain IV access.
4. Monitor respiratory rate, heart rate, BP and pulse oximetry, and temperature.
5. If **stable**:
   - History: onset and duration, sputum, past history, medications, allergies, smoking.
   - Examination: colour and perfusion, chest auscultation (focal signs), sputum, general clinical state.
   - Initial investigations: CXR, white blood cell count (WCC), blood cultures if temperature ≤38.5°C, sputum examination if purulent, ABGs (initially on O_2 if breathless).

Specific treatment

1. Continue oxygenation, monitored by pulse oximetry.
2. IV volume resuscitation if systemically septic.
3. Specific antibiotics for likely organism.

SPONTANEOUS PNEUMOTHORAX

This chapter deals only with spontaneous pneumothorax that occurs as a result of rupture of a superficial lung bleb or bulla in young, tall, thin patients, or in those with preexisting obstructive lung disease (asthma or CAL). Traumatic pneumothorax is covered in Chapter 14.

Spontaneous pneumothorax generally presents as sudden onset of chest pain together with shortness of breath, and may be recurrent. The pain is often unilateral but poorly localised.

The immediate threat to life occurs only if there is tension (rapid expansion, impeding venous return to the thorax and impairing cardiac output). While the mechanism of deterioration is ultimately circulatory, the patient will present with extreme or rapidly progressive respiratory distress.

Initial stabilisation (unless minimal symptoms)

1. Triage to acute treatment area.

2. Apply high-flow oxygen (assists resorption).
3. Obtain IV access.
4. Monitor respiratory rate, heart rate, BP and pulse oximetry
5. If **signs of tension** (extreme or rapidly progressive shortness of breath, sweating, anxiety, refusal to lie flat, poor peripheral perfusion), immediately decompress with 12-gauge cannula in second intercostal space, midclavicular line, while preparing for formal thoracostomy.
6. If **stable**:
   • History: previous episodes and treatment, preexisting lung disease, general health and function.
   • Examination: colour and perfusion, tracheal deviation, chest auscultation (often difficult to detect unless massive pneumothorax).
   • Initial investigations: CXR, inspiratory and expiratory; ABGs, initially on O_2 if breathless.

Specific treatment

Depends on size of pneumothorax together with clinical state (symptoms and lung function). Options include:

1. Conservative management as an outpatient

Suitable for well patients with no preexisting lung disease, mild symptoms and no hypoxia. Ensure reliable follow-up (serial CXRs and clinical review) and advise against flying/diving until fully resolved. If recurrent, consider referral for pleurodesis.

2. Aspiration (special device, or cannula and 3-way tap)

Suitable for moderate symptoms and pneumothorax of 20–40% and no underlying lung disease. If still inflated at 6 hours and patient well, may be discharged for outpatient management (see above). Less likely to succeed if recurrent or massive pneumothorax (<40%). If failure, may leave aspiration catheter device in place, or proceed to formal tube thoracostomy (see below).

3. Tube thoracostomy (intercostal catheter)

Insert (with adequate analgesia and local anaesthesia) in 4th–5th intercostal space, midaxillary line, and connect to underwater seal. Low suction may be required if resolution is slow.

PULMONARY EMBOLISM

While pleuritic chest pain is a common presenting symptom, these patients may present with shortness of breath, with or without pain, or with syncope. The diagnosis depends on a combination of predisposing factors, clinical features and diagnostic tests.

See also Chapter 9.

ACUTE LUNG INJURY (NON-CARDIOGENIC PULMONARY OEDEMA)

This range of conditions can be described as 'permeability' pulmonary oedema, where there is exudation of fluid into alveoli due to lung tissue inflammation or injury.

Common causes include pulmonary contusion, aspiration, toxic inhalation, heroin use and severe infection. The condition overlaps with adult respiratory distress syndrome.

Patients present with worsening shortness of breath, respiratory distress and worsening hypoxaemia. The CXR shows interstitial and airspace oedema (local or generalised), usually with normal cardiac size; it may show the underlying cause.

The wet, stiff lungs make gas exchange and ventilation difficult.

In the case of lung contusion, generally associated with rib fractures in major trauma, the severity of the lung injury may not become manifest for several hours, when the patient starts to decompensate and tire. This deterioration should be anticipated.

Initial stabilisation

1. Triage to resuscitation area.
2. Apply high-flow oxygen, with reservoir mask.
3. Obtain IV access (two large lines, if trauma).
4. Concurrently manage life-threatening conditions of airway or circulation.
5. Monitor respiratory rate, heart rate, BP and pulse oximetry. Check temperature.
6. If **rapidly worsening hypoxaemia**, assist oxygenation with bag-valve-mask and 100% O_2, and arrange for intubation and ventilation. (Ventilation, if required, should involve conservative rate and tidal volume, to avoid pulmonary barotrauma). CPAP may be useful if the patient is alert and there is no history of trauma.
7. If **stable**:
   - History: trauma, period of unconsciousness, inhalation of fumes, sputum, chest pain, underlying lung disease, drug use.
   - Examination: evidence of trauma, injection sites, pressure areas, focal lung signs.
   - Initial investigations: CXR, WCC, ABGs (on oxygen), urinary drug screen (if indicated).

Specific treatment

1. Maintain adequate oxygenation by whatever means required to maintain SaO_2 above 94% (see oxygen therapy). Monitor by pulse oximetry.
2. Steroids have not been found useful.

3. Management of the underlying cause (e.g. antibiotics for sepsis).
4. Careful fluid management, in ICU.

ANAPHYLAXIS WITH BRONCHOSPASM

An acute Type 1 hypersensitivity reaction (allergic reaction) may present with acute upper airway (lips, tongue) or lower airway (stridor, wheeze or bronchospasm). These patients are an acute life-threatening emergency requiring resuscitation, high-flow oxygen, IV access, bronchodilators and adrenaline (IV if hypotensive/shock, IM if well-perfused).

Standard therapy also includes corticosteroids, antihistamines and H_2 antagonists.

The patient must be closely observed and monitored until all symptoms are settled.

RECOMMENDED READING

Marx J, Hockberger R, Walls R, et al, eds. Rosen's emergency medicine: concepts and clinical practice. 5th edn. St Louis: CV Mosby; 2001.

Tintinalli JE, Kelen GD, Stapczynski JS. Emergency medicine: a comprehensive study guide/American College of Emergency Physicians. 6th edn. New York: McGraw-Hill; 2003.

| 14 | Assessment and management of major trauma |

Martin Duffy, Anthony J Grabs and Joanne Sheedy

Trauma in Australia and New Zealand is the leading cause of death in the first four decades of life. Fortunately, injury-related deaths have declined over the past 20 years, but they still continue to be a significant burden on health resources. The identification and management of seriously ill patients requires a coordinated approach that includes pre-hospital management, emergency management and definitive surgical care. The development of the Early Management of Severe Trauma Course and the Definitive Surgical Trauma Course, both available in Australia and New Zealand, has provided the platform for improved trauma management.

DEFINITION OF MAJOR INJURY

Numerous trauma scoring systems are used throughout the world in an attempt to define the severely injured patient. Unfortunately, all have their advantages and disadvantages, with one of their key problems being the need to collect data 'after the fact'. Scoring at the time of presentation may underestimate the severity of the injury and lead to under-triage. Major injury has previously been defined as having an injury severity score (ISS) in excess of 15, as it was associated with a chance of dying in excess of 10%. Most trauma centres would now define major injury as follows:

- ISS >15.
- Requirement for urgent surgery.
- Intensive care admission.
- Inpatient stay longer than 3 days.
- Head injury requiring assisted ventilation for longer than 24 hours.
- Death.

Patients with major injuries need to be triaged early, with activation of a coordinated trauma response from emergency, anaesthetics, intensive care and surgery.

PRE-HOSPITAL TRIAGE

Pre-hospital assessment and management by ambulance services now enable the initial triage of patients to regional or major trauma services. The overriding goal is to get the **right patient** to the **right hospital** at the **right time**. Patients meeting the following criteria should be considered as having potentially life-threatening injuries requiring the services of an appropriately designated trauma centre. These criteria are also used by many hospitals as triggers to activate a trauma team response for an incoming patient, and include:

1. Respiratory distress—rate <10 or >30, or cyanosis.
2. Systolic blood pressure <90 or no palpable radial pulse in children.
3. Reduced level of consciousness.
4. Serious trauma to any region of the body.
5. Burns (partial or full thickness) >20% in adults or >10% in children.

The definition of serious trauma to any body region includes:

1. Penetrating injury of:
   a. head,
   b. neck,
   c. chest,
   d. abdomen,
   e. perineum,
   f. back.
2. Head injury with:
   a. one or both pupils dilated,

   b. open head injury,
   c. severe facial injury.
3. Abdominal injury with:
   a. distension,
   b. rigidity.
4. Spinal injury with:
   a. weakness,
   b. sensory loss.
5. Limb injury with:
   a. vascular injury with ischaemia of limb,
   b. amputation,
   c. crush injury,
   d. bilateral femur fractures.

Effective communication between the pre-hospital personnel and the receiving hospital is paramount. The history of the injury and pre-hospital management is extremely important and this should be relayed via the MIST system, which is defined as follows:

M **M**echanism, e.g. fall, motor vehicle accident, pedestrian

I **I**njuries, e.g. abdominal tenderness, chest injury, fractured long bone

S **S**igns, e.g. pulse, systolic blood pressure, respiratory rate, conscious level

T **T**reatment, e.g. cervical spine immobilisation, oxygen, intravenous therapy, drugs

This information enables the trauma team to prepare and focus their attention on specific early interventions that may be life-saving for the given situation. For example, the multitrauma victim with abdominal injuries who remains hypotensive after 2 litres of intravenous fluids in the field will need uncrossmatched group O blood via a rapid warmer to be available on arrival and will probably require early transfer to the operating suite for definitive care.

It is often best to prepare for the incoming trauma patient by mentally working your way through the ABCs and thinking about what equipment/personnel may be necessary for each area of concern. Knowledge of the mechanism of injury enables some prediction of possible injury/injuries. Standard precautions are a must—goggles, mask, impervious gown and gloves. The early donning of lead gowns enables potentially crucial X-rays to be performed in a timely and appropriate fashion without significant interruption to resuscitation efforts once the patient arrives.

SYSTEMATIC ASSESSMENT AND MANAGEMENT

The care of the injured patient by a trauma team is somewhat different from traditional medicine, with diagnosis, investigations and management frequently occurring simultaneously and performed by more than one doctor. A team leader should direct the overall management, including:

- Primary survey.
- History.
- Resuscitation.
- Secondary survey.
- Definitive care.

When caring for the paediatric trauma patient, the priorities are the same as for the adult patient. Allowances must be made for the child's size and physiology but the approach to assessment and management is otherwise identical. Beware of differences in injury patterns and the child's ability to compensate. Don't forget the parents—modify your approach to include family in the resuscitation room.

Care of the pregnant patient follows a similar line. Again, allowing for differences due to the anatomic and physiological changes of pregnancy, assessment and management are the same as for the non-pregnant patient. Early use of fetal monitoring is important, but good care of the fetus equals good care of the mother, so remain focused on the following priorities as outlined for the adult patient.

PRIMARY SURVEY

During the primary survey you need to simultaneously identify and manage immediately life-threatening injuries. The priorities of the primary survey, in order, are:

1. Airway maintenance with cervical spine protection.
2. Breathing and oxygenation.
3. Circulation and control of external haemorrhage.
4. Disability: brief neurologic examination.
5. Exposure with environment control.

The primary survey needs to be continually repeated throughout the initial phase of management. The key to good trauma care is directed assessment, followed by appropriate and timely intervention and subsequent directed reassessment—the AIR (assessment, intervention, reassessment) approach.

Six key injuries that need exclusion during the primary survey can be remembered by the mnemonic At This Moment Find Ominous Conditions:

Airway obstruction

Tension pneumothorax

Massive haemothorax

Flail chest

Open pneumothorax

Cardiac tamponade

1. Airway maintenance with cervical spine protection

Patients with a decreased level of consciousness or inadequacy of protective reflexes are prone to airway obstruction and aspiration. All patients should be considered to have a cervical spine injury until proved negative—this has significant implications for airway management. The head and neck should be supported at all times, especially during logrolling. The first priority is to establish a patent and protected airway. This may require:

- The removal of blood, vomitus and foreign bodies by posturing, suction or Magill's forceps.
- Jaw thrust and chin lift manoeuvres.
- The insertion of an oropharyngeal/nasopharyngeal airway.
- Endotracheal intubation.
- Establishment of a surgical airway.

A high concentration of oxygen should be administered to **all** patients. Patients with a decreased level of consciousness associated with a traumatic brain injury should be considered for early endotracheal intubation.

Nasotracheal intubation is rarely required in acute management and should be performed only by staff experienced in the procedure. A surgical airway is indicated only if there is an inability to perform bag and mask ventilation or failure to intubate.

2. Breathing and oxygenation

Once the airway has been deemed patent and protected, the adequacy of ventilation should be assessed. This is achieved by:

- Exposure of the chest.
- Inspection for cyanosis, tachypnoea, chest movement and chest wall integrity.
- Palpation of the tracheal position, subcutaneous emphysema and chest wall integrity.
- Percussion.
- Auscultation for the presence and symmetry of air entry.
- Oxygen saturation and arterial blood gases.

The team should identify and provide immediate management for the following life-threatening injuries well before a mobile chest X-ray has been obtained:

- Tension pneumothorax
- Large haemothorax
- Large flail segment
- Open pneumothorax

However, an early mobile chest X-ray may provide vital warning of a potentially life-threatening chest injury not yet detected by clinical examination.

3. Circulation and control of external haemorrhage

The maintenance of adequate tissue perfusion, especially of the brain, is the primary objective of the circulation component of the primary survey. Hypotension is almost always due to blood loss in the trauma setting. You must **stop the bleeding**. This may simply require the application of pressure to a site of external haemorrhage or it may necessitate transfer to the operating suite for an immediate laparotomy.

Examination

Assessment of a patient's circulatory status does not require waiting for the blood pressure reading. Information gained from examination of the patient's pulse, skin and level of consciousness is enough to make immediate resuscitation decisions, and the only equipment required are your eyes and your fingers. Remember to interpret your findings in the context of each individual you are assessing—the young, fit male who can compensate well despite considerable blood loss versus the elderly woman with multiple comorbidities on numerous physiology-altering medications are two entirely different scenarios. Be wary of patients who are hypotensive in the supine position—they have lost in excess of 30–40% of their blood volume and will require urgent resuscitation (Table 14.1).

Table 14.1. Estimated fluid and blood losses based on patient's initial presentation (for a 70 kg patient)

	Class 1	Class 2	Class 3	Class 4
Blood loss (mL)	Up to 750	750–1500	1500–2000	>2000
Blood loss (% blood volume)	Up to 15%	15–30%	30–40%	>40%
Pulse rate	<100	>100	>120	>140
Blood pressure	Normal	Normal	Decreased	Decreased
Pulse pressure	Normal or increased	Decreased	Decreased	Decreased
Respiratory rate (breaths/min)	14–20	20–30	30–40	>35
Urine output (mL/h)	>30	20–30	5–15	Negligible
CNS/mental status	Slightly anxious	Mildly anxious	Anxious, confused	Confused, lethargic
Fluid replacement (3:1 rule)	Crystalloid	Crystalloid	Crystalloid and blood	Crystalloid and blood

Pulse
The pulse rate and character should be determined as an initial assessment of the circulatory status. Tachycardia with a small volume pulse is due to hypovolaemia until proven otherwise. Patients with systolic blood pressures less than 80 mmHg frequently have absent peripheral pulses.

Skin perfusion
Pale, cool, clammy skin with a capillary refill time greater than 2 seconds is an early indicator of hypovolaemia.

Level of consciousness
A decreased level of consciousness is an indicator of poor cerebral perfusion and again is presumed to be due to hypovolaemia until proven otherwise.

Priorities

a. Control of external haemorrhage
This may require direct digital pressure over a wound, suturing/stapling of briskly bleeding scalp wounds, the reduction of facial fractures and nasopharyngeal packing.

b. Establishment of intravenous access
Two large-bore cannulas (14- or 16-gauge) should be inserted, usually into the cubital fossa of each arm. In patients with severe upper limb or chest trauma, one large-bore cannula should be above the diaphragm and one below the diaphragm. Large-bore cannulas may also be placed in the subclavian or jugular position or into the femoral vein if necessary. Intraosseous needles can be used in children under 8 years old with life-threatening injury if venous access cannot be established within an appropriate time frame.

c. Resuscitation fluids
Warmed intravenous fluids should be given at a rate appropriate for the clinical situation at hand. Anticipate the need for transfusion early, as fully crossmatched blood takes at least 40 minutes to organise. Be prepared to use group-specific or uncrossmatched group O blood in urgent cases.

d. Stop the bleeding
Fluid resuscitation does not replace the need to control ongoing bleeding—get the patient to the operating suite at the **right time**.

Deteriorating haemodynamic status may be due to:

- Ongoing blood loss.
- Tension pneumothorax.
- Cardiac tamponade.

Immediate directed re-examination for tension pneumothorax and cardiac tamponade should be performed. Frequently neck veins will be collapsed in hypovolaemia. However, if the jugular venous pressure is raised this suggests increased intrathoracic pressure. Having clinically ruled out these two conditions, you are then faced with the challenge of determining the source of ongoing blood loss.

Major blood loss can occur from the following five sites:

- Chest.
- Abdomen/retroperitoneum.
- Pelvis.
- Long bone fracture/s.
- External haemorrhage.

Focus on these sites particularly when dealing with the trauma patient who remains hypotensive despite intravenous fluid resuscitation and other appropriate measures. It is imperative to remember that at this stage of the resuscitation determining the site of blood loss is far more important than trying to determine which specific organ is bleeding.

External haemorrhage can be visualised and then controlled with appropriate pressure. Long bone fractures can be determined by clinical examination and then splinted to limit further blood loss. Significant blood loss into the chest can be ruled out by clinical examination and with the aid of an early mobile chest X-ray. Likewise, significant blood loss from the pelvis can be ruled out by clinical examination and with the aid of an early pelvic X-ray. The abdomen/retroperitoneum is, by default, the only other site of blood loss left to contend with, and in the context of haemodynamic instability this usually means an emergency laparotomy is in order.

Always remember, however, that the patient may bleed into multiple sites simultaneously, making such an 'orderly' assessment difficult in practical terms. The role of bedside ultrasonography as an adjunct to the clinical examination in the trauma patient has been developing for many years throughout the world and is rapidly expanding in Australia, replacing diagnostic peritoneal lavage in many centres. It has the advantage of being rapid, safe, non-invasive and, most importantly, repeatable. The use of ultrasound in a directed and limited manner by performing a focused abdominal sonogram for trauma (FAST) examination is now commonplace. Its primary role is to look for free fluid in the abdomen by examining the hepatorenal, splenorenal and retrovesical regions. In the appropriate circumstances examination for fluid in the pericardial sac may also be carried out. It should be performed by an experienced team member and should not distract the trauma team from the other components of the primary survey. Remember, it is a rule-in test—if it is negative all bets are off.

4. Disability: brief neurologic examination

A decreased level of consciousness is due to hypoxia or hypovolaemia until proven otherwise. Beware of hypoglycaemia. However, once these issues have been addressed, the priority is to determine the presence or absence of an intracranial injury that requires urgent neurosurgical intervention.

The pupils should be assessed for size, symmetry and response to light and the patient's level of consciousness should be quickly assessed using the AVPU method, i.e. is the patient:

- **A**lert?
- responding to **V**erbal stimuli only?
- responding to **P**ainful stimuli only?
- **U**nresponsive?

The Glasgow Coma Score (GCS) may also be used to assess the level of consciousness at this stage, or can be deferred until the secondary survey is performed. In conscious patients, all limbs should be assessed for movement and sensation to detect possible spinal injury.

All patients with a GCS of less than 12 should have aggressive airway, circulation and breathing (ABC) management, including consideration for early intubation. This will enable controlled ventilation/oxygenation and allow the team to focus on the circulatory status, thus attending to two key factors responsible for adverse outcomes in traumatic brain injury—hypoxaemia and hypotension.

5. Exposure with environment control

Patients who have sustained a major injury should have all their clothing cut off without delay to allow adequate assessment of the entire body. Remember, however, that hypothermia kills trauma patients. Unless your resuscitation room has dedicated temperature control capabilities, as soon as your examination and any required procedures have been performed the patient should be covered. A warming mattress and a Bair Hugger may also be needed to control the patient's temperature.

HISTORY

A nominated member of the trauma team should obtain further information that will allow the acute event to be managed in the context of the patient's premorbid state. A simple way to cover most of the important areas is to use the AMPLE approach:

A **A**llergies

M **M**edications—particularly anticoagulants!

P **P**ast history—particularly diseases that alter clotting ability; pregnancy

L **L**ast food/fluid; last tetanus injection

E **E**vent details

This history may not be available directly from the patient and other sources may need to be questioned, e.g. pre-hospital personnel, relatives, friends, the local doctor, old medical records etc. In the unconscious patient always remember to look for a medical alert bracelet or any pertinent information on the person or in a wallet or handbag.

Mechanism of injury details are vitally important. Conceptually, injury is the result of a transfer of energy to the body's tissues. The severity of injury is dependent upon the amount and speed of energy transmission, the surface area over which the energy is applied, and the elastic properties of the tissues to which the energy transfer is applied. In the Australian setting, the most common cause is blunt trauma. Penetrating trauma, however, is on the increase. Common causes of blunt trauma include:

1. Motor vehicle crashes.
2. Pedestrian–motor vehicle accidents.
3. Falls.
4. Industrial accidents.
5. Assaults.

Specific injuries may be predicted from the mechanism of injury, which provides 'advanced warning' of possible injuries. It is a useful guide but remember that there are always exceptions.

1. Injuries in motor vehicle crashes

- Frontal impact—cervical spine fracture, anterior flail chest, traumatic aortic disruption, pneumothorax, myocardial contusion, ruptured spleen or liver, posterior dislocation/fracture of hip/knee.
- Lateral impact—cervical spine fracture, lateral flail chest, traumatic aortic disruption, pneumothorax, diaphragmatic injury, ruptured spleen or liver, renal injury, fractured pelvis.
- Rear impact—cervical spine injury.
- Ejection—increased risk of any injury.
- Rollover—increased risk of any injury.

Important information from pre-hospital personnel that provides some idea of the energy transfer involved includes details of the estimated speed, impact, damage to vehicle, entrapment, use of restraint devices, deployment of airbags etc.

2. Injuries in pedestrian — motor vehicle accidents

- Remember the injury triad—impact with the bumper, impact with the hood and windscreen, and subsequent impact with the ground.
- Bumper—lower limb fractures, fractured pelvis, torso injuries in children.
- Hood/windscreen—head injury, torso injuries.
- Ground—head injury, spinal injuries.

Again, pre-hospital information that gives some idea of the energy transfer involved is important.

3. Injuries in falls

- The predominant underlying mechanism of injury is deceleration.

- Important considerations include the height of the fall, the landing surface, and the position of the patient on impact.
- Injuries include head, spine, torso and multiple fractures (calcaneus, ankle, tibial plateau, hip and vertebral column).

4. Injuries in industrial accidents

- May be blunt or penetrating.
- Other mechanisms need to be considered—blast, thermal, chemical.
- Injuries will depend on the above mechanisms.

5. Injuries in assaults

- Unfortunately a common cause.
- May be blunt or penetrating.
- Determine the energy transfer—weapon, fists, stomping.
- Injuries will depend on the above mechanisms.
- Stabbings are low-energy injuries—severity determined by organs injured, e.g. major vascular injury versus muscle.
- Gunshot injuries vary in energy level—increased bullet velocity equals increased injuries secondary to cavitation.

RESUSCITATION

As the initial assessment is performed and airway and breathing issues are attended to, intravenous fluids should be given in volumes appropriate for the estimated extent of hypovolaemia. In general, hypotensive patients should have 20 mL/kg of warmed intravenous fluids infused rapidly. An adult patient who requires more than 2 litres of intravenous fluids and remains hypotensive should have blood as the next resuscitation fluid. Ideally, crossmatched blood should be given but group-specific or uncrossmatched group O blood may need to be given, depending on the patient's clinical status.

While placing intravenous lines, draw blood for the following investigations. Note that not all will be necessary in every situation.

- Full blood count.
- Electrolytes/urea/creatinine.
- Glucose.
- Liver function tests.
- Amylase/lipase.
- Coagulation studies.
- Group and hold/crossmatch.
- Blood alcohol level—including an appropriate sample for the police when required.
- Beta human chorionic gonadotrophin (HCG).

The timing of radiological studies will vary depending on the urgency of the situation. In major trauma patients, however, the early performance of a trauma series (chest X-ray/pelvis/lateral C-spine) is appropriate and usually is done as the team is performing the primary survey. The most logical order for the films is:

1. Chest X-ray—as an adjunct to 'B' and 'C' assessment.
2. Pelvis—as an adjunct to 'C' assessment.
3. Lateral C-spine. Because this film on its own will not exclude a C-spine injury, it may be delayed if necessary while continuing immobilisation measures.

During the resuscitation phase, a urinary catheter should be passed to assess urine output. A urinary catheter is contraindicated if there is blood at the external meatus, blood in the scrotum or per rectum (PR), the prostate cannot be palpated or is high riding. In general, a urethrogram is indicated in these circumstances and an urgent urological opinion should be sought. A suprapubic bladder catheter is an option in the presence of significant urethral trauma.

A nasogastric tube should be placed in all intubated patients and patients who have sustained significant abdominal trauma. This is to prevent gastric aspiration and the development of acute gastric dilation. In the presence of head or facial injuries the tube should be placed via the mouth.

The relief of discomfort is an important component of trauma care, and analgesia should be provided in an appropriate form and amount depending on the clinical state of the patient. In most circumstances this will equate to the provision of an intravenous opioid delivered in small aliquots and titrated to effect while monitoring for adverse events.

Consider tetanus immunisation and prophylactic antibiotics as required, depending on the circumstances.

The ongoing resuscitation status should be monitored by:

- Respiratory rate and effort.
- Pulse oximetry.
- Peripheral perfusion.
- Pulse rate/ECG rhythm.
- Blood pressure—with particular attention to pulse pressure.
- Glasgow Coma Score.
- Arterial blood gases (ABGs)—base deficit and lactate.
- Urine output.

Persistent haemodynamic instability should again raise the possibility of:

- Continued blood loss.
- Tension pneumothorax.
- Cardiac tamponade.
- Other conditions—e.g. myocardial injury, spinal cord injury etc.
- Equipment problems—e.g. blocked or displaced intercostal catheter, dislodged peripheral or central access resulting in extravasation of fluids, malfunction of ventilation equipment etc.

At this stage the trauma team leader should decide whether the patient should be transferred immediately to the operating suite for a resuscitative thoracotomy and/or laparotomy.

MANAGEMENT OF LIFE-THREATENING CONDITIONS

As previously stated, life-threatening conditions should be suspected and identified during the primary survey. The management of these conditions may be based in the emergency department or may require immediate transfer to the operating suite.

Tension pneumothorax

A 12- or 14-gauge cannula should be inserted into the second intercostal space in the midclavicular line as an initial treatment. This should be followed by an intercostal catheter in the fourth or fifth intercostal space just anterior to the midaxillary line.

Open pneumothorax

A large combine should be placed over the defect and secured in position with an op-site dressing. At the same time, a large intercostal catheter needs to be inserted to treat the now 'closed' pneumothorax and to prevent the possible development of a tension pneumothorax.

Massive haemothorax

A large intercostal catheter (minimum 28 Fr) should be inserted into the fourth or fifth intercostal space just anterior to the midaxillary line and directed posteriorly. An initial drainage of greater than 1500 mL should signal the team to consider early thoracotomy, especially in penetrating trauma.

Note: All intercostal catheters should be connected to an underwater sealed drain and have low wall suction applied. A stat dose of prophylactic antibiotics (a first-generation cephalosporin for the nonallergic patient) should reduce the risk of an infective complication.

Flail segment

Flail segments frequently result in inadequate ventilation/oxygenation and are prone to the collection of air or blood in the pleural cavity. Associated pulmonary contusions are the major cause of morbidity and can result in progressive deterioration in respiratory function. Adequate drainage of the pleural cavities should be ensured by a large intercostal catheter, otherwise the management remains largely supportive with adequate analgesia via an appropriate route (including such options as a thoracic epidural) and assisted ventilation/oxygenation (ranging from non-invasive techniques such as bi-level positive airway pressure—BiPAP—to endotracheal intubation).

Ongoing blood loss

These patients should be considered for early transfer to the operating suite for a resuscitative thoracotomy and/or laparotomy. If pelvic bleeding is suspected the application of a C clamp for pelvic stabilisation and early angiography should be considered.

Cardiac tamponade

The diagnosis should be suspected clinically and confirmed with focused assessment with sonography in trauma (FAST) if possible. Management focuses on adequate resuscitation and performing a left anterolateral thoracotomy to release the fluid within the pericardial sac. This should be undertaken by the most experienced trauma team member. Needle pericardiocentesis should be considered only in smaller hospitals if experienced staff are not available. Needle pericardiocentesis may be life-saving but rarely drains the pericardial sac adequately and is associated with significant complications.

Pulseless electrical activity

This is sometimes called electromechanical dissociation and in the context of trauma is usually caused by exsanguination, tension pneumothorax, massive haemothorax or cardiac tamponade. Pulseless electrical activity should be managed by immediate intubation, ventilation, bilateral chest drains, the administration of at least 3 litres of intravenous fluids and consideration for an open thoracotomy and pericardial release. This is of special importance in penetrating chest injuries.

SECONDARY SURVEY

The secondary survey is a detailed systematic head-to-toe examination in order to detect all injuries and enable planning of definitive care. This should not commence until the primary assessment and management have stabilised the patient. During the secondary survey all components of the primary survey should be repeated and the team should be responsive to any new findings. Unless the patient has been transferred immediately to the operating suite, the secondary survey should be undertaken in the emergency department.

1. **Head**. Assess the scalp for lacerations, contusions, fractures and burns. Examine the ears for haemotympanum and cerebrospinal fluid (CSF) leakage. Check the eyes for visual acuity, pupil symmetry and response to light, movements, lens injury; always check for the presence of contact lenses and remove them early.

2. **Face**. Assess for lacerations, contusions, fractures and burns. Check cranial nerve function. Examine the mouth for bleeding, loose teeth and soft tissue injuries.

3. **Cervical spine and neck**. Assess for tenderness, bruising, swelling, deformity, subcutaneous emphysema and tracheal deviation. Beware of carotid dissection.

4. **Chest**. Assess for evidence of rib fracture, subcutaneous emphysema, open wounds, haemothorax and pneumothorax. Check for evidence of myocardial injury, and perform a 12-lead ECG.

5. **Abdomen**. Assess for bruising of the anterior abdominal wall, distension, tenderness and guarding, rebound, rectal and vaginal examinations.

6. **Back**. All trauma patients need to undergo a logroll with cervical spine immobilisation to examine the entire length of the spine, looking for tenderness, bruising or deformity. This should be done early so that the patient can be removed from the spinal board, thus improving patient comfort and decreasing the risk of pressure injuries in patients with spinal cord injuries and altered sensation/awareness. A PR examination should be done at this time.

7. **Limbs**. All limbs need to be examined for fractures, lacerations, haematomas, peripheral pulses and neurological deficits. All fractures should be reduced and splinted and consideration given to intravenous antibiotics and tetanus prophylaxis.

SPECIFIC INJURIES

Head trauma

Traumatic brain injury is common. Unfortunately, despite this fact, there is a scarcity of good evidence in the literature upon which to base investigation and management decisions, particularly with regard to the mildly head-injured patient. It is important to determine at an early stage whether your facility can provide the appropriate care necessary for the patient's severity of injury or whether urgent transfer to another hospital will provide the best possible care.

Classification systems abound and all have their limitations, but the following GCS-based system is a useful guide:

- Mild head injury—GCS 14–15.
- Moderate head injury—GCS 9–13.
- Severe head injury—GCS 3–8.

See also Chapter 15.

Mild head injury

Fortunately the majority of patients you deal with will have only a mild injury, usually characterised by an awake patient who may have a history of a brief loss of consciousness and some degree of amnesia about events surrounding the injury. Often the history of loss of consciousness is unclear and despite information from bystanders and pre-hospital personnel it can be difficult to determine the true details of the event. In general, if there is a history of more than a momentary loss of consciousness, amnesia, significant headache or vomiting following the injury, a computerised tomography (CT) scan of the head should be performed. If the CT scan is normal, subsequent deterioration is unlikely and the majority of these patients can expect an uneventful recovery. The patient may be discharged to the care of a responsible adult, provided the home circumstances are adequate. Before discharge, a discussion with the patient and the carer regarding important symptoms and signs to look out for should take place—and this information should also be provided in written form by way of a head injury advice card.

Moderate head injury

Patients with this degree of head injury require more aggressive management and further investigation. Remember to keep in mind the different needs of patients, depending on where they lie on the disease spectrum. Early endotracheal intubation and controlled ventilation/oxygenation should be considered. Appropriately aggressive fluid resuscitation in the hypovolaemic patient is also vitally important. Having performed a primary and secondary survey and responded appropriately to the findings, the next priority is to determine whether a neurosurgically correctable lesion is present by proceeding to urgent CT scanning. Further management will depend on the findings, with a number of patients requiring urgent transfer to the operating suite for evacuation of a haematoma. The majority of other patients will require admission for ongoing neurological observations.

Severe head injury

Patients with severe head injury are fortunately in the minority. However, when faced with such a patient a coordinated team approach with meticulous attention to the prevention of secondary brain injury is paramount. Early notification of the neurosurgical team is important. The ABCs must be appropriately and aggressively resuscitated. Key points in the management include:

1. Endotracheal intubation with controlled ventilation/oxygenation. Before sedating and paralysing the patient, every attempt should be made to perform and document a limited neurological examination—the GCS and pupillary responses. It is important to note these findings in the context of the patient's blood pressure at the time because of its potential influence on cerebral perfusion/function. Also remember it is the best motor response that is the more accurate predictor of outcome.

2. Mild hyperventilation to a pCO_2 of 30–35 mmHg in the patient showing signs of raised intracranial pressure from an expanding haematoma—as a 'stop gap' until reaching the operating suite. The

patient's end tidal CO_2 should be monitored closely, having confirmed the accuracy of the readings by performing a formal arterial blood gas measurement.

3. Fluid resuscitation with normal saline, Hartmann's or blood (no glucose-containing solutions) as required to maintain a mean arterial pressure of greater than 90 mmHg in the patient suspected of raised intracranial pressure.

4. Mannitol 0.5–1 g/kg given as an infusion over approximately 5 minutes in the patient showing signs of raised intracranial pressure from an expanding haematoma—as a 'stop gap' until reaching the operating suite; frusemide may also be used, often in addition to mannitol.

5. Prophylactic anticonvulsants—at the discretion of the treating neurosurgeon—usually phenytoin 15 mg/kg administered intravenously at a rate no faster than 50 mg/min in adult patients.

The management of the head-injured patient with intercurrent hypotension can be a real challenge, and it is therefore important to keep a few key principles in mind:

1. Head injury + hypotension = worse outcome.
2. Determine the cause of the hypotension.
3. Treat the cause of the hypotension.

THEN

4. Treat the head injury.

Neck injuries

The accurate assessment and management of neck injuries is important not only because of the potentially devastating effects of cervical spine/spinal cord injuries but also because of the life-threatening potential of injuries to other vital structures such as the airway/larynx and vascular anatomy. A detailed search for swelling, expanding haematoma formation, subcutaneous emphysema, tracheal deviation, hoarseness, stridor and carotid bruits should be performed.

Key points in management

1. Ensure airway patency. Repeated examinations are essential and early intubation may be life-saving.

2. Blunt injury to vascular structures can be 'occult'. Maintain a high degree of suspicion and proceed to further investigation, e.g. ultrasound, angiography.

3. Beware of penetrating injuries. If the platysma is breached the right place for the patient to be further examined and treated is in the operating suite with on-table angiography facilities.

4. Clearing the cervical spine. Patients suffering blunt trauma who meet the following five criteria can be classified as having a low probability of cervical spine injury and can be cleared on clinical grounds. No radiological imaging is required if the patient has:

- Normal alertness.
- No intoxication.
- No painful, distracting injury.
- No midline cervical tenderness.
- No focal neurologic deficit.

Abdominal trauma

The abdomen is renowned for its reputation as an 'occult' source of blood loss in the trauma victim. Add to this reputation the poor sensitivity and specificity of the physical examination in this setting and it is not hard to see why investigation and management decisions can seem daunting. As stated previously, during the initial assessment of such patients it is important to keep in mind that it is more important to determine the site of bleeding than the specific organ injured. Remember the full 'extent' of the abdomen when assessing a patient—the anterior borders are the trans-nipple line superiorly, the inguinal ligaments and pubic symphysis inferiorly, and the anterior axillary lines laterally.

The most common mechanism of abdominal injury in the Australasian setting is blunt trauma, usually in the context of a motor vehicle crash. Penetrating abdominal trauma is on the increase though, and the differences in the biomechanics of low-energy versus high-energy injuries need to be taken into account. However, regardless of the mechanism, the initial assessment and management need to follow the same principles of airway, breathing, cardiovascular, drug therapy (ABCD).

Blunt abdominal trauma: key points in management

1. Remember that the physical examination is **unreliable**.
2. By a process of elimination the abdomen/retroperitoneum can be diagnosed as the site of blood loss—if it is not external, chest, pelvis or long bones, the abdomen/retroperitoneum is the only site left.
3. If the patient is haemodynamically stable, a CT scan is an appropriate investigation to confirm your clinical suspicion (Table 14.2).
4. If the patient is haemodynamically unstable do not go to CT—go to the operating suite!
5. For the patient 'in between' a FAST examination or a diagnostic, peritoneal lavage may be invaluable (Table 14.2).
6. Remember that a FAST examination can only rule in the presence of free fluid. If it is negative, all bets are off.
7. Be appropriately aggressive with resuscitation fluids—the **right** amount for the **right** patient at the **right** temperature.
8. **Stop the bleeding**—for some patients this will mean immediate transfer to the operating suite.

Penetrating abdominal trauma

Advice regarding resuscitation and imaging is as for blunt trauma (see above). Other important points include:

1. The entry wound can be a misleading predictor of the trajectory of penetration and potential underlying injury/ies—**do not** rely on it.
2. Anterior abdominal stab wounds with hypotension, peritonitis, or evisceration of omentum or small bowel require no further imaging or investigation—they need to go to the operating suite for a laparotomy.
3. Local exploration of stab wounds under sterile conditions and local anaesthesia may be performed by the skilled surgeon in stable patients, searching for a breach in the anterior fascia. If a breach is present the patient is at increased risk of an intraperitoneal injury, and common practice in Australia is to proceed to laparoscopy.
4. The value of repeated examinations should not be underestimated.

Thoracic trauma

The majority of chest injuries can be managed in the emergency department with the use of supplemental oxygen, an appropriately placed intercostal catheter and the judicious use of analgesics via an appropriate route. Hence it is important that doctors working in such an environment develop the skills to assess and manage these patients correctly.

Often when the patient arrives, the examination and chest X-ray are performed in the supine position, and allowances must be made for this in terms of examination technique and film interpretation. For example, percussion should be performed in an anterior to posterior direction for detecting the presence of a haemothorax—and the chest X-ray will have a generalised increase in radiodensity on the affected side as compared to the usual meniscus on an erect film. Watch out for the patient with a widened mediastinum on chest X-ray suspicious of a contained rupture of the

Table 14.2 Imaging in abdominal trauma.

	Ultrasound	Diagnostic peritoneal lavage	Computed tomography
Indication	Document free fluid if decreased BP	Document bleeding if decreased BP	Document organ injury if BP normal
Advantages	Early diagnosis; performed at the bedside; non-invasive; repeatable; 86–97% accurate	Early diagnosis; performed at the bedside; 98% accurate	Most specific for injury; 92–98% accurate
Disadvantages	Operator-dependent; bowel gas and subcutaneous air distortion; misses diaphragm, bowel and some pancreatic injuries	Invasive; misses injury to diaphragm and retroperitoneum	Cost and time; transfer to medical imaging department; misses diaphragm, bowel tract, and some pancreatic injuries

aorta—if you don't have cardiothoracic facilities, transfer the patient without delay so that further investigation and treatment can take place at the right hospital.

Keep in mind the presence of common intercurrent diagnoses that may impact on a patient's ability to cope with a chest injury, such as chronic airflow limitation and asthma, not to mention smoking status.

Given the important structures inside the chest, it is not surprising that patients can suffer a large number of possibly life-threatening injuries, including those previously discussed under the primary survey, as well as the following:

1. **Pulmonary contusion**. Commonly associated with many of the other injuries and is often the main cause of deteriorating lung function. Develops over hours to days. May require increasing supplemental oxygen, non-invasive ventilatory support or subsequent intubation/ventilation.

2. **Haemothorax**. Drainage via an appropriately sized and placed intercostal catheter is important, as noted previously. Transfer to the operating theatre should be considered in any patient who drains more than 1500 mL immediately or continues to drain more than approximately 200 mL/h for 2–4 hours.

3. **Simple pneumothorax**. There is some controversy about the management of some of these injuries, depending on such factors as the size of the pneumothorax, associated injuries, need for positive pressure ventilation, need for transfer to another facility, and coexistent respiratory diseases; most would still advocate drainage via an appropriately sized intercostal catheter.

4. **Blunt cardiac injury**. Suspect in the patient who remains haemodynamically unstable. There is no one clear diagnostic test—the ECG, cardiac markers, and other imaging modalities such as echocardiography are all adjuncts to the clinical examination.

5. **Traumatic aortic disruption**. Most patients die at the scene. If they survive to reach hospital, there is a window of opportunity to investigate and treat them at a facility with cardiothoracic capabilities. Signs to look for on the chest X-ray include a widened mediastinum, obliteration of the aortic knob, deviation of the trachea to the right, obscuration of the aortopulmonary window, depression of the left main stem bronchus, deviation of the oesophagus (nasogastric tube) to the right, widened paratracheal stripe, widened paraspinal interfaces, presence of a pleural or apical cap, left haemothorax, or fractures of the first and second ribs or the scapula. Early surgical consultation is important.

6. **Tracheobronchial tree disruption**. An unusual injury; patients usually die at the scene. Suspect if a large air leak persists after placement of an intercostal catheter for a pneumothorax. Early surgical consultation is important.

7. **Traumatic diaphragmatic injury**. Often missed; interpret X-rays with care. Early surgical consultation is important.
8. **Traumatic oesophageal disruption**. Rare; fatal if missed because of subsequent mediastinitis. Suspect if there is a left pneumothorax or haemothorax without a rib fracture, pain or shock out of proportion to the injury (usually a blow to the lower sternum or epigastrium), or if there is particulate matter in the intercostal catheter. Early surgical consultation is important.

Rib fractures

Having noted the above injuries, do not underestimate the significant morbidity and potential mortality associated with the most common of chest injuries—rib fractures! Important points in the management of this everyday problem include:

1. The ability of X-rays to detect rib fractures is poor—even if the films are read accurately!
2. If the patient has a good history and significant pain, fracture is probably the diagnosis.
3. The role of the chest X-ray is to help exclude complications such as a pneumothorax, haemothorax, pulmonary contusion, atelectasis, subsequent pneumonia.
4. It is clear from the above that 'rib views' are therefore not necessary.
5. The presence of intercurrent disease may influence management decisions.
6. Adequate analgesia that allows deep breathing and coughing is paramount to the successful management of patients with these injuries:
   • Start with simple oral therapy—paracetamol.
   • Add other oral options—non-steroidal anti-inflammatory drugs (NSAIDs)/tramadol/endone—being alert for respiratory depression.
   • Use parenteral therapy—tramadol/opioids—again being alert for respiratory depression.
   • The use of patient-controlled analgesia may be appropriate in many circumstances.
   • Consultation with the anaesthetic/pain management service with a view to other alternatives—intercostal blocks/epidural anaesthesia.
7. Paramedical services play an important role—physiotherapy.
8. Use non-invasive ventilatory support such as BiPAP early.
9. Closely monitor the patient's progress—respiratory rate and effort, pulse oximetry, ABGs.
10. Be prepared for the patient who despite the above measures continues to struggle—intubation with controlled ventilation/oxygenation may be necessary.
11. With few exceptions, elderly patients with fractured ribs require inpatient care.

Pelvic trauma

Pelvic injuries can range in severity from simple pubic rami fractures to unstable injuries with associated life-threatening exsanguination. It is important to appreciate the magnitude of force required to fracture the pelvis—and hence the high association with other potentially life-threatening injuries.

Three common mechanisms of injury are:

1. Anteroposterior compression, e.g. crushing injury.
2. Lateral compression, e.g. motor vehicle crash.
3. Vertical shear, e.g. fall from a height.

Be suspicious of significant pelvic injury with the above mechanisms and perform a careful clinical examination, noting any lower limb shortening or rotation (in the absence of a lower limb fracture) and any pain or movement on palpation of the pelvic ring. Compression-distraction of the pelvic ring should be performed **once only** as part of this examination, because of the risk of exacerbating any bleeding. The early performance of a pelvic X-ray as part of the trauma series will assist decision making.

Important points in management

1. Major pelvic disruption with haemorrhage should be suspected from the mechanism of injury, e.g. motorcycle crash, pedestrian versus car, fall from a height or a direct crushing injury.
2. Significant injuries are usually clinically apparent.
3. Be alert for and understand the potential for major blood loss—from the ends of fractured bones, from injured pelvic muscles and from the pelvic veins/arteries—and fluid resuscitate the patient appropriately.
4. Simple measures to control bleeding in the emergency department include:
   - Bringing the lower limbs back out to length with traction.
   - Internally rotating the lower limbs and strapping them together.
   - The application of a pelvic support/sling—this may be as simple as wrapping a sheet around the pelvis.
5. Early consultation with the orthopaedic team is paramount with regard to urgent fixation.
6. Occasionally embolisation via angiography is necessary—ideally done in the operating suite.

Always remember the possibility of associated urological injury. Suspicious examination findings include blood at the external urethral meatus, scrotal or perineal bruising, and an impalpable or high-riding prostate on PR exam (all contraindications to catheterisation, as previously noted). In the multi-injured patient with a significant pelvic fracture, the bladder and/or urethra may be injured. In this setting the urethra is more commonly injured above the urogenital diaphragm. The patient is often in 'retention'. The usual approach to management includes:

1. Assess and treat for other life-threatening conditions.
2. Perform a urethrogram and treat accordingly.
3. Suprapubic catheterisation in selected patients.
4. Urological consultation.

Musculoskeletal trauma

Musculoskeletal trauma is very common. Fortunately most injuries threaten neither limb nor life, although they can on occasion look very dramatic. It is important not to be distracted by the injury and to manage all these patients in an orderly fashion with meticulous attention to the ABCs first. Some important points in the management of such injuries include:

1. Musculoskeletal injuries that are potentially life-threatening need to be recognised early and managed appropriately.
   - **Major arterial haemorrhage**. These injuries may be as obvious as an avulsed limb or as subtle as the bleeding associated with a long bone injury or major joint dislocation. Do not blindly clamp open injuries—use direct pressure. Limb realignment and splinting are important measures which help reduce blood loss. Carefully assess the limb for the presence of distal pulses—absence equals arterial injury till proven otherwise. It is important to contact the surgical team early with a view to transfer to the operating suite for urgent exploration and/or angiography on the operating table.
   - **Crush syndrome**. Be alert for this potential problem in any patient who has had a significant portion of a limb trapped for a period of time. The associated rhabdomyolysis and release of toxic byproducts can lead to life-threatening hyperkalaemia, hypovolaemia, metabolic acidosis, hypocalcaemia and disseminated intravascular coagulation. Resuscitate the patient with large volumes of normal saline, aiming for a urine output of approximately 200 mL/h in an adult. Alkalinisation with sodium bicarbonate and the use of osmotic diuretics have also been advocated, although evidence is limited.
2. Most other injuries can be diagnosed and treated as part of the secondary survey.
3. Carefully examine the limb—skin integrity, colour, bruising, haematoma formation, neurovascular status, bony tenderness, function.
4. Be thorough—it is easy to overlook extremity injuries, therefore repeated examination is important.
5. Only proceed to imaging once the patient is stable and all life/limb threats have been addressed. Image the joints above and below the suspected fracture site.
6. Limb realignment and splinting reduces movement at the injury site, limits further bleeding, and reduces pain. Always re-examine the neurovascular status of a limb if you have performed manipulation or applied a splint.

7. Early elevation of the injured limb reduces oedema formation.
8. Provide adequate analgesia, usually in the form of intravenous opioids titrated to effect.
9. Consider tetanus and antibiotic prophylaxis for open injuries.
10. Always be on the alert for complications—any site where muscle is contained within a closed fascial space has the potential to develop compartment syndrome.

Compartment syndrome

1. A time-critical diagnosis—you have 4–6 hours at most to save the ischaemic contents of the compartment!
2. Potentially devastating if missed.
3. Commonly occurs in the leg, forearm, foot, hand, gluteal region and thigh.
4. Suspect the diagnosis in any patient who has pain greater than expected and that typically increases when the involved muscles are passively stretched—most of the other clinical signs are insensitive or develop late in the disease process.
5. Warning—the distal pulse is usually present!
6. Measure compartment pressures—greater than 35 mmHg in a normotensive patient is abnormal (lower pressures in the hypotensive patient may be significant). The trend in repeated measurements is generally more helpful than a one-off reading.
7. Treatment:
   • Release any constricting bandages, casts etc.
   • Urgent fasciotomy if no improvement.
   • Treat complications, e.g. rhabdomyolysis.

DEFINITIVE CARE

Definitive care in all trauma patients needs to be directed by the trauma surgeon or the team leader.
Definitive care involves:

• Specific investigations, e.g. CT scan of the head/chest.
• Consultation with specialty teams.
• Documentation of all injuries and treatment.
• Specific management plans from all appropriate teams.
• Definitive placement to appropriate specialty team.

Tertiary survey

The tertiary survey is a complete review of the patient performed within the first 24 hours of their admission to hospital aimed at detecting any further injuries or problems that may have been overlooked in the excitement of the initial resuscitation. It includes a further thorough head to toe clinical examination as well as a complete review of all investigations and treatments performed thus far.

Trauma service performance improvement

Care of the injured patient requires the services and skills of many different individuals. Trauma service performance improvement refers to the evaluation of the quality of care provided by a trauma service. Hospital-based performance improvement programmes generally focus on the following aspects of health care:

1. Safety—the extent to which risks and inadvertent harm are minimised.
2. Effectiveness of care—does the treatment/intervention achieve the desired outcomes?
3. Appropriateness—is the selected treatment/intervention likely to produce the desired outcome?
4. Consumer participation—engaging consumers in planning and evaluating health care services.
5. Efficiency—maximal total benefit is derived from the available treatments/resources.
6. Access—the extent to which an individual or population can obtain health care services.

Performance improvement in trauma relies on the continual efforts of the multidisciplinary trauma team to measure, monitor, assess and improve both processes and outcomes of care. Trauma performance improvement programmes are based on the following elements:

- A trauma registry/database to identify problems and the results of corrective actions.
- Multidisciplinary peer review of care, including morbidity and mortality analysis.
- Incident monitoring.
- Use of specific statistical methods for mortality analysis (e.g. Revised Trauma Score and Injury Severity Score combined—TRISS; A Severity Characterisation of Trauma—ASCOT).
- Classification of deaths and complications as preventable, potentially preventable, non-preventable.
- Clinical indicators to measure current practice against accepted benchmarks.
- Use of evidence-based clinical guidelines, protocols and pathways.
- Evidence of 'loop closure'—that is, evidence that the process or outcome needing improvement is remeasured following corrective action and that improvement is demonstrated.

Clinical practice guidelines and protocols

Clinical practice guidelines and protocols are outlines of accepted management approaches based on best available evidence and are designed to assist clinical decision making. Clinical pathways are multidisciplinary plans of best clinical practice for specified groups of patients with a particular diagnosis that aid the coordination and delivery of high-quality care.

Clinical indicators

Clinical indicators are measures of the process or outcomes of care. They are not designed to be exact standards but rather act as 'flags' to alert clinicians to possible problems in the system or opportunities for improvement. For clinical indicators to be effective they must be relevant and clearly defined. Development of a set of clinical indicators is iterative. Indicators are reviewed on an ongoing basis with reference to the usefulness of the data and the resources required to collect it. Trauma service indicators are used to monitor process and outcomes of care from the pre-hospital phase through to rehabilitation and discharge. Close analysis of data is required, as there may be valid reasons why an event occurs differently from an expectation.

Examples of trauma service clinical indicators are:

1. Proportion of patients with a documented GCS <9 who do not receive an endotracheal tube (ETT) within 10 minutes of documentation of that score.
2. Proportion of head-injured patients with a documented GCS <12 who do not have a CT scan of the head within 4 hours of arrival in the emergency department.
3. Proportion of trauma patients transported to hospital by ambulance (not entrapped at the scene) who have a documented scene time of >20 minutes.

Outcome measures

Historically, trauma services have focused on the issue of preventable deaths as the main outcome measure. Outcome analysis in trauma is slowly expanding. Trauma services are now beginning to analyse other outcomes such as morbidity, functional impairment, quality of life and patient satisfaction. Comparison of outcomes across different sites relies on use of standardised reliable outcome measures. Similarly, morbidity analysis requires tight definitions of problems with rate comparisons potentially confounded by demographic differences between hospitals.

A large number of measures exist for outcomes analysis in trauma. These include:

- Glasgow Outcome Scale (GOS) for head-injured patients.
- Disability rating scale (DRS).
- Short form (SF)–36 survey.
- Sickness impact profile.
- Hospital anxiety and depression scale (HADS).
- Functional independence measure (FIM).

CONCLUSION

The patient suffering multiple injuries is often a distressing sight and can at times seem like an overwhelming challenge to manage. By approaching care of such patients in a directed manner, prioritising the assessment and management of life-threatening injuries as outlined above, both you and your patients can look forward to the best outcomes possible. Appropriate and timely intervention is the key.

RECOMMENDED READING

American College of Surgeons Committee on Trauma. Advanced trauma life support program for doctors—student course manual. 6th edn. Chicago: American College of Surgeons; 1997.

American College of Surgeons. Trauma performance improvement: a reference manual. Online. Available: http://www.facs.org/dept/trauma/handbook.html; 2002.

Ferrera PC, Colucciello SA, Marx JA, et al. Trauma management—an emergency medicine approach. St Louis: Mosby; 2001.

Hoffman JR, Mower WR, Wolfson AB, et al for The National Emergency X-Radiography Utilization Study Group. Validity of a set of clinical criteria to rule out injury to the cervical spine in patients with blunt trauma. N Engl J Med 2000; 343(2):94–99.

NSW Health Department. 2001. The clinician's toolkit for improving patient care. 1st edn. Sydney: NSW Health Department; 2001.

NSW Health Department. Easy guide to clinical practice improvement. A guide for health professionals. Online. Available: http://www.health.nsw.gov.au/quality/files/cpi_easyguide.pdf: 2002.

St Vincent's Hospital trauma handbook. 4th edn. Sydney: St Vincent's Hospital; 2002.

15 Neurosurgical emergencies

Robert Edwards

This chapter covers a number of neurosurgical emergencies. Before examining each of these individually, it is instructive to consider some very important general principles and concepts which are relevant regardless of the actual pathology involved.

GENERAL CONCEPTS AND PRINCIPLES

Pathophysiology

There are many ways of classifying an insult to the brain. A useful way is to divide it into primary and secondary brain injury. This is most applicable in traumatic brain injury.

Primary brain injury

Primary brain injury is the injury that occurs at the time of the trauma. Interventions that impact on primary brain injury are obviously out of the immediate control of the emergency physician, but overall are very important and include public health measures aimed at prevention. Some measures that have reduced traumatic brain injury (TBI) include compulsory use of seat belts in cars and helmets for motorcycle riders and pedal cyclists.

Secondary brain injury

Secondary brain injury occurs after the initial injury and is due to sequelae of the original injury, such as raised intracranial pressure, hypoxia or hypotension. Its effects can therefore be either minimised or prevented with good management.

Cerebral perfusion pressure

Of major importance is maintenance of cerebral perfusion pressure (CPP). This is the pressure that drives cerebral blood flow and hence cerebral perfusion.

$$CPP = \text{Mean arterial pressure (MAP)} - \text{intracranial pressure (ICP)}$$

Normally ICP is between 5 and 10 mmHg. Autoregulatory mechanisms will maintain constant cerebral blood flow when the cerebral perfusion varies between 50 and 150 mmHg. In some patients, such as those with severe head injury, cerebral autoregulation may be lost. Any process that reduces MAP (e.g. hypovolaemic shock) or increases ICP (post-injury oedema, expanding intracranial haematoma or mass, hypercarbia) will compromise cerebral perfusion, leading to secondary brain injury.

Clinical features

Headache is a hallmark symptom of a neurosurgical emergency. As headache is a frequent complaint of patients presenting to the emergency department, the emergency physician is left with the problem of working out which headaches have a potentially life-threatening cause—which may not only be subarachnoid haemorrhage but also meningococcal disease or space-occupying lesion and raised ICP.

Unfortunately, the emergency physician cannot rely on the fact that conditions such as subarachnoid haemorrhage are relatively uncommon (12 cases per 100,000 per year), because these patients choose emergency departments, either through referral from their primary physician or self-referral.

The problem is which of these patients should be investigated with a CT scan and which should not. Tables 15.1 and 15.2 outline some criteria for CT scanning of both trauma and non-trauma patients respectively. Symptoms that indicate a headache is due to raised intracranial pressure are

Table 15.1 Indications for cerebral CT in mild head injury

GCS <15 at 2 hours after injury
Suspected open, depressed of base of skull fracture
Age ≥ 65
Vomiting (2 or more episodes)
Major mechanism of injury with significant force
Focal neurological signs
Persistent headache

Table 15.2 Indications for cerebral CT in non-trauma patients with headache

Focal neurological signs
Altered mental status
Age >60
Nausea and vomiting
Severe or sudden onset suggestive of SAH
Absence of other demonstrable cause for headache
History of cerebral tumour, warfarin

associated nausea and vomiting, headache worse on awakening in the morning and on lying down.

Glasgow Coma Score (GCS)

The GCS is a widely accepted scale for assessing alterations to a patient's level of consciousness. A score is given based on three components—eye opening, verbal response and motor response (see Table 15.3). In adults, the score achieved correlates well with the severity of the underlying condition. Maximum score is 15 and minimum is 3.

Herniation syndromes

The cranial cavity is divided into compartments by sheets of dura mater (the falx cerebri and tentorium cerebelli). The tentorium separates the cerebrum above from the cerebellum and brainstem below. Because of the rigidity and non-expansile nature of the cranial vault, significant increases in ICP can lead to herniation syndromes where the contents of one compartment herniate across an opening in these dural structures, causing specific neurological signs. The significance of a herniation syndrome is that ICP has increased beyond the capacity of the brain to compensate and death will ensue if emergent treatment is not undertaken. Table 15.4 outlines features of herniation syndromes.

Raised intracranial pressure will also lead to high blood pressure and bradycardia (Cushing response).

Table 15.3 Glasgow Coma Score

Assessment	Response	Score
Eye opening	Spontaneous	4
	To voice	3
	To pain	2
	None	1
Best verbal response	Alert	5
	Confused	4
	Inappropriate words only	3
	Incomprehensible sounds	2
	Nil	1
Best motor response	Obeys commands	6
	Localises pain	5
	Withdraws to pain	4
	Abnormal flexion	3
	Abnormal extension	2
	None	1

Table 15.4 Herniation syndromes

Syndrome	Pathology	Clinical features
Uncal herniation	Increased pressure above tentorium forces uncus of temporal lobe to herniate down past medial edge of tentorium, pressing on brainstem	Dilation of ipsilateral pupil (later bilateral), contralateral pyramidal weakness
Posterior fossa transtentorial herniation	Increased pressure below tentorium causes cerebellum and midbrain to herniate up	Miosis, loss of vertical eye movements, downward gaze
Cerebellotonsillar herniation	Cerebellum pushed down through foramen magnum	Miosis, paralysis, death

Management principles

The aims of treatment are to prevent any further brain injury, treat the underlying condition, minimise symptoms and optimise neurological and functional recovery. Emergency department management is concerned with the first three of these.

Airway, breathing and circulation

A patent airway is the first priority (see Chapter 2). Simple manoeuvres to maintain patency may prevent secondary brain injury from hypoxia. Airway protection is also important—patients with a GCS of 8 or less will not be able to protect their airway from aspiration or maintain a patent airway and need intubation. Adequate ventilation is required to avoid hypoxia and hypercarbia. Treatment measures vary from oxygen therapy by mask to full mechanical ventilation if required. Adequate CPP relies in part on a normal blood pressure. Hypotension should therefore be treated with volume expansion.

Specific manoeuvres to reduce ICP

A number of interventions can reduce ICP. These include:

- Adequate sedation and paralysis of intubated patient with neurosurgical emergency.
- Prevention of rise in ICP during rapid sequence intubation. Pre-treatment with lignocaine narcotic and a defasiculating dose of muscle relaxant prior to suxamethonium is recommended.
- Mannitol infusion (20%) 1 mg/kg. Mannitol decreases ICP through its osmotic effect of drawing water out of the brain. It causes osmotic diuresis. Indicated when there is severe increase in ICP (e.g. evidence of herniation syndrome, significant mass effect on computerised tomography, CT, or high ICP as measured by ICP monitor).
- Barbiturates. Bolus therapy with thiopentone can reduce increases in ICP. Should be given only when there is an ICP monitor to guide therapy.

Hyperventilation to lower than normal PCO_2 is not recommended, as this causes cerebral vasoconstriction and does not improve the outcome. In ventilated patients, target PCO_2 should be in the normal range.

The indications for surgery are discussed for each condition.

TRAUMATIC BRAIN INJURY (TBI)

TBI is a common emergency. It is a major cause of morbidity and mortality in Australia. Of all trauma-related deaths, TBI is a major factor in a significant proportion. For those who survive traumatic brain injury, some are left with neurological impairment that often requires lengthy rehabilitation and may result in inability to return to work. The social and financial costs of this morbidity are very high.

There are two specific areas that are challenging for the emergency physician. The first is diagnosis, particularly in so-called 'mild' TBI. The second is in the area of management, to ensure that secondary brain injury is prevented or minimised by timely and appropriate management.

Table 15.5 Pathological lesions seen in traumatic brain injury

Type of injury	Lesions
Skull fractures	Depressed
	Base of skull
	Linear
Cerebral contusion	
Haemorrhage	Intracerebral
	Subarachnoid
	Subdural
	Extradural
Diffuse axonal injury	

Classification and pathophysiology

There are different ways of classifying TBI. Each is useful in that there is some relationship to treatment and prognosis. Table 15.5 outlines a classification according to actual pathology of the injury. TBI can be classified according to severity based on GCS (GCS ≤8 severe, GCS 9–13 moderate, and GCS 14–15 mild or minor).

Morbidity and mortality arise either from the primary brain injury or from secondary brain injury. Secondary brain injury results from raised ICP caused either by swelling of the injured brain or from an expanding haematoma. It may also arise from hypoxia (caused by airway compromise or chest injuries) and hypotension (blood loss from associated injuries).

Assessment and diagnosis

Assessment should be performed according to advanced trauma life support principles, which use a prioritised and systematised approach (for general principles of trauma management, see Chapter 14).

The diagnosis of TBI per se is usually obvious from the history. However, the occasional patient presents with an altered state of consciousness without a definite history of trauma. In cases where the patient may have been drinking alcohol, it is sometimes misdiagnosed as alcohol or drug intoxication, and this classic misdiagnosis can have lethal consequences.

Where alcohol use and head injury coexist, always assume that any alteration in mental state is due to the head injury.

Clinical features

The severity of mechanism of injury, a history of loss of consciousness and the duration of loss of consciousness are important parts of the history. Did the patient regain consciousness? The patient may be experiencing symptoms such as headache, nausea and vomiting. There may be amnesia concerning the events around the time of injury, or for a period before the injury (retrograde amnesia). There may also be anterograde amnesia (inability to remember information acquired since the injury). This often manifests as the patient asking the same questions over and over again. On examination, local head trauma (lacerations, haematomas) may be present. The GCS should be measured (see Table 15.4). Focal neurological signs such as pupillary dilation with or without hemiparesis with increased tone and reflexes indicate an uncal herniation syndrome requiring emergent management. Where there is significant increase in ICP, the Cushing reflex will lead to hypertension and bradycardia.

Clues to a fractured skull base are cerebrospinal fluid (CSF) leak from nose, bilateral periorbital bruising (raccoon eyes), CSF leak from the ear, haemotympanum and bruising behind the ear (Battle's sign).

Investigation

Definitive investigation is a CT scan of the head. This should be done urgently for severe and moderate head injuries. For mild head injury (GCS 14–15), see Table 15.1. A mild or minor head injury may be defined as one where there is witnessed loss of consciousness, amnesia or witnessed disorientation in patient's with a GCS of 13–15.

Skull X-rays have become superfluous. Many would say the indications for a skull X-ray necessitate a cerebral CT scan. Those who advocate a place for skull X-rays for mild head injury do so in patients who do not have indications for CT, but few patients fall into in this group.

Blood tests such as white cell count (WCC) and haemoglobin are relevant but not diagnostic. Coagulation studies should be done if there is intracranial haemorrhage or if the patient is on anticoagulation.

Management

A systematic trauma approach that identifies and prioritises injuries is mandatory. As outlined above under 'General concepts and principles', this will allow immediate management of life-threatening problems such as airway obstruction, lack of airway protection, hypoxia, blood loss and hypotension, thus avoiding secondary brain injury. Specific management includes the following.

Measures to reduce ICP

The specific measures mentioned above are appropriate for all patients with severe TBI. Mannitol is usually reserved for those who have evidence of a herniation syndrome, evidence of mass effect on CT, or high ICP as measured on an ICP monitor.

Surgery

Surgery is required for drainage of extradural and subdural haematomas and may be required urgently if they are causing mass effect with raised intracranial pressure. Supportive therapy is required for contusions, subarachnoid haemorrhage and diffuse axonal injury. Surgery is also required for depressed skull fracture. In severe head injuries, insertion of an intracranial pressure monitor and monitoring of intraarterial blood pressure to direct therapy (see above) is aimed at reducing raised ICP. To maintain adequate cerebral blood flow, a CPP of above 70 is ideal.

Other acute treatments

Antibiotic therapy for base of skull fracture or open brain injury. If seizures occur during the acute phase, phenytoin intravenous loading is used to prevent further seizures.

Analgesia

In a setting where patients with TBI can be closely monitored and CT scanning performed, sensible use of narcotic analgesia to relieve headache and pain is indicated. Codeine is not a good analgesic and is associated with a lot of nausea. Carefully titrated doses of morphine are preferable. For patients able to swallow, paracetamol can be used. Aspirin is contraindicated because of its antiplatelet effect.

Minor head injury

Exclusion of more serious pathology (e.g. extradural) is the highest priority. Effective analgesia is required. Patients not having a CT scan (see Table 15.4 for indications) should be observed until they have been symptom-free for 4 hours. When discharged, these patients should be provided with written head-injury advice, outlining indications for review and further investigation. About a third of patients with so-called minor head injury experience disabling symptoms for several days to weeks after the head injury, including headaches, difficulty concentrating and dizziness. Patients should be warned about this.

SUBARACHNOID HAEMORRHAGE

Nontraumatic subarachnoid haemorrhage (SAH) is associated with major morbidity and mortality—50% of SAH patients either die or are permanently disabled as a result of the initial haemorrhage. Another 25–35% die of a later haemorrhage if left untreated. The size of this latter group suffering repeat haemorrhages can be minimised if there is prompt diagnosis and treatment.

Despite this, diagnosis of SAH is often missed or delayed. In two-thirds of cases, SAH is due to a rupture of a cerebral aneurysm.

Nontraumatic haemorrhage is usually due to rupture of a cerebral aneurysm. The commonest site is the anterior communicating artery.

Clinical features

Sudden onset of severe headache is the hallmark of subarachnoid haemorrhage. This is often associated with nausea, vomiting, and symptoms and signs of meningism (photophobia, neck stiffness). Neurological deficit ranges from none to coma. Absence of meningism or neurological signs does not exclude the diagnosis. The severity of SAH can be graded by the Hunt and Hess system (Table 15.6). There is an increased incidence in patients who have a family history of Berry aneurysm. Patients may occasionally exhibit effects of the aneurysm before it has bled, such as warning headaches and occasionally oculomotor nerve palsy (ptosis, dilated pupil, and diplopia with the eye in the down and out position).

Investigation and diagnosis

Cerebral CT scan will show subarachnoid haemorrhage in 95% of bleeds that occurred within the previous 24 hours. At 1 week post-bleed, the sensitivity is only 50%. Because the consequences of missed diagnosis of SAH are very serious, a lumbar puncture (LP) should be performed in those with a negative CT so that a false-negative CT can be picked up. The LP should be examined for the presence of blood (either macroscopic or microscopic). If red blood cells are present, it is difficult to differentiate a traumatic tap from a subarachnoid haemorrhage. The CSF should be examined for breakdown products of red blood cells (oxyhaemoglobin and bilirubin) by CSF spectrophotometry. Oxyhaemoglobin takes 2 or more

Table 15.6 Hunt and Hess classification of subarachnoid haemorrhage and outcome of patients according to grade[3]

Grade	Clinical features	Dead	Outcome- dependent	Independent
Grade I	Asymptomatic or minimal headache and slight nuchal rigidity			
Grade II	Moderate to severe headache, nuchal rigidity. No neuro deficit apart from cranial nerve palsy	7%	6%	87%
Grade III	Drowsiness, confusion, mild focal deficit	23%	13%	64%
Grade IV	Stupor, moderate to severe hemiparesis, possibly early decerebrate rigidity, and vegetative disturbances	44%	22%	33%
Grade V	Deep coma, decerebrate rigidity, moribund appearance			

hours to develop, but bilirubin takes 12 hours to develop. A traumatic tap can give rise to oxyhaemoglobin, but the presence of both bilirubin and oxyhaemoglobin peaks on spectrophotometry is indicative of SAH.

If either CT or LP is positive for SAH, the source of the haemorrhage must be found with a cerebral angiogram. CT angiography of the circle of Willis using intravenous contrast is a less invasive alternative that can identify aneurysms and AV malformations. It has not replaced conventional cerebral angiography but is useful in investigating patients with high clinical suspicion of SAH but who have equivocal or negative CT and LP.

Treatment

As with any emergency, care of the airway, breathing and circulation takes first priority. Definitive treatment is early surgery to clip the aneurysm to prevent rebleeding, which may be catastrophic. Spasm of cerebral vessels is a delayed complication of SAH that may lead to cerebral ischaemia. The risk of this can be minimised by using nimodipine, which should be started intravenously within 72 hours of the SAH. Control of blood pressure within normal limits is important.

SPACE-OCCUPYING LESIONS AND RAISED ICP

A number of nontraumatic conditions can give rise to raised intracranial pressure by enlarging in size and causing mass effect. These include tumours (primary and secondary tumours) and intracerebral haemorrhage (including posterior fossa haemorrhage). Subdural haematomas may occur without a definite history of trauma. Large cerebellar infarcts can be complicated by significant swelling, rapid increase in ICP and a herniation syndrome.

Clinical presentation of these lesions can vary greatly from just headaches with features suggestive of raised intracranial pressure to coma and herniation syndromes at the severe end of the spectrum.

The management of these conditions is guided by the principles outlined at the beginning of this chapter. Emergent surgery is required for haemorrhagic space-occupying lesions such as subdural haematomas and posterior fossa haemorrhages. Raised intracranial pressure from tumours is often responsive to treatment with bed rest and dexamethasone.

COMPLICATIONS OF VENTRICULAR DRAINAGE DEVICES

Blocked ventriculoperitoneal (VP) shunt

Patients with VP shunt not infrequently present to the emergency department with shunt problems. The commonest of these are shunt obstruction and shunt infection. It is important to recognise these complications when they occur, because if untreated they can lead to significant morbidity or mortality.

Clinical features

The patient will usually have a clear history of having had a VP shunt inserted. Often there is a history of a similar presentation in the past. Symptoms and signs are variable, but include one or more of the following: headache, decreased level of consciousness, ataxia, nausea and vomiting. On examination the patient may have a decreased level of consciousness and, in severe cases, focal neurological signs may indicate a herniation syndrome. Papilloedema may be present and paralysis of upward gaze may be seen. If a shunt reservoir is palpable, inability to empty it by pressing on it would suggest a distal obstruction; if it can be compressed but is slow to refill, this suggests a distal proximal obstruction.

A cerebral CT will demonstrate if there is any hydrocephalus. A normal CT, however, does not rule out a shunt malfunction.

Management

The general principles of management are as outlined for other neurosurgical emergencies, namely attention to the airway, breathing and circulation, and specific measures to reduce ICP. Definitive treatment is shunt revision.

SPINAL INJURIES

In everyday language the term 'spinal injury' is often used to describe any injury to the vertebral column or spinal cord, and as such can be ambiguous. Here, vertebral column injury refers to injury to any of the bones, joints and ligaments making up the vertebral column. This may or may not be associated with spinal cord injury, which refers to injury to the spinal cord itself.

Trauma to the vertebral column and associated injury to the spinal cord is a challenging problem from both diagnostic and therapeutic standpoints. The types of trauma that have a high risk of spinal injury include high-speed motor vehicle accidents (particularly if there has been ejection from the vehicle), diving injuries, rugby football injuries and falls. In the elderly, falls from a standing position can result in cervical spine injury.

Clinical features

The features of vertebral column injury are midline pain, particularly on attempted movement and local tenderness. It may or may not be associated with a spinal cord injury, which is manifest by neurological deficit. The neurological deficit can be classified according to function (motor, sensory or autonomic), its distribution (level and in partial cord lesions depending on which part of the body is affected) and whether the loss of function is complete or incomplete.

Diagnosis is difficult because clinical assessment alone is often not adequate in defining vertebral column injuries. Radiological assessment can be difficult both in interpretation of films and in detecting subtle abnormalities—plain X-rays can miss around 5% of cervical vertebral column injuries.

Assessment

Assessment has three aims: detection of a vertebral column injury, determination of stability of the vertebral column injury, detection of and assessment of the presence of a spinal cord injury.

Detection of a vertebral column injury

Clinical

In patients with trauma, the cervical spine should be immobilised until it can be 'cleared'. The cervical spine may be cleared clinically in patients who are lucid and alert, have no neck pain or midline neck tenderness, no neurological signs referable to the spinal cord, no significant distracting injuries, and in those who have not received large doses of opiate analgesia.

If the cervical spine cannot be cleared, then radiological assessment must ensue. It should also be remembered that of patients with a vertebral column injury, 5–7% will have a second injury.

Radiological

At a minimum, three views should be taken of the cervical spine. These are lateral, anteroposterior (AP) and odontoid peg (open-mouth) views. The sensitivity of each of these views for detecting a cervical spine injury are, respectively, 85–90%, 1–2% and 5%. The lateral view must show down to the cervicothoracic junction (C7 and at least upper part of body of T1). If it does not, a swimmer's view can be obtained to better show the cervicothoracic area. This view needs to show both the alignment and some detail of the C7/T1 area. For patients who have large shoulders and upper torsos, or who cannot physically be placed in the swimmer's position (one shoulder abducted), a CT scan may be required to image the cervicothoracic junction.

Other films may be useful in certain situations. Oblique views of the cervical spine can be used to evaluate the facet joints on each side. They can also be used as an alternative to the swimmer's view in imaging the cervicothoracic junction. Flexion and extension views are indicated to detect instability in an otherwise normal cervical spine with symptoms. Recent literature has questioned the value of flexion and extension views in detecting injuries not already seen on plain films.

Accurate interpretation of plain cervical spine films can be difficult and less experienced doctors should check their interpretation with an emergency physician. Table 15.7 outlines a system for reviewing cervical

Table 15.7 Checklist for assessment of cervical spine X-rays

- Quality of film. Includes all of C7 and at least part of T1.
- Alignment. Check for smooth continuity of four 'lines'. Anterior alignment of vertebral bodies, posterior alignment of vertebral, the spinolaminal line (junction of lamina and spinous process) and tips of spinous processes.
- Prevertebral soft tissue swelling. Best judged in upper cervical spine. 5 mm allowed at C2, 7 mm allowed at C4.
- Predental space (between dens and anterior arch of C1). >2–3 mm in adults and 4 mm in children.
- Relationship of adjacent vertebral bodies (e.g. movement of one body on another, angulation).
- Integrity of the elements of each vertebral body (e.g. loss of height, visible fracture lines, abnormalities in bony architecture).
- Facet joints between adjacent vertebrae (subluxation or dislocation).
- Integrity of posterior elements such as pedicles, laminae and spinous processes.
- Integrity of odontoid peg (on lateral and peg views).
- Subluxation of either atlantoaxial joint (on peg view).
- Alignment and integrity of all elements on anteroposterior (AP) film. Particularly look for alignment of spinous processes in midline and alignment of facet joints.

spine X-rays. Abnormalities may be non-specific and simply draw attention to the need for further imaging. See also Chapter 48.

Indications for computerised tomography (CT)
Technological advances in the design of CT scanners have greatly assisted the radiological assessment of the cervical spine. With high-speed scanners acquiring multiple slices at narrow distances, computerised reconstructions of the entire vertebral column are possible.

Computerised tomography is indicated in the following circumstances:

1. For better definition of abnormalities seen on plain film.
2. Further imaging in patients with significant symptoms (pain and tenderness) but normal plain films.
3. Imaging of C1/C2 in severely head-injured patients (high incidence of unrecognised injuries on plain films in such cases).
4. Inability to image adequately with plain films (e.g. C1/C2, cervicothoracic junction).

Magnetic resonance imaging (MRI)
CT scans are particularly useful for identifying bony injury. Clinical and radiological assessment as described above will pick up the vast majority of fractures and dislocations. MRI is better for identifying ligamentous injury, however, and is useful in the further assessment of known injuries or the investigation of spinal cord injury without radiological abnormality (SCIWORA).

Assessment of presence of spinal cord injury

The hallmark of spinal cord injury is the presence of neurological deficit referable to the spinal cord. Sensory, motor and autonomic modalities may be affected. An evaluation of motor tone, power and reflexes should be done. Initial screening sensory examination is with light touch or pinprick. If there is other evidence of neurological deficit, test temperature and proprioception (posterior column). When sensory loss is present, a sensory level below which sensation is lost can define the level of the injury. A working knowledge of the dermatomes of the body is required. It helps to remember that the junction of shoulder and neck is at C4, nipple at T4, umbilicus at T10, inguinal region at L1. When the patient is logrolled to examine the back, perianal and buttocks, sensory testing should be done, as well as assessment of anal tone. Sparing perianal sensation and anal tone may be evidence that the lesion is not complete and there may be some functional recovery.

Other clinical clues that suggest spinal cord injury are diaphragmatic breathing in high-mid to lower cervical spine injury (loss of intercostal power supplied by thoracic cord with intact diaphragm supplied by C4, 5 and 6). In males, priapism may be present owing to loss of sympathetic tone. There may also be hypotension and bradycardia as a result of loss of sympathetic vascular tone. Other causes of shock from trauma (haemorrhage, pericardial tamponade and tension pneumothorax) must be ruled out.

Whether or not the cord lesion is complete or partial is obviously vital for prognosis. Complete lesions have total loss of all three modalities (motor, sensory and autonomic). Partial lesions can have some residual function in any of the modalities. There are some syndromes with typical patterns of deficit indicating injury to certain parts of the cord (Table 15.8).

Determination of stability of vertebral column injury

The ability of the vertebral column to protect the spinal cord from abnormal movement and therefore injury should be evaluated. Ideally, this evaluation should be done by a spinal surgeon.

Table 15.8 Partial spinal cord syndromes

Syndrome	Part of cord affected	Motor	Sensory
Brown-Séquard	Hemisection of cord	Ipsilateral loss	Loss of ipsilateral proprioception, contrateral pain/temperature
Anterior cord	Anterior half of cord	Bilateral motor loss	Bilateral temperature loss. Intact proprioception/vibration
Central cord syndrome		Weakness in upper limbs, sparing of lower limbs	Loss of sensation in upper limbs, lower limbs spared

The vertebral column can be considered to consist of three structural components: namely the anterior, middle and posterior columns.[3] The anterior column consists of bone and ligaments from the anterior half of the vertebral bodies forward. The posterior column is made up of the neural arch (laminae and pedicles), spinous processes and posterior ligamentous complex. The remainder, the middle column, is from the posterior longitudinal ligament and posterior half of the vertebral body. If at least two out of three of these columns are disrupted, the injury is considered unstable.

Treatment

In the patient with multiple injuries, vertebral column and spinal cord injuries should be managed as part of a prioritised management plan that addresses other serious injuries in context (see Chapter 14 for general principles of trauma management). The consequences of injury to the spinal cord in a patient with an unstable vertebral column injury are of major life-changing significance for the patient. Precautions to prevent further injury to the cord should therefore be instituted from the beginning.

Interventions can be classified as those that stabilise the vertebral column and those that aim to minimise or improve cord function.

Immobilisation of vertebral column

Precautions to prevent movement of the vertebral column should be instituted until it has been cleared. Patient transfers should be carried out while maintaining the position of the vertebral column. In hospital, this means use of specialised lifting frames (e.g. Jordan frame) or techniques such as logrolling or spinal lifting. In each of these, a designated person needs to maintain the position of the cervical spine and monitor the manoeuvre.

Numerous orthoses are available to minimise vertebral column movements. There is no perfect splint that prevents all vertebral column movements, particularly in uncooperative patients.

Cervical collars restrict but do not completely prevent cervical spine movement. Soft collars are very poor at preventing movement. Hard collars (e.g. California stiff neck collar) are better. At a minimum, any patient with a suspected cervical spine fracture should wear a hard cervical collar and the transfer techniques outlined above should be used. 'Sandbags' may also be used for additional immobilisation. Imaging should be expedited, as prolonged periods in hard collars and lying supine without moving are uncomfortable and painful.

A number of 'extrication devices' are available to aid immobilisation of the patient with vertebral column injuries in the thoracic or lumbar spine (e.g. Kendrick extraction device). These consist of moulded plastic with a hard 'spine' that straps around the neck and torso. They are most appropriately used in the pre-hospital setting.

Airway management may be problematical. Mask ventilation has been shown to result in inadvertent neck extension. If intubation is required, a proven safe technique is in-line immobilisation of the cervical spine by a person assigned only to that task plus intubation by an experienced operator during rapid sequence induction.

Referral and supportive care

Patients with high cervical lesions may have respiratory muscle weakness, which may lead to respiratory failure. Therapy for this may vary from supplemental oxygen to mechanical ventilation.

Patients with spinal cord injury should also have a gastric tube passed and an indwelling catheter placed.

Early transfer to a specialised spinal unit within 24 hours of injury has been shown to affect outcome positively.

Early referral to a spinal surgeon (neurosurgeon or orthopaedic surgeon) should happen as soon as a diagnosis is made. Decisions regarding the stability of a vertebral column lesion should be made by the spinal surgeon. Additionally, patients may require long-term immobilisation with skeletal traction.

High-dose corticosteroids

The use of early high-dose methylprednisolone is controversial. Evidence of a benefit is limited to one large, prospective placebo-controlled randomised study,[4] in which patients with cervical spine injury were treated with 24 hours of methylprednisolone (30 mg/kg bolus followed by 5.4 mg/kg/h infusion). This failed to show any improvement in morbidity or mortality, but those treated within 8 hours showed a greater improvement in the return of motor ability (5 points) and sensation (2–3 points) as measured on a 70-point scale at 6 weeks and 6 months.

This validity of this study has been questioned because of the methods of statistical analysis employed, the functional significance of the measured motor and sensory improvements is unclear, and the results have not been confirmed in other trials.[5] The potential benefit must then be weighed up against the adverse risks of high-dose methylprednisolone.

REFERENCES

1. Stiell IG, et al. The Canadian head CT rule for patients with minor head injury. Lancet 2001; 357:1391–1396.
2. Coyne TJ, Stuart G. A two-year survey of aneurysmal subarachnoid haemorrhage. Med J Aust 1991; 154:506–509.
3. Denis F. The three-column spine and its significance in the classification of acute thoracolumbar spinal injuries. Spine 1983; 8:817.
4. Bracken MB, et al. A randomized controlled trial of methylprednisolone or naloxone in the treatment of acute spinal cord injury. N Engl J Med 1990; 322:1405.
5. Pointillart V, et al. Pharmacological therapy of spinal cord injury during the acute phase. Spinal Cord 2000; 38:71.

16 Aortic aneurysms, dissections and acute limb ischaemia

Michael Novy

Vascular emergencies presenting to the emergency department may occur for many reasons, both medical and surgical, and may present in many varied ways. Physicians working in the emergency department need to be aware of these conditions, which may present subtly. Failure to diagnose and treat appropriately may result in catastrophic outcome.

THORACIC AORTIC ANEURYSMS AND DISSECTIONS

A thoracic aortic aneurysm is usually caused by atherosclerotic plaques and is a completely different condition from a thoracic dissection, which is caused by a tear in the intima, secondary almost exclusively to hypertension. As the population ages, patients with thoracic aortic dissections are seen more frequently in emergency departments.

They may be classified into proximal or distal dissection by a number of different classification systems. The DeBakey system classifies dissections into Type 1 (the entire aorta is involved), Type 2 (only the ascending aorta is involved) and Type 3 (only the descending aorta is involved). The Stanford classification separates the dissections into Type A (involvement of the ascending aorta) and Type B (the descending aorta is involved).

Improved diagnostic tools are becoming more readily available, leading to increasing diagnosis of this condition. Careful history, examination and investigations, and early detection may lead to increased survival. However, despite advances in emergency medicine care, mortality remains at approximately 50%.

Although ruptured aneurysms and thoracic dissections are separate disease processes, their initial emergency department management is identical.

Causes

Atherosclerosis, hypertension, trauma, postcardiac catheterisation.

History

Presents classically with a sudden onset of severe chest pain, tearing in nature, radiating through to the back; the pain may also radiate to the neck, arms or abdomen. There may be an associated shortness of breath.

The patient may present with signs and symptoms of cerebral vascular injury.

There is often a past history of hypertension, smoking and hyper-cholesterolaemia, and the nature of these should be ascertained.

Examination

Classically, these patients look unwell, and are often diaphoretic. Hypertension is often present.

Comparative blood pressure readings of both arms is vital, and a difference of greater than 20 mmHg is a significant finding. Pulses may be decreased or absent in one of the upper limbs. There may also be a pulse differential between the upper and lower limbs.

Auscultation of the precordium may reveal a new aortic regurgitation murmur and there may also be decreased heart sounds due to tamponade. A third heart sound is sometimes heard.

Investigations

1. Bedside investigation should include blood pressure measurements on both arms and an ECG. The ECG may sometimes be difficult to interpret as it may sometimes show changes consistent with an acute myocardial infarction.
2. A mobile CXR should be ordered, as in most cases patients are too unstable to move to the radiology department for formal views. Classic changes associated with thoracic aortic injury include a widened mediastinum, a double aortic knob sign, left pleural effusion, capping of the apex, loss of the aortopulmonary window, depression of the left main bronchus.
3. Blood should be taken for a full blood count (FBC), urea electrolyte creatinine (UEC), and cardiac markers, and crossmatch should be organised.
4. Several types of definitive studies may be undertaken to confirm the diagnosis. If the patient is acutely unwell and haemodynamically unstable, the investigation of choice is a bedside echocardiograph. There is relatively high sensitivity and specificity for this investigation. Echocardiograph allows for visualisation of the injury and also gives some functional information regarding ejection fraction and decreased cardiac muscle contractility.
5. If the patient is haemodynamically stable, CT may be considered as the definitive diagnosis. The patient must be accompanied to the radiology department by a senior clinician and adequate monitoring and resuscitation equipment must be available.
6. With improving resolution of CT scanners and the increasing availability of CT angiogram, classic angiography plays a lesser role.
7. Magnetic resonance imaging (MRI) may be considered in the stable patient. Although the sensitivity and specificity of this modality are

both very high, the patient must be well enough to undergo this investigation.

Emergency department management

1. The patient's airway, ventilation and circulation should be managed concurrently with a team approach in an acute-care area of the emergency department.
2. Establish continuous cardiac and respiratory monitoring via a 3-lead ECG, pulse oximetry and non-invasive blood pressure monitoring. Invasive blood pressure monitoring via an arterial line should however be considered early.
3. Give supplemental oxygen.
4. Establish intravenous access via two large-bore cannulas, but use fluids judiciously.
5. Give adequate intravenous analgesia.
6. The patient is often hypertensive. Antihypertensives should be commenced to obtain a systolic blood pressure of less than 120 mmHg. Antihypertensive agents with a short half-life, such as sodium nitroprusside or short-acting beta-blockers, should be used, so that dosages may be titrated to achieve appropriate blood pressure readings.
7. Early involvement with the cardiothoracic team should be sought.

Disposition

Surgical intervention is more likely to be offered for patients who have a proximal dissection or a dissection involving the aortic valve. Mortality from this procedure is as high as 50% and it is important to discuss this with the patient and the family.

If it is decided to have surgical intervention, the patient should be taken to the operating room as soon as possible. Medical management should take place in a high-dependence or intensive care unit.

ABDOMINAL AORTIC ANEURYSMS (AAAs)

AAAs are found in approximately 2–4% of the population, but are far more commonly found in men over 65 years of age. The majority of patients who have a ruptured AAA die suddenly in the pre-hospital environment before the arrival of an ambulance or presentation to the emergency department.

AAAs that measure less than 4 cm in diameter are almost always benign and are unlikely to rupture. These are usually discovered as incidental findings during CT scan or ultrasound investigation or during screening for other diseases. These AAAs do not require acute intervention but need to be followed up via regular ultrasound. If the AAA increases in size by more than 0.5 cm in 6 months or if the AAA becomes larger than 5 cm, a surgical opinion should be obtained.

Patients who present to the emergency department with a leaking or ruptured AAA require prompt diagnosis and treatment, as survival decreases by approximately 1% with each minute after the event.

History

Patients with a leaking or ruptured AAA classically present to the emergency department with a sudden onset of severe abdominal pain, which is associated with syncope. The pain may radiate through to the back, into the flank region or into the groin. The pain may mimic the pain that is described with renal colic. This occurs when there is involvement of the renal artery and, with dissection of the artery, there may also be associated haematuria. In a patient over the age of 60, without a history of renal colic, the diagnosis of AAA rupture must always be excluded before the diagnosis of renal colic is made.

The patient may present with only syncope, as classical signs are present in only 30–50% of cases.

Past history of coronary artery, peripheral vascular disease or cerebrovascular disease should be obtained as well as information about the associated risk factors of smoking, hypertension, diabetes (DM) and hypercholesterolaemia, and family history.

Examination

If the AAA leaks or ruptures and is contained in the retroperitoneal space, vital signs may be normal and there may be very few clinical findings.

Patients classically present with a pulsatile abdominal mass—hypotensive and tachycardic. However, auscultation of the abdomen for bruits and palpation of the peripheral vessels should also be completed, as these are often abnormal and may be more common than a pulsatile abdominal mass.

Investigation

1. Bedside investigation should include an EG, initial pulse and BP, and oximetry.
2. If the patient has severe cardiovascular compromise, and there is high index of clinical suspicion of the diagnosis, then a focused assessment with sonography in trauma (FAST) study may be performed to confirm the presence of free fluid in the peritoneum. Surgical intervention, however, must not be delayed. A FAST study may have a false-negative if the rupture is solely retroperitoneal, but these patients are usually more stable and a definitive diagnosis may be obtained.
3. Full blood count, UEC, liver function tests (LFTs), amylase and crossmatch should be obtained.

There are several options available for definitive diagnosis:

1. Departmental ultrasound is non-invasive, but cannot determine involvement of branches of the aorta. Sensitivity may be decreased with obese patients or if large amounts of bowel gas are present.

2. Abdominal CT scan is useful for stable patients with a suspected AAA. It has a high sensitivity, allows visualisation of the retroperitoneum, and allows for assessment of involvement of the branches of the aorta. The patient must be stable and have continuous cardiovascular monitoring, and a trained medical escort during the CT scan.
3. MRI and angiogram are available but are rarely used for the acute diagnosis of an AAA rupture.

Emergency department management

The patient should be triaged to an acute-care area of the emergency department. A team approach should be used to manage and treat the patient's airway, breathing and circulation concurrently.

1. Supplemental oxygen.
2. Establish continuous cardiovascular monitoring via 3-lead ECG, non-invasive BP and pulse oximetry.
3. Establish IV access via two large-bore cannulas and commence fluid resuscitation.
4. Draw bloods as above.
5. Adequate intravenous pain relief.
6. Indwelling catheter (IDC).
7. Early surgical consultation.

Disposition

Early surgical intervention is essential in the unstable patient, as survival decreases approximately 1% per minute.

Stable patients with a rupture may be investigated as above, but should be taken to the operating theatre as soon as possible.

The patient should be followed up and monitored in an intensive care or high-dependency unit.

ACUTE LIMB ISCHAEMIA

Acute limb ischaemia requires rapid assessment and treatment in the emergency department and may often require ongoing surgical intervention. Failure to identify and treat this condition may lead to tissue necrosis and its associated complications.

Causes

Atherosclerosis, thrombosis, embolic diseases, trauma, misadventure with intravenous drug use (IVDU) resulting in arterial injection.

History

History is dependent on the particular cause. In acute limb ischaemia, time of onset of symptoms is critical. Previous episodes of events are important to document. Past history of clotting disorders, both of the patient and of family members, should be requested.

Patients presenting with misadventure of IVDU resulting in intraarterial injection should be asked what substance they have injected.

Examination

The affected limb may appear mottled or cyanosed compared with the other limb. The limb may feel colder, pulses may be decreased or absent. Objective examination of sensation may not reveal abnormalities until irreversible damage has been done, and as such should not be relied on as a sign.

Investigations

1. Bedside investigation should include an ECG, in particular looking for atrial fibrillation.
2. Ankle pressure indexes may be performed, looking for a difference between limbs.
3. Bedside Doppler studies may aid in the diagnosis.
4. FBC, UEC and coagulation studies should be performed.
5. Doppler ultrasound should be obtained to view the obstruction.
6. Angiography, if available, may be considered.

These investigations should not delay definitive treatment of the patient.

Emergency department management

Assess and manage the patient's airway and circulation concurrently.

1. Supplemental oxygen.
2. Position the limb at the level of the torso.
3. Establish intravenous access and commence appropriate fluid resuscitation.
4. Give adequate analgesia, such as morphine, in 2.5 mg aliquots.
5. Commence anticoagulation with heparin as per departmental protocol.
6. Obtain urgent surgical consultation with view to embolectomy.
7. Consider broad-spectrum antibiotic coverage if due to IVDU.

Disposition

Patients should have definite treatment in the operating theatre without delay.

Medical management should occur in a high-dependency unit.

COMPARTMENT SYNDROME

First described by Richard von Volkmann in 1881, compartment syndrome is caused by an increase in intracompartment pressure above that which allows blood flow to occur, which leads to tissue ischaemia. Compartment syndrome occurs more commonly in the lower and upper limbs, and less commonly around the shoulder girdle or gluteal region. Failure to recognise and treat this condition will lead to tissue necrosis, permanent loss of function and, if left untreated, renal failure, electrolyte abnormalities and death.

Causes

Trauma fractures, bleeding into an enclosed tissue space, external compression, vigorous exercise, small thrombotic or embolic events, and intramuscular injections.

History

In the conscious patient, there may be pain that appears to be greater than expected with the degree of injury. Pain may be difficult to distinguish in the presence of other injuries, such as fractures of long bones, but may be absent if there is an associated spinal cord injury. Compartment syndrome may also be associated with patients who have had prolonged periods of unconsciousness without movement, such as occurs with narcotic overdose. Collateral history from paramedics and relatives may be vital in this situation.

Examination

Classically the patient may present with the five Ps associated with ischaemia: pain, pallor, paraesthesia, paralysis and pulselessness. However, these are often late signs and irreversible damage to tissue may have occurred by this stage.

The affected limb or region may often feel firmer upon examination than the comparative region on the other side of the body. There may be distal paraesthesia. Pulse initially may be decreased or distal capillary return decreased, but these are both unreliable signs.

Investigations

1. Bedside investigations should include a BSL, urinalysis and ECG. Bedside ultrasound examining blood flow may be useful, but should not delay definitive management.
2. Lab work-up should include FBC, UEC (in particular, creatine kinase and arterial blood gases).
3. Urine microscopy may show urine myoglobin, but the absence of this does not rule out the diagnosis.
4. Examination of the affected compartment with a tonometer will allow for the direct measurement of pressure within the affected region.

Treatment

1. First address initial management of the whole patient, including airway, ventilation and circulation.
2. Correct positioning of the affected limb level with the torso (elevation of the affected limb will lower arterial pressure!).
3. Supplemental oxygen 15 L/min via non-rebreathing mask
4. Establishment of IV access and fluid resuscitation as needed.
5. Patient with severe compartment syndrome may have life-threatening hyperkalaemia with cardiac compromise, which may need to be treated initially.
6. Analgesia should be given intravenously as required.
7. Prompt involvement with the surgical team should occur.

Disposition

Once the diagnosis is suspected, prompt fasciotomy is the treatment of choice. Ongoing care should be in the high-dependency or intensive care unit to monitor and treat renal impairment and electrolyte abnormalities.

EDITOR'S COMMENT

In any patient with severe pain, especially if unrelieved by analgesia, worry and observe! It is the most common hallmark of a missed catastrophe and morbidity.

RECOMMENDED READING

Erbel R, Zamorano J. The aorta. Aortic aneurysm, trauma and dissection. Crit Care Clin 1996; 12(3):733–766.

Gomez-Jorge J. Aorta dissection. Online. Available: http://www.emedicine.com/radio/topic43.htm.

Hagan PG, Nienaber CA, Isselbacher EM. The International Registry of Acute Aortic Dissection (IRAD): new insights into an old disease. JAMA 2000; 283(7):897–903.

Hoover TJ, Siefert JA. Soft tissue complications of orthopaedic emergencies. Emerg Med Clin North Am 2000; 18(1):115–139.

O'Connor R. Aneurysms, abdominal. Online. Available: http://www.emedicine.com/emerg/topic27.htm.

Wallace S, Goodman S. Compartment syndrome, lower extremity. Online. Available: www.emedicine.com/orthoped/topic596.htm.

17 Musculoskeletal injuries and orthopaedic principles

Geoffrey Stubbs and David Sonnabend

OUTPATIENT FRACTURES (Geoffrey Stubbs)

The ease and quality of the reduction always parallels the quality of the anaesthesia. There is a 70% reduction in cost if the fracture can be successfully managed in the emergency department, and in children there is much less psychological stress. Many techniques are described (haematoma block, Bier's and mini-Bier's block, axillary/supraclavicular block, specific nerve block, e.g. femoral). All work well, provided the administrator is skilled in the technique required, knows the anatomy, understands the pharmacology and acts in a confident and unhurried manner. Sedation and base-line pain relief are valuable additions; consider midazolam (0.05–0.2 mg/kg IV), morphine (0.1–0.2 mg/kg IV) or fentanyl (1.0–5.0 µg/kg IV) to calm and relax the patient.

Gentleness and gravity always suffice. If the fracture needs force, then the mechanism is not understood.

Well-padded casts, accurate reduction, elevation and support should make the fracture sufficiently comfortable that simple analgesics such as paracetamol give adequate pain control. Pain beyond this level suggests some complication/complicating fracture.

Always split the cast or use non-continuous slabs. Swelling is unpredictable; splitting a cast later is distressing. Arrange for a follow-up cast check within 24 hours.

Check for the recognised complications of the fracture or anaesthetic technique before discharge. Ensure the patient/parent understands any warning signs.

The general rule for cast treatment of fractures is to immobilise the joint above and below the fracture. For distal forearm and ankle fractures, this means immobilising the elbow (long arm cast) and the knee (long leg cast). Often this is not done for good reasons, but you should be aware of those reasons and how they apply to the particular fracture you are treating.

Describing a fracture or dislocation

It is important that you are able to describe a fracture over the phone. A senior colleague's advice is only as good as the information you give. Take a little time and make some notes that answer these questions:

- Who has suffered the injury? A child, an athlete, an elderly person?
- What is their general condition? Is this an isolated injury or part of multitrauma? Is the patient comfortable or shocked, confused etc?
- Which bone has been broken?
- Where?
- In one or more places?
- Is there a complicating injury like nerve damage?
- Is the circulation distal to the fracture satisfactory? Warm with good peripheral pulses and capillary refill? Or cold, pale and pulseless?
- Is the skin broken? If it is, how big is the wound? Is it obviously contaminated with dirt etc? Are the soft tissues healthy or questionable? Is the skin stretched tight over the deformity?
- What have you done so far? Have you aligned the injured limb? Have you splinted the fracture to immobilise it? What pain relief have you given? What was the effect?

Fracture classification

There many classification systems. Most are used for outcomes assessment or as a guide to treatment options. For triage and initial care the following points are more helpful, as they relate to the immediate care decisions.

- Is the patient suitable for ambulatory care management?
- If yes, do you understand the fracture mechanics?
- Is the fracture a 'sleeper'? Is there anything about the fracture that may be more complicated or treacherous than it appears? Children's fractures often are, so a brief review of their classification is in order.

Salter-Harris classification of children's fractures

Type I, separation through the physeal plate

Children rarely suffer dislocations, as the growth plate represents a weak point near the joint. The same forces that in an adult would produce a ligament injury cause a separation at the physis in a child. The physeal plate and epiphysis stay as one unit, and the metaphysis and the rest of the bone as the other. The weak point is at the metaphyseal margin of the physeal plate where the zone of provisional calcification is being absorbed by osteoclasts. Immediately metaphyseal of this is the zone of osteoblastic new bone formation that adds length to the growing bone.

There are hidden effects in Type I fractures. The separation may not be noticed on the X-ray, since you expect a lucent line there. It is usually widened, but that is a very subtle point. The periosteum attaches to the perichondrial ring at the same place and at least part of this attachment will stay intact despite the injury. This allows the separated epiphysis/physis to snap back into place, leaving no obvious deformity on the X-rays. In adults, dislocations may do the same, also leaving normal-looking positions to the bones. As with adults, stress views may show quite alarming displacement. In children, the active bone generation zone adjacent to the separation plane will produce very rapid union. The early stages of callus formation are collagen generation, so the separation may quickly become painless and the child resume activity, but the plasticity of the callus allows deformity to develop and later mineralisation of the callus fixes the deformity. This is especially embarrassing, as the first X-rays may be passed as 'normal'. Worse, even if anticipated, a heavy and ill-supported cast may contribute. The following rule is useful: if the part is painful, the child won't use it and there is well-localised bony tenderness, a Salter-Harris Type I fracture is likely (see Figure 17.1). In the wrist and ankle, stress views are usually not required, providing the possibility that an ill-supported cast may cause deformity is considered. At the elbow and knee, the potential for mischief is much greater, since long arm and long leg casts make the distal limb heavier and make the potential for displacement greater than if there is no cast at all.

Type II

The plane of separation is mostly through the epiphysis as in a Type I, but a small metaphyseal fragment remains attached to the physis. This is the commonest type. Reduction can be very difficult if you visualise the fracture in just two dimensions. There is a twisting component, so the

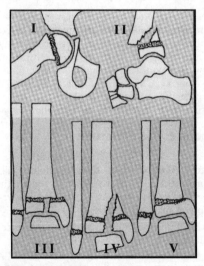

Figure 17.1 Epiphyseal plate injuries

Notes

1. The growth plate always 'goes' with the epiphysis, and fracture healing does not cross an intact growth plate.
2. Whenever the growth plate is broken, the potential exists for fracture healing to occur between metaphysis and epiphysis and produce secondary deformity. Hence Types III and IV require anatomical reduction (by surgery, if necessary).
3. In principle, joint surface congruity should be restored in any intraarticular fracture.
4. In Type V, the growth plate is crushed and stops growing. Later deformity results.

displaced metaphyseal fragment does not lie directly opposite the point it came from but is rotated and lies against an intact piece of the metaphysis. Just pushing won't get it back. Think of a key in a lock: it needs to be turned to the unlock position before it can be reduced. In distal forearm fractures, the metaphyseal 'key' is usually supinated in relation to the rest of the metaphysis, and the fracture needs to be reduced and held in supination. That means a long arm cast. That is just the more common situation, as most often a child falls forward on a pronated wrist. If the child fell backwards, everything is in reverse. There is no 'rule': each fracture presents is own puzzle.

Types III and IV

Both these fractures either cross the growth plate (III) or involve the joint surface (IV). The potential for increasing growth disturbance from even minor malunion is marked. Children will 'grow out' most malunions. Small children who have the most growth to do can 'grow out' malunions with Type I and II fractures that appear quite alarming, but with III and IV the malunion increases with each year of growth so small children need special vigilance. Treatment is by open reduction and temporary fixation.

Types V and VI

These are rare but nasty. Type V is a crush injury that directly damages part of the physis so badly that the cartilage cells are destroyed. Early union over this part of the physis occurs but the less crushed area recovers and continues to grow. It may not be recognised on the films as there may be no displacement at all. Type VI involves a direct injury to the perichondrial ring, so beware of deep wound over the physis.

Tip: Fax a tracing of the fracture to the consultant.

When to reduce the fracture

As noted with Salter-Harris Type II fractures, future growth will often remodel the fracture. Many other fractures near joints will also remodel. A pertinent question is therefore: do you need to reduce the fracture at all? It is a question that needs some experience to answer but there are guidelines to help you make the choice.

- The younger the child, the more growth will take place and hence the more remodelling.
- The closer the fracture is to the joint, the more potential for correction. Midshaft fractures do not remodel except in very young children.
- The remodelling occurs only in the normal plane of movement of the joint. At the elbow and knee (which is essentially anterior and posterior hinge) flexion and extension, deformities of 30° will model out, but varus and valgus deformities persist. Supracondylar fractures of the humerus are a real trial, not only because of the high likelihood of nerve and vessel injuries but because of the difficulty in assessing residual varus

and valgus deformity with the elbow flexed (the stable position to hold the reduction).

- The proximal humerus, on the other hand, is a forgiving site because of the nearly 360° motion of the shoulder.
- The wrist is also a fairly forgiving site and up to 30° dorsiflexion will grow out, together with lesser amounts of palmar, radial and ulnar tilt.
- Torsional deformities don't correct.
- Overlap does improve. End-to-end apposition of the bone is not essential—overlap of a couple of centimetres will grow out in the femur. The extra blood flow associated with fracture union stimulates physeal growth and femoral shaft fractures are close to perfectly self-correcting for length. The same for the humerus with 1–2 cm overlap. Overlap elsewhere is more of a problem, as the fracture is unstable in all three planes and hard to hold with a cast.
- Growth plate injuries get worse rather than better.

Tip: Assessing residual rotation (torsional) deformity in a midshaft fracture of the radius and ulnar is difficult. The bones are triangular in cross-section, so the cortical diameters should be the same immediately proximal and distal to the fracture. The second clue is the position of the radial tubercle. This points anterior if the forearm is supinated and appears as an oval marking within the proximal radial shadow on an anteroposterior (AP) X-ray. Make sure this film includes the hand, so that it can be assessed as an AP projection too. They should be in the same plane with the thumb on the radial side. In a lateral view, the radial tubercule will be a lump pointing in the same direction as the palm.

First aid

A lot can be done with a little thought.

1. Obviously, bent limbs are broken. The limb can be aligned by maintaining gentle traction for a minute or two. Your intention is not to reduce the fracture as such, but to get the broken ends more nearly in the correct place. That will remove tension from the nerves and blood vessels, which may be stretched across the fracture site. Circulation will be improved and relaxed nerves are more likely to recover.
2. Next splint the limb. The less movement, the less pain, and the easier it is to move the patient about. The splint need not be a full cast: a plaster front slab laid over a broken limb and bandaged on after drying will immobilise the fracture well enough for the patient to be X-rayed.
3. A sterile occlusive dressing should be put over the wound and left there. Whatever bacterial contamination has occurred so far is mild compared with the superbugs found in hospitals. You can't adequately clean and debride a compound fracture in the emergency department, so any poking and prodding is much more likely to contaminate the wound than to yield any useful information.

4. Attend to the patient's general needs. Analgesia, IV line, antibiotics, tetanus, splints and slings should all be done before X-ray.

X-ray tips

- Always get the whole of the bone on film.
- Two views at 90° are the minimum necessary. Two 90° obliques are better than an AP and an oblique but disorienting, since the projections will properly show the fracture without making clear just what has happened.
- The radiographer will take the views you ask for and cannot do better than that. The more information you give, the better the pictures: 'tender tip of lateral malleolus following inversion injury' will get the correct views from the radiographer and greatly assist the radiologist when the films are reviewed. Ankle views are no good for a foot fracture.
- The most useful X-ray sticks in the bag, so make sure you see them all.
- The pathology is usually under the identification label; Murphy was a radiographer!

Common problems

Scaphoid fractures and lunate dislocations

Suspect in all falls with 'normal wrist X-rays'. Painful ulnar deviation is the most helpful sign. Suspicious cases need a CT scan; this is the most reliable method of clarifying a borderline fracture. If a scaphoid fracture is in the proximal third, vertically oriented or more than 1 mm displaced, consider primary internal fixation. Watch for widening of the scapho–lunate interval: the scapho–lunate ligament may be torn and the resultant instability is a common cause of persistent wrist pain. Median nerve paraesthesia is associated with lunate dislocation. X-ray the other wrist if unclear. Rotational forces are the commonest cause of non-union in an undisplaced scaphoid fracture. A man can do heavy work in a conventional scaphoid-style cast, so consider extending the cast above the elbow.

Colle's fracture

Reduction is easy but difficult to maintain. The crushed osteopenic bone of the fracture allows for collapse at the fracture site as the swelling subsides. Do you really want to reduce this fracture or is the position acceptable as it is? The crushed cancellous bone can be pulled back into good alignment only by creating voids that the fracture will fall back into once the traction is reduced, so some collapse is very likely in the first weeks. Stopping this becomes complicated. It may need some kind of fixation, percutaneous pins, external fixateur and so on. Might these not create more long-term problems than a rapid malunion? Regular X-rays (weekly to start) should be taken to look for loss of position. Significant loss of position is an indication for fixation. Ulnar deviation is the key to good cast support. Excessive palmar flexion should be avoided as this does not aid fracture reduction; it increases swelling and discomfort, increases the likelihood of carpal tunnel syndrome and may be a factor in the high incidence of reflex sympathetic dystrophy. Consider a bone density study in older women. Always ask if the patient is on NSAIDs: there are reports that these delay bone healing.

Paired bone and greenstick fractures

Children's bones bend: this gives springiness to the fracture and the initial deformity will recur inside the cast. Midshaft fractures of paired bones are especially prone to this. The radius and ulna are the commonest sites but beware of the fractured tibia with an intact fibula. The smaller diameter of the fibula means it will bend considerably without actually breaking. The fractured bones can be pushed straight but the springiness will persist unless the manipulator breaks the other cortex (with a loud snap). In a pair of bones, one cannot be broken and displaced without something happening to the other. If the intact bone appears straight then it must be dislocated at its end. An intact radius with a fractured ulna is dislocated at the radiohumeral joint (Monteggia's fracture-dislocation), and an intact ulna with a broken radius is dislocated at the distal radioulnar joint (Galeazzi's fracture-dislocation). The radiohumeral joint is not dislocated if a line drawn along the shaft of the radius always intersects the capitellum in *every* projection.

Fractures around the elbow

These are the most difficult to sort out. If in any doubt, X-ray the other side. That is a good guiding principle for any point of uncertainty.

Supracondylar fractures of the humerus are very challenging. There is a high incidence of nerve injury, but fortunately this usually recovers. Brachial artery injury is the real worry. A careful check of the peripheral pulses is essential. In most cases, the pulse will return once the fracture is reduced. Vascular surgical advice is essential, even when a good pulse seems to be restored. All displaced supracondylar fractures should be admitted for neurovascular observation.

Hip fractures in the elderly

These are easily missed; the radiological signs of a non-displaced hip fracture are subtle. In osteopenic bone, the fracture may start as a stress fracture and become painful after an awkward movement. Falls are common causes of fractures, but not the only cause. Always suspect and if in doubt scan: a CT, MRI or bone scan will give the diagnosis.

Ischaemia

A cast that is too tight is a major cause of vascular impairment. Always split casts, but do not be deluded that this alone is sufficient. Ischaemia is characterised by disproportionate pain: a well-reduced and properly supported fracture is uncomfortable, not painful. Ensure the cast is split and you can see skin along the entire length. If the pain is not eased, a compartment syndrome is present. Adequate distal pulses may be present. Ischaemia occurs when the compartment pressure exceeds the capillary flow pressure. This is well below arterial pressure. Compartment syndromes are true emergencies as muscle death occurs in a few hours. A fracture need not be present; crush injuries can cause compartment syndromes in the absence of a fracture.

Ankle fractures

There are two key issues with ankle fractures. Is the talus centred under the tibia? If it is not, an open reduction and internal fixation is the nearly universal treatment, so splint the fracture accordingly and arrange for admission. If the talus is squarely under the tibia, is there any suggestion of potential instability? Ankle fractures usually involve fractures of both medial and lateral malleoli, but sometimes fractures of just one with marked swelling and tenderness around the other. The latter suggests a colateral ligament injury, and the talus may shift position in the early healing stage. Only healthy strong adults can manage non-weight-bearing casts. Most children and all elderly women will take some weight through their cast. Fixation of the fracture is often indicated to improve stability.

Ottawa rules

These are simple validated rules that make for sensible X-ray studies in adults. If the rules are followed, the likelihood of missing a significant ankle fracture is near zero.

An ankle X-ray series is necessary only if there is pain near the malleoli and there are either of the following findings:

1. Inability to bear weight both immediately and in the emergency department (four steps).
2. Bone tenderness at the posterior edge or tip of either malleolus.

A foot series is necessary only if there is pain in the midfoot and there are either of the following findings:

1. Inability to bear weight both immediately and in the emergency department (four steps).
2. Bone tenderness in the navicular or the base of the fifth metatarsal.

Midfoot and forefoot fractures

These may be much nastier than they at first seem. The foot has usually been pinned—for example under the wheel of a car—so there is some crushing component, which will lead to a lot of soft tissue swelling and perhaps a compartment syndrome.

Plasters

1. Always pad.
2. Always split.
3. Always arrange a plaster check the next day.

4. Always stress the need for immediate review if the fracture is disproportionately painful and/or swollen, the extremity is numb and/or discoloured, or the patient cannot move fingers/toes.
5. Immobilise the joint above and below the fracture.
6. It is impossible to immobilise the humerus without immobilising the shoulder: that indicates a body jacket! Perhaps a sling bound to the side would give more support to the fracture and do less harm?
7. Plaster is heavy, especially for small children. A heavy, unsupported cast slips and displaces the fracture. Adequate support of the cast is essential: always provide a sling for an arm fracture and insist that it be worn.
8. It is impossible to plaster finger fractures. Either the fracture is stable and in satisfactory position and so can be strapped to the adjacent finger, or it needs internal fixation.
9. Joints should be immobilised in the position of best function where any stiffness will do the least harm: the elbow at 90°, the wrist in slight dorsiflexion and ulna deviation, the metacarpophalangeal joints at 90° and the fingers straight.
10. The only position to immobilise the foot is with the ankle plantigrade.
11. Casts make comfortable supports for soft tissue injuries. Physiotherapy may be the best treatment once the pain and swelling settle, but it is always easiest for the therapist to start mobilisation from a functional position.

Slings

1. Rarely use a collar and cuff. The only fracture that may benefit is a midshaft humeral fracture. Subcapital fractures of the humerus do not benefit from the collar and cuff, which gives poor immobilisation and allows the impacted fracture to disimpact.
2. All shoulder girdle injuries need slings. A triangular bandage sling is for first aid only. The knot cuts into the neck. Switch to an envelope sling with a body binder as soon as possible.
3. Figure-of-eight bandages for clavicular fractures rarely work. To effect any reduction in the displacement, the figure-of-eight bandage needs to be uncomfortably tight and the patient needs to tighten it several times a day.
4. Children in long arm casts must be kept in slings, otherwise the cast will slip and displace the fracture. Ensure that parents understand this.
5. No patient in a sling can exercise the uninjured joints too many times.
6. Clavicular fractures usually do not require surgery, but if the overlying skin is dented or pierced, or the X-rays show the fracture tends to overlap by 2 cm or more, early orthopaedic review is indicated.

Top 12 missed fractures

1. Basilar skull.
2. Odontoid process.

3. Zygomatic arch and orbit.
4. C7 fracture dislocation.
5. Posterior dislocation of the shoulder.
6. Scaphoid, perilunar dislocation and scapholunate dissociation.
7. Sacroiliac fractures.
8. Undisplaced femoral neck fractures.
9. Dislocated hip with ipsilateral femoral fracture.
10. Tibial plateaux.
11. Any fracture near a joint when the same bone is broken elsewhere.
12. Metatarsal fractures in major lower limb injuries.

Fractures may be missed because of poor images, complicated X-ray shadows or when an obvious injury diverts attention.

Neck trauma

Get a lateral plain X-ray early in polytrauma patients. A normal lateral (that includes C7-T1) in a patient with negative physical exam and who is alert and not intoxicated is sufficient to exclude cervical trauma that may complicate the administration of a general anaesthetic.

Further studies are needed if there is:

- Loss of consciousness.
- Facial trauma.
- Immediate postaccident neck pain.
- Pronounced cervical muscle spasm.

Flexion/extension cervical sprain

Delayed onset neck soreness is very common after a road traffic accident (RTA). This may be thought of as a special form of delayed onset muscle soreness (DOMS), typically produced by eccentric single or multiple muscle contraction. The exact mechanisms of this type of pain are only just being clarified. Characteristics are:

- Delayed onset between 24 and 72 hours, paralleling increased creatine phosphokinase (CPK) secretion.
- Spontaneous resolution, much improved after 1 week, but effects noticeable for longer than 28 days.
- Some blocking with immediate NSAIDs, though this may be due to analgesic rather than anti-inflammatory properties.
- Experimental studies showing reproducibility with injected inflammatory mediators, and infiltration by inflammatory cells over 2–3 days following muscle injury.
- Temporary 20–40% diminution in maximum fibre tension.
- Greater resistance in conditioned muscles.

Significant injury can be excluded by flexion and extension views taken in the pain-free interval. Spontaneous recovery is usual; no specific treatment is required. Heat is soothing, rest and time off work may be needed, and

NSAIDs are best given before the onset of symptoms. Patients should be cautioned to expect this. Significant neck injury causes immediate pain.

Remember to take any neurological symptoms or signs very seriously. There can be spinal cord damage without a fracture or dislocation, i.e. X-ray and CT imaging are negative—an MRI helps.

Sports injuries

Quadriplegia can result from sports injuries; less serious injuries are common. Diving and horse riding are probably more likely to cause these injuries than football. The issue is deciding when it is safe to return to sport: many athletes underestimate the consequences of temporary problems like momentary arm weakness or electric shock-like pain ('burner'). These are guidelines for giving advice:

- Normal X-ray series including at least flexion and extension views.
- No pain or spasm.
- Full pain-free range of movement.
- Normal neurological examination.

Distinguishing neck and shoulder pain

Confusion between these is easy. The cervical and upper thoracic spine gives origin to the muscles that move the shoulder blade. Cervical pain radiates distally and excessive use of the shoulder blade to guard or compensate for glenohumeral pain results in fatigue of the scapular muscle. Here are some tips:

- Support the arm with a sling for a few minutes. If the source of pain is primarily from the shoulder, the neck will move comfortably.
- Examine the patient lying down, with the neck well supported. If the pain is primarily from the neck, the arm will move through a full range.
- Elderly patients especially, but any patient generally, will get scapula fatigue and neck pain if they are trying to support a heavy arm cast.
- Local tenderness along the medial border of the scapula may mean either neck or arm pain, but will ease in a few minutes if the shoulder is supported and the pain arises from the shoulder or arm.

Back pain

This is a sorting process. Most acute onset back pain occurs with everyday activity. The pain has a defined point of onset, say lifting, and a characteristic postural component, such as relief with lying down. The sufferer can usually find some comfortable position and the pain is reduced by simple analgesics. Neurological examination is normal. There is usually spasm with movement and bilateral restricted straight leg raising. But the sufferer is otherwise well.

The prognosis is benign; most back pain settles in a few days, and more than 90% of patients will recover within 6 weeks. There is no known therapy beyond common sense. The patient should rest in the most comfortable position, usually lying down. Simple analgesics should be taken regularly. Long-acting NSAIDs are useful as they give supplementary pain relief and are synergistic with paracetamol taken in regular divided doses. Strict bed rest is not required: many sufferers get more relief by changing posture. Light activity is allowed. Provided the history is uncomplicated, X-rays and blood tests do not clarify the diagnosis and are not indicated. Supplementary physical therapy or fringe medicine has not been shown to be of advantage. If intervention is desired this should be towards healthier life style, weight loss, regular exercises etc. Acute lumbar strain is an acceptable term, since it does not imply a specific pathology. Tears in the annulus fibrosus are the probable cause, but this is better thought of as a normal ageing phenomenon than as a disease. Acute on chronic patterns are usual. Acute but short-lived back pain occurs at infrequent and unpredictable intervals. With ageing, the sufferer is less likely to experience sudden incapacitating pain but more likely to get backache with constant posture, stiffness and reduced capacity to lift and bend.

Back pain becomes more complicated in the following circumstances:

- Pain lasts longer than 6 weeks.
- Pain occurs in a compensable circumstance.
- Pain is associated with a definable 'injury', a fall or RTA rather than just lifting.
- The patient is otherwise unwell.
- Pain is atypical, constant and unremitting rather than postural.
- Pain is associated with a clear dermatome pattern, numbness and/or with reflex changes.

Pain that is constant in nature, especially if the patient is unwell, suggests:

- Posterior abdominal source, penetrating peptic ulcer, low-grade pancreatitis, or abdominal aortic aneurysm.
- Spinal infection.
- Secondary tumour.

Infection usually starts in the intervertebral disc, destroys the disc and involves the adjacent portions of the vertebral bodies above and below. Tumours colonise the cancellous bone of the vertebral body and lead to collapse. The disc is usually spared and prevents spread to adjacent levels. A secondary tumour is unusual in the lamina, transverse and spinous processes of the vertebrae; destruction here is almost always from a primary bone tumour.

Aseptic disc destruction occurs in children. No organisms are cultured. The discitis resolves spontaneously. Immunodeficient people, including IV drug users, are very prone to spinal infection. Recovery of the organism is vital; antibiotics should be withheld until direct culture is obtained. Atypical organisms are common. Opportunistic infection is likely.

Pain associated with reflex changes and true sciatica (clear dermatome distribution) probably arises from a prolapsed intervertebral disc. Surgical assessment is required if:

- There is bladder or bowel disturbance, and/or saddle anaesthesia. This is the cauda equina syndrome and requires immediate assessment. Nerve root injury is likely to be permanent if symptoms persist beyond 24 hours.
- Reflex changes or anaesthesia is progressive, especially if weakness develops.
- There is no improvement in 3 weeks.

Ninety-five per cent of all disc prolapses concern L4-5 and L5-S1, so only three nerve roots are involved. L4 supplies the medial dorsum of the foot and tibialis anterior muscle (weak ankle dorsiflexion). L5 supplies the lateral dorsum of the foot and extensor hallucis longus (weak big toe extension, diminished EHL jerk). S1 causes plantar numbness, weak big toe flexion and diminished ankle jerk. Reliable additional signs include restricted unilateral straight leg raising, pain in the leg and foot on ankle dorsiflexion (Le Sage test) and pain in the opposite leg on straight leg raising of the comfortable leg. This is termed the cross-extension sign and is almost pathognomonic for massive disc prolapse.

It is worth remembering that at 2 years there is no difference between patients with intervertebral disc prolapse treated by laminectomy or treated by rest only.

When pain follows a clear injury:

- Structural lesions, like compression fractures, need to be assessed.
- Resolution is likely to be longer than 6 weeks; even minor compression fractures are uncomfortable for months.
- Legal claims may arise.
- Patients are reassured by a full early prognosis.

When the pain is work-related:

- A legal claim is likely.
- Uncertainty over the diagnosis translates into uncertainty about the prognosis.
- Early planning for return to work with a rehabilitation provider much increases the success rate for eventual return to work.

Caution is needed over the interpretation of results. Most plain X-ray changes are long-standing: the X-rays would have looked the same if taken before the index event. Co-relation of X-rays with the clinical findings, diagnosis and prognosis is very uncertain. CT and MRI scans have a high false-negative rate. Forty per cent of symptom-free adults show changes. The investigations do not give the diagnosis. In legal claims the investigations and reported results often propel the claim. Nothing beats a careful history and examination; all investigations need careful consideration in light of the clinical findings.

Limping child

The diagnosis may be made by answering simple questions.

1. Is the child sick?

Fever, malaise and listlessness suggest an infective process; raised WCC, erythrocyte sedimentation rate (ESR) and C reactive protein (CRP) confirm. Some acute onset primary bone tumours mimic this. Very young children may just be listless and not gaining weight.

Look for foci of infection and culture before starting antibiotics: stools if there is diarrhoea, throat swabs if there is an upper respiratory tract infection (URTI), direct swab for sores and blood cultures in rising fevers. Presumptive evidence of infection requires adequate blood levels of antibiotics to penetrate into bone and joints. Start IV antibiotics based on the best guess for likely sensitivities: URTI, diarrhoea or age under 2 years is more likely to include gram-negative organisms. In older children, gram-positive organisms predominate.

Is there a fluid collection? Pus should be drained. An ultrasound is helpful for all joints; perhaps the fluid can be drained for culture under ultrasound control.

Bone scans are sensitive and may help to localise but lack specificity. MRI is very useful. Accessible joints may be arthroscoped in larger children. The hip is a special case; high intraarticular pressures stop blood flow in the bone of the femoral head, leading to avascular necrosis and long-term complications. Arthrotomy is indicated in any failure to respond to antibiotics, or if diagnosis is delayed. Include inflammatory conditions like juvenile rheumatoid arthritis in the differential diagnosis.

2. Is the condition painful?

Refusal to walk or stand is often the presenting complaint. Try to find the point of maximum tenderness. Since osteomyelitis occurs in the juxtaphyseal metaphysis and the nearby joint may have a passive effusion, differentiating this from septic arthritis may be very difficult. Look for signs of trauma and if there is an unconvincing history consider a skeletal survey. Always consider the proximal joints: pain is often referred—slipped capital epiphysis often presents as knee pain.

3. What is the limp like?

- Short-stance phase antalgic limp: the stance phase of the painful limb is shortened, the normal limb hurries through with a short quick step to take the weight off the affected leg, and standing on the leg hurts. The gait pattern tells you the limb is painful but not where: the limb can be painful at any point from toes to hip.
- Painless toe-walking: tight tendo-Achilles, clubfoot, cerebral palsy or unequal leg length.

- Trendelenburg lurch (rolling shoulders): Perthes disease, congenital hip dysplasia, muscular dystrophy, and hemiplegic cerebral palsy.
- Circumduction (one leg lifted out to the side): unequal leg length, cerebral palsies, any cause of ankle or knee stiffness.
- High-stepping walk: cerebral palsy, myelodysplasia, Charcot-Marie-Tooth disease, Friedreich's ataxia.
- Can I learn more if I ask the child to hop (hip) or squat (knee), or tip-toe walk (foot and ankle)?

4. How old is the child?

- <4: toddler's fracture of tibia or foot, congenital dislocation of the hip, osteonecrosis of the navicular.
- 4–10: Perthes disease, transient synovitis hip or knee, osteochondritis of knee or ankle, Sever's apophysitis of the calcaneus, accessory tarsal navicular.
- >10: inflammation of the patella tendon (proximal, Sinding-Larsen-Johansson syndrome; distal, Osgood-Schlatter disease), chondromalacia patella, tarsal coalition (peroneal spastic flat foot), stress fracture, slipped capital epiphysis.

5. Are the parents reliable?

Could this be child abuse?

Limitations of investigations

- Plain X-ray changes are unreliable for 10–12 days in infection. A good lateral is essential to diagnose slipped capital epiphysis: the AP film may look normal.
- Bone scans have high sensitivity but miss some tumours.
- Ultrasound cannot distinguish between sterile and septic effusions but can show periosteal swelling and deep soft tissue swelling.
- WCC may be normal in 30% of children with osteomyelitis; the differential count is more reliable but not 100%.
- ESR rises within 24 hours; raised ESR is present in 90% of children with osteomyelitis but is non-specific. CRP rises and falls more quickly. WCC of >80,000 and polymorphonuclear count of >75% in joint fluid is strongly suggestive of infection.
- Rheumatoid arthritis (RA) latex is positive in less than 20% of juvenile rheumatoid arthritis (JRA).

COMMON DISLOCATIONS (David Sonnabend)

Shoulder

The young patient who presents to the emergency department with a painful shoulder after an injury may have dislocated the joint. Anterior dislocations, by far the commonest, present with the patient cradling one arm with the other, in considerable pain, with a hollow where the humeral head normally sits, and a prominence visible or palpable anteriorly, next to the coracoid process.

The diagnosis is best made by radiograph. The dislocation is often accompanied by a fracture, either of the greater tuberosity of the humerus (which is 'left behind', attached to the rotator cuff) or of the lower pole of the glenoid. A humeral fracture is easily seen on preliminary radiographs. A glenoid fracture may be difficult to pick, and should be sought on post-reduction films.

Reduction of the dislocation, by any of the well-described manoeuvres, should be performed under good analgesia and relaxation. If an initial attempt is unsuccessful, it is probably best to resort to general anaesthesia.

Medicolegally, it is important to check for axillary nerve palsy (deltoid paralysis and numbness over the deltoid insertion) before reduction is attempted, lest the clinician be accused of causing the nerve palsy by the reduction. Clearly, findings should not only be sought but also documented.

If the patient has suffered his or her first dislocation, early review by an orthopaedic service is important. Recent advances in shoulder bracing may prevent the otherwise often inevitable recurrent instability. In other cases, early arthroscopic repair can save the patient from a more complex and less reliable procedure later.

Posterior dislocations are rarer, and easier to miss. They usually occur as a result of the arm being forced backwards in a flexed, internally rotated and sometimes adducted position. The patient holds the arm internally rotated, and any active or passive external rotation produces severe pain. Plain radiographs need to be inspected carefully. The dislocation is obvious on lateral or axillary views, but on the standard AP view is easily missed. The humeral head does not drop inferiorly, as with anterior dislocation, and may not be much displaced medially. The tell-tale X-ray sign is a position of fixed internal rotation, with the bump of the greater tuberosity not visible on the film, and the humeral head appearing like a scoop of ice cream on the top of a cone. No patient should be sent home with a fixed internal rotation deformity of the shoulder without posterior dislocation being definitively excluded.

Reduction of posterior dislocations is relatively easy and rarely requires general anaesthesia, but recurrence is frequent and specialist advice should be sought early. As with anterior dislocations, plain radiographs should be carefully checked for any evidence of glenoid fracture. In both anterior and posterior scenarios, if doubt exists regarding the state of the glenoid, CT scanning is useful.

Shoulder dislocations in the older patient

Shoulder dislocation is accompanied by differing complications at different ages. While axillary nerve palsy and glenoid fractures are frequent in younger patients, extensive rotator cuff tears are common in older patients. If, following reduction and pain relief, an older patient has difficulty with shoulder flexion, abduction or external rotation, the diagnosis may not be that of axillary nerve palsy, and if the weakness persists for more than a few days some form of reliable imaging of the cuff should be obtained.

In the older osteoporotic patient, shoulder dislocations need to be treated with more respect, as forceful manipulation may fracture the humerus. This is particularly the case if the bone is already weakened by a fracture of the greater tuberosity. In the osteoporotic patient, gentle reduction under general anaesthesia and muscle relaxation is advisable.

Radial head dislocation

Dislocation or subluxation of the radial head needs to be suspected in various situations. Whenever there is a fracture of the ulna without any obvious injury to its paired bone, the radius, radial head dislocation should be sought both clinically and radiologically. The clinical signs are local tenderness over the radial head (just distal to the lateral epicondyle of the humerus) and local distortion of anatomy (with the radial head being prominent either anteriorly or posteriorly). Radial head dislocation alone is associated with marked loss of pronation and/or supination, but in the presence of an ulnar fracture this is difficult to test.

If there is uncertainty whether a radiograph shows the radial head to be dislocated or not, a straight line should be drawn along the shaft of the radius, through the middle of the radial head. If that line does not cross the centre of the capitellum, the radial head is displaced.

In young children, the so-called pulled elbow is due to subluxation of the radial head. It presents as pain over the lateral aspect of the elbow, and an unwillingness to move the joint. When it occurs for the first time in a particular child, the diagnosis may need to be made radiologically, using the 'line through the capitellum' technique described above. A gentle tweak into forced supination usually relieves the pain, but recurrences are common.

Dislocation of the patella

Lateral dislocation of the patella is common in knock-kneed adolescent girls with ligamentous laxity. It can of course also occur in other groups. It presents as a painful swelling over the lateral aspect of the knee, exquisitely tender, and associated with severe restriction of knee movement. If need be, the diagnosis can be confirmed with a skyline radiograph of the intercondylar notch. In recurrent cases, the patient is usually well aware of the diagnosis. Initial dislocations are most frightening and the possibility of an osteochondral fracture should not be overlooked. The dislocation is best reduced after pain relief, with the knee fully extended, by gently pushing the patella medially. The knee should then be wrapped straight, and orthopaedic advice sought.

Sternoclavicular dislocations

Dislocation at the medial end of the clavicle is uncommon but potentially catastrophic. The medial end of the collarbone may be displaced forwards (anterior dislocation) or backwards. In the latter case, the displaced bone may press on the adjacent trachea or large vessels. Discomfort in the sternoclavicular region, together with either hoarseness or shortness of breath, should ring alarm bells.

The diagnosis can be made provisionally by simple palpation of the area, using the manubrial notch and the contralateral sternoclavicular region as reference points. Specialised X-ray views of the area are difficult to perform and interpret, and any doubt is best resolved by a CT scan. If there is any concern in the emergency department regarding complications of a posterior sternoclavicular dislocation, surgical help (orthopaedic or cardiothoracic) should be sought at once. (Incidentally, the epiphysis at the medial end of the clavicle is the last in the body to fuse, and in patients under 25 years of age 'dislocations' are often transepiphyseal fractures. Irrespective, the approach is the same.)

While most posterior sternoclavicular dislocations can be treated electively, in peace and quiet, it is occasionally necessary to place a rolled towel between the patient's shoulder blades, causing retraction of the shoulders, to grasp the medial end of the displaced clavicle through the skin with a sharp clamp or towel clip and urgently pull the medial clavicle forwards (using local anaesthetic to the skin!).

Midfoot dislocation

The base of the second metatarsal extends further proximally than the bases of metatarsals I and III, which form a mortise around it. Sometimes the forefoot can shear off the midfoot. This so-called Lisfranc's fracture dislocation occurs in a straight line which includes the bases of metatarsals I, III, IV and V but curves (fractures) the base of the second. The MT II fracture is the key to recognising this often-missed injury, which usually requires surgical correction and stabilisation.

EDITOR'S COMMENT

This chapter does not attempt to cover the large spectrum of emergency department orthopaedics, so please rely on your clinical suspicions and if in any doubt get further advice.

Also, it has been said bones are not full of marrow but black ingratitude. It is easy to miss a subtle fracture! Always arrange to have patients followed up and inform them that no X-ray is 100% and you are not a radiologist. It will keep our indemnity costs down!

RECOMMENDED READING

Apley AG, Solomon L, Warwick D, Nayagam S. Apley's system of orthopaedics and fractures. 8th edn. New York: Oxford University Press; 2001. A comprehensive review of orthopaedics, related trauma and treatment.

Charnley J. The closed treatment of common fractures. Edinburgh: Churchill Livingstone; 1972. Simply the best explanation of the mechanism of fracture reduction and immobilisation. Very readable but out of print. Nevertheless, your library should have a copy.

Journal of the American Academy of Orthopaedic Surgeons. Also online, although there is an access fee for non-members. Available: http://aaos.org/wordhtml/journal.htm.

Rang M. Children's fractures. 2nd edn. Philadelphia: Lippincott; 1983. As good as Charnley and equally readable. This is still in print.

North American Spine Society. Algorithms for managing back pain. Online. Available: http://www.spine.org. Also try the American Academy of Orthopaedic Surgeons at http://www.aaos.org as an alternative. Just follow the prompts.

Salter RB, Harris WR. Injuries involving the epiphyseal plate. Journal of Bone Joint Surgery 1963; 45A:587–622.

18 Hand injuries

Bill Croker

Hand injuries are common in emergency departments. Meticulous assessment and management is crucial because preservation of function is critical to livelihood and recreation.

ASSESSMENT

Document:

1. Handedness.
2. Occupation.
3. Special interests (guitar, piano, model making etc).
4. Mechanism of injury: cutting, crushing, industrial, high-pressure injection, burn, bite.
5. Contamination.

6. Time of injury.
7. Specific symptoms—tingling, numbness, weakness.
8. Treatment so far.

EXAMINATION

Document:

1. Position of hand—noting variation of finger positions from usual 'rest' posture.
2. Location of injury:
   - Name fingers (not number).
   - Palmar (volar) or dorsal surface.
   - Radial or ulnar border.
3. Perfusion.

Nerve function—screening tests

Median nerve

1. Motor: abduction of thumb from the plane of the palm while palpating thenar eminence.
2. Sensory: volar surface—thumb, palm and radial two-and-a-half fingers. Dorsal surface—radial two-and-a-half fingers distal to proximal interphalangeal (PIP) joint.

Radial nerve

1. Motor: wrist extension.
2. Sensory: dorsal surface—radial two-and-a-half fingers proximal to PIP joint and dorsum of hand.

Ulnar nerve

1. Motor: adduction of fingers in extension (hold a piece of paper between fingers).
2. Sensory: ulnar one-and-a-half fingers and extension onto volar and dorsal surfaces.

Tendon function

Test each joint of fingers and thumb in flexion and extension. This will detect complete laceration only. Warn the patient about the possibility of delayed rupture. The exact posture of the injured part at the time of injury cannot be accurately known. Therefore inspect the base of the wound through the full range of movement of the adjacent joints. Testing flexor digitorum profundus (FDP) at the distal interphalangeal (DIP) joint requires the joint more proximal to be held in extension during flexion of the joint being tested. Testing flexor digitorum superficialis at the PIP joint requires all fingers except the one being tested to be held in extension to neutralise the mass flexor effect of FDP at the PIP joint.

TREATMENT
Initial treatment

1. Analgesia:
   * Digital block (avoid adrenaline).
   * Wrist block.
   * IV narcotics.
2. X-ray the injured part if there is a possibility of bony injury or foreign body.
3. Tetanus status (ADT).
4. Carefully clean open injuries and remove debris.
5. Antibiotics if extensive injury or compound fracture.
6. Elevate (pillow case sling from an IV pole if being admitted).
7. Keep fasted and commence IV fluids if surgery a possibility.

Splinting

1. The hand is splinted in a position to minimise the risk of stiffness after treatment: wrist extended (20°); metacarpophalangeal (MCP) joints flexed (70°) and fingers fully extended. This position keeps the collateral ligaments of the fingers at their maximal length.
2. Splint only those joints that need to be included for a particular injury.
3. Explain to the patient the importance of moving any joint not enclosed in the splint to minimise stiffness.

Hand therapy

Follow-up that involves a hand therapist ensures optimal outcome.

SOFT TISSUE INJURIES
Lacerations

1. Require careful inspection through full range of movement following local anaesthetic (without adrenaline). Document any sensory changes prior to anaesthetic.
2. Sutures, if required, should be 5/0 non-absorbable and are removed after 5–7 days—longer if over extensor joints, in the elderly or in patients on steroids.

Fingertip injuries

While usually not large, these can be very painful.

Small skin loss (smaller than a 5 cent piece)— without bone exposed

1. Anaesthesia.
2. Clean.

3. 'Wet' dressing (membrane).
4. Change every 2–3 days until healed (dressing clinic, LMO or home).
5. Elevate (hand above elbow) to reduce pain and swelling for first 2–3 days.
6. Refer to the hand/plastic/orthopaedic team according to your hospital's practice for outpatient follow-up.
7. Active and passive mobilisation to avoid stiffness after first 2–3 days.
8. Analgesia.
9. Review for infection (increasing pain, spreading redness, fever—a late manifestation).

Larger defect or with bone exposed

1. Refer to the hand/plastic/orthopaedic team according to your hospital's practice. Commence initial treatment.

Finger lacerations

Careful assessment for associated nerve and tendon injury. If present, appropriate referral. Otherwise suture as indicated.

Palmar lacerations

'No-man's land' is the zone from the midpalm to the PIP joint where the tendons of the flexor superficialis and profundus are enclosed together in tendon sheaths. Great care in assessment is necessary. Palmar skin is thick and difficult to suture. Anaesthesia is difficult to achieve with local infiltration for similar reasons. Request senior review.

NAILS

Nailbed lacerations

1. Meticulous repair is critical. It is not just cosmetic; poor technique results in a permanently split nail. Refer to the hand/plastic/orthopaedic team according to your hospital's practice for repair of laceration.
2. Preserve the nail; it can be used as a splint.
3. Commence initial treatments.

Subungual haematoma

With no injury to nail or surrounding nail margin

1. Drill through the nail in two or three spots with a 19-gauge needle spun between thumb and index finger to release blood.
2. Analgesia, elevate for 48 hours.
3. Associated undisplaced fractures are considered 'open' and treated with oral antibiotics.

With injury to nail or surrounding nail margin

Risk of nailbed laceration. Refer for review by the team.

Avulsion

Nails take 3 months to grow from nailbed to tip, delayed by a month if injured.

If the nail is avulsed there is a risk of nail bed laceration. Refer for review by the team.

TENDONS

Lacerations of the extensor surface overlying the PIP joint

Otherwise innocuous-looking lacerations of the extensor surface of the PIP joint can transect the central slip of the extensor mechanism with initial preservation of extensor function. However, a boutonnière deformity will subsequently develop if the tendon has been cut.

1. Refer to the hand/plastic/orthopaedic team according to your hospital's practice for exploration and repair.
2. Commence initial treatment.

Mallet finger

A mallet finger is an avulsion of the extensor tendon at its insertion into the distal phalanx. The patient is unable to fully extend the distal phalanx. It occurs when there is a sudden forced flexion of an extended finger (hit by cricket ball, basketball etc).

Without fracture

1. Splint in gentle hyperextension for 6 weeks—commercially available splints recommended.
2. Refer to the hand/plastic/orthopaedic team according to your hospital's practice for outpatient management.

With fracture

1. If there is a fracture involving more than 50% of the articular surface, this will need to be meticulously repaired. Refer to the hand/plastic/orthopaedic team according to your hospital's practice.
2. Commence initial treatment.

NERVE INJURIES

The digital nerves and arteries run in a bundle along the line joining the flexion creases of a flexed finger. Beyond the distal flexion crease the nerve breaks up into terminal branches which are not practical to repair. Some sensation will return anyway.

1. Lacerations proximal to the DIP joint causing sensory loss require exploration. Refer to the hand/plastic/orthopaedic team according to your hospital's practice.
2. Commence initial treatment.
3. Nerves regrow at a rate of 1 mm a day. After repair no guarantee can be given about return of function, which takes several months even when repair is successful. Commitment to physiotherapy is required to optimise outcome.

VASCULAR INJURIES

The ulnar artery is the dominant artery of the hand.

1. Control brisk bleeding with direct pressure—gauze and gloved fingers—to prevent exsanguination.
2. If bleeding persists when pressure removed, before exploration and definitive treatment apply an arterial tourniquet (blood pressure cuff inflated to 50 mmHg above systolic pressure for no longer than 20 minutes). Tourniquets are very painful and carry the risk of tissue ischaemia if left inflated too long.
3. A history of pulsatile bleeding dictates exploration of the wound to tie off both ends of the artery to prevent formation of a pseudoaneurysm.
4. Refer to the hand/plastic/orthopaedic team according to your hospital's practice.
5. Commence initial treatment.

SPECIFIC INJURIES
Burns

Burns of the hand represent a 'special area' injury and should be discussed with the regional burns injury unit.

1. Commence initial treatment—generous analgesia.
2. Superficial partial-thickness dorsal surface burns (classically scalds or fat burns) should be reviewed at 24 hours to ensure correct initial assessment and then can be treated with analgesia, elevation and daily dressings by LMO or dressing clinic.

Electrical injuries

Initial assessment can be misleading, as the full extent of injury may not be apparent at first.

1. Perform a very careful neurovascular examination.
2. Refer to the hand/plastic/orthopaedic team according to your hospital's practice.

Infections

1. Suspect foreign bodies.

2. Pain on passive stretch suggests tendon sheath infection or compartment syndrome.
3. If not septic and no suggestion of tendon sheath infection, commence oral antibiotics, splint and review in 24 hours (earlier if there is any sign of deterioration).
4. Otherwise, refer to the hand/plastic/orthopaedic team according to your hospital's practice.
5. Commence initial treatment, particularly early antibiotics.

Felon

A felon is an abscess of the pulp of the distal phalanx which requires drainage to prevent complications.

1. Paronychia.
2. Infection of the tissues around the fingernail.
3. Digital block.
4. Soak the finger in warm water for about 10 minutes.
5. Blunt dissect under the skin fold to open the abscess.
6. Irrigate.
7. Pack.
8. Analgesia, antibiotics, elevate and review in 24 hours.

Bites

Bites have a high rate of infection.

1. If simple, superficial and seen in under 8 hours, with no evidence of involvement of underlying structures:
   • Irrigate copiously.
   • Debride as necessary.
   • Consider delayed primary closure.
   • Elevate.
   • Immobilise.
   • Review at 24 hours to ensure no infection.
2. 'Bites' due to punching injuries should be X-rayed to ensure there are no teeth fragments in the wound.
3. For all other injuries (complex or deep lacerations, involvement of underlying structures or delayed presentation), refer to the hand/plastic/orthopaedic team according to your hospital's practice.
4. Commence initial treatment.

Crush injuries

Crush injuries cause extensive soft tissue damage, without necessarily causing any bony injury. Initial assessment may reveal minimal external evidence of injury. Contained bleeding and tissue oedema resulting from the crush injury can cause progressively increasing pressure resulting in tissue ischaemia—the compartment syndrome.

1. History should be extended to include mechanism of crush, duration of compression and areas subjected to the compressive forces.
2. Examination in particular for signs of the compartment syndrome: pain out of proportion to the injury, pain on passive stretch of the compartment, tense feel to the compartment and distal paraesthesia. Pulses are normal until very late in the evolution of the compartment syndrome.
3. Refer to the hand/plastic/orthopaedic team according to your hospital's practice for observation and possible fasciotomy.
4. Commence initial treatment.
5. Treat associated injuries as appropriate (lacerations, fractures or dislocations, arterial injuries).
6. Strict elevation and hourly limb observations to detect early signs of compartment syndrome.

High-pressure injection injuries

1. Industrial accidents involving injection into the hand are referred to the hand/plastic/orthopaedic team according to your hospital's practice for observation and possible fasciotomy.
2. Commence initial treatment.

Hydrofluoric acid burns

Hydrofluoric acid in various cleaning products produces ongoing tissue damage and intense pain often without much external sign of injury.

Specific treatment is calcium, which can be administered by a variety of routes. Refer for treatment to the hand/plastic/orthopaedic team according to your hospital's practice.

BONY INJURIES

Phalanges

Fractures with rotational deformities

1. Assess for the presence of any rotational deformation by getting the patient to touch the thenar eminence with all fingers simultaneously. If the injured finger is twisted, a rotational deformation is present.
2. Digital block.
3. Correct rotational deformation.
4. Buddy-strap finger (gauze between fingers to minimise rubbing).
5. Elevation, analgesia, active and passive movement of fingers to reduce stiffness.
6. Refer to the hand/plastic/orthopaedic team according to your hospital's practice for outpatient follow-up in about 1 week to ensure no delayed deformity.

7. If rotational deformation, or more than 10° of angulation, persists after reduction, refer to the hand/plastic/orthopaedic team according to your hospital's practice for accurate reduction and fixation.

Fractures without rotational deformities

If no rotational deformity is present, buddy-strap, elevate until acute pain settles and then use hand normally, provide analgesia and refer to LMO for review.

Fractures involving joint surfaces

1. Refer to the hand/plastic/orthopaedic team according to your hospital's practice for accurate reduction and fixation.
2. Commence initial treatment.

Dislocations

1. Digital block.
2. Reduce dislocation, usually by gentle traction. If unsuccessful, try increasing the deformation (i.e. if dorsal dislocation, hyperextension before traction).
3. Buddy-strap finger (gauze between fingers to minimise rubbing).
4. Elevation, analgesia, active and passive movement of fingers to reduce stiffness.
5. Refer to the hand/plastic/orthopaedic team according to your hospital's practice for outpatient follow-up in about 1 week to assess for instability and continued hand therapy.

Compound fractures

1. Refer to the hand/plastic/orthopaedic team according to your hospital's practice for washout, reduction and closure.
2. Commence initial treatment.

Fracture of the fifth metacarpal neck

1. Provided angulation of this common 'punching' injury is less than 45°, a simple dorsal back slab for 3–4 weeks will usually provide sufficient support. Refer to LMO for review to ensure fracture doesn't slip.
2. Otherwise refer to the hand/plastic/orthopaedic team according to your hospital's practice for reduction.

OTHER INJURIES

Game keeper's thumb

Forced abduction of the thumb (as in skiing) results in rupture of the ulnar collateral ligament of the thumb. Complete rupture may require surgery.

Assess for tenderness over the ulnar border of the MCP joint. If present, treat with a scaphoid plaster and refer to the hand/plastic/orthopaedic team according to your hospital's practice for outpatient follow-up in about 1 week to reassess and for continued hand therapy.

Amputations

1. Refer to the hand/plastic/orthopaedic team according to your hospital's practice for consideration of reimplantation.
2. Commence initial treatment.

Care of the amputated part

1. Carefully clean.
2. Wrap in gauze moistened with sterile saline.
3. Place in plastic bag in an ice bath.
4. X-ray the amputated part.

EDITOR'S COMMENT

Hand and finger injuries are very common but require extra knowledge and care to avoid functional problems.

RECOMMENDED READING

Semer NB. Practical plastic surgery for nonsurgeons. Philadelphia: Hanley & Belfus; 2001.

McRae R. Practical fracture treatment. 4th edn. Edinburgh: Churchill Livingstone; 2001.

19 Urological trauma and emergencies

Phillip C Brenner

RENAL TRAUMA

Initial assessment

1. **Penetrating.** <15% of all renal trauma, usually gunshot or knife.
   a. Will usually be explored for associated injuries.
   b. CT with contrast necessary (or intravenous pyelogram—IVP, if CT not available) to ensure contralateral kidney function and to assess disruption of urinary collecting system.
2. **Blunt.** 85% of all renal trauma. Most will be conservatively managed.

Indications for radiological imaging

1. Gross haematuria.
2. Microscopic haematuria as well as:
   a. Hypotension (systolic <90 mmHg) any time since accident.
   b. Suggestive injury:
      - Fall >3 m, flank bruising.
      - Direct blow.
      - Deceleration injury >60 km/h.
   c. Suggestive associated injury:
      - Fractured lumbar vertebrae.
      - Fractured lower ribs.
3. Microscopic haematuria alone is followed up electively with IVP to exclude pre-existing disease (e.g. polycystic kidney).

Type of imaging

CT with contrast. Look for:

1. Contralateral functioning kidney.
2. Delayed or absent function in affected kidney.
3. Contrast extravasation.

Management

General

1. Blood and fluid replacement.
2. Assess associated injuries.
3. Conservative for stable patients with functioning kidney and minor extravasation only.

Surgical exploration—acutely

1. Unstable patient due to haemorrhage.
2. Major extravasation due to shattered or bisected kidney.
3. Renal pedicle disruption.
4. Continued subacute haemorrhage.
5. Urinoma with sepsis.

Ureteric injury or pelviureteric disruption

Rare except in children. This is typically a deceleration injury. Diagnosed on IVP.

Rupture of bladder or posterior urethra

This is usually due to a fractured pelvis. Occasionally a stab wound or seat belt injury will rupture a full bladder.

Seat belt or knife wound

1. Associated injuries may need to be explored.
2. Cystogram (see below) is performed.

3. Minor extraperitoneal rupture may be managed with catheter drainage alone.
4. Major extraperitoneal or intraperitoneal rupture must be repaired.

Fractured pelvis

1. The patient is often shocked and requires resuscitation.
2. There is a tender mass suprapubically which may be a pelvic haematoma or a full bladder.
3. There may be blood at the urethral meatus.
4. Urinary retention is usually the rule, but urine may have been passed and should be examined for blood.

Management of stable patient

1. If there is no blood at the meatus, a 16 Fr or 18 Fr catheter may be gently passed. If there is no macroscopic blood, no further imaging is necessary.
2. If there is blood at the meatus, a urethrogram is performed.
   a. Commonly a complete rupture of the prostatomembranous urethra will be seen. This will require exploration or suprapubic diversion. There is often associated rupture of bladder—ultrasound will identify a full bladder.
   b. If the urethra is intact, the catheter is advanced into the bladder and a formal cystogram is performed.
3. Cystogram—350 mL water-soluble contrast are instilled unless extravasation is seen. The bladder is drained and post-drainage films are examined for extravasated contrast.
4. Limited extraperitoneal rupture may occasionally be managed with catheter drainage, but most major extraperitoneal and all intraperitoneal leakages are explored and repaired.
5. IVP must be performed to exclude associated ureteric or renal injury.

Management of unstable patient

In an unstable patient who is going to laparotomy with blood at meatus:

1. A gentle attempt to pass a catheter should be made by experienced staff.
2. If the catheter enters the bladder, a limited IVP and cystogram should be performed as time permits.

Surgical management

Surgical management will be to repair bladder, place suprapubic diversion and attempt to stent urethral disruption with urethral catheter.

Rupture of bulbar urethra

This is due to a fall-astride injury, e.g. onto the crossbar of a bicycle, cutting the bulbar urethra between the pubic bone and bar. There is:

1. Blood at the meatus.
2. 'Butterfly' bruising in perineum, and scrotal swelling.
3. Urinary retention.

Treatment

1. Retrograde urethrogram to establish whether tear is complete.
2. Suprapubic stab cystotomy for drainage.
3. Incomplete tears—a catheter will be passed under X-ray control to try to stent the urethra.
4. Complete tears need surgical exploration and reanastomosis, either at time of injury or when bruising settles.

Renal colic

Clinical presentation

1. Severe flank pain radiating around to groin, testis or labia.
2. Patient rolls around, unable to find comfortable position, sweats and may be pale, sometimes vomits.
3. Low stones present with ill-defined lower pain and extreme desire to pass urine with empty bladder. (May present with 'retention' but there is no urine in bladder.)
4. Microscopic or macroscopic haematuria is present in over 90% of cases.
5. Stone will be seen on X-ray in 85%. *Note:* Ureter runs across tip of transverse processes of L2–L5, upper and lower sacroiliac joint and next to ischial spine. Ureteric orifice is medial, near coccyx.
6. Patient has often had renal colic before. In older patients with first episode, aortic aneurysm should be suspected.

Initial assessment

1. Exclude: (a) peritonitis (rigid abdomen); (b) fever; (c) urinary retention.
2. Administer analgesia: (a) IV morphine (b) antiemetic metoclopramide or prochlorperazine; (c) indomethacin 100 mg suppository; (d) hyoscine 20 mg IV may help less severe pain.
3. Dipstix for haematuria.
4. Plain X-ray of kidney-ureter-bladder (KUB).
5. If pain settles patient may be discharged to have outpatient **non-contrast CT** and referral to a urologist.

Indications for admission

1. **Absolute**: (a) ongoing or unrelieved pain; (b) fever >37.5°C; (c) anuria or serum creatinine >0.20 mmol/L; (d) known solitary kidney.
2. **Relative**: (a) stone >8 mm seen on KUB; (b) diabetes; (c) background renal compromise; (d) re-presentation with pain.
3. If admitted, **non-contrast CT** is performed on semi-urgent basis. If serum creatinine >0.15 mmol/L, do ultrasound.

Notes on renal calculi

1. Stones
   <5 mm—90% likelihood of passing without intervention.
   >10 mm—10% likelihood of passing spontaneously.
2. Renal calculi
   <2 cm are often treated with lithotripsy.
   Larger renal calculi will best be cleared with percutaneous nephrolithotomy.
3. Ureteric calculi
   Most will pass spontaneously.
   In lower half of ureter, may be removed with ureteroscope.
   In upper half are pushed back into kidney for lithotripsy.

Urinary retention

1. Acute retention most commonly occurs in elderly men.
2. The patient complains of severe pain and inability to pass urine.
3. Bladder is palpable and percussible.

Common causes

1. Primary prostatic obstruction.
2. Urethral stricture.
3. Bladder neck stenosis, following transurethral resection of prostate.
4. Recent instrumentation.
5. Clot retention.

Treatment

1. Attempt to pass soft 16 Fr or 18 Fr catheter.
   a. Measure and note volume of retention.
   b. Send urine for culture and sensitivity.
   c. Urinalysis.
2. Clot retention.
   a. If postoperative, heavy haematuria or suggestion of clots—attempt to pass 22 Fr, three-way irrigating haematuria catheter.
   b. If unable to pass urethral catheter, place suprapubic catheter; introducer to be used only by experienced staff.
3. Suprapubic catheter.
   a. Check for lower abdominal scar that may be tethering bowel.
   b. Check for anticoagulant (warfarin) therapy.
   c. Infiltrate spot two finger breadths above pubis in midline with local anaesthetic.
   d. Confirm presence of full bladder by passing 22-gauge spinal tap needle—urine must be demonstrated before passing trocar of suprapubic catheter.
   e. Pass trocar at right angle to skin.

TESTIS AND EPIDIDYMIS

Torsion

Testicular torsion is commonest at puberty: 75% of cases are under 20 years of age. It rarely occurs in a normal testicle. Predisposing causes are congenital and developmental abnormalities of the testicle.

Presentation

1. Sudden onset of agonising testicular pain, nausea and vomiting.
2. The testicle is swollen and exquisitely tender.
3. The cord is short and the testicle drawn up.
4. Pain is increased by elevation of the testicle.

Treatment

1. Urgent surgical exploration—testicle is untwisted and, if viable, orchidopexy is performed.
2. Gangrenous testicles are removed. Orchidopexy should be carried out on the unaffected testicle to prevent future torsion.

Acute epididymo-orchitis

This must be distinguished from torsion.

Presentation

Severe pain and swelling of the testis and epididymis is often associated with recent prostatitis and urethritis, instrumentation of the urethra and open prostatectomy. Pyrexia may be present. The testicle and epididymis are swollen and tender. There is often a secondary hydrocele.

Investigations

1. Urinalysis for leukocytes and nitrites.
2. Microscopy and culture of urine.
3. Doppler ultrasound to demonstrate normal blood flow within testis.

Treatment

1. Antibiotics, bed rest and scrotal support.
2. Mild cases as outpatients, with ciprofloxacin 500 mg twice daily or amoxycillin/clavulinic acid duo forte.
3. Severe cases as inpatients, with ampicillin and gentamicin.

Scrotal trauma

1. Testicular rupture, as evidenced by severe swelling and bruising, must be explored. Ultrasound is mandatory if conservative management is considered.
2. Soft tissue swelling or pampiniform plexus trauma may be managed conservatively.

Phimosis

Inability to retract foreskin. May result in ballooning of foreskin, retention, and underlying pus (balanitis).

Treatment

Urgent circumcision. In some circumstances an incision of foreskin only may be performed in the emergency department. This is done on the dorsal aspect (dorsal slit) with local infiltration or penile block.

Paraphimosis

The foreskin has been retracted and is unable to be replaced, causing swelling of glans. Often occurs after catheterisation when the foreskin is left retracted.

Treatment

Gentle prolonged pressure on glans may reduce swelling enough to reduce foreskin; surgical intervention is necessary if foreskin cannot be reduced.

Priapism or prolonged erection

Causes

1. Arterial—self-injection with prostaglandin or papaverine.
2. Venous—haematological disorders: e.g. sickle cell trait, leukaemia, antipsychotic medication, neoplasm or trauma.

Presentation

1. Idiopathic—prolonged painful erection, may be associated with difficulty voiding.
2. If arterial, glans will be engorged; in venous obstruction glans is soft.

Treatment

1. Oral pseudoephedrine 60 mg is effective in mild cases where self-injection is cause.
2. More severe: 23 Fr butterfly into corpora cavernosa—aspirate 25–30 mL blood; note if blood is bright red (arterial) or dark (venous stasis).
3. Leave butterfly in.

If erection recurs, aspirate further 25 mL and administer *either* ephedrine 1mL 30 mg/mL diluted with 9 mL normal saline in 0.5 mL doses until erection subsides, monitoring blood pressure, pulse and ECG, *or* adrenaline 1 mL 1:10,000 diluted with 9 mL normal saline in 0.5 mL increments.

Fractured penis

Traumatic rupture of the corpus cavernosum.

Presentation

The patient hears a loud snap like the breaking of a glass rod, associated with a direct injury to the erect penis. The penis collapses immediately and develops a large swelling on the affected side. On rare occasions the urethra may be ruptured.

Management

Urgent admission to hospital for the surgical repair of the ruptured corpus cavernosum.

Complications

Some 50% of patients will remain impotent.

COMMON POSTOPERATIVE PROBLEMS

Extracorporeal shock-wave lithotripsy (ESWL)

1. Most commonly, patients will present with pain and haematuria and will require narcotic analgesia only.
2. Plain X-ray of kidney-ureter-bladder (KUB) is relevant to establish size of stone fragment that is passing down ureter, or presence of Steinstrasse (series of stone fragments in a line).
3. Measure diameter of largest fragment in millimetres.
4. Fever >38°C is an absolute indication for admission and indicates an infected, obstructed system requiring decompression by a double-J stent or nephrostomy.
5. Anuria or raised creatinine due to bilateral disease or solitary kidney is similarly an emergency requiring admission.

Treatment

1. Morphine IV.
2. Metoclopramide or prochlorperazine, rectal indomethacin 100 mg (if no history of peptic ulcer).
3. Buscopan IV.
4. Urinalysis for blood, and for microscopy, culture and sensitivity.
5. Plain X-ray (KUB).
6. If pain-free, discharge with indomethacin suppositories 100 mg twice daily (if no history of ulcer) and Panadeine Forte.

Prostate biopsy

This is performed in the office under ultrasound control. Needle is passed transrectally and hence is prone to sepsis, which may be life-threatening.

Complications

1. **Sepsis**. Patients with any fever >37.5°C must be admitted for intravenous ampicillin and gentamicin (or ciprofloxacin if allergic to

penicillin). Take three blood cultures and urine culture, and transfer to intensive care unit if there are signs of hypotension or anuria.

2. **Haematuria**. Only requires treatment if it precipitates retention or is massive. Use a 22 Fr three-way irrigation catheter.

3. **Retention**. Usually due to pre-existing prostatism. Pass a small (14 Fr or 16 Fr) Foley catheter. If this is not possible, use a small suprapubic stab catheter (12 Fr).

RECOMMENDED READING

Gillenwater JY, et al. Adult and pediatric urology. Vol. 3. St Louis: Mosby Year Book; 2001.

McAninch JW, ed. Traumatic and reconstructive urology. Philadelphia: WB Saunders; 1996.

MacFarlane MJ. Urology for the house officer. 2nd edn. Baltimore: Williams and Wilkins; 2000.

20 Burns

Linda Dann

Skin is the largest organ in the body, approximating 15% of body weight and 4.9 square metres in an adult. It has a number of functions, which correspond to the rationale of management and the potential complications of burns:

- Protection from the environment (infection).
- Temperature control (hypothermia).
- Fluid control (dehydration).
- Energy control (need for increased caloric intake).

The majority of burns occur in the home and affect mainly young men and those at the extremes of age.

TYPES OF BURNS

- Thermal.
- Chemical.
- Electrical.
- Radiation.

Specific other factors

- Eyes: chemicals, flash burns, molten metal.
- Extremes of age (<5 or >65 years).
- Airway/lung injury: blast injury may be fatal if untreated.
- Hands/feet/perineum.
- Circumferential burns of limbs or torso.
- Burns crossing joints (especially flexor surfaces).
- Deliberate abuse.

ASSESSMENT OF THE BURNS PATIENT

1. History of patient, including any chronic conditions that may affect wound healing such as steroid use, diabetes etc. Tetanus status.
2. History of the events surrounding the injury, including:
   - time of injury (fluid requirements assessed from this time)
   - location of event (in open air, in closed room etc)
   to give an indication of concomitant injury, including carbon monoxide or toxic fume inhalation, blast injury, trauma from fall etc.
3. Full examination to exclude other injury.
4. Assessment of the depth and extent of the burn injury using standard protocols such as Wallace's Rule of Nines or the Lund and Browder chart (Figure 20.1).

ASSESSMENT OF DEPTH AND EXTENT OF BURN

There are two methods of assessment of the extent of burns:
1. Wallace's Rule of Nines chart—varies with age: good for quick assessment.
2. Lund and Browder chart—allows for age variation: more accurate.

Depth of burn

Terms such as first, second and third degree have been largely replaced by the the terms superficial, partial thickness and full thickness.

Superficial

This refers to epidermal reddening, e.g. sunburn. Extremely painful, no blistering, skin is red and heals spontaneously without scarring. Not counted in extent of burn.

Partial thickness

Subdivided into superficial and deep:
- **Superficial partial thickness.** Red or pink with mild blistering as it involves dermis. Extremely painful but heals spontaneously.
- **Deep partial thickness.** May be initially red, then white. Involves deep layers of dermis and is extremely painful. May require skin grafting to prevent infection and scarring.

Full-thickness burns

Involve all layers of skin including blood vessels, nerve endings, hair follicles and the dermis. As a result, they are insensate, dry, white, translucent or even charred. All but the smallest will require skin grafting.

GENERAL MANAGEMENT

First aid

Remove the victim from the source of injury. Ensure adequate oxygenation if there is any possibility of blast injury, smoke or toxic fume inhalations, stridor, hoarseness of the voice or evidence of soot around the mouth or nose. Any burned patient removed from an enclosed space may be assumed to have airway injuries even when no burns are evident. Adherent material should not be removed at this stage.

Analgesia

Superficial and partial thickness burns are extremely painful. In minor or localised burns, application of cold water (for at least 30 minutes) and dressings alleviates pain. Simple oral analgesia may be required at home. Inability to control pain is an indication for admission, particularly in children.

In more severe cases, initial management includes narcotic analgesia. Narcotics should be given intravenously and liberally: e.g. morphine 0.1 mg/kg initially, then titrated to response. Large doses are often required.

Thermal burns

Application of cool water (not ice) to minor burns for a minimum of 30 minutes may alleviate pain and reduce the severity of the injury. This is of no value if applied more than 3 hours after the injury. If burns are extensive, there is a risk of hypothermia. Unburned areas should be kept warm with thermal blankets where possible.

Chemical burns

Copious amounts of water for at least 20–30 minutes are required to effectively dilute chemicals in the first instance. There is a risk of further injury from the dilute chemical run-off. Showers and removal of contaminated clothing may have occurred in the workplace. Specific antidotes, if available, can be used after this initial treatment (see below, 'Hydrofluoric acid').

Dressings

For small, superficial partial thickness burns, a variety of dressings have been suggested including Vaseline gauze, transparent dressings and other

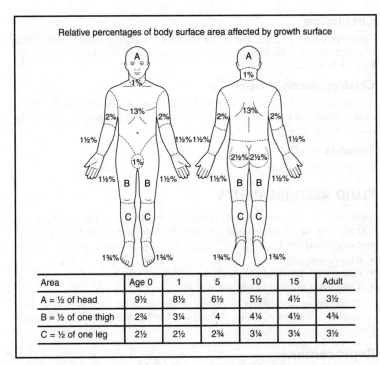

Figure 20.1 Lund and Browder chart: estimation of extent of burn

closed 'burns' dressings. Silver sulphadiazine is generally not recommended for outpatient care as it may become a potential source of infection after 24–48 hours. Dressings alleviate pain of irritated nerve endings by reducing exposure to air and clothing.

Other factors

Airway/lung injury/inhalation injury

This includes carbon monoxide and toxic fumes such as cyanide. Supplemental oxygen is required for all but minor burns and in all patients in whom there is actual or suspected inhalation injury (include patients with no evidence of burn but where there has been a fire in an enclosed space). Intubation may be required early in patients with cyanosis, respiratory distress, stridor or hoarseness. Anticipate lung injury or swelling of the airway if facial burns are evident.

Circulation

Where possible, IV lines should be inserted through unburned skin. Fluid requirements may be high in extensive burns at 2–4 mL/kg/% burn in the first 24 hours.

Gastrointestinal tract

Gastric stasis or ileus can be assumed in all cases of >20% burns. Except in minor burns, all patients should be nil orally until assessed regarding the need for urgent surgery.

Tetanus status

The usual protocols apply.

FLUID REQUIREMENTS

Significant fluid resuscitation after burns is required to maintain circulating volume and an adequate urine output. Volume losses can be anticipated and calculated from:

- Patient weight.
- Extent of burn (body surface area—BSA).
- Time from original burn injury.

There are a number of formulae available. The recommended fluid replacement and maintenance from the 1996 NSW Health Burns Transfer Document are given here.

Replacement

In the first 24 hours after burn injury: 2–4 mL × kg × %burn BSA Hartmann's solution. Half of this amount in the first 8 hours and the remainder over 16 hours.

Maintenance

1. **Adult.** Replacement plus 2–3 litres daily maintenance fluid. Add potassium as required in maintenance for losses due to muscle/skin damage.
2. **Child <30 kg.** 4% dextrose + N/5 saline **or** 3.75% dextrose + N/4 saline according to weight. See Table 20.1.

Table 20.1 Fluid requirements for children by weight

Weight increments	Maintenance fluid rate
0–10 kg	100 mL/kg/24 h
11–20 kg	Add 50 mL/kg/24 h
>20 kg	Add 20 mL/kg/24 h

Urine output

1. **Adult.** Aim for 0.5–2 mL/kg/h.
2. **Child.** Aim for 1 mL/kg/h if <30 kg.

ADMISSION AND TRANSFER TO SPECIALISED BURNS UNIT

Referral criteria to specialised burns unit

1. Deep burns involving 10% BSA or more in adults or 5% BSA or more in children.
2. Burns involving the face, hands, feet, perineum, flexor joint surfaces.
3. Any inhalation injury.
4. Burns with associated injury, major pre-existing disease or suspected child abuse.
5. Significant chemical or electrical burns.

Admission criteria to general or plastic surgery unit

1. Uncontrolled pain, particularly in young children.
2. Burns greater than 1–2% BSA full thickness, 15% BSA (adult) or 10% BSA (children) partial thickness.

SPECIFIC BURNS

Electrical: lightning, high voltage and domestic

Skin resistance varies with moisture content, thickness and cleanliness. There may be extensive damage of underlying tissue while there appears to be minimal skin damage. As a result, the extent of burn is often underestimated. Entry and exit wounds may be present. The effects of electricity are determined by:

1. Type and amount of current.
2. Pathway of current.
3. Duration and area of contact.
4. Resistance of the body.
5. Voltage.

The physiological outcomes for various levels of contact over 1 second are well documented:

- 1 milliampere (mA) is the threshold for perception.
- 10–15 mA cause sustained muscle contraction (tetany).
- 50–100 mA can cause respiratory paralysis and ventricular fibrillation.
- >100 mA cause sustained myocardial contraction.

Broken bones can result from tetany or, in the case of high-voltage contact, from being thrown away from the source. Neurological sequelae are common complications of electrical injury.

Chemical

Copious washing for at least 20–30 minutes is required before use of any specific antidote. The severity of chemical injury is related to a number of factors:

1. pH of the agent.
2. Concentration of the agent. Some concentrated chemicals may produce heat when diluted, leading to thermal as well as chemical injury.
3. Length of contact time.
4. Volume of the agent.
5. Physical form of the agent.

Acids generally produce coagulation necrosis by denaturing protein. This leads to the formation of eschar, which tends to prevent further penetration of the acid. Alkalis act both by denaturing protein and by fat saponification (liquefaction necrosis). As a result, there is no barrier to further penetration and the damage may be more severe.

Hydrofluoric acid (HF)

This is one of the strongest inorganic acids. Used mainly in industry (e.g. car detailing, glass etching), the commonest exposure is to the hands and fingers. HF penetrates deeply before dissociating to free hydrogen and fluoride ions. The hydrogen ions are corrosive. The fluoride ions (tissue chemical burn) combine with calcium and magnesium to form both insoluble and soluble salts. Systemic fluoride ion poisoning from severe HF burns can lead to hypocalcaemia, hypomagnesaemia, hyperkalaemia and sudden death. Symptoms of tissue destruction and necrosis may be delayed. Initial treatment utilises topical calcium gluconate gel. In severe cases, calcium gluconate may need to be injected subcutaneously or intravenously.

SPECIFIC OTHER FACTORS

Circumferential

Circulation may be distally compromised in peripheries due to eschar. Reduced chest wall movement with hypoventilation is possible with circumferential burns to chest. Escharotomy may be required. Note that eschar is full-thickness and therefore pain-free.

Flexor surfaces of joints

Early prevention of contractures is required.

Hands, feet and perineum

These are specialised skin areas with a high risk of circulatory compromise leading to the development of scars and subsequent deformity.

Child abuse

Any suspicious burns, especially those with unusual appearance or in unusual places. The commonest burn injury in children is scalding.

Eyes

The eye is more resistant to acid than alkali. Copious washout, including eversion of the eyelids, is required to dilute the chemical before administering any specific antidote. Solid particles must be removed from under the eyelids (especially powdered alkali), as this may lead to corneal scarring and opacification. Molten metal should be left to cool before removal by an ophthalmologist.

Flash burns

From arc welding, these are acute corneal burns, which generally heal without sequelae within 24 hours. The onset of symptoms is delayed for several hours and they are extremely painful. Topical local anaesthetic may be required initially to examine the eye but should not be used as treatment. Beware of metallic foreign body overlooked on examination.

Extremes of age

In general, the larger the burn and the older the patient, the less chance there is of survival. A child has a relatively large surface area in the most common burns, such as scalds, increasing the risk of complications.

Airway/lung injury

If not immediately evident, blast injury, carbon monoxide or other toxic chemical inhalation and burns to the upper airway are potentially fatal injuries if overlooked and untreated. A chest X-ray is required in any patient in whom airway injury is suspected.

Other concerns

Any other concerns can always be discussed with local burns unit medical staff.

RECOMMENDED READING

Cox, R. Burns, chemical. Online. Available: http://www.eMedicine.com; 2001.
Edlich, R. Burns, electrical. Online. Available: http://www.eMedicine.com; 2001.

NSW Health Department. Management guidelines for people with burn injury. Sydney: NSW Health Department; July 1996.
NSW Health Department. Transfer guidelines for people with burn injury. Sydney: NSW Health Department; July 1996.
Plantz, S. Burns. Online. Available: http://www.eMedicine.com; 2001.

21 Lacerations and minor emergency department surgery

Michael Ardagh and Paul Gee

The purpose of good wound care is to restore structural and functional integrity to tissues and to facilitate healing without infection.

Wounds can be classified simply as clean or contaminated. They can be isolated injuries or one aspect of a patient with multiple injuries. The most frequently injured body parts are fingers, hands, scalp and face, and the groups treated most frequently are young males and elderly females.

ASSESSMENT

Primary survey

A primary survey identifies threats to life or limb requiring immediate treatment. The dramatic appearance of a wound should not distract you from other more life-threatening injuries.

A brief assessment from the bed end should establish whether the patient needs urgent support of airway or breathing first. In conducting the circulation assessment, ongoing haemorrhage should be controlled and fluid resuscitation commenced if required.

Almost all external haemorrhage can be controlled with direct manual pressure and elevation. A common mistake is to apply additional dressings to an actively bleeding wound. This is a good way to hide ongoing blood loss. A dedicated person applying direct pressure with a small gauze pad is the best haemostat.

A sphygmomanometer cuff can also be used on extremities to control distal bleeding. The cuff should be inflated to at least 30 mmHg higher than systolic blood pressure and should be left inflated only long enough to allow a better assessment of the wound.

Uncontrolled sources of haemorrhage may require urgent surgical consultation. The distal part of an injured limb may become ischaemic as a result of deformity or direct vascular injury. Early reduction of a bone or joint deformity and early identification of a vascular injury may save the limb.

Secondary survey

History

Once the patient is stabilised, a thorough secondary survey can be conducted. A proper history, including time and mechanism of injury, will influence management. Blunt lacerations may have a component of crushing. Tissues devitalised in this way are far more prone to subsequent infection. Whether an injury was intentional (assault or self-inflicted), accidental or occupational has medicolegal implications.

Delays of more than 6 hours in seeking treatment make wound infections much more likely. Medication history is important. Warfarin and aspirin may make haemostasis difficult and anti-inflammatories in general will retard healing. Ascertain tetanus immunisation status. Known allergies will affect the choice of antibiotics if required. Chronic conditions such as diabetes and renal failure will alert you to the risk of delayed healing.

Examination

In addition to assessing the features of the wound, the examination will also be directed towards identification of injuries to important underlying structures. A three-step approach should be applied:

1. Suspicion in the light of knowledge of the anatomy (reference to an atlas may be necessary).
2. Assessment of distal function.
3. Exploration of the wound cavity.

The location of any wound should elicit suspicion of injury to underlying structures. In limbs, the important structures are nerves, vessels, tendons and muscle. The hypothesis of deeper injury can be tested by assessing distal function. Nerve function should be tested and the results documented. After verifying normal nerve function, local anaesthetic can be used for analgesia. It is much easier to perform an examination of function if the patient is comfortable.

Two traps can snare the unaware:

1. **Lacerations to the dorsum** of any digit may divide the central slip of the extensor expansion. The patient will still be able to actively extend the digit but the slip needs repairing or late rupture and disability may occur. This is best assessed by direct vision of the wound while the joint is put through a range of motions. The lacerated central slip should come into view when the joint is put into the position it was in when the injury occurred.
2. The second trap is a patient with a **palmar aspect digit, wrist or forearm laceration**. The superficial digital flexor (FDS) tendon may be

divided but if the deep flexor (FDP) is intact, the patient will still be able to actively flex the digit. Specific testing of FDS or careful exploration can expose these injuries. FDP flexes the distal interphalangeal joint. FDS flexes the proximal joint and this can be assessed by passive hyperextension of the other fingers and asking the patient to actively flex the finger under examination. An intact FDS will allow the patient to flex the finger at the proximal joint with little or no flexion at the distal joint.

All wounds should be examined carefully and any recesses explored thoroughly (with the exception of neck wounds through the platysma and abdominal wounds that extend deep to the peritoneum). Exploration of wounds near joints should be performed while passively moving the limb or digit through a range of motions. This will expose deep muscle or tendon injuries that may not initially be apparent to inspection. Foreign bodies, especially clay soils, greatly increase the risk of wound infection, and missed foreign bodies greatly increase the risk of litigation.

MANAGEMENT

Anaesthesia and analgesia

Many options are available. Local infiltration of the wound into the layer just deep to the dermis is the easiest and most commonly used method. This plane is best accessed from below the wound edge, not through intact skin. To reduce the pain of injection, use a 30-gauge or 27-gauge needle and inject the local anaesthetic slowly (over 10 seconds). Plain bupivacaine is a good choice, as onset of action is as fast as other agents, but its duration of action is longer. Local anaesthetics containing adrenaline will decrease wound bleeding during the repair but they are associated with higher rates of infection. Avoid adrenaline-containing local anaesthetics if possible, and definitely do not use adrenaline near end arteries (digits, penis, ears and nose).

Regional blocks are an excellent alternative to local infiltration. They are associated with a lower wound infection rate and do not distort the tissues, thereby allowing accurate approximation. You will never regret taking the trouble to learn regional block skills. Digital, median, radial, posterior tibial and sural nerves are all easily accessible nerves on the extremities. On the face, supratrochlear, supraorbital, infraorbital and mental nerves can be anaesthetised easily.

Young children

Minor procedures on young children are often major endeavours. It helps to get senior advice early and to plan the intervention with military precision.

Anxiolysis should accompany effective analgesia. The presence of the child's carer is reassuring to the child and generally accepted as beneficial to all parties. Carers should be given a clear understanding of what they are likely to witness subsequently. They should not be forced to stay if uncomfortable and should be allowed to leave if events become too distressing. Further anxiolysis can be provided with selective use of nitrous oxide inhalation or sedation (for a discussion of drugs and the conduct of a procedural sedation, see Chapter 2). This should be followed by effective analgesia/local anaesthesia. When all else fails, general anaesthetic can be the best option for repairs of complex lacerations or with recalcitrant children.

Wound preparation, irrigation and debridement

Aseptic technique is important so as not to introduce more pathogens to an already compromised tissue bed. Wash your hands, use powder-free sterile gloves. Cleanse the intact surrounding skin with an antiseptic solution such as chlorhexidine or dilute iodophor (avoid near eyes!).

Remove obvious particulate material. Once the cavity has been explored adequately, the wound should have pressurised irrigation. This can be easily accomplished with a 19-gauge cannula tip (or needle) on a 20 mL syringe loaded with saline. Cleansing is complete when the wound looks free from visible contaminants and the exposed tissue is pink and viable. Debridement can be used sparingly if wound edges are very ragged or still contaminated despite cleansing. This can be accomplished with sharp surgical scissors and a number 15 scalpel blade. Retain as much viable skin as possible, as gaping wounds are difficult to close. The hand (especially the palm) has minimal redundant skin and therefore minimal debridement should occur here. If significant debridement appears to be needed, refer to a hand surgeon. Debridement of facial wounds should also be minimal, as the skin of the face has good reparative qualities and the cosmetic implications may be significant.

Wound closure

Early wound closure may be undesirable in the wound at high risk of infection (grossly contaminated, more than 6 hours old, or with crushed or devitalised tissue), and in wounds with significant swelling. These can undergo delayed closure or be left to heal by granulation. However, for most clean wounds, immediate closure gives the best results and can be accomplished in a number of ways. The common options available for wound closure are sutures, tapes, tissue adhesive (glue) and staples.

Superficial clean lacerations can be closed with tapes or tissue adhesive as long as they are not under significant tension. Areas of skin under tension gape wide open when cut. When wound glue is used, multiple thin applications are better than flooding the wound. Remember the glue is for 'welding' the surface edges and does not go in the wound. Gluing eyebrow lacerations in children often ends in glued eyelids, so do not attempt this unless you are familiar with this method of closure. A smear of KY jelly can prevent glue from running onto skin you do not wish to glue.

Table 21.1 Sutures and their use

Location	Suture	Size	Removal (days)
Face	Nylon monofilament	5-0	5
Scalp	Nylon	3-0, 4-0	10
Intraoral	Braided absorbable	4-0, 5-0	7, if required
Digits	Nylon	4-0, 5-0	7
Nailbeds	Chromic gut	5-0	5–7, if required
Torso and limbs	Nylon	4-0	10
Back and knees (high-tension areas)	Nylon	3-0, 4-0	14

Suturing has been the gold standard for wound closure for hundreds of years. The best closure requires preparation and attention to detail. You should get the patient to lie down. You should ensure good lighting and good-quality surgical instruments. Assemble all the equipment you may require, including comfortable seating for yourself, and allow adequate time to perform the procedure. The manual technique of suturing and knot-tying is best learned by demonstration, supervision and practice, so is beyond the scope of this text.

The best cosmetic result when using sutures is obtained with nylon monofilament sutures and early removal. Braided absorbable sutures incite an inflammatory response in skin. This increases scarring, so this suture type has limited utility for external closure. Absorbable sutures such as dexon or vicryl are useful for repairing subcutaneous structures and intraoral mucosa.

Table 21.1 shows sutures used for different locations.

Antibiotics and tetanus immunoprophylaxis

Grossly contaminated wounds (especially those that cannot be well cleaned or that are subject to delayed presentation), hand injuries and all bite wounds will usually require prophylactic antibiotics for 48 hours, with reassessment of the wound at that time. A regimen covering streptococci and beta-lactamase-producing staphylococci is usually chosen, such as penicillin and flucloxacillin or amoxycillin with clavulanate. Anaerobic cover may also be required, especially after bite wounds.

Tetanus immunoprophylaxis is required if the patient does not have current immunity. In addition to active immunisation with tetanus toxoid, passive immunisation with tetanus immunogobulin may be required if the patient has not previously been immunised and the wound is high-risk. For guidelines for the management of tetanus-prone wounds, see Table 43.5.

Follow-up care

Wounds should be routinely checked and redressed at 48 hours. Patients should be given written instructions regarding after-care and complications to watch for.

SPECIAL WOUNDS
Facial lacerations

Facial lacerations present a challenge to the surgeon. Obviously, the aim of any repair is to obtain the best cosmetic result possible. You cannot undo the damage already done, but with good technique you can reduce the subsequent scarring. Refer to a plastic surgeon if the wound is complex, large or if appearance is of significant importance to the patient. Eyelid lacerations involving the tarsal plate should be referred.

Damage to important structures like the facial nerve, parotid and nasolacrimal ducts should not be missed! Lip lacerations should be assessed carefully. They often require three-level closure. The orbicularis muscle and intraoral mucosa should be closed in layers with 4-0 absorbable suture. The skin should be closed with 5-0 or finer nylon and there must be accurate alignment of the vermilion border.

Facial wounds rarely get infected. For the first week, application of a thin film of intrasyte gel to the wound line will stop the wound sticking to the patient's pillow. If the wound is perpendicular to a wrinkle line it will have a tendency to gape, even after suture removal. To reduce skin tension, apply wound tape across the scar and instruct the patient to keep reapplying tape for up to 3 months. This will prevent stretching and enlargement of the immature scar tissue.

It is valuable to give the patient (or parent) a realistic expectation of the process of healing. Wounds are often an obvious pink/red for some months and the long-term result may not be apparent until the scar blanches. Any undesirable scar can potentially be revised at a later date by a plastic surgeon.

Bites
Animal bites

These are often associated with significant crush and tearing. The wounds also receive a heavy inoculation with bacteria, so are very prone to infection. The wound should be vigorously irrigated as soon as possible. Wounds on the face can usually be closed. Intravenous amoxicillin with clavulanate should be given early if wound closure is considered (erythromycin or doxycycline are acceptable alternatives). All other wounds are best left open for delayed closure or healing by secondary intention. Large or complex lacerations may have a large amount of devitalised tissue, and this may not become apparent for 24–48 hours. Unless the bite wound is minor and well cleaned, prescribe 48 hours of prophylactic antibiotics and review at 48 hours.

Puncture wounds should be left open after cleansing and mupirocin ointment applied three times daily. All bite wounds need close follow-up as the development of infection can be catastrophic.

Human bites

These are often associated with delayed presentation. The most common form of this is the 'fight bite', where incisor or canine teeth penetrate the skin of a closed fist during a punch. The puncture may extend into the metacarpophalangeal joint and cause a septic arthritis. Any suspicion of extension into joint or sign of infection should prompt immediate antibiotics. If the presentation is delayed or infection is clinically present, refer to a hand surgeon for a joint washout.

Scalp wounds

Scalp wounds have the potential to bleed profusely, but direct digital pressure and prompt closure will reduce overall blood loss. Combing the hair back from the wound will allow inspection, and the hair can be held back with KY jelly. Clipping the hair just at the wound margin will make knot-tying easier and prevent hair from falling into the closure. Irrigate thoroughly and, if necessary, repair the galea with absorbable suture. Closure of the skin using 2-0 nylon taking 'large bite' interrupted stitches is quick and stops bleeding. Tying off individual vessels is almost never required with this technique. If the wound is long and cleanly cut, surgical stapling is an even quicker option.

Plantar puncture wounds

Trying to irrigate a small clean puncture wound will cause more damage than the original injury. Leave these wounds open and apply mupirocin three times daily.

Road rash

Dirt and asphalt are ground into the skin, causing abrasions. Topical 2% lignocaine jelly can be used as an anaesthetic and debriding agent for small areas. Alternatively, infiltration or regional block will provide guaranteed anaesthesia and will allow a brisk scrubbing with a surgical scrub brush or sterile toothbrush. Covering the wound with an alginate dressing promotes haemostasis and soaks up exudate. The dressing can be painlessly removed at follow-up. Special areas may require general anaesthetic.

MINOR SURGERY: ABSCESS DRAINAGE

Care should be taken in selecting which abscesses to drain. Perianal and natal cleft abscesses usually require surgical treatment under general anaesthesia. Breast infections may require an ultrasound scan to establish whether a collection of pus is present. Consult a senior before considering drainage of any abscess on the face.

If an abscess is fluctuant and threatening to burst through the skin, drainage will hasten its resolution. Sometimes it is unclear whether there is pus collected in an area of cellulitis. Gentle aspiration with an 18-gauge needle may resolve the question.

Incision and drainage of abscesses is a painful procedure. The relatively acidic environment of the abscess reduces the effectiveness of local anaesthetic. A good strategy is to pre-treat the patient with nitrous oxide or intravenous morphine and warn that there may be temporary discomfort. Bupivacaine should be injected into the roof of the abscess. Make an incision at least two-thirds the diameter of the abscess and break down any loculations within the abscess. Irrigate the cavity until the saline effluent appears relatively clear. The cavity will bleed, so be prepared to apply digital pressure for 10 minutes. Gently insert an alginate rope or sheet into the mouth of the cavity to allow further drainage. Tightly packing ribbon gauze into the abscess cavity is painful and no longer recommended! Cover the wound with dressings that will absorb copious exudate. Prescribe antibiotics to cover *Staphylococcus* and *Streptococcus* if there is surrounding cellulitis. Drained abscesses initially require daily dressings and review.

RECOMMENDED READING

Trott AT. Wounds and lacerations. 2nd edn. St Louis: Mosby; 1997.
Eriksson E. Illustrated handbook in local anaesthesia. 2nd edn. London: Lloyd Luke; 1979.
Roberts JR, Hedges JR. Clinical procedures in emergency medicine. 3rd edn. Philadelphia: WB Saunders; 2004.

22 Analgesia and sedation in the emergency department

John Vinen

Emergency physicians should be competent in the management of pain. The early relief of pain is a right and an expectation when a patient presents to the emergency department. The management of pain is often compromised by misunderstandings, myths, prejudice and inappropriate reliance on inflexible cookbook formulas. Good patient care demands effective pain relief; failure to effectively manage pain is a failure in the quality of care.

Many patients presenting to the emergency department in pain, including those transported by ambulance, remain in pain on arrival.

Time from arrival or triage to analgesia is one of the areas of current focus in the improvement of the quality of care in emergency departments. Studies have demonstrated that delayed and sub-therapeutic pain relief remains a problem, with a median of 58 minutes or more for time-to-analgesia.

A range of strategies, including nurse-initiated analgesia, have been implemented in order to achieve the time-to-analgesia benchmark of 20 minutes.

Time-to-analgesia will be influenced by many factors, including the patient's triage category. Patients in severe pain should be allocated triage category 2 (to be seen by a doctor within 10 minutes of arrival) to ensure that analgesia is administered early. Alternatively, where nurse-initiated analgesia is available, patients in pain may be allocated lower triage categories, unless their condition requires otherwise.

ASSESSMENT OF PAIN

A visual analogue scale (VAS) in centimetres may be used to evaluate the patient's subjective sensation of pain (Figure 22.1).

Alternatively, a numerical rating scale (NRS) from 0 to 10 (0 = no pain, 10 = worst possible pain, see Table 22.1) has been demonstrated to

No pain   Unbearable pain

| 0 | 1 | 2 | 3 | 4 | 5 | 6 | 7 | 8 | 9 | 10 |

Figure 22.1 Visual analogue scale for assessment of pain

Table 22.1 Suggested analgesia for acute pain in adults based on the VAS or NRS

Pain score	Suggested analgesic
1–2	Paracetamol PO ii tabs
3–4	Paracetamol and codeine 8 mg PO ii tabs
5–7	Paracetamol and codeine 30 mg PO ii tabs or Tramadol 50–100 mg IVI
8–10	Morphine IVI

correlate closely with the VAS in measuring pain, with the VAS and the NRS having almost identical minimum clinically significant differences.

Pain response is unique to each individual. A good guide to adequate analgesia is the dozing patient who opens the eyes when his or her name is called.

In the evaluation of acute pain, a difference in the VAS of <20 mm is unlikely to be clinically significant (see Kelly AM).

THE RATIONAL USE OF ANALGESICS AND SEDATIVES

A large number of pharmacological agents exist, each with their own indications, contraindications, modes of action and routes of administration. In order to select the correct agent, an understanding of the principles that determine the use of analgesics and sedatives in the emergency department is required.

Always refer to the drug's product information (PI) before prescribing or administration.

Guiding principles

1. Rapid onset of action is required.
2. Agents need to be effective, i.e. potent.
3. Judicious intravenous administration, either bolus or by an infusion (titration to effect desired), is the most effective way to achieve the desired result.
4. Duration of effect is important.
5. Concurrent administration of a sedative enhances patient comfort and cooperation.
6. A good understanding of the agent's adverse effects is essential to safe use.
7. Resuscitation skills, including airway management, together with a full range of resuscitation equipment, are essential to deal with the occasional situation that occurs as a result of excessive sedation or an allergic reaction.
8. Administration of oxygen via mask or nasal cannula with monitoring by oximetry should be considered. Patients with known respiratory and cardiovascular disease should be given supplemental oxygen and their oxygen saturation should be monitored; cardiac monitoring may also be necessary.

Pharmacological agents

Simple analgesics

Acetylsalicylic acid (aspirin) with or without codeine, and paracetamol with or without codeine, are commonly used for mild pain. Both are also used as antipyretics; in addition, aspirin has an anti-inflammatory action.

Table 22.2 Adult sedatives, analgesics and muscle relaxants

Drug	Dose	Frequency	Route
Analgesics			
Paracetamol	600 mg	Every 6 h prn (as necessary)	Oral
Morphine	0.1–0.2 mg/kg	Every 4 h titrated to response	IVI
Pethidine	1.0–2.0 mg/kg	Every 4 h titrated to response	IVI
Fentanyl	2.0–3.0 g/kg		IVI
Codeine phosphate	10–60 mg	Every 4–6 h	Oral
Tramadol	50–100 mg	Every 4–6 h max, 600 mg/day	Slow IVI or IMI
	50–100 mg	max 400 mg/day (300 mg day in elderly) 2–4 times daily	PO
Sedatives/muscle relaxants			
Diazepam	0.1–0.3 mg/kg		IVI
Midazolam	0.1–0.2 mg/kg	A total dose of <5 mg is usually adequate	IVI, IMI
Orphenadrine citrate	60 mg		IV or IM
Non-steroidal anti-inflammatory drugs (NSAIDs)			
Aspirin	325–650 mg	Every 4 h prn	Oral
Ibuprofen	200–400 mg	Every 4–6 h	Oral
Indomethacin	25–50 mg	2 or 3 times daily up to 150–200 mg/day	Oral
Naproxen	250 mg	Every 6–8 h	Oral
Sulindac	200 mg	Twice daily	Oral
Ketorolac	15–30 mg	6–hourly	IMI

Non-steroidal anti-inflammatory drugs (NSAIDs) are other commonly used analgesics. NSAIDs are more potent analgesics than paracetamol and aspirin. Table 22.2 lists the commonly used agents and their properties.

Narcotics and opioid analgesics

Natural and synthetic opioids are the most commonly used analgesic agents in the emergency department. Opiates should be administered IV and titrated to desired effect. Onset of action is rapid. They may also be administered IM or subcutaneously (SC). Respiratory depression, nausea and vomiting are the most common side effects. Supplemental oxygen and oximetry monitoring should be used in patients with cardiac and lung disease. Cardiac monitoring may also be necessary. Anti-emetics should be used concurrently, except in children under 10 years of age because of the high incidence of extrapyramidal reactions.

Opiates should not be withheld because of a perceived risk of addiction. The dangers of addiction have been exaggerated. Respiratory depression can be reversed by the opioid antagonist naloxone (0.8–2.0 mg IV repeated as necessary). *Note:* Naloxone has a short half-life compared with narcotic analgesics. Repeat doses may be required.

Morphine should be used in preference to pethidine because:

- Duration of action of pethidine is shorter.
- Pethidine has no additional analgesic benefit.
- Pethidine has a similar side-effect profile to morphine, including bronchospasm and increased biliary pressure.
- Pethidine is metabolised to norpethidine, which is associated with toxic effects, especially seizures, particularly in association with renal dysfunction.
- Pethidine has a range of serious interactions with other drugs.
- Pethidine is the most commonly abused medical narcotic because of its euphoric effects.

As morphine and pethidine increase biliary pressure by causing spasm of Oddi's sphincter, caution is advised in using them for biliary colic. Morphine also releases histamine, resulting in 'morphine itch', a distressing side effect.

Tramadol is frequently used as an alternative to morphine and pethidine because it lacks their addictive properties. It can be administered orally, IMI or IVI. Dose reductions are required in patients with hepatic or renal dysfunction.

Skeletal muscle relaxants

These drugs are used to treat pain due to ligamentous strains, tension myalgias and radiculopathies in combination with rest, splinting and application of heat. Drugs in this group include orphenadrine citrate and benzodiazepines such diazepam and midazolam.

Nitrous oxide (N₂O)

A colourless gas with a sweet taste and odour, this is a good analgesic agent frequently used as a 50% N_2O mixture with 50% oxygen (Entonox). It is often used by supervised self-administration. Analgesia occurs within 20 seconds, peaking in 1–2 minutes. It also has potent sedative and anxiolytic properties. It can cause euphoria, dysphoria, drowsiness, light-headedness and nausea.

Contraindications include the presence of gas-containing cavities, especially a pneumothorax.

Sedating agents

Benzodiazepines are commonly used in the emergency department, usually in combination with an opioid to treat pain, most commonly during procedures requiring sedation and muscle relaxation (reduction of dislocations and fractures, cardioversion). Hypoventilation, airway obstruction and apnoea can occur with even small doses, particularly in the elderly.

   Midazolam has ideal properties for use during procedures requiring short-term sedation because of its short half-life. The dose of midazolam is 0.01–0.15 mg/kg (titrated cautiously to response). Flumazenil, a benzodiazepine antagonist, can be used to reverse the sedative effects of benzodiazepines. It is particularly useful after procedures where midazolam has been used, in order to speed up recovery. The dose is 0.2 mg followed by 0.1 mg increments up to a total of 1 mg: the usual dose is 0.3–0.6 mg. Care should be taken not to produce an acute benzodiazepine withdrawal syndrome. Seizures may occur as a result of its use.

Ketamine

Ketamine is a dissociative anaesthetic. It induces a state of analgesia, amnesia and unresponsiveness to noxious stimuli while at the same time preserving airway and breathing reflexes. With care, it is a safe alternative to general anaesthesia for minor procedures on children in the emergency department. Ketamine should be administered only by staff with advanced airway and resuscitation skills. Patients should be fasting for at least 3 hours and fully monitored during the procedure. For doses and effects, see Table 2.1 (p 16).

LOCAL ANAESTHESIA

Intravenous regional anaesthesia (Bier's block)

A rapid and effective technique suitable for fracture reduction and extremity wound repair. The technique requires the use of a double blood pressure cuff, drainage of blood from the limb and IV administration of prilocaine (2.5 mg/kg). Prilocaine, because of its high level of tissue binding, is safer to use than lignocaine.

Local infiltration

Lignocaine, with or without adrenaline, is the agent of choice for the majority of local anaesthetic procedures in the emergency department. (*Note:* Adrenaline should not be used in situations where end arteries are involved: i.e. fingers, toes, nose, ears, penis.) A 0.5–1.0% solution is recommended, and when adrenaline is used it should be used as a 1:200,000 solution. The size of the needle and the speed of injection are important in minimising pain associated with the injection of the local anaesthetic agent. Buffering lignocaine with the addition of sodium bicarbonate (1 mEq/mL per 10 mL lignocaine) decreases the pain associated with lignocaine infiltration. A 25-gauge needle should be used, at least with the initial infiltration, with the rate of injection being as slow as possible. The dose of lignocaine should not exceed 3 mg/kg for plain lignocaine and 7 mg/kg for lignocaine with adrenaline. Care should be taken to avoid intravascular injection.

Topical application

EMLA patches or cream can be used to anaesthetise small areas in children. They are frequently used in preparation for insertion of an intravenous cannula or lumbar puncture. EMLA is a mixture of 2.5% lignocaine and 2.5% prilocaine. An occlusive dressing should be used. EMLA should not be applied to mucosal surfaces. The major disadvantage of EMLA in the emergency department is that it takes at least 60 minutes to achieve adequate analgesia.

Local anaesthetic blocks

A variety of peripheral nerve blocks are possible. Nerve blocks are generally less painful than local infiltration, especially in sensitive areas, including the palm and sole. A useful block is a femoral nerve block, which is used for analgesia (usually in combination with a narcotic) for fractured shaft of femur. Either lignocaine or bupivacaine individually or in combination are used for femoral nerve blocks.

The dose of lignocaine in adults is 20 mL 1% with adrenaline (not more than 7 mg/kg).

A combination of 10 mL lignocaine and 10 mL 0.25% bupivacaine with adrenaline (maximum of 2 mg/kg)—plain and adrenaline-containing solutions can be used for rapid onset and long duration of action.

NON-PHARMACOLOGICAL METHODS

Patients presenting to the emergency department in pain focus on the painful stimuli in what is to them an unfamiliar, threatening environment. Establishing a patient–doctor relationship and reassuring the patient at the same time lessens anxiety and fear, and can also mitigate the patient's reaction to pain. The initial encounter with the patient sets the tone for the rest of the patient–doctor interaction; reassurance and empathy go a long way towards managing the situation.

Elevation, the application of ice to the injured area and splinting are effective analgesic techniques, especially for traumatic limb injuries. Using these techniques either singly or in combination can reduce or even obviate the need for pharmacological analgesic agents.

PAEDIATRIC ANALGESIA AND SEDATION

Children have an exaggerated response to painful stimuli. Adequate analgesia and sedation are essential in managing children in what to them is a terrifying environment. Verbal reassurance and parental assistance and distraction are important, but in most situations pharmacological intervention will be required. As with adults, the treating doctor must be adept in advanced airway management and life support.

The assessment of the degree of pain in children can be difficult. Children as young as 5 years have been shown to be capable of using the visual analogue scale (VAS). Recently the usefulness of a coloured analogue scale (CAS) and a facial affective scale (FAS, see Figure 22.2) were assessed. Both scales have numerical values on the reverse side to assist in documenting the severity of pain. Almost all children are easily able to use both the CAS and VAS. A visual analogue scale, facial affective scale or a colour analogue scale should be used in assessing and monitoring pain in children.

Approach to the child

Non-pharmacological techniques, including distraction, reassurance, elevation, application of ice and splinting, are just as important in children as in adults. Children lend themselves to alternate routes of analgesic/

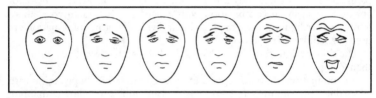

Figure 22.2   Facial affective scale to help children indicate the severity of their pain

Table 22.3 Paediatric sedatives and analgesics

Drug	Route	Paediatric dose (mg/kg)	Maximum dose (mg)
Aspirin*	PO	10–15 q4h	975
Paracetamol	PO	10–15 q4h	975
Morphine	IV, IM	0.1–0.15 q3h to q4h	10
Pethidine	IV, IM	0.1–2.0 q3h to q4h	100
Diazepam	IV PR	0.05–0.2 titrate over 3 min to desired effect 0.5	10
Midazolam	IV, IM IN, PR PO	0.01–0.15 0.2–0.4 titrate over 3 min to desired effect in 0.02 mg/kg increments 0.5	4
Ketamine **	IV, IM	1 (slow bolus)	3

IM Intramuscularly	IV Intravenously	PO Orally
PR Rectally	IN Nasally	

* Remember Reye's syndrome in young children. Do not use aspirin for children under 12 years of age.
**Pre-administration of atropine (10 µg/kg–100 µg minimum, maximum 500 µg IV).

sedative drug administration: oral, nasal, topical and rectal. The easiest manner of drug administration in children is transmucosally (either orally, nasally or rectally). While the effect of a drug administered this way is less predictable, and higher doses are required compared with parenteral administration, it is a very effective and useful way of administering drugs to apprehensive children (Table 22.3).

Intranasal (IN) midazolam has been found to be easy to administer, well tolerated, safe and effective for the sedation of children.

No one drug is ideal for all situations—a combination of agents may be required to produce the desired effect. Consideration should be given to using a general anaesthetic in operating theatres if a prolonged or difficult procedure is required.

PATIENT MONITORING

Monitoring of a patient's vital signs (pulse rate, blood pressure, respiratory rate, level of consciousness) and oximetry should begin before and continue throughout the recovery phase. The intensity of monitoring will depend on the level of sedation/analgesia, pre-existing illness (cardiac or respiratory disease) and the patient's general condition.

PATIENT DISCHARGE

Full recovery should take place before discharge. Discharge criteria are given in Table 22.4. Patients, or their parents in the case of children, should be given both verbal and written instructions (Table 22.5).

Table 22.4 Discharge criteria after sedation and analgesia

Verbal
- Return to baseline verbal skills.*
- Can understand and follow directions.
- Can verbalise, including correct diction.

Motor
- Return to baseline muscular control function.*
- If an infant, can sit unattended.
- If a child or adult, can walk unassisted.

Sensory
- Return of sensation and muscle function where a nerve block has been used.

Mental
- Return to baseline mental status.

Other
- Patient, or responsible person with patient, should be able to understand emergency department discharge instructions about specific conscious sedation and/or analgesia.

* These items may need to be modified to account for the patient's visit to the emergency department.

ANALGESIA IN SPECIAL SITUATIONS

There are a number of common clinical situations in the emergency department where a combination of agents is commonly required to achieve the desired analgesic and sedative effect (Table 22.6).

Analgesia can safely be administered in patients with acute abdominal pain without affecting the physical examination findings.

Table 22.5 Paediatric discharge instructions

Your child has been given a sedative or pain medication as part of his/her emergency department visit today. Medications of this type can cause a child to be sleepy, less aware, not to think clearly, or be more likely to stumble or fall. Because of this you should watch your child closely for the next 8 hours.

In addition, please observe the following precautions:

- No eating or drinking for the next 2 hours. If your child is an infant he/she may be fed half a normal feed 1 hour after discharge.

- No play that requires normal childhood coordination, such as bike riding, skating, or use of swings or monkey bars for the next 24 hours.

- No playing without adult supervision for the next 8 hours. This is especially important for children who are normally allowed to play outside alone.

- No baths, showers, cooking or using possibly dangerous electrical devices (such as curling irons) without adult supervision for the next 8 hours.

- If you notice anything unusual about your child or have any questions, please call the emergency department immediately.

Table 22.6 Emergency department approach to analgesia in special situations

Indication	Analgesic(s) of choice	Adjuncts
Cardioversion	IV fentanyl IV midazolam	
Renal colic	IV morphine	Indomethacin suppositories PR
Headache	PO soluble aspirin plus metoclopramide 10 mg IV Chlorpromazine 12.5-25 mg IV/IM Sumatriptan 6 mg IM	IV morphine
Fractured shaft femur	IV morphine or IV pethidine	Femoral nerve block

Ophthalmic pain due to ciliary muscle spasm	Topical tropicamide* and/or
	  IV morphine or
	  IV pethidine or
	  Oral analgesics
		Cyclopentolate Hydrochloride*
		Homatropine Hydrobromide

IM Intramuscularly   IV Intravenously   PO Orally   PR Rectally
*Contraindication: glaucoma.

EDITOR'S COMMENT

Many studies show that the management of pain relief in the emergency department could be improved, in both timeliness and effectiveness. Strategies to give the patient pain relief at triage are appropriate and humane.

RECOMMENDED READING

Australian College for Emergency Medicine. Guidelines for the implementation of the Australian triage scale in emergency departments. Online. Available: http://www.acem.org.au/oren/documents/triageguide.htm.

Bijur PE, Sliver W, Gallegher EJ. Reliability of the visual analog scale for measurement of acute pain. Acad Emerg Med 2001; 8:1153–1157.

Fry M, Holdgate A. Nurse-initiated intravenous morphine in the emergency department: efficacy, rate of adverse events and impact on time-to-analgesia. Emerg Med 2002; 14:249–254.

Kelly AM. Setting the benchmark for research in the management of acute pain in emergency department. Emerg Med 2001; 13:57–60.

Priestly SJ, Taylor J, McAdam CM, Francis P. Ketamine sedation for children in the emergency department. Emerg Med 2001; 13:82–90.

Victorian Medical Postgraduate Foundation. Analgesic guidelines. Melbourne: Victorian Medical Postgraduate Foundation; 1995.

23 Patient transport and retrieval

Christopher F Gavaghan

Some clinicians take a fairly casual approach to patient transport, often delegating it to nursing staff, ambulance staff or hospital transport services without much further thought. The perils of doing this can be driven home to you in ways you may never imagine, particularly in this era of high litigation and medical indemnity costs. Careful attention to the relatively straightforward issue of patient transport can and does pay dividends that will protect you and your patients from adverse outcomes.

Patient transport covers the whole range of patient types and conditions and is necessarily very variable, depending upon the circumstances in which you find yourself and the resources you have immediately available at your own institution. This can be as simple as organising to send a patient from your emergency department to the radiology suite for a plain radiograph, through to the mounting of a fully fledged retrieval of a multitrauma patient from a small institution with few personnel and little in the way of sophisticated resources back to a major tertiary centre for definitive care.

Patient transport and retrieval has a long history of involvement with aviation and military conflicts dating back to World War I. With the ever increasing sophistication of aircraft and ongoing world conflicts, this association has developed through World War II to the Korean and Vietnam wars. The aircraft have changed and the pure military emphasis has been diluted by a growing number of civilian aeromedical retrieval services. In Australasia there are a number of different models of service provision. Few are purely hospital-based; some are operated by police, ambulance or other government agencies and some by private contractors. Most operate with medical attendants supplied to the air operators by the health services involved in the care of the patients they transport. The level of medical attendant varies depending upon the service and the condition of patients. Generally there are physician–nurse, physician–paramedic or nurse–paramedic combinations of staffing. There is little substantial literature to determine what constitutes the best aeromedical flight crew configuration, despite a number of publications.[1]

There are, however, common elements in the requirements of patient transport across this spectrum of scenarios. It is a sound general principle that, whenever a patient is moved from one point to another after entering a health system, the treating doctor who requests that transport has a responsibility to ensure that the level of care the patient receives is at least at a minimum safe standard throughout. Ideally there should be an escalation of the level of care from the point of first contact and thereafter. Such a hierarchical system underpins the very nature of our health system with involvement of increasingly more specialised staff and facilities.

This chapter will focus on the transport of the critically ill patient and the concept of medical retrieval.

In 1996 the Faculty of Intensive Care, Australian and New Zealand College of Anaesthetists (FICANZCA) and the Australasian College for Emergency Medicine (ACEM) released a revised version of a document detailing the minimum standards of transport of the critically ill.[2] This was and still is a very useful policy document and has been used by many retrieval services around this country to improve the level of patient care during medical retrieval and patient transport.

INDICATIONS FOR PATIENT RETRIEVAL

In most hospitals in Australia there are limits to the range of services that are available on campus. In rural locations this is particularly true, especially for neurosurgery and cardiothoracic surgery. These subspecialty disciplines are often required in the acutely traumatised patient. Some rural facilities may not even have the capacity to perform advanced imaging techniques such that definitive diagnoses (e.g. subdural haematoma) may not be able to be precisely diagnosed. In these instances, transport may be necessary not only for treatment but also for diagnostic purposes. Immediately this points to two general indications, diagnostic and therapeutic.

Diagnostic indications

Diagnostic indications will largely depend on the nature of the patient's illness. For example, a patient with an undifferentiated decreased Glasgow Coma Score (GCS) secondary to trauma, even without a neurosurgically treatable condition, will need a retrieval for CT scan if it cannot be performed on site. Likewise a patient who has a widened mediastinum after trauma will need imaging to define the state of the aortic arch and will need retrieving if the imaging cannot be performed on site. The list of diagnostic indications would be extensive and is influenced by whatever level of service is available at your institution.

Therapeutic indications

Similarly, therapeutic indications are determined principally by the nature of the patient's illness and the level of service at your institution. In these circumstances, the interventions will be determined after appropriate diagnostic investigations have been carried out. Many of these therapeutic measures can be discussed with referral hospital centres to determine the need and timeframe of such treatments to allow a rational approach to the patient's management, while making the most efficient use of resources and at the same time ensuring the best outcome for the patient.

Shortage of beds

Another indication for retrieval that is becoming increasingly common in these times of economic pressures on health services and increasing demand for intensive care (ICU) beds is the shortage of ICU beds at all levels of hospital. In these circumstances the drivers for this need are often a shortage of funds and nursing staff to adequately run an ICU bed. These issues are nonetheless frequently the cause of having to arrange retrievals. In many cases such retrievals can be arranged within the same urban area but sometimes they require significant travelling distances and time.

ORGANISING A MEDICAL RETRIEVAL

Irrespective of the indication, the keys to arranging and securing a successful patient transport or retrieval are thorough preparation and clear communication.

Preparation revolves around the planning for what is likely to occur to any particular patient, given the variables of the natural condition of the illness suffered as well as the mode of transport that is likely to be used. In many instances, the likely sequelae of particular diseases or illnesses are predictable and preparation will involve the steps that are necessary to try to prevent these sequelae, or at least treat them if they do occur (e.g. pneumothoraces in chronic airways disease).

Preparation for transport/retrieval will vary to some extent because of variables related to the transport mode. This is particularly evident in aeromedical transport, where special physiological changes are introduced into the equation, such as changes in gas pressures and volume with altitude.

Note: Atmospheric pressure equals 47 mmHg at a pressure altitude of 63,000 feet. This means that above a pressure altitude of 63,000 feet body fluids will boil as body water tries to saturate the atmosphere to a partial pressure of 47 mmHg! Fortunately this is not of any concern, as all aeromedical retrievals will occur below 40,000 feet, even on commercial jets.

PRACTICAL TRANSPORT ISSUES

Contact with receiving institution

When a patient is to be retrieved to another hospital, the first step—after determining the real nature of the patient's condition—is to communicate with the receiving hospital medical staff, most often at a tertiary centre, to ascertain their preparedness to accept the patient. Not only must the accepting inpatient team (e.g. neurosurgeons) be contacted, but it is also necessary to confirm that the receiving hospital has the appropriate bed available (e.g. an intensive care bed). There is little joy in having a neurosurgical patient accepted by a particular team only to find that there is no bed for the patient.

At the same time that the inpatient team is advising about their ability to accept the patient, information should be sought about any specialised treatments that they advise to be initiated at your own hospital before transport. This advice may be forthcoming from either the accepting team or a retrieval consultant. A retrieval consultant will usually be available for advice by phone through the agency that you would normally use to transport your patients. Such a person is usually a senior clinician who has been (and may still be) involved with retrievals of patients at all stages and who will be able to advise on most matters pertinent to patient transport as well as facilitating bed finding through involvement of other services.

Retrieval organisations

Most parts of Australasia have a coordinating organisation or structure for overseeing the conduct of retrievals. This will most often involve the ambulance services of the various states or territories in which the patient is being treated. Such a system is not only appropriate but also one that is enshrined in legislation concerning the movement of patients (e.g. Ambulance Act). These organisations must be contacted as soon as possible after the patient has been stabilised and consideration has been given to arranging a retrieval, otherwise nothing will occur in a coordinated fashion.

Ideally these organisations will initiate most of the retrieval process for you once you have given details of the patient's condition and destination hospital.

Coping with a different environment

It is vital to bear in mind that irrespective of the mode of patient retrieval (i.e. road, fixed-wing or helicopter), the environment in any of these vehicles is distinctly different from a hospital emergency ward or ICU. The first and most obvious difference is the size of the area to work in. The second and perhaps most obvious is that the platform is moving relative to the ground. Consequently the facility of doing procedures to a patient, should the need arise, is significantly reduced. This means that all the usual things that you might otherwise think are unnecessary, such as a urinary catheter, will become necessary. Oxygen tension and gas pressures are affected by altitude. According to Boyle's law, hollow viscus gases will change their volume and pressure with altitude. A simple measure such as instilling sterile water into an endotracheal cuff rather than air can avoid many of these concerns but they need to be considered first.

It is necessary to anticipate these changes both for convenience and for avoidance of injury to the patient. It is a distinctly different prospect to try to insert a nasogastric tube into a patient in the back of a moving ambulance or helicopter than to do the same procedure in a hospital bed where you have adequate light, oxygen, suction and above all a stable platform to work on.

Apart from the issue of a moving platform, which all modes of patient retrieval will involve, there are several other factors peculiar to retrieval that must be anticipated. Thermoregulatory issues must be taken into consideration. There can be significant alterations in temperature, with altitude changes compounding the fact that a patient must be moved from a situation where there is most likely functional air-conditioning to one in which there may not be. This is gradually being addressed as motor vehicle and aviation systems are becoming more sophisticated. Consequently, a patient must be covered appropriately to ensure normal body temperature is achieved and, perhaps more importantly, core temperature must be monitored regularly throughout the transport.

Monitoring and therapeutic options

Some other factors that need to be considered are the reliability and safety of monitoring and therapeutic options during the course of the retrieval. In particular, non-invasive oscillometry for blood pressure determinations tends to be unreliable in machines subject to large-scale altitude and pressure changes and/or significant vibration influences (e.g. in helicopters and fixed-wing aircraft). Under such circumstances, if the patient's condition warrants, invasive blood pressure monitoring should be the preferred method.

Similarly, the use of pulse oximetry is sometimes unreliable owing to movement artefacts or excessive ambient light interfering with the infrared sensor device. Often during the transfer of cardiac patients, concerns can arise over the safety of electrical cardioversion or defibrillation on board an aircraft in flight. There has been little in the way of published literature to define this but Dedrick et al[3] did a survey of 79 helicopter programmes in the United States, of which 69 (87%) had defibrillated in flight without incident (the others not having had to do so). There have certainly been cases where patients requiring cardiac pacing have been transported by air in this country without adverse aircraft effects. Additionally, patients who have recently undergone treatment with thrombolytic therapy have been transported by aircraft without ill effects.[4] It is also not unusual for some of the larger hospitals to request transport of their cardiac patients with invasive intraaortic balloon pumps to other cardiac services. These last points demonstrate the level of sophistication that is possible in the current practice of medical retrieval.

HOW TO PREPARE FOR A RETRIEVAL

The most effective preparation is to anticipate that if something can go wrong, it will. With this in mind, a number of steps can reduce the stress that both the patient and you will experience.

Securing the airway

It is safe to assume that all but the most alert and cooperative patients will have their airway definitively secured. In this case, a cuffed endotracheal tube, securely tied at an appropriate length, is the gold standard. At the same time, a decompressing gastric tube (oral or nasal) on free drainage, also securely tied, should be inserted. Both of these should be checked for proper position by a chest X-ray.

While securing the airway, an end-tidal carbon dioxide monitor should be used in all intubated patients during retrieval. This serves a dual purpose. Firstly, it ensures proper ventilation is occurring and secondly it alerts the medical attendant to any disconnection by a clear and unambiguous visual display on a monitoring device.

Pneumothoraces

Any pneumothoraces, confirmed before transportation, should be drained definitively with a thoracostomy tube and one-way valve drainage device (e.g. Heimlich valve). This is preferable to an underwater seal drainage device, which is prone to spillage and potentially leaking air back into the thoracic cavity. If spinal immobilisation is deemed necessary, a vacuum mattress is a good option in combination with a cervical collar and/or sandbags to the head as well as taping across the forehead.

Venous access

Good venous access is the next most important consideration. Central line access, while desirable, is not always essential. What is important is that the attendant has a readily accessible injection port close by his or her hand for the administration of medications. At least two moderate to large venous cannulae should be inserted for transport, taped securely and with functionality confirmed. As mentioned above, a non-invasive blood pressure cuff has significant limitations, so an invasive arterial line is preferred for all but the most stable patients.

Other considerations

Good-quality cardiac electrodes should be applied and taped over for security. A pulse oximeter should be applied and a reliable trace obtained. This should also be taped into position and re-checked then covered with a sheet or towel to reduce ambient light interference. A urinary catheter should be inserted in all patients being retrieved. A temperature-monitoring device is used or available (e.g. tympanic, bladder or central line device).

RETRIEVAL PROCESSES

Once a retrieval team arrives, a number of processes need to occur. Obviously the patient must be stable enough to move onto the retrieval stretcher. The actual process of moving a patient onto a retrieval stretcher is one that is often associated with change in clinical condition. Once moved, the patient must be carefully checked as well as all tubes and monitors for proper function.

Retrieval stretchers are necessarily smaller than hospital beds. Occasionally this will be problematic. Most ambulance stretchers in Australia are rated to take only 150 kg and occasionally a patient exceeds this limit. This then becomes a weight and space issue. However, in the majority of cases the patient can be transferred onto the retrieval stretcher and monitoring applied.

Retrieval teams will provide their own monitoring equipment in most instances. What is important at this stage is that the monitors that are to be used during the retrieval are fully charged, cables to various monitoring devices coiled and tied and that the patient is covered appropriately to minimise heat loss. Ideally the monitors and/or ventilator are attached to a bridge system that sits over the patient and faces the attendant, who can see all parameters and adjust all ventilator controls. All drug infusions are best administered either by syringe pump or by infusion pump, rather than by gravity alone. These controls also should be within easy reach of the attendant.

In any retrieval vehicle there is a lot of movement, and distraction is a real factor: alarms that might easily be heard in an emergency department

Table 23.1 Simplified checklist for retrieval

Stages	Patient status	Airway	Breathing	Circulation	Drugs	Extras
1. Retrieval indicated & ambulance notified 2. Bed available at receiving hospital	Awake, stable, cooperative	Natural	O_2 by mask	IV × 2	Analgesia +/- sedation, other drugs	IDC +/- NGT
3. Receiving hospital team accepts patient 4. All info with patient	Obtunded, unstable, uncooperative	Intubated	Ventilated	IV × 2 +/- CVL Arterial line	Analgesia, sedation, relaxants, +/- inotropes, others	IDC, NGT

or ICU can be overlooked. It is necessary to have some system of flagging alarms so that they can be detected early. Some aeromedical systems have a hard-wired alarm connection to allow monitor alarms to be heard through the aircraft headsets. Most road ambulance vehicles unfortunately do not have this system, but the ambient noise in these vehicles is not as loud. Lighting systems in retrieval vehicles vary greatly, so it is best to complete all procedures in hospital where light conditions are ideal rather than in the back of a transport vehicle.

Once all of the above has been attended to and the patient is loaded and stable, the retrieval can occur. What is most important next is to alert the receiving hospital of the departure of the team and the expected time of arrival to destination. The retrieval team should be given all relevant paperwork, results, X-rays and patient details to hand on to the receiving hospital staff. By ensuring that the receiving hospital has been reliably informed and that all the appropriate accompanying information is with the patient, you will smooth over the process for any future referrals you may have to arrange and be serving the patient's best interest simultaneously.

Table 23.1 summarises these steps in simplified form.

REFERENCES

1. Thomas SH. Aeromedical transport. Online. Available: http://www.eMedicine.com; May 2001.
2. Faculty of Intensive Care, Australian and New Zealand College of Anaesthetists and Australasian College for Emergency Medicine. Minimum standards of transport of the critically ill. Policy document; 1996.

3. Dedrick DK, Darga A, Landis D, Burney RC. Defibrillation safety in emergency helicopter transport. Ann Emerg Med 1989; 18(1): 69–71.
4. Kaplan L, Walsh D, Burney RE. Emergency medical transport of patients with acute myocardial infarction. Ann Emerg Med 1987; 16(1):55–57.

24   Mass casualty, chemical, biological and radiological hazard contingencies

Jeff Wassertheil

Fortunately, incidents involving mass casualties are infrequent. However, they have the potential to overwhelm normal health resources with very little notice. Because of this, it is important that contingencies are developed, tested and ready for immediate implementation. Such contingencies outline the responsibilities for overall medical control, coordination and effective casualty management in major emergencies and disaster situations. They include the procedures for triage, first aid and resuscitation, some of which require modification when resource availability needs to be rationed.

Response plans must provide a framework for coordination of transporting injured or incident-affected individuals to appropriate treatment sites. Plans must incorporate procedures to enable the presence of medical, nursing and first aid personnel to provide care at the scene of a mass casualty incident.

At a hospital level, plans need to be developed, implemented, rehearsed and evaluated. This enables hospitals that are often full to manage a large number of patients in excess of their usual workloads or capacities and, in certain circumstances, victims with special or specific needs.

Incorporation of public health resources and interventions is integral to providing guidance and procedures where hygiene, sanitation, communicable disease or biological hazards potentially exist. Contingencies must provide an interface for concurrent activation of recovery plans. Access to appropriate and timely psychological support for victims and care providers is included in both early and ongoing recovery phases. The overall objective is to mitigate diasters by participation in event planning and medical and emergency service activation and training.

PHASES OF A DISASTER

The phases of disaster management are prevention, preparedness, response and recovery.

Prevention

The prevention phase concentrates on strategies that minimise the severity of an incident. It aims to cushion the severity, reduce the effects, minimise adversity and contain the impact of a disaster. Prevention strategies also include incorporation of lessons learned from previous experiences.

Preparedness

Effort in optimal preparedness promotes effective and optimal resource allocation and consumption. This phase occurs with an expectation that the plan will at some time need to be activated. Preparedness occurs from within and outside the health service.

Planning includes both providers from within and stakeholders from outside the health service who would be expected to respond in accordance with emergency management contingency plans. Local community stakeholders—such as the police, ambulance and the fire department—as well as public health and recovery agencies should be included on health service planning committees. Likewise, health service representation should be included on local council, shire or regional planning committees.

As highlighted under prevention, the recommendations from previous operational debriefings, adverse incidents or experience are woven into response plans.

Response

The response is the activation of personnel and other resources in accordance with the predetermined plan to respond to multicasualty external disasters.

Recovery

Recovery contingencies are implemented and provide for the short- and long-term recovery of the community (victims and helpers) affected by the disaster. This includes the health service staff, and the repair and re-instatement of physical resources, consumables and services.

ADMINISTRATIVE AND LEGISLATIVE MANDATES

Each state or territory has legislative a framework under which counterdisaster planning for response and recovery to emergency situations throughout Australia takes place. Separate state emergency recovery plan arrangements, designed to meet long-term assistance to people and communities, are activated during the response phase of an incident to provide early commitment of resources.

Very broadly, these legislative frameworks provide for:

- Disaster planning and response coordination of activities throughout the state to be enacted by the chief commissioner for police or nominated deputies.
- Roles and responsibilities of control and support organisations and agencies for various types of emergencies or disasters.
- The state body for health to be the coordinator of agencies involved in providing recovery actions in communities following major emergencies and disasters.

Accordingly, under these arrangements, the police and the various state or territory emergency service organisations severally develop the non-medical component of the state disaster emergency management plans. Under the various state emergency response arrangements, the health departments have statutory responsibility to provide the necessary planning and response required to deal with matters associated with the general health of the community and to provide medical and hospital services required as a result of a major emergency or disaster.

MEDICAL RESPONSE PLANS, OR MEDICAL DISPLAN

Medical Displan is an organisational framework plan that outlines the roles and responsibilities of the various participating medical and health responders, and provides the necessary integrated procedures for altering and mobilising medical and health personnel, for establishing onsite medical control and for definitive treatment of casualties. The concept is that all arrangements and procedures made within Medical Displan are applied from the smallest to the largest incident with a build-up of medical coordination and medical and health resources as necessary, following the general pattern of normal daily operational procedures wherever possible. Medical Displan takes part in contingency planning and has a presence at major events where potential public threat is perceived to exist. Action can be taken in the absence of a declared disaster in order to provide protection from personal liability, and compensation is available for injury to volunteers not covered under other insurance arrangements while training for or participating in emergency response activities.

Medical Displan representation through medical and health participation in all local, regional and state Displan committees is mandatory to ensure integrated effective response can be provided in times of emergency.

Components of Medical Displan

Agencies or organisations responsible for health

The principal role of the health department is to deal with matters associated with the general health of the community and to provide health and medical services required as a result of a major emergency or disaster.

The health department ensures coordination of:

- Provision of hospital and medical services.
- Provision of transport and hospitalisation for the injured or sick.
- Supply of medical and first aid teams.
- Setting up medical centres and casualty clearing posts.
- Provision of disease control and other scientific and pathological services required.
- Health and scientific survey teams.
- Public health information, advice and warnings, to control and support agencies and for release to the affected communities.

The health department has direct responsibilities as the control agency for:

- Infectious disease outbreaks.
- Contaminated foodstuffs and water.
- Chemical, biological and radiological (CBR) substance releases.

It is also the support agency for all incidents, and includes advice to all combat, support agencies and to the general public in hazardous material, chemical, biological, radiological and nuclear incidents.

Acute health sector

The senior medical adviser manages the internal administrative functions of Medical Displan, in support of a medical coordinator group that includes both metropolitan and rural doctors who are appropriately trained in emergency management.

The senior medical adviser also manages the emergency operations centre when activated, in support of the medical coordinator squad. In addition, the adviser assists with the distribution of mass casualties to hospitals, and in times of major emergencies will provide briefings via the health department to the appropriate minister.

Emergency operation centres (EOCs)

EOCs will be activated when a major support effort is required to assist with onsite and central medical coordinator response activities. For longer-term recovery assistance, EOCs are essential to coordinate the physical, medical and mental health activities required to assist ongoing needs of communities and public health issues.

Public health agencies

In emergencies where public health is threatened, the health department, local government public health medical practitioners and environmental health officers provide the necessary expertise to preserve general healthy living standards. All work within the framework of the health department public health sector for preventing and controlling outbreaks of communicable diseases, and for the preservation of acceptable standards for safe drinking water and foodstuffs.

Ambulance service

This provides:

- 24-hour operational communications to initiate and instigate the necessary alerts and mobilisation of medical coordinators, hospital medical teams and casualty-receiving hospitals in major emergencies.
- The initial setting up of a medical controlled area incorporating a casualty collecting post (CCP) and casualty cleaning stations and for triage and treatment onsite until a joint medical command post is established.
- Assistance with onsite decontamination of people exposed to toxic or microbiological hazards.
- Transportation of casualties to appropriate hospitals.
- Coordination of first aid service responses until the establishment of a medical command structure.

Medical coordinator organisation

This group of doctors provides the necessary medical control and coordination of resources at the disaster scene and centrally for the distribution of casualties to appropriate hospitals. It also provides, through the health department EOC when established, other medical and health resources such as mental health professionals and public health and environmental health staff, and for additional medical and nursing staff to supplement facilities.

Pre-hospital medical coordination/disaster scene

Area medical coordinator (AMC)

The AMC is responsible for onsite medical coordination of all medical and health resources required and for the command of all health responders. The AMC is responsible for:

- In conjunction with the ambulance coordinator, establishing an effective medical controlled area (casualty collecting post and medical command post) and liaising with the police coordinator and other emergency services.
- Providing frequent and accurate assessment of the casualty status to a central medical coordinator, usually based at the ambulance communications centre.
- Assessing the onsite conditions and if necessary initiating, through the central medical coordinator, the setting up of an interim casualty clearing station or designating a triage hospital where transport of injured persons from the scene or local area may incur significant delays.

- Assessing the requirement for relief of or for further medical teams at the scene, for further fist aid support and whether psychological services may be needed.

Central medical coordinator (CMC)

The CMC is located in the ambulance communications centre. The CMC's role is to:

- Initiate and arrange distribution of casualties to appropriate hospital facilities, in conjunction with an ambulance commander—the concept is to distribute casualties to as many hospitals as practicable to avoid facility overload.
- Alert and mobilise medical teams and other medical and health responders to the disaster scene.
- Liaise and request activation of health department emergency operation centres at state and regional level if necessary, and provide situation reports at frequent intervals to the EOC and to request further assistance.
- Instigate stand-down of the various medical and health responders as appropriate after consultation with the onsite medical coordinator and other emergency service authorities.

Site medical control

The disaster site medical procedures in place for establishing early medical control for the proper triage, treatment and transportation of casualties are initially provided by officers of the first responding ambulance vehicle. These officers carry out the roles of:

1. Casualty collecting officer—to assess numbers and types of casualties, to carry out a reconnaissance of the area and select an area suitable to set up a casualty collecting post, to report findings to ambulance control and to commence triage of casualties.
2. Transport control officer—to establish suitable access and turn-around for ambulance vehicles, and to report this information to ambulance communications centre for further incoming response vehicles.

As an AMC or ambulance commander arrives onsite, further assessments will be made and a joint medical command post established. All incoming medical responders report to the command post where tasks within the CCP are allocated. Further medical assistance required onsite is requested through the central medical coordinator to avoid convergence and duplication of resources.

The medical services provided onsite will be limited initially, using the principle of doing as little as possible, as simply as possible, as quickly as possible and to as many as possible.

Life-saving procedures, such as airway management, immediate decompression of tension pneumothorax, arrest of haemorrhage, fracture stabilisation and relief of a pain where necessary, may be the limit of medical assistance when medical resources are few. Thus effective triage or classification of casualties by a casualty collecting (ambulance) officer (CCO), medical officer or team leader from a medical team is essential.

Triage and reverse triage

Triage generally implies direction of clinical resources to the most seriously ill or injured by a trieur or triage officer. In a mass casualty situation, demand may be in excess of resources availability. It is neither ethical nor practical to classify clearly non-salvageable victims as top priorities. Given this, two methods of field or mass casualty triage are employed, depending upon the number of casualties and the availability of clinical resources. The two methods of triage—SIEVE and SORT—are used at different phases of casualty management at disaster sites.

SIEVE

This triage method is used during the initial phase of managing mass casualties. It focuses on determining which patients will survive and channels resources to moving that cohort of patients from the scene to a casualty clearing post or station. Triaging in this manner is a repeated process to ensure refinement of urgency stratification and to respond appropriately to the ongoing evolution of a casualty's injury complex and consequent physiology. See Figure 24.1.

Casualty assessment is based on the findings of a primary survey. If casualties are ambulant, they are initially regarded as walking wounded and are directed or escorted to a casualty clearing post. If not ambulant, a triaging primary survey is performed. This looks at the airway, respiratory rate and capillary refill. Treatment is limited to the institution of simple, life-saving, primary survey manoeuvres. These are:

- Airway clearance by manual or other available methods.
- Decompression of a tension pneumothorax by needle thoracostomy.
- Control of external haemorrhage.
- Appropriate positioning of unconscious patients or patients with head, chest, abdominal pelvic or spinal injuries.

Casualties must be re-triaged on the basis of response, injury pattern and likely prognosis. If critically injured or ill patients are unresponsive to these measures and unlikely to survive, they become second priority casualties. This is sometimes known as reverse triage.

A standard clinical reasoning scheme for triage is outlined in Figure 24.1. SIEVE triage categories are as follows:

1. **Top priority patients** are those who are severely injured and in need of urgent emergency care. They are those in whom there is actual physiological embarrassment. Treatment is generally urgent, quick, simple and minimal in an endeavour to stabilise before priority transportation. They are patients who are deemed as able to be saved but will die or suffer major disability if not treated (Table 24.1).

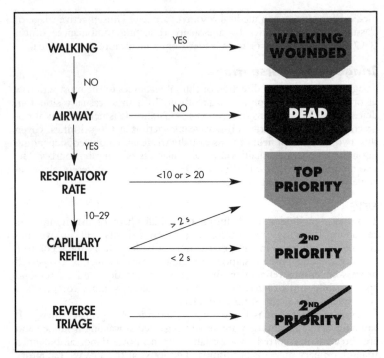

Figure 24.1 Approach to triage using the SIEVE method

Table 24.1 Triage groupings and criteria for mass casualty situations

Group	Priority	Criteria
Group 1	Red–priority 1	Severely injured but salvageable. In need of urgent medical care. Urgent resuscitation and transportation required.
Group 2	Yellow–priority 2	Significant injuries and condition stable. Treatment can wait or patient is unlikely to live and extensive medical care will jeopardise the survival of other casualties.
Group 3	Green–minor injuries	Casualty ambulant (walking wounded) and hospital admission unlikely. Uninjured, psychologically disturbed persons included in this category.
Group 4	Black–deceased	Medical officer is required to certify death on card. Body becomes the responsibility of police/coroner's office.

2. **Second priority patients** are those who may have significant injuries but in whom airway is not problematic and who have normal respiratory or perfusion status assessments. They constitute most of the injuries that are time-critical on a pattern of blunt injury. The implication of being stratified as a second priority patient is that transfer to and treatment at hospital is required.

3. **Second priority patients with a black stripe**. A black stripe may be drawn on a second priority tag by a trieur. This indicates that injuries sustained are likely to be incompatible with survival and that extensive medical treatment will jeopardise the survival of other casualties. An example is a patient with 90% burns when there are many patients with survivable injuries. Such casualties require a decision to be made to transfer to hospital as third priority or die at scene.

4. **Dead.** These are deceased individuals. They need to be certified as dead in the history section of the triage tag by a medical practitioner. The deceased become the responsibility of the police and the state coroner. They are generally transferred to a mortuary area onsite.

5. **Walking wounded patients** are divided into those who require physical first aid and those who require mental health first aid. In both instances, this could be provided at the scene in a field hospital or similar setting and the patient is then discharged to appropriate continuing care providers.

6. **Plain walking wounded tag.** These are casualties either with physical injuries or who are medically unwell. They are those who have sustained minor injuries or have non-time-critical medical problems unlikely to require hospital admission.

7. **Walking wounded tag with black stripe.** This tag identifies casualties with acute mental health problems due to psychological trauma or stress. In general, these casualties are suitable for urgent defusing or counselling, preferably onsite. Ongoing care can be planned for a later time.

SORT

This triage method is the more formal risk stratification or triage system that identifies the urgency with which most emergency health workers are familiar. SORT identifies time-critical patients and assists in scheduling optimal allocation of available resources. If used in the initial triage, this mode of triage is applicable for incidents involving only a small number of casualties. It is more commonly used on admission to casualty collecting posts or field hospitals.

This method of triage is consistent with the Australasian Triage Scale and triage practices taught in emergency management of severe trauma (EMST), emergency life support (ELS) and advanced paediatric life support (APLS) courses (see Chapter 25). It is identical to the practices employed by ambulance, first responder and other emergency medical services personnel for determining the time-critical patient. It is a repeated process that is dependent upon traditional ongoing patient observation.

SORT can also be implemented using the revised trauma score to rank physiological embarrassment and allocating an ordinal score.

Further refinement of triage can be assisted by attention to the pattern of injuries or mechanism of injuries. However, in a trauma-related mass casualty incident, a considerable number of patients may be classified as time-critical on mechanism of injury alone (see Chapter 14). Close observation of this latter group is necessary. Although these patients are of lower priority owing to normal physiological parameters or the absence of an identified pattern of injury, they are victims of major trauma, have sustained major forces and are at risk of significant and occult internal injury.

First aid services

First aid services can be provided by several different organisations. The common ones are St John Ambulance Australia and Australian Red Cross. These may be complemented by other first aid providers such as the Australian Ski Patrol Association, Royal Life Saving Society or Surf Life Saving Australia, depending on the circumstances. First aid agencies are often activated by the ambulance service. Several states have first aid subplans to assist with delineation of command structure, roles and responsibilities.

The principal role of first aid organisations is to assist with minor injuries where the setting up of separate treatment centres are necessary to cope with walking wounded. First aid teams generally work under the direction of a medical coordinator or ambulance commander in casualty collecting posts or holding areas or in field hospitals.

Hospital external disaster or emergency management plans ('Respond Brown')

All public hospitals are required to have external disaster plans to cope with mass casualties directed to hospital facilities for treatment. Public hospitals are required to develop, implement and test contingencies for the reception of mass casualties. This is a requirement both of legislature and of the Australian Council on Healthcare Standards. Some private hospitals participate in counterdisaster planning activities. These generally assist with walking wounded and second priority patients.

Such plans may also include the procedures for providing a trained and equipped medical team for casualty treatment at a disaster site. The provision of medical teams may reduce the emergency department effectiveness. Consideration is given to replacing or providing a team from another facility if the responding hospital is to continue to be a major casualty-receiving hospital.

Certain first aid organisations such as St John Ambulance and the defence forces are also able to provide medical teams on request. Some base hospitals in rural regions also have the capability to provide such teams, with smaller hospitals having a reduced capability.

Planning, exercises and review of plans

All participating agencies integral to Medical Displan response have subplans to ensure effective response is available when required. Integrated medical response planning with other emergency services takes place at all levels, addressing various hazards that exist. The exercising and testing of plans takes place at frequent intervals and as necessary following planning reviews.

Health service emergency management plans

The role of a health service in responding to external incidents will be dependent upon the size and scope of health care services usually offered. Health services that offer acute, subacute and long-term care as well as community outreach health care are more able to manage demand and overflows. Smaller hospitals can contribute by providing care to patients or casualties not requiring intensive resources or by assisting in decanting convalescing patients from other acute services, thus freeing resources to receive disaster victims.

Phases of the external disaster plan

In general the phases of an external disaster emergency management plan are alert, standby, activation (declared or action), stand down and debrief.

Alert

Notification of a possible disaster may be made by one of the emergency services, a media enquiry or a member of the public. Sometimes the alert is raised when ambulant victims present for treatment before any other notification. A chemical or biological exposure may be suspected when several patients present with similar symptoms or clinical syndromes over a short time.

All notifications or alerts should be validated. Occasionally, emergency services may need to be alerted by the health service after a number of patients have presented with a clinical syndrome suggestive of an exposure. Food poisoning and chemical exposures are examples of the latter.

When the alert has been validated, an emergency control officer or similarly authorised person initiates the response plan.

Standby

Standby advises the health service that an external incident has occurred which may impact on hospital resources and services. During this phase, designated officers assess resources. Current staffing levels, any imminent shift changes and any extra staff that would be required in such a situation are noted. Bed availability is estimated.

An emergency control centre (ECC) is established in the designated area. The ECC becomes responsible for the management of all aspects of the external disaster as it affects the hospital.

Staff must access action cards or documents and become familiar with their roles during the various phases of the emergency management response. Staff not covered by specific action cards continue normal duties.

Notification is dependent upon the nature of the incident. For example, with a chemical hazard it may be decided not to advise the senior surgical staff.

Activation (declared or action)

Access to hospital beds

The following are principles to guide creation of bed capacity. It is desirable to accommodate all the disaster victims in one area or receiving ward. The following groups of patients are considered for discharge or transfer to less acute facilities. These are:

- Electives with non-life-threatening conditions.
- Patients for routine investigation.
- Postnatal patients more than 24 hours postpartum.
- Stable patients undergoing long-term treatment.
- Stable postoperative patients >36 hours after the time of operation.
- Patients able to be accommodated by a 'hospital in the home' program.

Emergency department response

Aim

The aim of the emergency department is to rapidly assess and stabilise patients and then clear them from the department as soon as possible. If the external disaster is limited, with no possibility of further casualties, a full patient assessment could be completed in the emergency department in keeping with usual practices.

Call-in and notifications

Key clinical staff, clinical departments and management staff placed on standby are advised of the escalation. Clinical staff are initially summoned to the emergency department and prepared to receive casualties.

Consulting space access

Emergency department clinical staff should endeavour to discharge patients by expediting treatment, disposition, completion of clinical procedures and return of investigation results. Where possible, patients able to be managed in different environments, such as in general practice, could be directed to those services.

Triage and triage officers

It is preferable for the triage role to be undertaken by a senior doctor experienced or knowledgeable in the SORT and SIEVE methods of disaster triage. There is an also ongoing obligation to continue triage of non-disaster patients. It may be elected to simply use the Australasian Triage Scale with reverse triage of expectant cases designated as urgent.

Clinical records

Previously compiled standard clinical histories should be used for all disaster victims. The disaster labels should be retained within the clinical records.

Clinical zones

In order to coordinate clinical care and depending on the size of the department and the anticipated workload, the emergency department can be divided into different zones with separate teams of clinical staff. Other clinical areas such as outpatients could be set up as satellite emergency departments to manage overflow ambulatory care patients.

Medical staff

It is preferable for emergency department doctors to be allocated to work in specific zones.

Additional medical officers may be requested through the emergency control centre.

In trauma incidents, a surgeon should remain in the emergency department for immediate referrals and assessments. That surgeon is responsible for prioritising patients for theatre.

An anaesthetist assists with urgent airway intervention, referrals and pre-operative assessments.

Junior medical staff may be used to manage ambulatory patients in designated satellite areas.

A doctor, preferably with three or more years' experience, or a senior nurse may be allocated to the care of extremely severely injured patients with low probability of survival—the expectant category. Intensive efforts to resuscitate these patients may jeopardise the survival of large numbers of other casualties because of an excessive drain on resources. Supportive and palliative care only should be given, until resources are available to commence more vigorous resuscitation, if appropriate.

Nursing staff

Emergency department nursing staff roles generally parallel those of the medical staff. Their role focuses on the nursing aspects of patient care and the management of the designated emergency department zones or other designated areas. Nurses receive and assess patients, and assist with the examination and treatment of patients.

Senior nursing staff allocate nurses and clerical support staff to the designated areas and assist the triage officer in resource allocation.

Table 24.2 Hospital-wide services necessary for external disaster plans

Executive management	Linen and waste
Emergency department	Food services
Receiving and non-receiving wards	Engineering & facilities department
Main operating suite	Security
Medical imaging	Traffic control
Laboratory services	Mortuary services
Pharmacy services	Management of disaster victims' families
Supply & materials department	Community relations and media management
Central sterilising supply department	Volunteers
Environmental services	

A particular focus is the availability of extra equipment, sterile stock and medications.

In-hospital responses

Management of in-hospital responses and executive management issues are beyond the scope of this chapter. However, Table 24.2 identifies the other departments and resource areas contributing to the overall response.

Site medical teams

Some health services are expected to provide site medical teams to work in casualty collecting posts and in field hospitals. These teams assist in the rescue, triage and treatment of disaster victims. The roles vary depending on the magnitude of the disaster, numbers of casualties and types of problems.

The team may consist of seven people—team leader, two additional doctors, three emergency nurses and a patient services assistant. The exact nature of this team will depend upon the personnel available and the nature of the disaster to which the team has been called. In general, it is desirable to have the most experienced personnel possible on this team. Thus, they should be recruited from the senior medical staff and nursing staff of three or four years' experience following qualification.

Stand down

The cessation of the response and return to usual operations is initiated by the ECC. The response may conclude on advice from the disaster site or a Medical Displan coordinator through the ambulance communication centre. However, the response plan may require ongoing activation until pressure on the health service or hospital resources has subsided and normal activities can be resumed.

The stand down mechanism may be total or progressive. Progressive stand down can be initiated when certain areas are no longer required to function under response plan conditions.

Debriefing

There are two types of debriefing, operational debriefing and psychological debriefing. The latter has two components. Immediate debriefing is a defusing of staff. The second is formal counselling offered for ongoing symptoms.

Operational debrief

A formal operational debrief, involving key participants and heads of departments, should be conducted within 1 week. This debriefing examines the incident and the organisational response. Reports are prepared for the external disaster committee. Recommendations in this report will form the basis of revisions to the health service's external disaster plans.

Defusing

Defusing is the immediate attention to the psychological needs of staff. This provides staff with an opportunity to express their feelings and thoughts about the episode.

Counselling

Counselling aims to assist staff with long-term distress suffered as a consequence of the disaster response. These services are generally provided by employee assistance programs or may be accessed through the various departments of health.

CHEMICAL, BIOLOGICAL AND RADIOLOGICAL HAZARDS

The approach to chemical, biological, radiological (CBR) exposures is similar in principle to multicasualty trauma incidents, whether exposed victims are single casualties, several or within the context of mass casualties. The prime difference is the need to prevent contamination and/or infection of rescuers, health providers and the community. The approach aims to provide optimum care while maintaining safety for other patients and staff. A second broad aim is to effectively decontaminate patients before they enter the emergency department. It focuses on a sequence of actions and interventions that admits decontaminated casualties to emergency departments. A further aim is the expedient identification of causal agents that may enable specific treatment.

Acute recovery incorporates the restoration to usual functions of areas used for decontamination. It includes management of contaminated items for cleaning and inspection by hazard management or public health agencies. Where applicable, non-disposable medical equipment is cleaned and retuned for regular use. Some contingency plans contain specific equipment kits reserved for use in CBR incidents.

In the field, the sequence begins with identification of casualties, proceeds to isolation, decontamination, triage, treatment and transport to hospital. Emergency department contingences are similar. However, treatment may need to commence before or concurrently with decontamination. The main risk for hospitals is the arrival of contaminated or infected individuals before a CBR incident has been recognised or advised, with consequent contamination of the emergency department and, potentially, the whole health facility.

Features of CBR and nuclear hazards

CBR and nuclear substances potentially cause harm to human health. Incidents with these substances often generate vapours, fumes, dusts and mists. Hazardous wastes can pollute waste streams, causing a threat to public health, safety or the environment. They can also be invisible.

CBR hazards can be infectious, toxic, mutagenic, carcinogenic, teratogenic, explosive, flammable, corrosive, oxidising and radioactive, and may cause immediate and/or long-term health effects. Exposure may result in poisoning, irritation, chemical burns, sensitisation, cancer, birth defects or organ disease of the skin, lungs, liver, kidneys and nervous system. The severity of the illness or disease depends on the nature of the substance and the dose absorbed.

Detailed information on all the hazards, their properties, effects and treatment is beyond the scope of this chapter. The following is a broad overview.

Mode of presentation

Education of all staff in recognising a contaminated or CBR-hazard-exposed person is necessary in order to minimise the risk of emergency department exposure and contamination. Self-presentation before notification by emergency services agencies is common in chemical incidents. Occasionally, emergency services may be unaware of the incident. In this situation the health service has a system initiation function. In biological incidents, there is often a trickle followed by an epidemic flood of patients. Radiological incidents may involve burns, the consequences of initial radiation illness or the management of ongoing radioactivity.

An uninformed public, presentation of the worried well and an uncertainty or lack of knowledge by community-based doctors and health providers compound the emergency department impact. It has been estimated that the ratio of worried well to affected victims is 10:1.

Chemical agents

Nerve agents

Nerve agents are organophosphates. They block acetylcholinesterase inhibitors, causing a cholinergic crisis. Examples include Tabun (GA), Sarin (GB) and VX.

Blistering agents

These irritate the epithelial surfaces by direct contact. The skin and mucosal surfaces are the target tissues. The mustard agents and lewisite are examples of this group.

Incapacitating agents

This group causes short-term disabling physical and/or mental effects by affecting higher cortical function. It includes central nervous system depressants, stimulants and hallucinogens. To qualify for membership of this group, agents must be potent, last hours to days, not be potentially lethal at effective doses and have no long-term adverse sequelae. LSD and 3-quinclidinyl benzoate (BZ) are examples of incapacitating agents. BZ is an anticholinergic agent.

Blood agents—the cyanides

These agents impair cellular function by uncoupling oxidative phosphorylation.

Pulmonary/choking agents

Choking agents impair the respiratory system by irritating the respiratory tract mucosa and alveolar epithelium. These can produce a spectrum of illness from minor irritation to acute respiratory distress syndrome. Examples include chlorine (CL) and phosgene (GC).

Biological hazards

These are varied. Illness is usually of insidious onset. Because early symptoms may be non-specific, especially when patients may be prodromally unwell, early recognition can be difficult. Once the community is aware, workload is increased. Patient load will include those with non-specific symptoms, worried patients with usual clinical features of a non-exposure-related illness and those with unusual symptoms or clinical signs needing diagnostic refinement.

Patients exposed to microbiological agents may be recognised when a number of patients present with unusual similar symptoms or clinical signs. Alternatively, an influx of patients with similar symptoms may present with diagnostic refinement identifying a common broad illness such as pneumonia with isolation of an unusual causal agent. Other dilemmas include when to immunise and when to definitively treat. These decisions must be made in conjunction with infectious diseases physicians and public health agencies. Rationalisation of available therapeutic substances is a logistic problem. The principles of managing this issue are no different from those of disaster triage and reverse triage. However, within this context, development of inclusion and exclusion criteria is more relevant. The impact of the espouser on hospitals is likely to increase the workload of laboratory facilities in initial identification and ongoing examinations for isolation of infective agents or bacterial endotoxins and exotoxins.

Radiological hazards

Two broad questions need to be asked when considering radiological exposure. Has the patient been irradiated? Is the patient radioactive? Irradiation alone can cause life-threatening illness. The latter additionally poses a risk to rescuers and ongoing careers.

All forms of ionising radiation can cause illness. Alpha particles generally have poor tissue penetration. They are of significance if ingested, inhaled or have contacted open wounds. Gamma rays penetrate tissues directly affecting cells. Neutrons cause effects indirectly. Human tissue provides some resistance to beta particles, thus decreasing impact and only causing tissue damage when they have penetrated cells. Bone marrow and gastrointestinal mucosa are the tissues at most risk. Injuries may be caused by a single radiation exposure, exposure to high levels of fallout and repeated exposures.

Acute radiation syndrome involves four phases: prodrome, latent period, manifest illness, and death or recovery.

Prodrome

Initial symptoms often appear within 6 hours of exposure. Symptoms include nausea, vomiting, anorexia and general malaise. Treatment is largely symptomatic and supportive. A 48-hour lymphocyte count and chromosomal analysis of lymphocytes for dicentric fragments are predictors of likely bone marrow suppression and haemopoietic syndrome.

Latent period

This phase is a variable symptom-free period of hours to weeks.

Manifest illness

In this, definitive radiation illness and its complications become evident. Four clinical syndromes are described: haemopoietic, gastrointestinal, vascular and cerebral.

The symptoms of the gastrointestinal syndrome are similar to those of the prodrome phase, with additional problems of diarrhoea, fever and gastrointestinal haemorrhage. Bowel perforation and septicaemia are complications of severe illness. Treatment is supportive with intravenous fluid resuscitation, dehydration and parenteral nutrition.

The haemopoietic syndrome is the effect of bone marrow suppression with increased susceptibility to infection, haemorrhage and occasionally anaemia. Treatment is generally supportive. Platelet transfusion may be necessary for thrombocytopenia-associated haemorrhage or if surgical intervention is required. Sepsis must be energetically treated. Wounds should be closed as soon as possible. Infected or devitalised tissue should be excised. Early skin grafting of burns prevents opportunistic infection. Other blood products to enhance immunocompetence may be considered as clinically indicated.

The vascular syndrome is due to vascular bed dilation and capillary leaking. Shock occurs as a result of volume loss and poor vascular resistance, due to stimulation of acute inflammation and release of vasoactive humoral mediators causing peripheral vasodilation.

The cerebral syndrome comprises nausea, vomiting, cardiovascular instability, confusion, ataxia, seizure and loss of consciousness. There is a high mortality within 24–48 hours.

Recovery/death

Death or recovery over several weeks are sequelae of the illness.

Goals of emergency department management of CBR exposure

The emergency department goals are to:

- Protect staff from toxic exposure.
- Rapidly assess and treat immediately life-threatening problems.
- Decontaminate.
- Determine the identity of the hazardous materials or chemical agents and provide specific treatment as indicated.
- Prevent cross-contamination of staff, visitors and other patients.
- Restore the clinical environment to normal functions following the incident.

Personal protective equipment (PPE)

The use of PPE for staff treating contaminated patients is the single most important line of defence against airborne agents. It prevents cross-contamination, and provides a physical barrier and respiratory protection.

There are various safety standards of protective equipment. Hospitals generally require Safety Standard C equipment.

Isolation areas

CBR plans must include the availability of an isolation area. In some instances, this may be a physical structure that has been developed in keeping with appropriate standards that have been incorporated into new or renovated facilities. In other circumstances, the isolation area may be makeshift or portable. Decontamination takes place within or immediately adjacent to the isolation area.

Hot zone

The hot zone is an area of contamination. For practical purposes, this is an isolation area for dealing with contaminated casualties. In selecting an appropriate area for the hot zone, consideration needs to be given to wind direction, slope for run-off, access to water and drainage, ability to provide screening for privacy, traffic management, and proximity to the emergency department.

Warm zone

The warm zone is a buffer area between hot and cold zones to minimise cross-contamination.

Cold zone
This is a clean, non-contaminated area.

Decontamination corridor
The decontamination corridor traverses the warm zone. Decontamination is functionally a one-way sequence and process. Contaminated casualties enter the hot zone, pass through the decontamination process, and exit into the cold zone, before definitive treatment within the emergency department.

Contaminated area and hot zone issues

Life-saving equipment required in this area will be out of service until decontaminated. All patient clothing and personal belongings are bagged and labelled. All items used and present in the hot zone must be decontaminated before reuse or, in the case of personal belongings, returned to owners. Specialist cleaning may be required.

Decontamination requires the availability of showering facilities. Screening is necessary for patient privacy. The area must be well ventilated. If necessary, ventilation may need to be enhanced using portable industrial exhaust fans.

In makeshift or portable situations, the contaminated hot zone, the uncontaminated cold zones and the emergency department should be easily identifiable and taped off to prevent accidental cross-contamination.

Contaminated waste and patient belongings are double-bagged, a red ('dirty') label is attached and the bag is placed in a yellow contaminated waste bin. Extreme care should be taken with patient clothing and valuables. These must be clearly labelled as they may be the only form of patient identification and may be required for forensic evidence.

Specimens that may cause cross-contamination through the normal means of transport must be transported in a safe manner. This may require specimens to be transported in labelled, sealed containers via a courier.

Decontamination

Decontamination aims to remove substance and stop ongoing exposure. Decontamination requires the removal of clothing and showering with copious amounts of water. If there is any doubt about contamination, then the person must be decontaminated. This also applies to emergency services personnel.

For safety reasons, only those staff designated as members of the decontamination team wearing full PPE are permitted to decontaminate patients. If protective respiratory equipment is required, only staff trained in the equipment are to be deployed.

The following is a guide to effective patient decontamination:

1. It is preferred that males and females be segregated.

2. The patient stands on a plastic sheet and removes clothing and personal belongings. These are wrapped in the sheet and placed in a bag. The bag is placed in a second bag. Identification and red contaminated labels are attached.
3. Patients proceed to decontamination showers. Copious amounts of water and soap are used. Liquid, flour and disposable wipes and tissues may be required to remove thick liquid before showering.
4. Following decontamination, patients move through the warm zone or corridor to the 'clean area' or cold zone. The patient is dried and clothed in a standard examination gown. Once externally decontaminated, the patient has a green external decontamination tag or armband applied and is moved to the triage area.

Specific decontamination issues

1. A contaminated appendage can be washed without wetting the whole body.
2. Skin is washed down for 5 minutes with copious amounts of soap and water.
3. Open wounds require gentle scrubbing or irrigation for 5–10 minutes with lukewarm water.
4. Eye exposures require irrigation of eyes with sterile normal saline for 15–30 minutes.
5. Contaminated facial and nose hair and ear canals are to be gently irrigated with frequent suctioning to ensure removal of contaminants.

Substance identification

Substance identification is necessary for correct decontamination and for providing medical treatment specific to the substance.

Chemical substances may be identified using:

- Hazmat or product advice sheets.
- Computerised databases, e.g. Poisindex.
- Dangerous goods guide.
- Poisons Information Centre: phone number 13 1126 (Australia-wide).

A biological agent may have been identified and advised by the state public health agency. If a biological agent is suspected, identification strategies should be planned in conjunction with health service clinical microbiologists or infectious diseases physicians. Forewarning of and close liaison with laboratory medicine is required.

Radiation hazard identification may have already been advised by relevant public health and environment protection agencies. However, local nuclear medicine departments, especially those associated with radiotherapy treatment centres, may initially be of assistance. It is preferable that a radiation physicist assist with onsite assessment of patients and the local environment for radioactive contamination.

Staff roles

It is essential that all staff members are familiar with their roles in a chemical, biological or radiation incident/disaster. The roles are similar to those identified for response to traumatically injured mass casualties.

The triage nurse or officer remains 'clean' adjacent to the triage station.

The senior doctor in charge remains in the cold zone and allocates medical personnel to specific duties and areas, such as to isolation and decontamination. Doctors allocated to the hot zone must be familiar with the PPE, equipment and procedures for decontamination and treatment. The doctor in charge endeavours to determine substance identification and specific treatment.

The role of the nurse in charge of management of nursing and clerical resources parallels that of the senior doctor. A specific responsibility is to ensure the decontamination area is screened off for patient privacy, clearly marked, signposted and isolated to prevent cross-contamination.

Decontamination teams

A decontamination unit consists of two teams, each with a minimum of three staff: doctor, nurse and patient services assistant. One team triages using either SIEVE or SORT methods and where appropriate clinically manages time-critical patients in need of emergency care. The second team concentrates on decontamination procedures.

Colour-coded role-specific action cards outlining team roles should be worn around the neck.

Men with full beards will not be able to obtain an accurate seal from the respirator and thus cannot participate in a medical decontamination team.

Clean-up and decontamination of hot zone equipment

Hot zone equipment may be separated into two groups, a chemical/disaster box and supplementary equipment, as outlined in Table 24.3.

Non-disposable hot zone equipment requires cleaning. Specialist cleaning may be necessary. These items should be double-bagged and labelled with a red contaminated label.

Disposal of consumables, cleaning of equipment and restoration of decontamination areas to usual activities will vary among hospitals depending on the set-up. Issues include:

- Chemical disposal of any contaminated waste water.
- Cleaning or disposal of contaminated clothing and contaminated disposable protective clothing.
- Cleaning of the shower and hot zone areas. Cleaning staff may need access to PPE.
- Cleaning of contaminated equipment.

Table 24.3 Suggested equipment lists for decontamination areas

CHEMICAL DISASTER BOX EQUIPMENT

- Personal protective equipment—disposable barrier suit, overshoes, nitrile gloves and respirator with disposable filter and air hose
- CBR procedure manual
- Liquid soap, flour, disposable wipes or tissues
- Clear bags for double-bagging of contaminated clothing and linen/black pen to write contents of bag (e.g. linen, patient's clothing, disposable equipment)
- Plastic sheet
- **Red CONTAMINATED** tags and **Green DECONTAMINATED** tags
- **Red CONTAMINATED** patient labels and **Green DECONTAMINATED** patient labels.
- Special specimen-carrying container for contaminated specimens
- Nozzle for hose
- Hazard signs and tape to identify isolation zone

OTHER EQUIPMENT

- Hoses to connect to external outlets (depending on decontamination zone design)
- Dressing trolley for laying out resuscitation equipment
- Patient trolley(s)
- Portable oxygen and suction
- Transport resuscitation bag—adult and paediatric
- Defibrillator
- Portable BP cuff & sphygmomanometer
- Portable otoscope
- Towels, gowns to use after decontamination shower, warm blankets
- Clean trolleys for decontaminated patients
- Dirty linen skip

- Emergency department staff may be able to clean equipment if this can be done safely. If not, specialist cleaning may be required.
- Disposable equipment will need to be replaced. This includes PPE equipment such as suits, gloves, overshoes and respirator hoods.
- Government agencies responsible for environment protection are notified if hazardous chemicals have entered the sewers or stormwater drainage system.
- Particulate matter removed from radiation exposure victims may need to be stored in lead-lined bags or sealed containers.

Staff decontamination

Staff should remove and dispose of personal protective equipment and clothing only when contaminated 'dirty' area clothing and linen has been double-bagged and trolleys and other equipment used in this area have been decontaminated.

Clinical and related wastes

The underlying principles for the treatment and disposal of clinical and related wastes are the health and safety of personnel, the public, and the minimisation of overall environmental impact.

Clinical wastes include sharp items and human tissue wastes. Related wastes include cytotoxic, pharmaceutical, chemical and radioactive wastes. Ultimate disposal of wastes will be dependent on their nature and national, state or local regulations governing the disposal of hazardous substances.

Wastes need to be segregated according to their category, bagged, packaged or containerised. Segregation practices need to facilitate the ongoing maintenance of safe waste movement and transport.

Plastic bags are used for the collection and storage of clinical and related wastes, other than sharps. They must be of sufficient strength to safely contain the waste class they are designated to hold. They need to conform to colour-coding and marking. If moist sterilisation is to be used for decontamination, bags must be suitable for that purpose. Bags may be filled only to a maximum of two-thirds of their capacity or to a maximum weight of 6 kg. This allows for secure final closure and unlikely tearing of the bag. Bags may be secured only with closure devices that do not have sharp protuberances such as staples or exposed wire ties.

Rigid-walled containers are used for collection of sharp items. Containers such as mobile garbage bins should be resistant to leakage, impact, rupture and corrosion. These containers should be inspected after each use to ensure that they are clean, intact and without leaks. Any containers shall have interiors of smooth, impervious construction to contain any spillage and to facilitate inspection, cleaning and sanitisation. Rigid-walled containers must be appropriately colour-coded and securely closed, but not necessarily locked, during transport.

The key consideration for clinical and related wastes storage is their safe containment in a vermin-proof, clean and tidy area. Storage requirements will depend on the volume and type of clinical and related wastes to be contained and the mode of waste treatment to be employed. Procedures will also be dictated by the logistics of waste treatment methods and the requirements of disposal facilities.

Waste segregation is maintained during the movement and handling of wastes. If waste is mixed or loses identification during movement, it must be treated at the highest level of contamination. Movement of wastes through patient care areas should be avoided. Industrial trolleys should be used to move clinical wastes contained in plastic bags or non-mobile rigid-walled containers.

Chemical exposure register

A chemical exposure register may be managed by the fire brigade or an appropriate hazmat management agency. However, hospital staff may be required to manage this.

All staff, including visiting emergency service personnel, and patients involved in contaminated areas must be listed on the register. The minimum details required in the register include name, hospital record number, designation and injuries sustained. Contact details of involved staff are recorded to ensure timely access if additional follow-up is required.

A tag stating the person has been exposed to a radiation, biological, or chemical hazard and the substance involved is attached to the patient in the form of a wristband. It is worn for a predetermined time, usually 48 hours in the case of a chemical exposure.

RECOMMENDED READING

American College of Emergency Physicians website. Available: http://www. acep.org.

Australasian College for Emergency Medicine website. Available: http://www. acem.org.au.

Beeching NJ, Dance DAB, Miller ARO, Spencer RC. Biological warfare and bioterrorism. BMJ 2002; 324:336–339.

Degg S. Chemical burns. Toxic chemical incidents. A symposium conducted at the Australia Disaster College, Mt Macedon, Victoria, 1997.

Emergency Management Australia. Emergency management practice manual 2: safe and healthy mass gatherings. 1st edn. Australian emergency manuals series, part 3. Emergency Management Australia; 1999.

Emergency Management Australia. Emergency management practice manual 3: health aspects of chemical, biological and radiological hazards. Provisional edn. Australian emergency manuals series, part 3. Emergency Management Australia; 2000.

Evison D, Hindsley D, Rice P. Chemical weapons. BMJ 2002; 324:332–335.

Hodgetts TJ, Mackway Jones K, eds (Advanced Life Support Group). Major incident medical management and support, the practical approach. 2nd edn. London: BMJ Books; 2002.

Tan GA, Fitzgerald MCB. Chemical biological radiological (CBR) response: a template for hospital emergency departments. Med J Aust 1997; 177:196–199.

Victorian and South Australian Metropolitan fire brigades protocols.

Acknowledgments

Part of this chapter was developed from the following documents:

Canestra J, Jones S, Wassertheil J, Johnstone R, eds. Frankston Hospital External Disaster Committee, Respond Brown—external disaster plan. Victoria: Peninsula Health; 1999.

Jones S, Smith M, eds. Hazardous substance management. Victoria: Peninsula Health; 2000.

The section on radiation illness was largely developed from: Holmes JL and Mark PD. Nuclear incident medical management. In: Emergency management practice manual 3: health aspects of chemical, biological and radiological hazards. Provisional edn. Australian emergency manuals series, part 3. Emergency Management Australia; 1999.

25 The seriously ill: tips and traps

Gordian W O Fulde

It is the purpose of every emergency department to assess, resuscitate, diagnose and treat, both definitively and symptomatically, the patients who walk or are wheeled through the door.

The ultimate responsibility for this belongs to the medical officer. In order to cope when faced with a variable number of patients whose conditions vary in severity, an organised approach is essential.

There must be triage (sorting). This is often done by a specially trained nurse whose sole duty is triage. The triage nurse must have immediate access to the medical officer for life-threatening situations or decision-making help. The triage nurse should be sited so that each patient (arriving by ambulance or walking) is assessed on arrival and directed to the appropriate area in the department where necessary care can be provided. Triage nurses can now order X-rays and give analgesia (including narcotics) in order to expedite care of the patient.

Throughout Australia the following national triage scale is used:

Category	Must be seen
1 (major trauma, cardiac arrest)	Immediately
2 (chest pain)	Within 10 minutes
3 (stable abdominal pain)	Within 30 minutes
4 (sprains, minor lacerations)	Within 60 minutes
5 (minor problems, e.g. ear wax)	Within 2 hours

Patients are seen according to their triage rating. It is a guide only, so beware: categories 3 and 4 can be sicker than 1 or 2 and may need to be upgraded urgently.

The emergency physician should use a priority problem-oriented approach and make clear decisions. For the leader of the team of medical officers, nurses, clerical staff, radiographers, porters and many others who are often needed to attend a sick patient, this approach is imperative. The physician must assess, resuscitate and manage the patient and the patient's relatives. As a rule, decision-making is harder in the case of patients who are not critically ill. Such patients should be assessed and managed with emphasis on early symptomatic relief and reassurance.

In attending to the many problems encountered in an emergency department, rely on good clinical commonsense in order to avoid pitfalls. At all times, play it safe. Be suspicious of any complication. The patient must be managed in as close to an 'ideal' fashion as possible. Distractions such as work pressure or the many other difficulties faced in emergency

Table 25.1	
EMERGENCY DEPARTMENT 10 COMMANDMENTS	
1	IF IN DOUBT, ASK. This includes asking medical, nursing, clerical and paramedical staff
2	NO PATIENT IS TO BE DISCHARGED FROM THE EMERGENCY DEPARTMENT UNLESS THE EMERGENCY REGISTRAR/CONSULTANT KNOWS ABOUT IT. Especially if sent in by an LMO.
3	BE SAFE. • Universal protective measures • Safe shoes • Sharps disposal • Immunisations up-to-date • Know 'needlestick' protocol • Know location of wall-mounted alarms • Wear personal duress alarms
4	IF YOU SUSPECT PROBLEMS, GET HELP EARLY.
5	SEE PATIENTS IN THE ORDER THEY APPEAR ON THE EDIS SCREEN and COMPLETE EDIS INFORMATION.
6	ALWAYS CONSIDER ANALGESIA. GIVE ANALGESIA EARLY VIA THE MOST APPROPRIATE ROUTE (INTRAVENOUS UNLESS SPECIFICALLY CONTRAINDICATED).
7	WHILE ON DUTY IN THE DEPARTMENT, BEHAVE AS YOU WOULD LIKE A DOCTOR TREATING YOUR OWN FAMILY TO BEHAVE.
8	TREAT EVERYBODY EQUALLY: • Socially • Medically • Be thorough and polite
9	WRITE NOTES GOOD ENOUGH TO USE IN A COURT APPEARANCE. DOCUMENT CLEARLY IN YOUR MEDICAL NOTES. Including discharge instructions and whom notified
10	BE TIDY. • Appearance • Identification • Names: your name should be legible; patient's name on history and medication charts • Do not leave X-rays out of packets. Give back private X-rays etc. • Keep consultation rooms clean • Put used trays and sharps away • Doctors, keep your office tidy • Cot bed sides up when you leave patient

departments (e.g. bed shortages) should play no major role in individual management. Of course, good written documentation is essential as evidence of what was done and why.

RED LIGHTS—BEWARE

For all of us there are red warning lights that alert us to potential pitfalls:

- **Representations to the emergency department**. Think it through again, do not just accept the last diagnosis.
- **Patient sent in by other healthcare professionals**, e.g. GPs, community nurses. They are asking for your and the hospital's help.
- **Repeated questions or protests**, e.g. the patient, a mother, anybody that keeps telling you 'they are sick' or 'this is not normal for the patient'. This is a key indicator of pathology occurring.
- **Triage categories 3 and 4** are often quite sick (especially if old).
- **Check vital signs frequently yourself** (BP, pulse, respiratory rate, temperature, blood glucose level, coma scale, oximetry).
- **Unpleasant patients (with or without difficult relatives).** *Never* vary your standard approach and management. Document all. This also applies to VIPs and friends. Always be polite, not rushed, try to sit down, get eye contact and listen.
- **Hand-over patients.** Make sure you have the whole story and plan. In the United States this patient group features highly in court cases.
- **Poor history, poor examination.** History and examination are cornerstones of the diagnosis. If you are unable to get good facts, be very careful and conservative, and worry.
- **Investigations are never 100% accurate.** Even if a test is very expensive, do not worship it, it makes mistakes. Many tests confirm a diagnosis, but do not fully exclude it. Look at the whole clinical picture.
- **Urgent treatment** (see Law 1, below). Sometimes you must treat on suspicion, now! For example, tension pneumothorax, bacterial meningitis, narcotic overdose, hypoglycaemia. Early pain control may also be needed.
- **Pain.** Always listen to the patient, go through all details of the pain (avoid leading questions!). This way you will probably get the diagnosis. Treat pain very early. Beware if pain is severe and unrelieved.

DECISION-MAKING TIPS

In the emergency department we are all seeing older, sicker, more complicated patients. You must focus on:

- What made the patient come to hospital?
- Are all the vital signs OK?
- Do I need extra help, extra information (old notes, general practitioner, specialist advice)?
- Problems—plan of management.

An important question is 'Does the patient need admission to hospital?' This is better approached from the other perspective: 'Is it safe or appropriate to send the patient home?' If the answer is to be 'yes', the patient must be able to cope alone. Is there anyone to help; can the patient take necessary medications; prepare and eat meals and go to the toilet? Also, can the patient survive any likely complication of the medical condition? The fact that the emergency department was excessively busy at the time and the hospital was full will not be at all useful as an excuse in a legal inquiry or a court case relating to the management of an individual who was inappropriately sent home. Always err on the side of safety, and if you are not sure what to do get the most senior medical officer possible involved in the decision-making. Always write details in the notes of what was decided, by whom and why.

An equally important aspect of management relates to the discharge of the patient. Usually some follow-up, by a local doctor, specialist or outpatients department, is indicated. This must be organised and noted in the patient's record.

IMPORTANT 'LAWS'

Law 1: All patients are trying to die before your eyes

You must always think in terms of worst-case scenarios: e.g. cardiac infarcts, meningitis, subarachnoid haemorrhage, pulmonary embolism. This is even more vital where early specific treatment will cure and prevent death. It may seem dramatic but if you treat or exclude these serious illnesses early, the further management of the patient is often very straightforward. Remember, medicine is best geared to treat the serious illnesses and society expects us to get these right.

Law 2: Call for help early!

The team approach for complicated emergencies, such as trauma and cardiac arrest, should be activated early. Early involvement of intensive specialists, those responsible for definitive care, is imperative. Never be reticent to ask for more help: a 'routine' case of acute pulmonary oedema is enough work for two doctors in the initial resuscitation phase. Always aim for the hypothetical optimum care scenario: i.e. pretend that the patient is a loved relative.

If the patient is critical and unstable, call the arrest team before it happens. The patient is much more likely to do better if you prevent the crash. Thus, if there is any problem with:

Airway	Care prevents death
Breathing	Noting oximetry, respiratory rate
Circulation	Early and adequate resuscitation
Consciousness	Even GCS 15 can be seriously ill

the patient should be in a resuscitation area with sufficient doctors and nurses. The 'drama' phase lasts only a few minutes and staff can return to their other patients as soon as you have control of ABCs.

Law 3: Be flexible

Many sick patients defy any discrete label or have a diagnosis backed up by clearly abnormal tests. Follow your clinical impression, keep looking and be prepared to be surprised and change your management direction. If in doubt, observe.

Do not feed the lawyers

1. See above.
2. Never openly criticise colleagues or management—you rarely have all the facts, let alone know the other side's reasons.
3. Respect the effort of the healthcare workers. Do not talk shop (i.e. the imperfect world of health care and mistakes or problems) in public. It makes it worse for everybody. If there are problems, use the system/process to improve it, i.e. be constructive—there is always someone to discuss a problem and give advice on how to tackle it and achieve improvement.
4. Always find out early what the patient, relatives, GP etc expect or want, especially if it is not clear what the problem is or why they came. You will make a lot of people happy with your service, even if it is only an explanation of why you cannot meet their immediate perceived need. You will also save a lot of time and expense.

26 Neurological emergencies

Donald S Pryor

COMA OR IMPAIRED CONSCIOUSNESS

Causes

1. Lesions of the brainstem.
2. Mass lesions causing secondary pressure on the brainstem.
3. Diffuse disease affecting the whole cortex bilaterally as well as the brainstem: e.g. trauma, epilepsy, meningitis, drugs, metabolic abnormalities including hypoglycaemia.

Initial assessment

Ensure vital functions are maintained.

1. Clear airway.
2. Assist ventilation if necessary.
3. Pulse and blood pressure—note that slow pulse and high blood pressure result from raised intracranial pressure.

History

Available information may be limited and a telephone call to family, neighbour, general practitioner, workplace, police etc. can be invaluable.

Examination

1. Document level of consciousness in terms of the Glasgow Coma Score (see Table 15.3, Chapter 15).
2. Palpate skull and neck, particularly for signs of trauma. Test for neck stiffness and Kernig's sign.
3. General examination:
   a. Respiratory pattern—obstruction or inhalation signs or diagnostic clues like Cheyne-Stokes or central hyperventilation.
   b. Deep body temperature—an axillary thermometer will usually grossly underestimate severe hypothermia or hyperthermia.
   c. Signs of intravenous drug use, malnutrition, chronic liver or renal disease, cyanosis, pallor or purpura.
   d. Urine analysis—catheterisation may be indicated to obtain urine for testing. It may also be indicated to monitor urinary output and for nursing reasons. As well as looking for glucose and ketones, consider saving the first urine for microscopy and drug screening.
4. Eye movements: these test brainstem control mechanisms and cranial nerves III, IV and VI.
   a. Position of eyes at rest may show a defect: failing to turn to the haemiplegic side in a hemispheric lesion; the opposite way in a pontine lesion.
   b. Functioning system: twitching of the eyes to the twitching side in focal fitting, ocular bobbing indicating a pontine lesion.
   c. Reflex movements:
      • Oculocephalic (doll's head), the eye movements induced by sharply turning the head.
      • Oculovestibular (ice-cold caloric testing) causing conjugate deviation to cold stimulus.
5. Pupils: size and reaction to light of each pupil may demonstrate third cranial nerve lesion of transtentorial herniation or brain death; small pupils indicate a pontine lesion.

   a. Drugs like atropine, high-dose barbiturate and hypothermia can fix and dilate the pupils. Opiates constrict them.

   b. Do not be tricked by mydriatic eye drops put in by another doctor.

6. Fundi—papilloedema (may be difficult to confirm or exclude); usually indicates raised intracranial pressure.

   a. Preretinal (subhyaloid) haemorrhage usually means subarachnoid haemorrhage.

   b. Hypertensive or diabetic retinopathy.

7. Motor signs: after noting posture and movements check:

   a. Tone—classically increased in central nervous system (CNS) lesions (upper motor neurone) but with acute CNS damage decreased tone is usual.

   b. Tendon reflexes—classically increased in CNS lesions; may be absent or reduced with an acute lesion.

   c. The plantar responses—may initially be absent rather than extensor.

Note: Decerebrate posturing may be confused with purposive movements. Drug effects and hypoglycaemia may mimic focal neurological lesions.

Investigations and management

Initial investigations

1. Blood count, electrolytes, glucose, urea, creatinine, liver function tests, calcium.
2. Blood and urine drug screen.
3. Arterial blood gases and pH.
4. Cerebral CT scans and chest X-ray.
5. ECG and monitoring.

Initial management

1. Attend to ventilation and oxygenation.
2. Treat circulatory failure. Establish a reliable venous access line.
3. Test blood glucose level to exclude hypoglycaemia.
4. Naloxone 0.4 mg intravenously, up to 2 mg over 10 minutes, if there is evidence of narcosis such as respiratory depression or pinpoint pupils.
5. Give 100 mg thiamine IV if there is uncertainty as to the cause of coma or any suspicion of chronic alcoholism.
6. Treat fits (see below).
7. Raised intracranial pressure is usually an indication for immediate neurosurgical consultation. Treatment to gain time for definitive surgery may be with:

   a. Passive hyperventilation to a PCO_2 of about 35 mmHg.

   b. Mannitol 20% (0.5–1.0 g/kg) by intravenous infusion over 20 minutes has an immediate effect which persists for hours.

    c. In proven cerebral tumours dexamethasone 12 mg IV—effect not apparent for hours, but has the potential for long-term use.
8. Monitor neurological signs half-hourly with the Glasgow Coma Score.
9. General care of coma patient for airway, hydration, urine output, temperature control, chest physiotherapy, skin pressure areas—regular turning—eyes, mouth.

Specific investigations

1. Electroencephalography (EEG) is particularly useful in continuous partial epilepsy, metabolic coma, herpes simplex encephalitis and drug withdrawal states.
2. Lumbar puncture (LP). Clinical signs of raised intracranial pressure such as impaired consciousness level, papilloedema or focal neurological signs contraindicate lumbar puncture without first seeing the cerebral CT scans.

EPILEPSY

Fits are usually self-limiting and no urgent drug treatment is needed.
    During fits (Figure 26.1):

1. Immediate care should be directed to minimising injury from burns, cuts, falls or drowning.
2. Observe the features of the fit. Classification as generalised or partial etc depends on the description and influences management. Pseudoseizures are common and are often hard to recognise.
3. Turn semi-prone and clear airway as soon as tonic phase and clonic movements cease.
4. Do not put anything between the teeth during a fit, because:
    a. The cyanosis often present is due to cessation of respiration rather than airway obstruction.
    b. You probably cannot prevent damage to the tongue (which always heals).
    c. You may cause broken teeth (which do not heal).
    d. You risk bitten fingers.

After the fit:

1. Is there a history of fits?
2. If there is a history, check the medications—what anticonvulsants have been prescribed? What anticonvulsants have been omitted? Take blood for anticonvulsant assay and blood glucose.
3. Advise maintenance anticonvulsant dosage until return to the doctor responsible for long-term management.
4. If there is no history of fits, first-ever fit patients deserve other relevant blood tests such as blood count, biochemistry, serology, drug screen or even porphyrins.

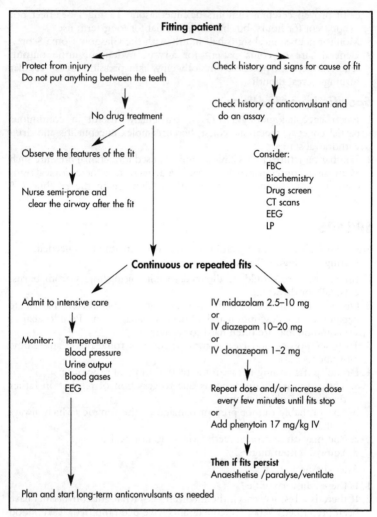

Figure 26.1 Management of the fitting patient

Prolonged or frequent fitting (status epilepticus)

Partial seizures may be prolonged or frequently recurrent without major hazard. Major generalised seizures lasting more than 5–10 minutes or recurring rapidly are life-threatening. This situation demands prompt and adequate IV drug therapy, monitoring and support. Arrange transfer to an intensive care area while commencing drug treatment. Establish IV access and give:

1. Midazolam 2.5 mg IV with repeated bolus doses up to 10 mg (0.2 mg/kg for a child). IM or intranasal administration can be used if venous access is difficult. Alternatives to midazolam are:
   - Diazepam 10–20 mg by slow IV bolus, repeated if necessary (child 0.1–0.25 mg/kg).
   - Clonazepam 1–2 mg bolus IV (child 0.25–0.5 mg bolus).
2. If necessary add phenytoin 17 mg/kg IV at no more than 50 mg/min (if not already taking phenytoin). For a child 20 mg/kg IV at no more than 25 mg/min. Do not use by IM injection.
   - Alternative to phenytoin is fosphenytoin.

Then:

3. Anaesthetise (thiopentone), paralyse and ventilate the patient in an intensive care area. Do not allow fits to continue for hours while giving low or moderate doses of various anticonvulsant drugs.
4. Monitor temperature, oxygenation, acidosis, hydration, urine output, serum electrolytes and EEG.
5. Review possible causes for the fits and adjust maintenance therapy as after a single fit (above).

CEREBROVASCULAR DISEASE

Stroke is either cerebral infarction or haemorrhage. CT scans clearly show haemorrhage immediately but the signs of infarction are usually delayed for several hours. Subarachnoid haemorrhage can be considered separately.

A sudden neurological deficit in someone aged over 60 years is likely to be a stroke. However, examination of the clinical features to attempt to predict the site of the lesion (e.g. brainstem or hemisphere) and the pathology (infarct or haemorrhage) may lead to an alternative diagnosis or help to reveal a treatable cause (such as infective endocarditis or thrombotic disorder).

Transient ischaemic attack is artificially defined according to the duration of the symptoms and needs to be managed as for ischaemic brain injury causing infarction.

Cerebral infarction

Evaluation

1. Clinical localisation of the lesion:
   a. Cortex—dysphasia, sensory inattention—embolism likely.
   b. Internal capsule—pure motor haemiplegia—hypertensive lacunar infarction likely.

    c. Brainstem—bilateral motor signs, sensory loss, vertigo/nystagmus, coma, ataxia, cranial nerve signs—vertebrobasilar system disease.
2. Clinical diagnosis of pathophysiology:
    a. Is it intracranial arterial occlusion due to atheroma, hypertension, diabetes? *or*
    b. Neck vessel disease with embolism—carotid bruit? *or*
    c. Embolism from the heart—e.g. atrial fibrillation, prosthetic valve, infective endocarditis, recent myocardial infarction?

Investigations

Except in the very ill or very old patient, cerebral CT scans are indicated. Perform full blood count (FBC), erythrocyte sedimentation rate (ESR), electrolytes, creatinine, blood glucose level, cholesterol, urinalysis, ECG and chest X-ray. Infarction is best shown on CT scans a few days after onset. Scans can be delayed until then, or repeated then, to document the extent of the lesion. The need for contrast scans depends on the individual case.

    Perform transthoracic echocardiography and carotid Doppler ultrasound studies. Transoesophageal echocardiography may be needed as well.

    Magnetic resonance imaging (MRI) and magnetic resonance angiography can replace CT scans and carotid ultrasound when available. MRI can show infarction immediately after a stroke and can identify a new from an old infarct. Small lesions and brainstem lesions invisible in CT scans can be seen with MRI.

Treatment

1. Monitor the **blood pressure** but do not treat hypertension during the first 24 hours after a cerebral infarct. Rapid blood pressure reduction is known to be hazardous at this time and is not known to be of any benefit except in the presence of other complications, such as hypertensive encephalopathy or left ventricular failure. The perfusion pressure to ischaemic brain in the hours following an infarct may depend on systemic hypertension. Established drug treatment for hypertension should be continued. Acute blood pressure elevation may denote raised intracranial pressure
2. **Hydration.** Until it is established that swallowing is safe, a 'nil by mouth' order is applied. IV fluids without glucose are given to correct dehydration at presentation and provide maintenance fluid and electrolytes. Planning of oral intake or IV or nasogastric fluids and feeding needs daily review.
3. **Bladder catheterisation** may be needed to assist nursing care of pressure areas.
4. **Emotional support** and added encouragement from nurses and relatives, as well as the company of other patients in the ward, should be considered.
5. **Passive and active limb movements** can be commenced immediately.

6. **Subcutaneous heparin and compression stockings** are usually used for prophylaxis against venous thrombosis.
7. **Reduction of raised intracranial pressure** is rarely indicated.

Fibrinolysis

Intravenous (within 3 hours of the onset) or intraarterial fibrinolytic treatment is being used in many centres.

Preventing further infarction

1. Treat the underlying cause if possible:
   a. Low-dose aspirin—100–150 mg per day—should be given immediately. Additional antiplatelet therapy with dipyridamole or clopidogrel can be considered after the first few days.
   b. Anticoagulation with heparin or warfarin should not be given in the first few days for fear of haemorrhagic transformation of the infarct. Warfarin is protective in the long term with atrial fibrillation and in other cardiac disease-causing embolisms.

Cerebral ischaemia (transient ischaemic attack—TIA)

This subgroup with little or no infarction deserves the same prophylactic management with at least the same urgency as bigger strokes. Hospital admission may be needed to avoid any delay. Prompt CT scans, neck and heart ultrasound studies and blood tests, as listed above for cerebral infarction investigations.

The clinical diagnosis of TIA is intended to identify patients with platelet or cholesterol microemboli arising in neck vessel atheroma. These attacks last only a few minutes. The World Health Organization (WHO) definition of 'less than 24 hours' duration' lacks clinical or pathogenic significance.

Diagnostic mistakes are more likely than with completed stroke. A history of transient monocular visual loss is very suggestive of carotid artery stenosis.

Listen for a carotid bruit. Look for microemboli in the retinal vessels.

Stroke in evolution

In this subgroup the neurological deficit worsens under observation, lending great urgency to any prophylactic therapy. Management is the same as for other patterns of cerebral ischaemia. Heparin is often used but its value is not established.

Cerebral haemorrhage

This is less common than infarction. Severe headache, marked hypertension or existing anticoagulant therapy may suggest haemorrhage, but the clinical signs do not distinguish from infarction.

Evaluation

1. Clinical localisation as for infarction. Sudden vertigo before losing consciousness may indicate cerebellar haemorrhage.
2. Acute haemorrhage is easily recognised as a radiodense area in CT scans. Clinically, infarction and haemorrhage are not distinguishable.
3. Hypertensive intracerebral haemorrhage will usually be in the internal capsule/striatum or pons. Intracerebral haematoma from a berry aneurysm will arise from near the circle of Willis and peripheral haematomas suggest amyloid angiopathy.

Investigations

Prompt CT scans are needed to confirm diagnosis and localisation. Perform FBC, ESR, electrolytes, creatinine, blood glucose level, ECG and chest X-ray (CXR). MRI and contrast cerebral angiography may be needed to define suspected aneurysm or arteriovenous malformation.

Treatment

1. Control blood pressure with caution. Do not suddenly lower blood pressure as cerebral perfusion may be compromised.
2. Hydration: nil by mouth until swallowing is safe. Give IV fluids. Fluid restriction may be needed, as syndrome of inappropriate antidiuretic hormone secretion (SIADH) is common.
3. Care of pressure areas; bladder catheter if needed.
4. Emotional support and encouragement from nurses and relatives and the company of other patients in the ward should be considered.
5. Passive and active limb movements can be commenced immediately.
6. Raised intracranial pressure may need specific treatment. Surgical drainage may be life-saving for cerebellar haematoma. It is of no certain benefit in intracerebral hemisphere haematomas.

Subarachnoid haemorrhage

Sudden onset of headache with meningism is classical but any new headache should be suspected of being a subarachnoid haemorrhage. It is often due to a ruptured berry aneurysm and sometimes to a vascular malformation.

Even without meningism, drowsiness, coma, confusion, vomiting or focal signs (such as hemiparesis or dysphasia) suggest subarachnoid haemorrhage. Absence of physical signs such as papilloedema or neck stiffness cannot exclude subarachnoid haemorrhage. Migraine is not a likely diagnosis in a first-time severe headache.

Evaluation

Document level of consciousness and any focal neurological signs that can result from a major intracerebral haematoma in addition to the subarachnoid blood or spasm of the affected arteries with resultant ischaemia.

Papilloedema may be present. Preretinal (subhyaloid) haemorrhage is virtually diagnostic. A cranial bruit may indicate an arteriovenous malformation. Hypertension, polycystic disease and aortic coarctation are associated with berry aneurysms.

Monoamine oxidase therapy or illicit drug use may result in acute hypertension with subarachnoid haemorrhage.

Investigations

Cerebral CT scans usually show the blood and may indicate the cause, but small amounts of blood will not be detected. Negative scans can result in the first few hours after the bleed or after more than 24 hours.

FBC, ESR, electrolytes, creatinine, blood glucose level, ECG and CXR are relevant.

Lumbar puncture may be necessary if CT scans do not provide a diagnosis. There is a small risk of coning in the absence of focal signs when intracranial pressure is raised. Small numbers of red cells or xanthochromia cannot be diagnosed without lumbar puncture. Delay for 6–12 hours from the onset will minimise false-negative findings.

Angiography will be necessary if surgical treatment is possible and its timing will be planned with the neurosurgeon. SIADH, temporary hyperglycaemia and cardiac tachyarrhythmias may complicate the bleed.

Treatment

1. Relieve headache and restlessness. Use diazepam for sedation, narcotic analgesia for headache.
2. Keep blood pressure down until the aneurysm is clipped.
3. Restrict fluids to 1200–1500 mL per day.
4. Antispasm drug treatment (nimodipine) is usual.
5. Monitor neurological signs.
6. Bed rest in dark quiet room.
7. Surgical obliteration of the aneurysm or excision of or embolisation of an arteriovenous malformation is safest, if possible.

HEADACHE

Raised intracranial pressure

This can cause only mild or moderate headache even when coning and death are imminent. Headache is provoked by coughing, straining or bending.

Headache, vomiting and papilloedema are the cardinal features, but each may be absent, despite high pressure. The absence of papilloedema does not exclude raised intracranial pressure.

Bradycardia and arterial hypertension are signs of raised intracranial pressure.

Finally, shift of brainstem and associated structures results in:

1. Drowsiness and coma.

2. Third nerve palsy—fixed dilated pupil, ophthalmoplegia.
3. Sixth nerve palsy.
4. Hemiplegia.
5. Decorticate or decerebrate postures.
6. Respiratory arrest.

Investigations

1. Urgent CT scans.
2. FBC, electrolytes and creatinine.

Treatment

1. Urgent neurosurgery for extradural or subdural haematoma or other obstructive or mass lesions. All medical services should be capable of creating burr holes in an emergency.
2. Mannitol 20% IV: 200–300 mL over 20 minutes has immediate effect, which persists for hours.
3. Passive hyperventilation to a PCO_2 of 35 mmHg.

Meningitis

Headache with fever suggests meningitis and there may be vomiting, photophobia, neck pain or stiffness, confusion, coma, irritability or fitting.

Examine for neck stiffness and Kernig's sign; purpura or hypotension in meningococcaemia; sources of infection, e.g. middle ear, sinusitis, cerebrospinal fluid (CSF) leak; or viral infection like mumps or mononucleosis.

Immune deficiency states will totally change the bacteria likely to be responsible.

Investigations

1. FBC, ESR, electrolytes, creatinine, blood glucose and CXR.
2. Blood cultures.
3. Nose, throat and ear swabs.
4. Viral cultures, viral antibody titres.
5. Cerebral CT scans may be obtained before an LP is performed. Focal neurological signs or features of raised intracranial pressure are all contraindications to LP without knowing current CT scan findings.
6. An LP is needed to confirm the diagnosis and to identify and culture the organism. It is dangerous in the presence of raised intracranial pressure.

Treatment

Give IV antibiotics as soon as the possibility of bacterial meningitis is realised. Do not wait for CT scans or LP. (Blood cultures or CSF bacterial antigen tests may assist when antibiotic treatment has rendered the CSF negative to Gram's stain and culture.)

1. Ceftriaxone 2 g IV every 12 hours (children 50 mg/kg/day).

2. Appropriate antibiotic for known organism/sensitivity, e.g. benzylpenicillin 1.2–1.8 g every 4 hours (children 350 mg/kg/day) IV for meningococcus or pneumococcus.
3. Obtain swabs and treat contacts of meningococcal and *H. influenzae* meningitis.
4. Treat disseminated intravascular coagulation, adrenal failure, SIADH and other complications.
5. Steroid therapy may have a protective role in the immediate treatment of bacterial meningitis and in tuberculous meningitis.

Encephalitis

Clinical features

Headache and fever with neurological signs or fits suggests encephalitis.

There is overlap between meningitis and encephalitis.

Encephalitis is mostly viral. Sometimes the specific virus can be identified from associated clinical features (e.g. mumps, rabies) or from laboratory tests, cultures and antibody titres, or from the epidemiology (e.g. Murray Valley encephalitis).

Only herpes simplex encephalitis demands early diagnosis, as treatment is life-saving.

Immunocompromised patients can present with parasitic or fungal as well as viral infections, e.g. *Toxoplasma*, cytomegalovirus, progressive multifocal leukoencephalopathy.

Beware of acute adrenocortical failure, which may simulate encephalitis.

Investigations

1. FBC, ESR, electrolytes, creatinine, blood glucose level and CXR.
2. Viral cultures and antibody titres.
3. Cerebral CT scan.
4. EEG.
5. Lumbar puncture—cells, protein, glucose, viral cultures and antibody titres, and polymerase chain reaction (PCR) for herpes simplex virus.

Treatment

Specific treatment is not available except for herpes simplex encephalitis, which responds to acyclovir 10 mg/kg in IV infusions every 8 hours for 10 days. Each dose must be infused over not less than 1 hour. This drug should be commenced urgently on suspicion of herpes simplex encephalitis: i.e. clinical encephalitis with cells in the CSF—do not wait for characteristic CT scan or EEG features to develop.

Subarachnoid haemorrhage

This should be considered in any new headache as the diagnosis is often missed. (See above under 'Cerebrovascular disease', and Chapter 15.)

Migraine

Major but temporary neurological signs may result from migraine, causing diagnostic problems, e.g. aphasia, hemiplegia.

Investigations will be normal and should be planned to exclude diseases which may be suggested by the clinical features—subarachnoid haemorrhage, meningitis etc.

Although not life-threatening, migraine causes great suffering. It is difficult to assess in the emergency situation.

When the diagnosis is secure, treat as listed below with oral or injected anti-emetics, simple oral analgesics and/or NSAIDs or oral or nasal triptans. Also parenteral sedation (e.g. diazepam) can be useful. Narcotics should not be used.

Treatment

1. Soluble aspirin 600–900 mg for an adult, repeat 4-hourly *or* paracetamol 1–1.5 g 4-hourly, up to 4 g/day.

Then add, if necessary:

2. Metoclopramide 10 mg or domperidone 20 mg orally.
3. For nausea or vomiting give prochlorperazine 12.5–25 mg rectally or 5 mg orally *or*
   parenteral metoclopramide 5–10 mg.
4. NSAIDS can be an alternative:
   - naproxen sodium 750 mg orally *or*
   - ibuprofen 800–1200 mg orally *or*
   - ketoprofen 100 mg rectally

If previous experience with these measures has failed:

5. sumatriptan 50–100 mg orally *or*
   sumatriptan 10–20 mg intranasally *or*
   naratriptan 2.5 mg orally *or*
   zolmitriptan 2.5–5 mg orally

If previous experience with these has also failed, consider:

6. dihydroergotamine 0.5–1 mg SC or IM *or*
   sumatriptan 6 mg SC.

Ergotamine is not listed here, as it needs to be given before the headache is established and after emergency presentation it is too late. Note that repeated doses of ergotamine or concomitant use of macrolide antibiotic can cause serious vasospasm. Rebound headache in overuse of ergotamine can be a problem. Ergotamine and a triptan should not be used within 24 hours of each other.

Giant cell arteritis (temporal arteritis)

This disorder needs urgent diagnosis and steroid treatment. It occurs in older people (over 50 years) and headache may be the only symptom. The

ESR is usually high. Clinical or histological evidence of superficial temporal artery disease may be absent.

Investigations

Urgent ESR and temporal artery biopsy.

Treatment

If the clinical diagnosis is likely, commence steroid therapy with prednisone 75 mg orally. The first dose of steroids can be given before the temporal artery biopsy to avoid delay. Reduce the dose rapidly to 25 mg/day and arrange for long-term therapy.

Acute glaucoma

May present with headache and vomiting.

Other

Very many other diseases of the ears, eyes, nose, sinuses, teeth and temporomandibular joints may cause head pain.

PARAPLEGIA

Acute paraparesis or paraplegia is an emergency, as any delay in treatment may cause irreversible spinal cord damage. Obviously mild or early cord lesions due to compression are most likely to benefit from prompt diagnosis and decompression and just such cases are more likely to be misdiagnosed.

Clinical features

Motor

Weakness in the legs presents as difficulty walking. There is a pyramidal pattern of weakness (flexors and abductors more than and before extensors). Spasticity may be present.

Tendon reflexes are increased with extensor plantar responses but in an acute cord lesion upper motor neurone signs may be absent. There may be flaccid paralysis with absent reflexes (spinal shock).

Flexor spasms can be mistaken for voluntary movements.

Sensory

Numbness or paraesthesias start in the feet regardless of the level of the lesion. Only when the damage has progressed will a distinct sensory level clearly indicate the segment of cord involved.

In spinal cord disease look for the highest abnormal signs. Minor abnormalities in the arms or a Horner's syndrome indicate that the disease is in the neck, when most of the deficit may still be in the legs.

Autonomic

Careful interrogation is often necessary to reveal significant symptoms in early cord lesions.

1. Constipation—insidious changes in bowel habit occur in subacute or chronic lesions.
2. Urgency of micturition is often admitted only after leading questions. Retention of urine in severe lesions is revealed by a palpable bladder. The retained volume should be recorded if a catheter is passed. Retention with overflow (palpable bladder and large volume on catheterisation or ultrasound) should not be confused with simple incontinence.
3. Erectile impotence may be revealed only on specific enquiry.

Investigations

1. FBC, ESR, electrolytes, creatinine, liver function tests (LFTs), CXR and plain X-rays of cervical and thoracic spine.
2. Myelography or MRI is urgent if there is any possibility of cord compression.
   a. The myelogram must extend to the foramen magnum if the compression is not apparent lower—even without clinical features of a high cord lesion.
   b. Make sure the radiologist knows the possible levels for the lesion. The cord ends opposite the first lumbar vertebra (L1), so clinical upper motor neurone signs mean disease in cervical or thoracic spinal canal, and radiological signs in the lumbar and sacral spine are probably not relevant.
   c. Make sure the CSF obtained is examined by the pathology laboratory.
3. CT scans can show the lesion, particularly if the exact level is known, but MRI or myelography is needed to exclude any compressive lesion. CT scans, after contrast has been injected for myelography, may contribute details of the lesion.
4. Magnetic resonance imaging replaces myelography in spinal cord disorders if it is available.

Treatment

Emergency surgery to decompress the cord is the important measure to consider.

Bladder care is also an urgent matter. Failure to relieve retention by catheter will damage the bladder. Leave an indwelling catheter draining.

Nursing and medical care is a specialised problem, and transfer to a special unit should be arranged without delay in acute or severe paraplegia.

CONFUSION
Clinical features
Document conscious state, behavioural and emotional disturbance, impairment of thought processes, disorientation, confabulation, delusions, hallucinations.

Differential diagnosis
Exclude focal cerebral disorder—especially dysphasia.

Acute confusion

1. Systemic infection—pneumonia, septicaemia.
2. Cerebral infection—meningitis, encephalitis, acquired immuno-deficiency syndrome (AIDS dementia complex).
3. Epilepsy—post-ictal, complex partial or absence status.
4. Metabolic—hypoglycaemia, uraemia, hepatic failure, hypercalcaemia.
5. Cerebral hypoxia—systemic hypoxia, hypotension, hyperviscosity.
6. Subarachnoid haemorrhage.
7. Cerebral tumour—including subdural haematoma.
8. Post-traumatic concussion.
9. Transient global amnesia.
10. Endocrine: hypothyroidism, hyperthyroidism, hyperglycaemia, hypoglycaemia, acute adrenocortical failure.
11. Toxic—alcohol (Wernicke's, delirium tremens), barbiturates and sedatives, anxiolytics, antiparkinsonian drugs, illegal drugs.
12. Deficiency states—thiamine, vitamin B_{12}.

Chronic confusion

1. Dementia—Alzheimer's disease.
2. Vascular disease—multi-infarct dementia.
3. Cerebral tumour—including subdural haematoma.
4. Chronic encephalitis/meningitis—viral, syphilitic, AIDS.
5. Communicating hydrocephalus.
6. Metabolic—uraemia, hepatic, electrolyte disturbance.
7. Endocrine—hypothyroidism.
8. Toxic—drugs, alcohol, Korsakoff's psychosis.
9. Pseudodementia due to psychiatric disorder.

Acute-on-chronic confusion

Usually an underlying dementia complicated by infection, drug toxicity or psychosocial disruption.

Management

1. Neurological and general physical examination.
2. Exclude infection in lungs or meninges, hypoxia.
3. FBC, ESR.
4. Electrolytes, creatinine, blood glucose levels, liver function tests, calcium, HIV, syphilis test (VDRL).
5. Midstream urine (MSU), blood cultures.
6. CXR, arterial blood gases/pH.
7. Vitamin B_{12}, folate, thyroid function.
8. Drug screen—urine and blood.
9. IV thiamine 100 mg.
10. EEG.
11. Cerebral CT scans or MRI.

RECOMMENDED READING

Adams RD, Victor M, Ropper AH. Principles of neurology. 7th edn. New York: McGraw-Hill; 2001.
Longmore JM. Oxford handbook of clinical medicine. 5th edn. New York: Oxford University Press; 2001.
Therapeutic guidelines: neurology. Version 2. 2002.

27 Gastrointestinal emergencies

Greg McDonald

The aim of emergency department assessment of patients with gastrointestinal emergencies is rapidly to detect and stabilise those patients requiring urgent surgical or procedural intervention. In pursuing this aim, the processes of assessment, investigations appropriate to the disease and management should be followed in an orderly and purposeful manner and must be performed simultaneously in the seriously ill.

ACUTE ABDOMEN

The priorities of treatment of the 'acute abdomen' follow the aims above. Having excluded a life-threatening cause of abdominal pain and resuscitated the patient as needed, decide whether in-hospital investigation and management is required. It should be remembered that up to one-third of patients with abdominal pain seen in the emergency department will have a final diagnosis of 'abdominal pain of uncertain cause'.

Assessment

History

Who is your patient? Age and sex are two important aetiological factors. Patients over the age of 65 years are twice as likely as younger patients to require surgical intervention.

Gynaecological disorders obviously need to be excluded in women, particularly in their child-bearing years. Women are also more likely to have a final 'uncertain' diagnosis. Previous medical and surgical histories and a drug history will give important clues to diagnosis and need to be considered for operative fitness.

When did the pain start? Acute onset of severe pain implies vascular events, perforated viscus or renal colic. Inflammatory causes tend to arise more slowly.

Where is the pain? Has it moved? Initial visceral pain is usually diffuse and in the midline. Later somatic pain localises better to the site of pathology.

What is the pain like? The colicky pain of bowel obstruction is typically episodic and gripping, with pain-free intervals. In the case of biliary and renal colic there is a constant pain rising to a crescendo. Constant severe pain indicates advanced or serious illness. Remember, only two-thirds of patients with acute surgical conditions have a 'typical' history of illness.

Which other symptoms accompany this illness? The onset of nausea and vomiting after the onset of pain suggests surgical illness. Constipation is non-specific but absolute constipation (neither faeces nor flatus) indicates bowel obstruction. Diarrhoea, jaundice, haematuria, haematemesis or melaena lead to specific diagnoses.

Examination

General

Appearance is apprehensive and motionless with peritonitis, unsettled and agitated with colicky pain, and pale and 'Hippocratic' with advanced disease. Check temperature, hydration, pulse and blood pressure (with postural drop).

Abdomen

1. Inspection—rigid • distended or scaphoid • visible peristalsis • operative scars.
2. Palpation—guarding • diffuse or local tenderness • rebound tenderness. (*Note:* 'Rebound' is not pathognomonic of peritonitis. It gives a false-positive in up to one-quarter of patients and is an observer-dependent sign. Cough and percussion tenderness are often more reliable.)

3. Percussion—local peritonism • air • fluid • masses • organs. *Note:* Loss of liver dullness with pneumoperitoneum.
4. Auscultation—peristaltic noises coinciding with colic in small bowel obstruction • diffuse increased bowel sounds in gastroenteritis • silent abdomen or occasional tinkling sounds in late bowel obstruction or diffuse peritonitis.

Special signs
1. Murphy's sign in cholecystitis • Rovsing's, psoas and obturator signs in appendicitis • Cullen's and Grey Turner's signs in pancreatitis • costo-vertebral tenderness with pyelonephritis or perinephric abscess.
2. Hernial orifices/scrotum and testes should never be forgotten.
3. Rectal examination is also mandatory • blood (bright, melaena or occult) • diffuse or local tenderness • masses • prostatomegaly.
4. Pelvic examination: incorrect and uncertain diagnoses occur much more frequently in women. A careful vaginal examination will help differentiate pelvic pathology. (*Note:* Cervical excitation is a classic sign of ectopic pregnancy and pelvic inflammatory disease but is an observer-dependent sign.)

OTHER SYSTEMS

Exclude non-abdominal pathology causing abdominal pain, e.g. pneumonia, pulmonary embolus and myocardial infarction. Assess operative fitness.

Investigations

Immediate
1. Urine—urine analysis • microscopy and culture* • pregnancy test*.
2. Blood—haemoglobin • haematocrit (PCV) • white cell count and differential • electrolytes, urea and creatinine • amylase/lipase*, blood gases* • group and hold serum/crossmatch (if operation likely).
3. Stool—occult blood.
4. Organ imaging—abdominal X-ray, supine and erect • chest X-ray, erect.

Semi-urgent (with appropriate indications)
1. Blood—liver function tests • coagulation studies.
2. Stool—smear and culture.
3. Organ imaging—abdominal ultrasound/CT scan • intravenous pyelogram • angiography.
4. Endoscopy—proctosigmoidoscopy • panendoscopy.

Value of investigations
All investigations should be used as adjuncts to clinical assessment—they do not make the diagnosis for the clinician.

If appropriate.

1. **Pregnancy** should be considered and excluded in all women of child-bearing years with acute abdominal pain. White cell count is non-specific unless a marked neutrophilia (over $20 \times 10^9/L$) is present. It is often a late manifestation of significant pathology.

2. **Serum amylase** is frequently elevated in a variety of surgical conditions. Levels greater than three times normal strongly suggest pancreatitis. Lipase is more sensitive and specific for pancreatitis and is the test of choice for this disease.

3. **Abdominal X-rays** are a poor tool for diagnosing non-specific abdominal pain, but are valuable in confirming specific and serious pathology. Bowel obstruction, paralytic ileus, caecal and sigmoid volvulus have typical findings. A paucity of bowel gas may be the only clue to mesenteric infarction. Don't forget to check the psoas shadows, the size and shape of solid organs, for calculi and for air in the biliary tree. Avoid abdominal X-rays in pregnancy if possible.

4. **Erect chest X-ray** will detect subdiaphragmatic free air, exclude pulmonary pathology and help preoperative assessment. Free air will be absent in about 20% of perforated peptic ulcers. Massive pneumoperitoneum suggests colonic perforation. The chest X-ray is the definitive investigation for Boerhaave's syndrome (oesophageal rupture).

5. **Abdominal ultrasound** is usually indicated for right upper quadrant pain and cholelithiasis, obstructive uropathy, pelvic pathology, suspected abdominal aortic aneurysm (in stable patients) and abdominal masses. Pelvic ultrasound is essential for the diagnosis of gynaecological and pregnancy-related diseases.

6. **Intravenous pyelography** is rarely indicated urgently in nontraumatic renal disease but is used semi-electively in renal colic and haematuria.

7. **CT scanning**. Spiral non-contrast CT is the initial test of choice for renal colic. Double-contrast CT is useful in diagnosing many acute surgical conditions, e.g. acute pancreatitis, intraabdominal abscess, intraabdominal trauma.

8. **Proctosigmoidoscopy** is a diagnostic tool in bright rectal bleeding, rectal mass and colitis, and is therapeutic in sigmoid volvulus.

9. **Panendoscopy** is indicated urgently in life-threatening upper gastrointestinal tract (GIT) bleeding and semi-electively in stable patients with suspected peptic ulcer or other inflammatory conditions of the upper GIT.

Management

Surgical emergency

Examples of a surgical emergency include perforated viscus, advanced peritonitis, mesenteric infarction and strangulated bowel.

Common indications for laparotomy

1. **Physical findings**. Diffuse or spreading rigidity • tense or progressive distension • increasing or severe localised tenderness and peritonism • tender abdominal mass with high fever or sepsis • equivocal clinical signs with: septicaemia; uncontrolled bleeding; suspected mesenteric ischaemia; deterioration with conservative treatment.
2. **Radiological findings.** Pneumoperitoneum • gross or progressive bowel obstruction • free contrast extravasation • suspected abscess on ultrasound/scan.
3. **Endoscopic findings**. Perforation or uncontrolled bleeding.

Preoperative treatment

1. Airway.
2. Breathing—oxygen by mask.
3. Circulation—intravenous access and appropriate blood tests • volume resuscitation • urinary catheter.
4. Analgesia should be given after medical assessment is complete and definitive treatment is established. Small increments of intravenous narcotics greatly benefit the patient and do not significantly alter findings with severe pathology.
5. Antibiotic prophylaxis is required with diffuse peritonitis or if infective pathology is suspected. Ampicillin, gentamicin and metronidazole is the usual combination therapy for intraabdominal sepsis.
6. Preoperative preparation—nasogastric tube • operative fitness • consent.

Surgical admission

Some conditions for which admission to hospital for conservative treatment, observation and semi-elective operation is appropriate are discussed later.

Emergency department observation and discharge

Patients with mild or equivocal tenderness, minor or no laboratory abnormalities and whose condition settles can be discharged for follow-up in the community, after observation in the department. Certain diagnoses, e.g. uncomplicated renal or biliary colic and peptic ulceration, are discharged in most cases for further investigations and referral.

SPECIFIC SURGICAL CONDITIONS

Acute appendicitis

This is the most common general surgical emergency. Most problems occur with extremes of age, <5 and >60 years, mostly due to atypical presentation and late diagnosis.

Assessment

1. Typical history is vague periumbilical pain, anorexia, nausea, vomiting, pain migration to right iliac fossa, fever. This occurs in only about half of cases.
2. Beware mesenteric adenitis in children and diverticular disease/caecal carcinoma in adults.
3. Clinical features—mild/moderate pyrexia • anorexia • McBurney's point tenderness and peritonism with or without mass • ruptured appendix will often have a quiet peritonitic abdomen with few localising signs.
4. Perform rectal and vaginal examinations to exclude pelvic pathology.

Investigations

1. Relatively clear-cut appendicitis—no investigations are required, other than for preoperative assessment if needed.
2. Uncertain diagnosis—urine analysis/MSU to exclude urinary tract infection • white cell count is moderately raised (10–15×10^9/mL with left shift) and is often a late indicator • AXR/CXR rarely necessary: perform only if you suspect another diagnosis or complications.
3. Ultrasound is useful in evaluating right iliac fossa pain in children and female patients if the diagnosis is uncertain.
4. Contrast helical CT is more sensitive than ultrasound and may reveal alternative diagnoses.

Management

1. Surgery as soon as practical. Overnight delay in the stable patient does not significantly worsen outcome.
2. Suspected perforation—urgent surgery.
3. Prophylactic antibiotics reduce infective complications. They should be given in the emergency department if peritonitis or abscess is suspected or if surgery will be delayed. Otherwise antibiotics can be given at induction of anaesthesia.
4. Mass/phlegmon—intravenous antibiotics and fluids • nil by mouth • ultrasound/CT scan • operation at surgeon's discretion.
5. Uncertain diagnosis—non-specific clinical findings and investigation results. Admit • nil by mouth • intravenous fluids • analgesia • close review • ultrasound/CT scan.

Acute cholecystitis

Assessment: clinical features

1. 25% of women and 12% of men have gallstones.
2. Past history of fat intolerance, eructation and flatulence.
3. Right upper quadrant pain becoming constant and severe.
4. Mild fever and tachycardia; mild icterus in 10% of cases.
5. Tender right upper quadrant with positive Murphy's sign.

6. Palpable gallbladder in about one-third of cases.
7. Empyema—toxic/shocked, high spiking temperatures.
8. Local perforation—progressing fever, symptoms and signs. Local mass and peritonism.
9. Free perforation—general peritonism.
10. Cholangitis • common duct stone • right upper quadrant pain • jaundice • fever/rigors.

Investigations

1. Urine analysis—bilirubin; exclude renal pathology.
2. White cell count—moderate neutrophilia is usual. Marked neutrophilia suggests complications.
3. Liver function tests—bilirubin >60 mmol/L suggests common duct obstruction.
4. Abdominal X-ray is often not helpful but may be ordered to exclude other pathology and complications.
5. Ultrasound demonstrates stones, debris within the gallbladder, wall thickening, masses or abscesses.
6. HIDA isotope scan may be used if the ultrasound is non-diagnostic, e.g. acalculous cholecystitis.
7. Operative fitness assessment, e.g. ECG, CXR, Hb, renal function.

Management

Uncomplicated biliary colic

Discharge home for outpatient investigation and referral if: pain resolves • no significant local signs • normal laboratory investigations.

Cholecystitis/cholangitis

1. Admit to hospital.
2. Nil by mouth and intravenous fluids.
3. Analgesia.
4. Antibiotics intravenously (ampicillin/gentamicin).
5. Ultrasound, usually within 24 hours.
6. Endoscopic retrograde cholangiopancreatography (ERCP) if obstructing bile duct stone.
7. Early cholecystectomy when condition settles.

Advanced/complicated disease

Examples of this are empyema, abscess, free perforation, septicaemia.
1. Rapid stabilisation and assessment.
2. Antibiotics (ampicillin, gentamicin and metronidazole or equivalents).
3. Urgent cholecystectomy or cholecystostomy.

Diverticular disease

Fifty per cent of people over 40 years of age have diverticulae.

Assessment

1. Previous history—irregular bowel habit • diffuse, non-specific lower abdominal pain.
2. Diverticulitis—fever • altered bowel habit • left iliac fossa (LIF) pain and tenderness with or without local peritonism • LIF or pelvic mass.
3. Diverticular abscess—toxic • palpable mass.
4. Free perforation—generalised peritonitis.
5. Bleeding (see 'Lower GIT bleeding' below).

Investigations

1. Urine analysis and midstream urine (MSU).
2. White cell count.
3. Occult blood.
4. Sigmoidoscopy.
5. Abdominal X-ray is usually non-specific, but will reveal perforation, local or generalised ileus or large mass.
6. Ultrasound/contrast CT scan to distinguish abscess.

Management

1. Diverticulitis—admit • nil by mouth • intravenous fluids • intravenous antibiotics (second-generation cephalosporin).
2. Complicated/severe disease (e.g. advancing peritonitis)—as above • triple antibiotic regimen (ampicillin/gentamicin/metronidazole or equivalent) • urgent surgery.

GASTROINTESTINAL BLEEDING

Upper GIT bleeding

Aetiology

1. 50% peptic ulceration.
2. 25% erosive gastritis/oesophagitis/duodenitis.
3. 15% oesophageal varices.
4. 5% Mallory-Weiss syndrome.
5. 5% others (tumour, blood dyscrasias etc).

Note: 30% of patients with known varices will bleed from other non-variceal causes.

Assessment

History

1. Amount and nature of bleeding (haematemesis/melaena).
2. Symptoms of occult bleeding.
3. Drug history—alcohol • non-steroidal anti-inflammatories • steroids.
4. Past GIT disease/other conditions.

Examination/immediate intervention

1. Airway.
2. Breathing—oxygen by mask.
3. Circulation—pallor/shock • pulse/blood pressure with postural drop • intravenous access: one or two large-bore cannulae with pump set.
4. Blood for haemoglobin • haematocrit • crossmatch • electrolytes • urea/creatinine • coagulation studies • liver function.
5. General—evidence of chronic liver disease and hepatic encephalopathy • abdominal examination including rectal exam with or without proctoscopy • cardiorespiratory status.

Investigations

1. Nasogastric tube for:
   a. Stable patients as a diagnostic tool if upper GIT bleeding is occult.
   b. Profuse haematemesis to empty stomach prior to endoscopy.
2. Panendoscopy is the definitive investigation and in many cases an effective immediate treatment of upper GIT bleeding. Urgent panendoscopy (within 12 hours) should be performed in cardio-vascularly unstable patients and on those with profuse or persistent bleeding. Information about the aetiology, site and prognosis of the bleeding is gained.

Management

1. Volume resuscitation with colloid and/or blood and/or clotting factors.
2. Close monitoring of vital signs, hourly urine output and haemoglobin/haematocrit. Central venous pressure (CVP) monitoring should be used in the cardiovascularly unstable patient and patients who are elderly or have cardiorespiratory disease.
3. Urgent panendoscopy on high-risk patients with: shock • blood requirements greater than 5 units • serious underlying disease • recurrent bleeding, especially if over 60 years of age.

Non-variceal bleeding

Eighty per cent of cases will settle spontaneously; 20% will require intervention for recurrent bleeding within 48 hours.

Poor prognostic endoscopic findings in non-variceal bleeding are: gastric ulcer, especially lesser wall • posterior site in duodenum • visible vessel • sentinel clot or black spot in ulcer base.

1. Further management:
   a. Notify a surgeon of high-risk patients, either on clinical criteria or endoscopic finding.
   b. Commence proton pump inhibitors: orally in most cases, intravenously in the seriously ill. There is evidence that bleeding recurrence will be reduced.
2. Definitive treatment:
   a. Endoscopic haemostasis.

b. Surgery.

c. Angiographic haemostasis (if high surgical risk).

Variceal bleeding

Poor prognostic factors include large blood requirements (over 4 units), active bleeding at endoscopy and Child's category C patients (advanced hepatic failure). Further management:

1. Endoscopic banding or sclerosis is 90% effective in controlling variceal bleeding. Balloon compression prior and/or simultaneously aids sclerotherapy.

2. Sangstaken-Blakemore/Minnesota tube—careful placement by an experienced person is necessary. Endotracheal intubation beforehand is preferred. Careful observation of position and balloon pressures with deflation at 24 hours minimise traumatic complications. About 50% of patients will rebleed within 24 hours.

3. Octreotide—lowers azygous vein blood flow in patients with portal hypertension. Dosage is 50–250 µg bolus and infusion of 50–250 µg/h.

4. Vasopressin infusion at an initial dose of 0.2–0.4 units/min controls variceal bleeding in about two-thirds of cases. Side effects include hypertension, nausea/vomiting and ischaemia of myocardium, bowel or skin. Terlipressin is a synthetic analogue that seems more effective with fewer side effects. Intercurrent vasodilator infusion (glyceryl trinitrate or nitroprusside) may be necessary to reduce complications.

(*Note:* Both points 3 and 4 are temporary measures with similar efficacy and a high incidence of rebleeding after cessation.)

5. Angiographic embolisation.

6. Transjugular intrahepatic portosystemic shunt (TIPS).

Lower GIT bleeding

Causes of profuse bright per rectal bleeding are: angiodysplasia • diverticular disease • polyps • carcinoma/colitis/solitary ulcer • Meckel's ulcer in children.

Note: Bright or maroon rectal bleeding can occur with profuse upper GIT bleed.

Assessment

History, examination and immediate intervention are as for upper GIT bleeding. Note that a high urea/creatinine ratio (>100:1) suggests an upper GIT site of bleeding.

Investigations

1. Sigmoidoscopy should be performed as the initial investigation.

2. Nasogastric tube for exclusion of upper GIT bleeding, if suspected, and/or preoperative preparation.

3. Radioisotope red cell scan or mesenteric angiography should be performed urgently if bleeding persists. A negative scan indicates bleeding rate less than 0.1 mL/min (see below, 'Further management').

Note: Barium studies have no role in the immediate assessment of severe lower GIT bleeding.

Management

1. Volume resuscitation.
2. Monitor vital signs, urine output, haemoglobin/haemocrit with or without CVP.
3. Notify surgeon.
4. Bleeding stops spontaneously in 75% of cases with conservative treatment. If bleeding is profuse or recurrent, undertake further management.

Further management

1. Negative isotope scan—semi-elective colonoscopy and/or other investigations.
2. Positive isotope scan (i.e. active bleeding)—further urgent investigation and/or treatment required.
3. Angiography—selective arterial catheterisation is 60% successful in identifying the bleeding site and allows treatment with vasopressin (temporary) or embolisation.
4. Colonoscopy has variable efficiency in brisk acute bleeding and requires experienced hands.
5. Surgery should be undertaken when the bleeding site is known and/or the above two modalities have not controlled the haemorrhage.

ACUTE PANCREATITIS

The causes of acute pancreatitis are: gallstones or alcohol (75%); idiopathic (20%); and other (5%).

Assessment

History

1. Aetiological factors.
2. Acute epigastric pain through to back associated with nausea and vomiting.

Examination/initial intervention

1. Airway.
2. Breathing oxygen by mask.
3. Circulation—shock • pulse, blood pressure with postural drop • intravenous line.
4. Blood for lipase/amylase • haemoglobin/haematocrit • electrolytes • urea/creatinine • calcium • glucose • liver function tests • arterial gases • coagulation studies • group and hold.

5. Abdominal examination—temperature, jaundice • epigastric tenderness with or without mass • local/diffuse peritonism • Cullen's (peri-umbilical) and Grey Turner's (flank) signs in haemorrhagic pancreatitis • paralytic ileus • subcutaneous fat necrosis.
6. Cardiorespiratory examination, especially to exclude complications.

Poor prognostic indicators

Ten per cent of patients have severe necrotising pancreatitis, which also may become secondarily infected. Clinical and radiological scoring can select those patients with more severe disease requiring ICU admission and consideration for CT guided drainage or surgery.

1. Ranson's criteria:
   a. Immediate—age >55 • hyperglycaemia • leukocytosis • LDH • AST.
   b. Two days—drop in haemoglobin/haematocrit • shock • hypo-calcaemia • hypoxia • azotaemia (elevated urea).
   c. Score ≥ 5 suggests serious illness.
2. APACHE score.

Investigations

1. Amylase—level more than three times normal confirms the diagnosis in the great majority of cases. Lipase is more sensitive and specific and is the test of choice.
2. Abdominal X-ray—exclude perforated peptic ulcer. Look for: pancreatic calcification/gallstones • ascites. 'Sentinel loop' is non-specific.
3. Chest X-ray—raised left hemidiaphragm • pleural effusion • atelectasis • adult respiratory distress syndrome (ARDS).
4. ECG to exclude myocardial infarct.
5. Ultrasound should be performed within 24 hours to exclude gallstones, pancreatitis.
6. CT scanning with contrast is indicated within 48 hours to assess severity.

Management

1. Volume resuscitation.
2. Supplemental oxygen.
3. Monitor observations, urine output with or without CVP.
4. Nasogastric tube for severe cases or if gastric dilation or ileus, otherwise nil by mouth.
5. Analgesia—parenteral narcotics after diagnosis is established.
6. Insulin infusion if blood sugar level >15 mmol/L.
7. Observe for other complications—shock/acidosis • acute tubular necrosis • ARDS/disseminated intravascular coagulation (DIC) • haemorrhagic pancreatitis • pancreatic abscess.
8. Early nutritional support—nasojejunal or parenteral.
9. CT-guided aspiration if abscess suspected. Laparotomy has up to 40% mortality.

10. Initial trials with platelet activating factor (PAF) antagonists suggested reduced mortality, but later trials have not confirmed any benefit.

HEPATIC FAILURE— PORTOSYSTEMIC ENCEPHALOPATHY

Fulminant

Encephalopathy, jaundice, hepatic foetor, multiple system complications.

Aetiology

1. Viral hepatitis.
2. Paracetamol overdose/CCL_4.
3. Drug reactions (eg. isoniazid, halothane, methyldopa).

Acute-on-chronic

Stigmata of chronic liver disease, jaundice, ascites, encephalopathy.

Aetiology

1. Alcoholic cirrhosis.
2. Chronic active hepatitis.
3. Postnecrotic.
4. Infiltrative.
5. Other.

Precipitating causes of encephalopathy

Fulminant

Encephalopathy from cerebral oedema is the hallmark of the disease. Coma has an 80% mortality. Can be exacerbated by the conditions listed below.

Acute-on-chronic

1. GIT bleeding (especially upper). Elevated urea/creatinine ratio is suggestive. This accounts for about 25% of cases.
2. Constipation.
3. Increased protein load.
4. Azotaemia/volume depletion—hepatorenal syndrome.
5. Hypokalaemia/alkalosis.
6. Hypoxaemia/hypoglycaemia.
7. Infection, including spontaneous bacterial peritonitis in ascites (usually coliforms or pneumococcus).
8. Ethanol, sedatives, opiates.

Assessment

History
1. Alcohol and drug history.

2. Rapidity of onset of symptoms.
3. GIT bleeding.

Examination/immediate intervention
1. Airway.
2. Breathing—oxygen by mask as necessary.
3. Intravenous access.
4. Blood for: haemoglobin/haematocrit • coagulation studies • electrolytes/urea/creatinine • calcium/phosphate/magnesium • blood sugar level • liver function tests • arterial blood gases • viral serology, drug screen, group and hold as necessary.
5. Dextrose—hypoglycaemia needs to be rapidly excluded and treated.
6. Encephalopathy—GCS • mini-mental state • Star chart • asterixis (flap).

Further examination
Foetor • evidence of chronic liver disease/ascites • liver/spleen/rectal examination • cause of likely decompensation, including rectal exam • complications (e.g. bleeding, cardiorespiratory, infectious disease, alcohol withdrawal).

Investigations
1. Septic work-up, including ascitic tap.
2. Arterial blood gases.
3. Serum ammonia (does not correlate well with severity of illness).
4. Occult blood.
5. Chest X-ray.
6. ECG.
7. CT scan and EEG to assess encephalopathy/oedema and exclude other pathology.
8. Liver biopsy in some cases.

Management
1. Treat precipitating causes, e.g. GIT bleeding, constipation, volume depletion, electrolyte abnormality, infection.
2. Reduce protein absorption—low protein diet (20–40 g/day) • oral lactulose (30–45 mL q8h) • oral neomycin (4–6 g/day) and metronidazole (250 mg q12h).
3. Other nutritional support, e.g. carbohydrates, zinc, magnesium.
4. Flumazenil to reverse intercurrent benzodiazepine ingestion. Bromocriptine may have a role in chronic encephalopathy.
5. Patients in coma will need endotracheal intubation and ICU transfer.
6. Consider radiographic occlusion of spontaneous portosystemic shunts if the patient is not responding to medical management. Surgical shunts (e.g. TIPS) may also be reversed.
7. Liver transplant in selected patients.

RECOMMENDED READING

Surgical-tutor. A free online educational student resource for undergraduate and postgraduate surgical examinations. Available: http://www. surgical-tutor.org.uk.

Marx JA, Hockberger RS, Walls RM, Adams J, eds. Rosen's emergency medicine: concepts and clinical practice. 5th edn. St Louis: Mosby; 2001.

Way LW, et al. Current surgical diagnosis and treatment. 11th edn. Norwalk: Appleton & Lange; 2001.

28 Poisoning and overdosage

Paul Preisz

Poisoning and overdosage are common clinical problems. While the diagnosis may sometimes be obvious, toxicology also forms an important part of the differential diagnosis for many patients with a wide variety of clinical presentations. Paediatric poisonings may be purely accidental or they may indicate non-accidental injury. Adult presentations may also be accidental or they may be associated with a range of psychiatric disorders and attempted suicide. Underlying drug addiction may be involved.

Table 28.1 Basic protocols in the management of overdosed patients

Safety of staff and other patients

- Precautions against contamination if indicated
- Appropriate setting and security staff if required
- Weapons search if indicated

Resuscitate

- Airway and breathing
- Haemodynamics
- Temperature

Antidotes and treatments

- Dextrose 25 g, thiamine 100 mg, naloxone 2 mg
- Oxygen
- Specific antidotes and treatments (see Table 28.4)

At present the majority of adult overdosage presentations in Australia involve alcohol, psychostimulants, benzodiazepines, sedatives, antidepressants or opiates, although a wide range of other drugs may be taken. Often more than one substance is present, and alcohol is the most common additional drug (Table 28.1).

ASSESSMENT

Assessment, basic resuscitation and supportive care will be the most important factors in the care of most patients, although specific antidotes and treatments are indicated in some cases.

History, including drugs ingested, is useful but unreliable. Details regarding the circumstances of the overdose are important and family, friends and the patient's usual doctor may need to be contacted. Many overdoses involve a drug prescribed to the patient, a relative or friend. Physical examination should begin with thorough assessment of ABCs, followed by a search for signs of recent injection and/or evidence of complications (e.g. aspiration, rhabdomyolysis). Alternative or additional diagnoses (e.g. trauma, sepsis) should also be explored.

Certain findings are helpful in establishing a diagnosis (e.g. pupils, perfusion and posture). Close monitoring and frequent reassessment are required.

A number of syndromes have been described, recognition of which may give a clue to the type of substance ingested (Table 28.2).

Investigations are tailored to suit the individual setting, and at the minimum in a sick patient should include:

- Full blood count.
- Urea, electrolytes, blood sugar level (BSL) and creatinine.
- CXR.
- ABG.

- βHCG if female.
- Paracetamol level.
- ECG.
- Troponin.
- Urinalysis.

Other investigations are guided by the clinical circumstances:

- Drug screen on urine or gastric aspirate. (Often this is not routine as it does not affect immediate management, but it is essential to have a specimen including blood for later assay if the condition remains serious.)
- Specific drug assays and levels, e.g. blood alcohol level, carbon monoxide, alcohol, paracetamol, digoxin, iron, lithium, gamma hydroxybutyrate (GHB).
- Measurements of liver and renal function.
- Creatine phosphokinase (CPK), urine myoglobin, others as indicated.
- Other X-rays, e.g. abdominal for ileus, perforation, radiopaque pills (e.g. iron), drug couriers.

See also Table 28.3.

MANAGEMENT

While resuscitation and supportive care form the mainstays of management, some specific manoeuvres can also be used to decrease drug absorption, to enhance drug elimination and to alter or negate the effects of toxic drugs or metabolites. A careful decision must be made as to whether the potential benefits of such additional treatment outweigh the added risks involved. Gastric lavage and the administration of activated charcoal in particular may confer no significant benefit in a relatively stable patient with a likely non-life-threatening overdose, particularly if the patient has presented late.

Decreasing drug absorption

Non-gastric

Many substances can be absorbed topically, most notably the organo-phosphates. Clothing should be removed and the body surface extensively washed. Staff must take precautions to avoid contaminating themselves.

Gastric

Food and other substances

The presence of food or other substances in the stomach may affect the absorption of a drug; however, this can be unpredictable. Altering gastric pH may be useful in some settings, e.g. instilling bicarbonate into the stomach after iron poisoning. Dilution of some caustic substances with milk, water or saline may also be considered as a first-aid measure.

Emesis

Emesis is used, particularly in children presenting early (<1 hour), although its efficacy has been questioned. Ipecacuanha syrup (Ipecac 6%) is the most useful agent. It should be given with at least 250 mL water, and a delay in its onset of action (up to 30 minutes) can be expected. Contraindications include: airway not secured; ingestion of low-viscosity hydrocarbons (e.g. petrol) or caustic agents;

Gastric lavage

This is also contraindicated when the airway is compromised, and in those who have ingested low-viscosity hydrocarbons or caustic agents. Treatment is more likely to be effective if begun early (<1 hour) using a large-bore (36 Fr) orogastric tube. Having aspirated the stomach contents via the tube, 1 mL/kg tepid water (normal saline in children) is instilled and then removed. This is repeated until at least 5 litres have been used and the return is clear. To avoid accidental fluid overload, lavage is stopped if there is a net loss of 500 mL or more.

Charcoal

Activated charcoal has a large surface area and high adsorptive power. It is a fine, black, odourless powder which is insoluble, but readily forms a suspension in liquids. The dose required depends on the amount of drug

Table 28.2 Syndromes identified in poisoning and overdosage

Syndrome	Features	Examples
Hyperthermia	Increased core temperature	Cocaine, PCP, neuroleptics, salicylates, tricyclics, serotonin uptake inhibitors
Hypothermia	Decreased core temperature	CNS depressants, exposure
Cholinergic	Defecation/urination, meiosis, bradycardia, emesis, lacrimation, secretions	Organophosphates, toxic mushrooms
Anticholinergic	Dry eyes/mouth/skin, urinary retention, decreased bowel sounds, mydriasis, hyperthermia, delirium	*Amanita muscaria*, anticholinergic drugs
Sympathomimetic	Hypertension/tachycardia excitation/tremor/convulsions	Cocaine, amphetamines, xanthenes, stimulants
Opiate	Decreased level of consciousness, meiosis, hypoventilation, hypotension	Heroin, methadone, codeine
Serotonin syndrome	Autonomic instability (fever, sweating, tachycardia, hypertension, mydriasis), altered mental status (confusion, agitation, hyperactivity, ataxia), neuromuscular abnormalities (hypertonia—symmetrical esp. legs, tremor, hyperreflexia)	Paroxetine

Table 28.3

Common differential diagnoses

Toxicity overdosage
Metabolic—e.g. hyper- or hypoglycaemia, hyponatraemia
Trauma
Stroke
Sepsis—either general (e.g. septicaemia or UTI) or neurosepsis (e.g. meningitis, encephalitis)
Tumour

Tests may be required to exclude alternative or additional diagnoses in some patients
Septic screen including LP
Cerebral CT

Table 28.4 Charcoal adsorption by drugs

Drugs poorly adsorbed by charcoal	Drugs well adsorbed by charcoal
Iron	Amphetamines
Lithium	Morphine
Cyanide	Aspirin
Caustics	Paracetamol
Methanol	Barbiturates
Ethanol	Digoxin
Malathion	Benzodiazepines
Ethylene glycol	Cocaine

to be adsorbed; optimally this ratio should exceed 10:1. A starting dose of 50–100 g is usual. Activated charcoal binds a large number of substances to varying degrees (see Table 28.4). Insoluble non-ionised drugs are usually well bound.

Charcoal may be given as a drink to those patients awake enough to cooperate or it may be instilled via a nasogastric or orogastric tube. The airway must have adequate tone, patency and protective reflexes, as vomiting and aspiration may occur. Note that any orally administered therapy will also be inactivated. Repeat doses should be considered when treating patients who have ingested drugs that undergo enterohepatic recirculation, or that can be drawn out of the circulation, such as theophylline, salicylates, digoxin and benzodiazepines. A cathartic such as mannitol 20% (50–100 mL) may be given orally at the same time for the first dose, to remove the absorbed drugs and to prevent ileus, although frequent loose motions may cause fluid and electrolyte disturbances. For repeat doses, normal saline should be used as a vehicle for the charcoal.

Whole-bowel irrigation

This may be used to remove drugs that are not adsorbed by charcoal, although the volume of fluid involved is several litres, and this in itself may cause problems. Precautions regarding airway protection should be observed.

Drug couriers

Drug couriers may have ingested large quantities of potentially dangerous drugs. The packets may be visible on plain abdominal X-ray. A laxative is sometimes useful. All such patients must be closely monitored, as complications include leakage of drugs with subsequent toxicity, mechanical obstruction or even perforation. Surgical intervention is infrequently required. Ethical and legal issues may arise and it is advisable to have a departmental policy in place for such cases. (See Chapter 50.)

Enhancing drug elimination

Supportive therapy

Supportive therapy is important, especially adequate hydration, in allowing effective elimination of some drugs, e.g. lithium.

Haemodialysis

Haemodialysis should be considered in the setting of a toxic drug with a relatively long half-life. It is most effective if the drug is water-soluble, has a molecular weight of less than 500, is not highly protein-bound and does not have a large volume of distribution. In practice, haemodialysis is uncommonly used except in critically ill patients in the following groups:

1. Renal failure, uncorrectable fluid overload or biochemical disturbance.
2. Severe poisonings with some toxins, e.g. ethylene glycol, salicylates, lithium, methanol.

Other

Other techniques such as haemoperfusion, plasma exchange etc have limited specialised application.

Drug manipulation and specific antidotes

Under some circumstances supportive therapy is supplemented by specific management.

Specific toxins and syndromes

Opiates

Opiate overdosage involves general central nervous system (CNS) depression, specific respiratory centre depression and marked cardiovascular depression:

- Pinpoint pupils (often but not always).
- Respiratory depression.
- Coma.
- Hypotension.

May be complicated by aspiration, rhabdomyolysis, compartment syndromes, renal failure or pulmonary oedema. All patients should be encouraged to stay for adequate assessment, as complications may not be immediately apparent.

As the half-life of many opiates far exceeds that of naloxone (especially methadone: 15–25 hours), patients should be kept for observation and further therapy if required. Note also that methadone may not be detected by some urine drug tests and that high doses of naloxone may be needed.

Apart from precipitating acute withdrawal in some opiate-dependent patients, naloxone is generally safe, even in high doses. Counselling and rehabilitation should always be offered and education should include advice not to inject alone, not to consume multiple other drugs or alcohol with heroin, not to inject a new batch without a sample test dose and to reduce the dose of heroin if there has been a period of abstinence.

Table 28.5 Specific antidotes and treatments

Drug	Specific therapy/antidote
Opiates	Naloxone
Paracetamol	N-acetylcysteine
Digoxin	Digoxin antibodies
Heparin	Protamine
Warfarin	Fresh frozen plasma and vitamin K
Organophosphates	Atropine and pralidoxime
Heavy metals	Chelating agents
Iron	Desferrioxamine
Benzodiazepines	Flumazenil
Carbon monoxide	Oxygen (hyperbaric)
Beta-blockers	Glucagon, isoprenaline, pacing
Chloral hydrate	Beta-blockers

Paracetamol

Paracetamol is found in many compounds, and adult toxicity can occur after ingesting 10 g or even less, with few early specific features. This dose may be much lower in the presence of preexisting hepatic disease. In therapeutic doses, 60–90% is conjugated to sulphates and glucuronides. However, when this pathway is overwhelmed the toxic metabolite N-acetylbenzoquinonimine (NABQI) rapidly depletes hepatic glutathione.

Initial presentation may be non-specific, with nausea, vomiting, shock and confusion progressing to coma, and hepatic and renal failure. The prothrombin time (PT) is a useful predictor in the early stages and, unless essential, fresh frozen plasma (FFP) is withheld to assist in monitoring progress. All overdoses (and any sick patient presenting a diagnostic dilemma) should have a paracetamol screen and level. Levels taken within the first 4 hours of ingestion may not be reliable and should be repeated 4 hours later. All patients with clinical evidence of toxicity, or those whose serum level approaches the threshold where toxicity is likely, should be treated with an intravenous infusion of NAC (N-acetylcysteine) even if presenting late (>24 hours after ingestion) as well as receiving supportive care and decontamination. (See Appendix K2: Rumack-Matthew nomogram of paracetamol toxicity.)

Cerebral oedema, renal failure (acute tubular necrosis—ATN), metabolic acidosis, hypoglycaemia, thrombocytopenia and fulminant hepatic failure may occur, and urgent consideration to liver transplantation should be given where this is available. Criteria include encephalopathy (grade 3 or 4) and long-term prognosis (psychiatric and medical concomitant illnesses).

Digoxin

Digoxin is a commonly prescribed medication and many plants, such as oleander and lily of the valley, also contain cardiac glycosides. Digitalis is a positive cardiac inotrope as it inhibits cardiac Na/K ATPase which leads to an accumulation of Na+ inside cardiac cells, providing more substrate for the Na/Ca exchange pump and subsequent elevation in intracellular calcium. Digoxin has complex actions with multiple cardiac effects, including enhanced atrial automaticity and increased AV nodal blockade

Elderly patients may have impaired renal function and may take other medications that can increase digoxin levels or precipitate toxicity, e.g. diuretics. Hypokalaemia, hypomagnesaemia and hypothyroidism all worsen toxicity. Symptoms of digoxin toxicity include bradycardia (or less commonly tachycardia), nausea, vomiting, confusion and diarrhoea.

Supportive therapy includes correcting any electrolyte abnormalities. While hypokalaemia worsens toxicity, hyperkalaemia is a marker of severe toxicity. Note that digoxin-induced hyperkalaemia should not usually be treated with calcium (see physiology above).

Bradyarrhythmias may require atropine or even temporary pacing.

For tachycardias use phenytoin, amiodarone or lignocaine. If defibrillating tachyarrhythmias, use the minimum possible energy charge. Severe poisoning warrants administration of digoxin antibody therapy (F antibodies at about 1.6 vials/mg of digoxin ingested) given intravenously over 30 minutes. Hypokalaemia may develop after Fab therapy.

Iron

Iron poisoning toxicity is related to the amount of elemental iron ingested and can cause gastric, pulmonary and hepatic injury as well as severe metabolic acidosis and mitochondrial poisoning, resulting in deranged energy metabolism. Different formulations of iron contain varying amounts of elemental iron: toxic effects of iron may occur at doses of 10–20 mg/kg elemental iron.

Phase 1 occurs during the first 6 hours after ingestion and is associated with GI haemorrhage, vomiting, diarrhoea and abdominal pain. This is predominantly due to direct local corrosive effects of iron on the gastric and intestinal mucosa. Early hypovolaemia may result from GI losses and contribute to tissue hypoperfusion and metabolic acidosis. Convulsions, shock and coma may complicate this phase if the circulatory blood volume is sufficiently compromised.

Phase 2 occurs 6–12 hours after ingestion and is usually associated with an apparent improvement in symptoms, especially when supportive care is provided during Phase 1.

Phase 3 begins 12–24 hours following ingestion. Ferrous iron is converted to ferric iron and an unbuffered hydrogen ion is released. Iron concentrates intracellularly, particularly in mitochondria, and disrupts oxidative phosphorylation, resulting in lipid peroxidation and free radical liberation. This worsens the metabolic acidosis, resulting in cell death and tissue injury. Gastrointestinal fluid losses lead to hypovolaemic shock and further acidosis. Cardiovascular symptoms include decreased heart rate, decreased myocardial activity, decreased cardiac output (due to a decrease in myocardial contractility) and increased pulmonary vascular resistance.

Phase 4 occurs 2–6 weeks after ingestion and is characterised by late scarring of the GI tract, causing pyloric obstruction or hepatic cirrhosis.

The diagnosis can be confirmed by seeing tablets on X-ray and by serum iron levels. These are predictive, with 4-hour plasma levels of 145 μmol/L in an adult (90 μmol/L in a child) indicating severe poisoning.

The mainstay of treatment is intensive supportive care and desferrioxamine (±bicarbonate) given by IM injection (less preferred) or IV at 15 mg/kg/h. Serum levels should be monitored (also check the urine for iron–desferrioxamine complex). Gastric lavage is unlikely to be effective because iron tablets are relatively large and sticky, and generally hard to remove. Whole-bowel irrigation has been used to speed the passage of undissolved iron tablets through the GI tract, e.g. with a polyethylene glycol electrolyte solution administered orally or via nasogastric tube. Continue irrigation until the repeat X-ray findings are negative or the rectal fluid appears clear.

If a patient does not develop symptoms of iron toxicity within 6 hours of ingestion, iron toxicity is unlikely to develop.

Benzodiazeprine

Benzodiazepine overdosage may present with drowsiness, slurred speech, and ataxia. Hypotension, respiratory and airway problems are not usually severe unless other drugs or medical problems are superimposed. Treatment is with supportive care and sometimes decontamination, usually with good results. Intravenous injection of crushed and dissolved tablets can result in severe vasospasm and later ischaemia and/or infection.

Flumazenil rapidly reverses benzodiazepine actions and may shorten the stay in hospital (and obviate need for transfer to the intensive care unit) but may not improve ultimate outcome. There is a risk of unmasking toxic effects of co-ingested drugs, of precipitating seizures in some patients with underlying epilepsy (or in those who have ingested drugs which in themselves cause fitting, such as tricyclics) or of precipitating acute benzodiazepine withdrawal in some patients. Flumazenil has a rapid onset of action but its half-life is much shorter than most benzodiazepines, so repeated doses are often required.

Carbon monoxide

Carbon monoxide is liberated during household fires as well as from car exhausts and domestic gas. It avidly binds haemoglobin and cytochromes, and causes tissue hypoxia by interrupting electron transport in mitochondria as well as competing with oxygen to bind to Hb. Organs which are most sensitive to oxygen deprivation (brain and heart) are most at risk, and problems may manifest late in seemingly initially well patients.

Tissue hypoxia is present without cyanosis. The described 'cherry red' discolouration is an uncommon and late sign of severe toxicity.

Urgent oxygen therapy at highest possible concentration is indicated, including intubation and ventilation with high FiO_2. Hyperbaric therapy is considered in the event of any neurological disturbance (headache, confusion, drowsiness) or cardiac effects, or if the carboxyhaemoglobin level is high (i.e. >20%) at any time, although efficacy has been questioned. *Note:* PaO_2 may be normal.

Sequelae include central nervous system (CNS) damage, e.g. frontal lobes, cerebellar or midbrain injury. Parkinsonism has been described. Cardiac ischaemia may result in cardiac failure or arrhythmias.

Tricyclic antidepressants

Tricyclic antidepressants have multiple toxic effects. First-generation drugs (e.g. amitriptyline, imipramine) are the most cardiotoxic. Anticholinergic effects include fever, convulsions, tachycardia and ileus. Peripheral vasodilation from alpha blockade may cause marked hypotension. Type 1a cardiac effects include QT and QRS prolongation and may lead to torsades de pointes ventricular tachycardia. Neurological eye signs and long tract signs may be present. Convulsions, coma, respiratory depression and hypoxia are possible. Renal failure has been reported.

Meticulous supportive therapy is required, including volume loading and care to maintain normal pH. $NaHCO_3$ should be used if significant ECG changes or acidosis are present, although the exact mechanism of benefit is debatable. Magnesium or amiodarone may be effective in managing torsade. Seizures can usually be controlled with IV diazepam. Physostigmine has been used for treatment of toxicity but carries high risk (seizures and asystole) and should be used only by experienced clinicians for severe refractory toxicity.

During the recovery phase, agitation and hallucinations may occur. Recovery in the absence of complications is often rapid (48 hours or less).

Salicylates

Salicylates are found in a number of preparations (e.g. oil of wintergreen) and ingestion may be associated with significant toxicity. Early signs include sweating and vomiting, followed by epigastric pain, tinnitus and blurred vision. Salicylates stimulate the respiratory centre and may cause respiratory alkalosis (in adults), although ultimately a metabolic acidosis will supervene. Renal potassium loss may be significant and hyper- or hypoglycaemia and hyper- or hyponatraemia may occur. Pulmonary oedema may be non-cardiac, and CNS abnormalities include confusion and hyperthermia, seizures and coma. GI bleeding is uncommon.

Fluid and electrolyte resuscitation and supportive care are most important (avoid overload and excess sodium), and intravenous bicarbonate to keep the urine pH above 7.5 is indicated. Multiple doses of oral charcoal can be used.

In severe poisoning (i.e. salicylate level >1000 mg/mL (7.25 mmol/L), haemodialysis should be considered.

Amphetamine and related drugs

Psycho-stimulants

Psycho-stimulants are becoming a far more common clinical problem, sometimes with multiple presentations from a single large event or venue. Cocaine may be injected, ingested, sniffed, smoked or absorbed from any mucosal surface. CNS stimulation may cause confusion, seizures or hyperthermia. Peripheral effects include tachycardia and hypertension. Transient ischaemic attacks, strokes, cerebral oedema and psychosis may occur. Arrhythmias and myocardial infarction (sometimes late) have been reported, as well as rhabdomyolysis and acute renal failure. Supportive care may include sedation with benzodiazepines, as well as management of complications. Exclusion of associated or alternative medical diagnoses is important and cerebral CT may be indicated. MDMA (ecstasy) and amphetamine may be ingested, injected or inhaled. Clinical presentation and management may be similar to that of cocaine; cardiac arrhythmias may cause sudden death. Electrolyte disturbances (hyper/hyponatraemia) and hyperpyrexia can occur. 'Ice', or metamphetamine, is very potent and has a half-life of many hours.

GHB (or 'liquid ecstasy') and derivatives usually ingested are associated with a dramatic fall in loss of consciousness (LOC), airway tone and respiratory drive in the presence of relative bradycardia and normo/hypotension, and sometimes with vomiting and other symptoms. Intubation and supportive care may lead to recovery within hours.

Serotonergic agents

Serotonergic agents such as selective serotonin reuptake inhibitors (SSRIs: fluoxetine, sertraline) and serotonin release inhibitors (venlafaxine) may lead to toxicity if ingested as an overdose, particularly if the patient's ability to compensate for increased CNS serotonin levels is impaired (e.g. co-ingested monoamine oxidase inhibitors—MAOIs). Amphetamine derivatives (see above) can potentially cause a serotonin syndrome. Serotonin influences multiple organ systems via a range of central and peripheral receptors.

The serotonin syndrome is usually diagnosed by the presence of autonomic disturbances, typically sweating, fever, tachycardia, tachypnoea, hypertension, nausea, diarrhoea or pupillary dilation, as well as neuromotor findings including rigidity or tremor, lack of coordination, restlessness or seizures and behavioural disturbances such as agitation, anxiety or confusion. Three or more of these findings are usually present and other diagnoses such as sepsis and malignant neuroleptic syndrome should first be excluded.

Onset may be several hours after ingestion and mild cases resolve with supportive and symptomatic care (diazepam, fluids, cooling). Severe toxicity may be treated with cyproheptadine (an antihistamine/ antiserotonergic agent), chlorpromazine and sometimes dantrolene. For severe hypertension, nitroglycerine (via nitric oxide-mediated down-regulation of serotonin) may be useful. Nitroprusside has also been used.

Organophosphates

Organophosphates are found in a range of products, such as insecticides, and are toxic because of their cholinesterase-binding properties, resulting in a severe cholinergic syndrome with salivation, bronchorrhoea, sweating, abdominal cramps, diarrhoea and fasciculations. At higher doses muscle paralysis, bradycardia and asystole can occur. Toxicity can occur through ingestion, inhalation or skin absorption.

Treatment is by decontamination (wash if topical, aspirate if ingested): staff should take care not to come into contact with contaminated material. Atropine in high doses may be needed and pralidoxime (bolus 1 g IV over 5 minutes then 0.5 g hourly) should be used in severe poisoning. Plasma cholinesterase levels should be monitored.

Ethylene glycol

Ethylene glycol (found in solutions such as antifreeze) is now an uncommon but dangerous poison seen with suicide attempts or as an alcohol substitute. Its metabolites are highly toxic and death may occur with ingestion of 30 mL or less. Clinical signs include drowsiness and ophthalmoplegia, loin pain, haematuria and renal failure. Coma and cerebral oedema, heart failure and cardiovascular collapse may occur. Gastric aspiration/lavage should be performed and an ethanol infusion commenced. Acidosis is treated and intensive supportive therapy maintained. Haemodialysis may be required in some cases.

Methanol

Methanol is found in a number of industrial chemicals and can be ingested, inhaled or topically absorbed. It is rapidly metabolised by alcohol dehydrogenase to formaldehyde, which is then oxidised to formic acid. Neuro- and ophthalmic toxicity (seizures, coma, blindness), as well as pancreatitis (abdominal pain, vomiting) and hypoglycaemia may occur.

Treatment involves supportive therapy, gastric aspiration and lavage (if presentation is <2 hours from ingestion), as well as fluid, electrolyte and acid–base management. Ethanol 10% in 5% dextrose IV infusion should be commenced and serum levels and arterial pH should be monitored. Severe toxicity (more than 30 mL ingested or serum level >500 mg/L), marked refractory acidosis, blindness, coma or renal failure are indications to consider haemodialysis.

Paraquat

Paraquat is a highly toxic liquid herbicide that causes severe gastrointestinal ulceration and scarring as well as progressive and often fatal pulmonary interstitial fibrosis. Cardiac, renal and hepatic failure have also been reported. Intensive support and resuscitation should be commenced. However, oxygen actually worsens the pulmonary toxicity so FiO_2 should be kept as low as feasible. Gastric lavage followed by fuller's earth via a nasogastric tube is the current treatment of choice, although significant ingestion (as little as 15 mL) is often fatal.

EDITOR'S COMMENT

Please freely contact the Poisons Information Hotline, a nationwide free call: 13 1126. This hotine can help with its comprehensive database and on-duty toxicologist—often an emergency physician.

RECOMMENDED READING

Bersten AD, Soni N, Oh TE, eds. Oh's intensive care manual. 5th edn.
    Edinburgh: Butterworth-Heinemann; 2003.
Katzung BG. Basic and clinical pharmacology. 9th edn. New York: Lange Medical
    Books/McGraw-Hill; 2004.
National Guideline Clearinghouse website: http://www.guideline.gov/.
Tintinalli JE, Ruiz E, Krome RL (American College of Emergency Physicians).
    Emergency medicine: a comprehensive study guide. 6th edn. New York:
    McGraw-Hill; 2003.

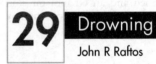

29 Drowning

John R Raftos

EPIDEMIOLOGY

Approximately 350 Australians die from drowning each year. Groups at increased risk are:

- Males (80% of all drownings).
- Young adults aged 15–29 years (25%).
- Children aged 0–4 years (22%).
- Overseas tourists (4.7%).
- Indigenous Australians, especially toddlers (4.2%).
- Epileptics (3%).

Fifty per cent of childhood drowning deaths occur in domestic swimming pools; 15% occur in the ocean; 15% occur in lakes, rivers, storm drains; and 15% occur in the bathtub, buckets and puddles. Adults drown more frequently in the ocean, lakes, rivers and drains but may also drown in the bathtub and in domestic pools. Alcohol use is associated with 50% of adult drowning.

PATHOPHYSIOLOGY

The principal injury and the cause of death and disability in drowning is cerebral hypoxic injury. Treatment aims to optimise cerebral perfusion and oxygenation so that additional brain injury does not occur.

Other primary drowning injuries include:

1. Lung injury (interstitial pulmonary oedema, pneumothorax, pneumo-mediastinum).
2. Circulatory compromise due to the effects of hypoxia on the heart and due to fluid shifts.
3. Hypothermia.

Secondary injuries in drowning include:

1. Additional cerebral injury due to failure to institute cardiopulmonary resuscitation (CPR) in the field or to control systemic oxygenation, cerebral blood flow and cerebral oedema in the emergency department.
2. Respiratory infection and/or aspiration pneumonitis.
3. Adult respiratory distress syndrome, renal failure, disseminated intravascular coagulopathy, multiple organ failure.

OUTCOME

It is not possible to predict the outcome of drowning patients who present unconscious. Indicators of poor prognosis include:

1. Prolonged submersion.
2. Delayed or no CPR.
3. Need for CPR in the emergency department.
4. Unreactive pupils.

However, individuals with all of these features may survive without disability.

Resuscitation must continue for at least 30 minutes after body temperature has been raised above 32°C. Longer resuscitation has been advocated for children and for profoundly hypothermic patients.

Drowning patients who present conscious should survive without neurological deficit.

MANAGEMENT

The primary aim of treatment for drowning is to minimise cerebral injury. This is achieved by restoring cellular perfusion and oxygenation as rapidly as possible and by maintaining these at optimal levels without dips (see Figure 29.1).

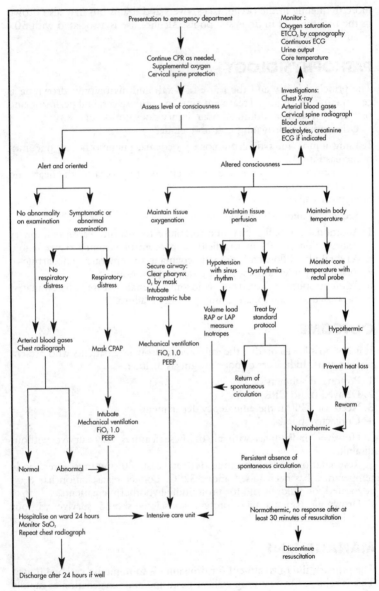

Figure 29.1 Flow diagram of the management of the near-drowned patient in the emergency department

Management of the unconscious near-drowning patient

If no resuscitative efforts have been initiated and there is apnoea or no cardiac output, continue or commence CPR:

1. Airway:
   a. Urgent endotracheal intubation is the preferred technique for airway management. Before intubation, the airway should be cleared and supplemental oxygen should be given.
   b. Cervical spine protection. About 0.5% of drowning patients have proven cervical spine injuries and these patients can usuallly be identified by a suggestive history. Apply a hard cervical collar if in doubt.
2. Breathing:
   a. Unconscious drowning patients should be paralysed, intubated and ventilated.
   b. Ventilation should aim to reverse hypoxia and acidosis.
   c. FiO_2 should initially be 1.0.
   d. Maintain $PaCO_2$ between 30 and 35 mmHg to optimise cerebral blood flow.
   e. Use positive end-expiratory pressure (PEEP) to treat pulmonary oedema and improve oxygenation.
   f. Decompress the stomach early with an intragastric tube to treat gastric distension from gasping and CPR.

   Barotrauma may occur as a result of ventilation, especially in young children, and tension pneumothorax should be suspected if there is unexpected hypotension, hypoxia or difficulty with ventilation.
3. Circulation:
   a. Venous access.
   b. Treat dysrhythmias (including asystole, AF, VT, VF) according to standard protocols.
   c. Hypoxia, hypercarbia and acidosis cause myocardial depression and should be treated by ventilation. $NaHCO_3$ should be used only when in extremis.
   d. Hypotension may require volume loading (NS or Hartmann's), inotropes, or both.
4. Thorough history:
   a. Past medical history should be taken from family if available. History of epilepsy, cardiovascular disease, cerebrovascular disease, or drug or alcohol abuse should be sought.
   b. A clear description of the drowning event is essential. This should include duration of submersion, timing of CPR and return of spontaneous circulation (ROSC), and breathing. Potential for other injury such as cervical spine or head injury should be assessed.

Decompression injury should be suspected if there is a history of ascent from a depth greater than 2 m.

5. Rewarm:
   a. Remove wet clothing. Dry the skin. Wrap the patient in aluminium foil to prevent further heat loss. Warm blankets over the aluminium foil are useful.
   b. Intravenous fluids should be warmed to body temperature.
   c. Ventilation circuits should contain a humidifier and air warmer.
   d. Neonates and young children lose heat rapidly and special care should be taken to ensure that they do not lose heat during treatment.
   e. Profound hypothermia (core temperature below 32°C) may require warm gastric or peritoneal lavage or even cardiopulmonary bypass.

6. Cerebral resuscitation:
   a. Maintain optimal cerebral perfusion.
   b. Maintain optimal oxygenation.
   c. Ventilate to a $PaCO_2$ between 30 and 35 mmHg.
   d. Elevate head of bed by 15° to 30° if systemic blood pressure is adequate.

7. Glasgow Coma Score (GCS): record the initial GCS and repeat at half-hourly intervals.

8. Investigations:
   a. Blood count, electrolytes, creatinine.
   b. Chest X-ray and cervical spine X-ray.
   c. Cerebral CT only if there is suspicion of cerebrovascular accident (CVA) or head injury.
   d. ABGs.
   e. ECG if there is dysrhythmia or suspicion of any preexisting cardiac disease.

9. Monitoring:
   a. Continuous ECG.
   b. SaO_2 by pulse oximetry.
   c. End-tidal carbon dioxide concentration ($ETCO_2$) by capnography.
   d. Non-invasive blood pressure.
   e. Continuous core temperature by rectal or bladder probe.
   f. Invasive blood pressure monitoring if blood pressure or oxygenation are problems.
   g. Right atrial pressure (RAP) or left atrial pressure (LAP) monitoring if hypotension is persistent.
   h. Urine output.

10. Procedures:
    a. Peripheral intravenous catheter.
    b. Endotracheal intubation.
    c. Intragastric tube.
    d. Urinary catheter.
    e. Central venous cannula if indicated.

f. Arterial cannula if indicated.

g. Swan-Ganz cannula if indicated.

Management of the conscious near-drowning patient

Patients who present awake (GCS >13) after a drowning incident should survive without neurological deficit. These patients can, however, have significant lung injury, cardiac dysfunction or hypothermia. All patients who describe a drowning incident, however apparently trivial, should be thoroughly examined and should be observed in hospital for 24 hours.

Management consists of:

1. Supplemental oxygen by mask.
2. Monitor ECG and arterial oxygen saturation (SaO_2).
3. History and focused examination of the cardiovascular, respiratory and nervous systems.
4. Investigation:
   a. Blood count, electrolytes, creatinine.
   b. Chest X-ray.
   c. ABGs.
5. Treat respiratory distress:
   a. Usually due to interstitial lung oedema. Pneumothorax should be suspected if refractory to treatment.
   b. Mask continuous positive airways pressure (CPAP) often obviates the need for intubation and ventilation.
   c. Small doses of loop diuretic may be of benefit.
   d. Small pneumothoraces frequently can be treated by observation unless positive intrathoracic pressures are to be used.
6. Treat cardiovascular compromise, which may be due to dysrhythmia, myocardial depression, or fluid shifts. These should be treated by standard protocol.
7. Rewarm.
8. Hospitalise and observe: pulmonary oedema and seizures may occur up to 24 hours after the accident in conscious drowning patients. All conscious survivors should be hospitalised and have respiratory and neurological observation for 24 hours.

MANAGEMENT POINTS

1. There is no evidence that prophylactic antibiotics or steroids are of benefit in the management of drowning.
2. There is no functional difference in the management of salt water and fresh water drowning or in 'dry' and 'wet' drowning.
3. Children tolerate cerebral hypoxia somewhat better then adults, partly because their brains are less differentiated.

4. The diving reflex (reflex bradycardia and rerouting of blood to brain and heart in response to contact of cold water with the face) offers some young children (under 5 years) a degree of protection from drowning.
5. Teaching children under the age of 4 to swim ('waterproofing') may not be beneficial.
6. Sudden cerebral cooling by immersion in icy-cold water provides a degree of cerebral protection. There are few circumstances in Australian conditions where water is cold enough to offer this protection.
7. Aggressive cerebral resuscitation, including intracranial pressure monitoring, osmotic diuretics, induced hypothermia and barbiturate coma, has not been associated with improved mortality or morbidity in drowning.

PREVENTION

Clinicians should be active advocates for preventative measures, which should focus on initiatives such as fencing of domestic pools, awareness of the link between alcohol and drowning, continuous adult supervision of children around water (including the bath), water safety education, education of epileptic and diabetic children and adults, use of personal flotation aids (life-jackets) and widespread public knowledge of CPR.

RECOMMENDED READING

Edmonds CW, Lowry C, Pennefather J, Walker R. Diving and subaquatic medicine. 4th edn. Oxford: Butterworth–Heinemann; 2002.

Mackie IJ. Patterns of drowning in Australia, 1992–1997. Med J Aust 1999; 171:586–589.

Olshaker JS. Near drowning. Emerg Med Clin North Am 1992; 10:339–350.

Waugh JH, O'Callaghan MJ, Pitt RW. Prognostic factors and long term outcomes for children who have nearly drowned. Med J Aust 1994; 161:594–599.

30 Envenomation

Shane Curran and Thomas McDonagh

Australia is home to many venomous creatures. Australian animals that cause envenomation in humans include snakes, spiders, octopuses, fish and other marine creatures. The distribution of venomous creatures is wide, and each region has its own pattern of envenomation. Local knowledge is very important and local expert knowledge can be invaluable.

Not all patients bitten by venomous creatures will suffer envenomation. Antivenom is not indicated in all cases. Every case needs to be assessed individually. First aid should not be removed if antivenom and treatment facilities are not immediately available. In the envenomed patient, multiple ampoules of antivenom are often necessary.

Resources that are available to you include the local emergency physician or the on-call toxicologist, who can be contacted via National Poisons Information (tel. 13 1126) and can advise on the management of patients with possible or definite envenomation.

SNAKEBITE

Australia is home to a number of the most venomous snakes in the world. Snake venom is a complex mixture of substances. Australian snakes produce venoms that have a range of clinical effects, including neurotoxic (presenting as progressive paralysis), myotoxic (causing rhabdomyolysis and subsequent renal failure), or severe coagulation disturbances and haemolysis (Table 30.1).

Snakebite is a medical emergency. Patients presenting following possible snakebite should receive urgent assessment and management. Patients who have significant envenomation may initially appear well.

The majority of snakebites will not result in significant envenoming, and so will not require antivenom. This is because many snakebites are 'dry

Table 30.1 Clinical effects of Australian snake venom

	Defibrination coagulopathy	Anticoagulation	Paralysis	Myolysis	Renal failure
	Low fibrinogen Raised FDP/XDP	Normal fibrinogen Normal FDP/XDP			ATN
Brown snake	+++				+
Tiger	+++		++ presynaptic	+++	+
Taipan	+++		+++ presynaptic	+++	+++
Mulga snake (King brown)		++	++	+++	+
Sea snake				+++	
Death adder		+	postsynaptic		
Redbellied black snake	Venom is low in potency and small in volume—no major complications				

bites' where no venom is injected. The amount of venom injected by a snake depends on snake maturity, fang length, venom yield, snake temperament, the number of bites and the time since the snake's last meal. Overall, fewer than one in four patients require antivenom.

First aid: the pressure-immobilisation technique

Snake venom spreads via the lymphatics. The pressure-immobilisation method of first aid prevents spread of the venom via the lymphatics and can prevent clinical envenomation. It involves applying a firm, broad bandage, commencing at the site of the bite, and then applying the bandage over the entire limb, extending both proximally and distally. The pressure is the same as that used for a sprained ankle. A splint is then applied to the limb, to immobilise the limb and reduce muscle contraction to further reduce lymphatic spread of the venom. The patient is then kept as still as possible and transported to hospital.

The pressure-immobilisation technique can prevent clinical envenomation if applied early and correctly. Both the limb and the patient should be kept still. The bandages are kept in place until facilities are available to treat clinical envenomation. This may mean transporting a patient to a hospital with a supply of antivenom. If deterioration occurs when the bandages are removed, then the bandages should be reapplied.

It is important not to wash the site of the bite, as it contains traces of venom which are important for identifying the snake type.

If a patient arrives following a possible snakebite and has had no first aid but is well with no signs of envenoming, there is no need to apply the pressure-immobilisation technique.

If a patient arrives with symptoms of envenomation and does not have a bandage applied, then one should be applied.

Table 30.2 Use of the pressure-immobilisation technique of first aid (Adapted with permission of Australian Venom Research Unit)

Pressure-immobilisation is recommended for:	Do not use pressure-immobilisation first aid for:
All Australian venomous snakebites, including sea snake bites	Redback spider bites
Funnelweb spider bites	Other spider bites, including mouse spiders, white-tailed spiders
Box jellyfish stings (if possible)	Bluebottle jellyfish stings
Bee, wasp and ant stings in allergic individuals	Other jellyfish stings
Blue-ringed octopus bites	Stonefish and other fish stings
Cone snail (cone shell) stings	Bee and wasp stings in non-allergic individuals
Australian paralysis tick envenomation	Bites or stings by scorpions, centipedes, beetles

Venom detection kit (VDK)

The venom detection kit developed by the Commonwealth Serum Laboratories (CSL) is important in the management of the patient with snakebite. The venom detection kit can detect minute amounts of snake venom, and is used to determine which family of snake the venom came from.

The venom detection kit does not indicate that a patient has been envenomed. It also does not determine that a patient should be given antivenom. It does, however, indicate which antivenom to use, once the decision to give antivenom has been made. The decision to give antivenom is a clinical decision based on symptoms, signs and pathology testing.

A swab of the bite site is best for venom detection, as this is where venom is present in highest quantities. A window can be cut in the bandages overlying the bite site. When the swab has been taken, the bandage is reapplied.

Urine is the next best for venom detection, since Australian snake venoms are excreted in the urine. Blood or serum is not used.

The venom detection kit is used by trained laboratory staff and the procedure takes about 20 minutes to complete.

Antivenom

Antivenom is the definitive treatment for a patient with systemic envenomation and its administration can reverse the clinical effects of envenomation. The treatment of envenomation following snakebite involves the administration of adequate quantities of the appropriate antivenom.

Antivenom is produced by CSL from antibodies that have been harvested from horses injected with subclinical doses of snake venom toxins. Because the antibodies are obtained from the horse serum, there is a risk of anaphylaxis, allergic reaction or delayed serum sickness. Before administration, therefore, preparations should be made to treat a possible anaphylactic reaction. Currently premedication with adrenaline is not recommended.

Antivenom is given intravenously, and multiple ampoules may be necessary. Monovalent antivenom is indicated if the type of snake is known, when the venom detection kit determines the type of antivenom to be given, or in areas where the occurrence of snakes is limited to specific snake types. Monovalent antivenom is preferred as it is less expensive, is a smaller volume of foreign protein and has fewer side effects.

Polyvalent antivenom contains antibodies to venom of all groups of snakes. It consists of a large volume, is expensive, but is used when treatment with antivenom is indicated, the snake type is unknown and the venom detection kit procedure is negative or will take too long to perform.

In certain areas a mixture of monovalent antivenoms, based on the local prevalence of snake types, may replace polyvalent antivenom.

The dose of antivenom is dependent on the dose of venom injected by the snake, not on the size of the patient, which means that children require the same amount of antivenom as adults do.

Laboratory testing

Laboratory tests are vital for the assessment of patients possibly bitten by a snake. They should have blood taken for:

1. Coagulation—activated partial thromboplastin time (APTT), prothrombin time (PT), fibrinogen level, D-dimer/fibrinogen degradation products (XDP), platelet count.
2. Creatine kinase.
3. Renal function.
4. Electrolytes.
5. Urine should be tested for myoglobin and blood.

If there is no access to a laboratory then a whole blood clotting time can be performed to determine the presence of coagulopathy. To perform a whole blood clotting time, 5–10 mL blood is placed in a clean, plain glass test tube and allowed to stand. The time to clotting is measured and is normally less than 10 minutes. A prolonged time indicates coagulopathy.

Laboratory tests may be normal initially and will need repeating. If all tests are normal then the first aid bandages should be removed and pathology tests repeated after 2–3 hours. Onset of coagulopathy may be delayed and blood tests should be repeated.

Signs and symptoms

Local signs of snakebite may vary from obvious bite marks, with local pain and swelling, to a trivial puncture or scratch. The absence of bite marks does not exclude significant snake bite.

General symptoms include non-specific symptoms such as nausea, headache, abdominal pain and collapse. Specific symptoms may include muscle pain, bleeding sites and muscle weakness. In an emergency, it may be possible to determine the snake from the clinical and laboratory effects. It is advisable to seek expert advice before administering antivenom.

Disposition

Admit and observe all cases of possible snakebite. Patients should be checked frequently for signs of envenomation, and blood tests should be repeated, even if normal initially. Urine should be tested again for blood and myoglobin. The patient should be observed for early signs of paralysis: e.g. ptosis, diplopia and dysarthria.

Patients who receive multiple doses of antivenom should also be given doses of steroids to prevent serum sickness.

All patients with brown snake bite should be admitted for 24 hours.

SPIDER BITES

Redback spider (*Latrodectus hasseltii*)

Redback spiders are common throughout Australia, in urban areas, in and around houses, gardens, sheds, rubbish piles and discarded objects. It is the female spider that is responsible for envenoming.

Only one-fifth of bites will result in significant envenoming. Only people with significant envenoming receive antivenom.

The redback bite is usually felt as an initial mild sting, with no signs of a bite at the site. Fifteen minutes to 1 hour later the bite site may become painful. The pain can become severe and extend to the regional lymph nodes. Following this, pain may extend to the whole limb and abdomen, and headache may occur. There may be nausea, malaise and hypertension. An area of sweating may develop surrounding the bite site. The patient may be sweating profusely and this may be generalised or localised to the bite site, or in an area remote from the bite.

If there is clear evidence of envenoming, then redback antivenom is given. The decision to treat is a clinical one; there are no tests to assist in the diagnosis.

Redback antivenom is given by intramuscular injection. This can be repeated in 1 hour, if there is incomplete reduction of symptoms, or if symptoms return. No premedication is required, but facilities to treat anaphylaxis should be at hand.

Redback antivenom can be useful for relief of symptoms up to days after the initial bite. The need for multiple doses is not uncommon. Advice should be sought if multiple doses of antivenom are needed.

Funnelweb spider (*Atrax* spp.)

There are at least 35 species of funnelweb spiders, but only one is known to cause death in humans. It is the Sydney funnelweb (*Atrax robustus*), which has a restricted range that includes the Sydney and Gosford regions. Other types are found over a wider range along Australia's eastern seaboard.

Following a bite from the Sydney funnelweb, death can occur within an hour. The effects are a bite that is usually painful, followed by perioral tingling, fasciculation of the tongue, profuse sweating, lacrimation and salivation, then skeletal muscle fasciculation and spasms. Hypertension and tachycardia usually occur and there may be rapid onset of pulmonary oedema.

First aid is with the pressure-immobilisation technique. Definitive treatment is with Sydney funnelweb antivenom. Multiple vials of antivenom, usually two to four, may be necessary, as well as resuscitation with airway control and ventilation.

All Sydney funnelweb spider bite patients should be admitted for close observation.

White-tailed spider (*Lampona cylindrata*)

The white-tailed spider is a common hunting spider that is often found in houses. Definite bites from this spider may cause some local pain and inflammation but are usually mild or moderate. The evidence linking the white-tailed spider to necrotic ulcers is limited, and research has failed to show that its venom causes significant skin damage.

Necrotic arachnidism

Many spiders can cause a bite that may be painful and mildly inflamed locally. In some patients, the skin may ulcerate. These small ulcers usually heal without specific treatment. The development of skin bites that ulcerate and develop necrosis is usually only tenuously linked to a spider bite. Often there is a painful area of skin that is found in the morning after a presumed bite, and this may later ulcerate.

A number of overseas spiders, such as the recluse and fiddleback spiders, are implicated in causing necrotic skin ulceration and systemic illness.

There is little evidence to suggest that any single species of Australian spider is the cause of necrotic toxic damage. In many cases, the cause of the tissue damage is a secondary bacterial infection.

Management includes adequate debridement of the wound, microbiological specimens as necessary and antibiotics if required.

MARINE ENVENOMATION

Box jellyfish or sea wasp (*Chironex fleckeri*)

The box jellyfish is one of the most venomous creatures in the world. It is found in the coastal waters of northern Australia, and is most commonly encountered in the summer months. Its tentacles contain stinging cells called nematocysts that contain venom and a spring-loaded harpoon. On contact with a victim, the nematocyst releases the coiled harpoon, which pierces the skin and releases the stored venom. Victims may discharge further nematocysts as they attempt to remove the tentacles that still contain intact stinging cells.

Clinically, there is severe localised pain, and local skin changes range from painful erythema to full-thickness skin necrosis. Typically there are linear red welts that may go on to blister and ulcerate. Confusion, agitation, and collapse with respiratory or cardiac arrest can occur. Onset of envenomation may be very rapid and death can occur in 5 minutes. The venom contains cardiotoxic, neurotoxic and dermatotoxic compounds.

The extent of envenoming is dependent on the area of skin that comes into contact with the tentacle. An area of tentacle contact of 10% of the total surface area is potentially lethal.

Immediate first aid is vital. Any undischarged nematocysts can be inactivated by applying large volumes of household vinegar (dilute acetic acid). Antivenom is available and can be given by intramuscular injection.

Box jellyfish antivenom is indicated for all but minor stings. One to three vials are administered by intramuscular injection as soon as possible in severe stings. Antivenom is given intravenously in the hospital setting.

Early administration of antivenom may result in reduced pain and reduces skin necrosis and scarring.

Irukandji (*Carukia barnesi*)

The irukandji is a small jellyfish, about 2 cm in diameter, found in coastal waters of northern Australia

The sting of the irukandji is moderately painful, with little skin damage, but within 30 minutes onset of systemic envenoming may occur, with severe abdominal and back pain, nausea and vomiting, and muscle or joint pain. Sweating and agitation occur, and the patient is hypertensive and tachycardiac. Symptoms are thought to be due to catecholamine release.

Treatment includes analgesia, and antihypertensive treatment may be required, in which case alpha-blocking drugs (phentolamine) may be used.

No antivenom is available to treat irukandji envenomation. The best form of first aid is currently unclear.

Portuguese man-o'-war, or bluebottle (*Physalia* spp.)

The Portuguese man-o'-war, or bluebottle, occurs throughout Australian costal waters, where it is often found washed up on beaches. It has a typical bright blue appearance.

The bluebottle causes a painful sting with localised discrete weals and surrounding erythema. A line of redness with raised weals or blisters is typical. Systemic symptoms are uncommon but comprise nausea, vomiting, headache and abdominal pains. Deaths have not been reported following bluebottle sting.

Treatment consists of removing the tentacles with forceps. Vinegar is not recommended. Analgesia is indicated, as are ice packs and local anaesthesia.

Blue-ringed octopus (*Hapalochlaena* spp.)

A bite from the blue-ringed octopus may be painless and difficult to see, and so may go unnoticed. The bites occur when the octopus is handled, and is in contact with the skin. The victim will usually report handling a small octopus in or around a coastal rock pool.

The saliva of the blue-ringed octopus contains a potent neurotoxin, tetrodotoxin, which causes a rapidly progressive flaccid paralysis, followed by respiratory failure and hypotension.

First aid involves applying a pressure-immobilisation bandage. There is no antivenom and treatment is based on maintaining supportive treatment. Respiratory support with ventilation may be required for a few days, until the effects of the toxin wear off.

Sea snakes

Sea snakes are found predominantly in the tropical waters of northern Australia. All are potentially dangerous to humans, but very few sea snake bites of significance occur.

Sea snake venoms contain postsynaptic neurotoxins and myolysins. Victims may therefore develop paralysis, with ptosis and diplopia, or muscle pain, weakness and myoglobinuria, and hyperkalaemia and renal failure may occur secondary to muscle breakdown. Coagulopathy is not a feature of sea snake bite.

Treatment is with the pressure-immobilisation technique of first aid. Sea snake antivenom is available and is used for neutralising venoms of all species of sea snakes. Sea snake venoms are not reliably detected by the venom detection kit.

Stonefish

The stonefish is responsible for a painful sting that usually occurs when wanderers step on it in shallow water around reefs and rock pools.

Most stonefish stings occur when the fish is stepped on and the spines inject venom, which causes instant and severe pain. Local swelling follows, which may be marked. Dizziness, nausea, hypotension and pulmonary oedema may rarely occur.

First aid involves immersing the limb in hot water. The water should not be hot enough to cause a scald. Analgesics are usually required. Local regional anaesthesia may help in providing analgesia.

Antivenom is available if there is significant envenoming, and is indicated if there is severe local pain. The number of ampoules to be given is related to the number of puncture wounds from the venomous spines.

TICK BITES

Ticks most commonly cause a local skin reaction, consisting of irritation and pruritus. Multiple bites may cause a rash. The most dangerous ticks are those that cause paralysis, belonging to the *Ixodes* species. The common paralysis tick is found along eastern Australia.

Tick paralysis occurs due to a presynaptic neurotoxin that occurs in the saliva of the *Ixodes* ticks. The toxin causes a progressive flaccid paralysis. Tick paralysis often occurs in children and presents as an ataxic gait with malaise and lethargy. The weakness may progress even after removal of the ticks.

A thorough search should be conducted to find all ticks, including scalp, ear canal and genitals. Ticks are removed by using tweezers on either side of the embedded mouthparts. Care is taken not to squeeze the body of the tick or more of the toxin can be injected. Care is also taken not to break off the mouthparts that may remain embedded in the skin.

The paralysis is treated with tick antivenom along with appropriate supportive care.

CENTIPEDES AND SCORPIONS

None of the species of centipedes or scorpions found in Australia is dangerous to humans. These species may cause a painful bite, but the pain does not usually last long. Systemic symptoms are unusual and are not usually severe.

RECOMMENDED READING

Australian Venom Research Unit website. Available: http://www.pharmacology. unimelb.edu.au/avruweb/index.htm.

Clinical toxinology website. Available http://www.toxinology.com.

CSL snake venom detection kit: technical information. Melbourne: Commonwealth Serum Laboratories.

Sutherland SK, Tibbals J. Australian animal toxins. 2nd edn. Melbourne: Oxford University Press; 2001.

White J. Bites and stings. Current Therapeutics 2003; 43(2):8–45.

White J. CSL antivenom handbook. 2nd edn. Melbourne: Commonwealth Serum Laboratories; 2001.

White J. Snakebite and spiderbite: a management protocol for NSW. Sydney: NSW Health Department; 1998.

31 | Electrical injuries

Gordian W O Fulde

Electrical injuries are frequently seen in the emergency department.

There are two main peaks of incidence, the first in early childhood— usually the result of domestic accidents—and the second in 20–50-year-olds, with a preponderance of males, reflecting occupational injuries.

The wide spectrum of injuries results from the multiple possible causes —the current itself, the heat generated, the explosion if any, or trauma from muscle contractions or falls. Later sequelae can include damage to the eyes with the formation of cataracts, and to the central nervous system with personality changes.

PHYSICS

Electricity is the flow of electrons from higher to lower potential. Direct current (DC), from sources such as car batteries or defibrillators, flows in one direction. Domestic alternating current (AC) switches to and fro at 50–60 cycles per second (hertz).

Lightning contains approximately 10×10^6 volts and a current of 10,000–200,000 amperes. However, as the result of the incredibly brief time (microseconds to milliseconds) involved in a lightning strike, the final amount of current is much less than expected.

The basic electrical injury potential rests with two laws:

Ohm's law   Current (amps) $= \dfrac{\text{Voltage}}{\text{Resistance}}$

Joule's law   Heat generated $= \text{Current}^2 \times \text{Resistance}$

Much of the precise pathophysiology to organs is, however, still being researched, particularly in the case of lightning. Listing tissues in order of increasing resistance (nerves, blood vessels, muscle, fat, tendon, bone) only partially explains the reported patterns of electrical injury. Dry skin has a very high resistance (100,000 ohms) but the resistance of moist skin is only 1000 ohms. The absorption of energy, usually heat, markedly influences the damage to that structure because veins thrombose early. The injury potential of lightning provides a particularly large and fascinating arena for research.

The preaching of prevention, especially of electrical injuries, is the duty of every emergency physician.

Lightning injuries can be markedly decreased by taking measures to prevent ourselves from becoming conductors, and by not being near obvious conductors.

In an emergency situation, the safety of the rescuer cannot be overemphasised. Wherever possible, rescue should be undertaken only by trained professionals. A downed power line near an accident victim can suddenly snake, or the ground around it can be live. Power should be turned off at the source and then be tested before any risks are taken. Victims frozen to an electrical contact will let go or fall back immediately the power is off. Wetness (such as rain, baths or pools) combined with electricity brings major hazards and should never be underestimated.

When faced with a patient who has experienced electrical injury, emergency physicians must think of 'worst-case scenarios', as electrical injuries often affect multiple systems and may well be covert. It is essential to keep an open mind as to causation, and to carefully explore the possibility of serious concomitant disease.

The standard approach to an unconscious or critically ill patient must always be employed. This includes neck immobilisation and exclusion of causes such as hypoglycaemia, overdose, cerebrovascular accident or trauma. This approach is particularly important in view of the fact that the prime treatment modality for the electrically injured is support of systems while waiting for, and attempting to avoid, complications.

LIGHTNING INJURIES
Epidemiology

Given the frequency of lightning strikes (8 million a day) to the earth's surface, it is not surprising that the mortality from strikes (estimated in the United States at about 200 per year) exceeds that of all other natural disasters. Those who enjoy outdoor recreation, such as golfers and hikers, are the main group of people affected. Solo people who are struck by a solitary lightning strike make up 70% of the recorded mortality. Most fatalities (about 70%) are recorded between midday and 6 pm.

Deaths occur five times more frequently in the country than in urban areas. The summer storm season is associated with the highest mortality. The annual mortality is decreasing in all recording countries.

Three major predictors of mortality are: cardiac arrest at the time of injury, cranial burns (five times increased) and leg burns.

In order to avoid lightning, there are some simple measures which should be followed.

1. Stay indoors during a storm, or seek shelter in a building or car (not a convertible).
2. Avoid contact with any metal such as golf clubs, umbrellas, tent poles, gates, roofs or hair clips.
3. Do not stand next to or under the tallest object in sight such as a tree, pole or haystack.
4. Avoid being in a group—split up so that someone can call help if necessary; give CPR.
5. Do not stand with your feet apart, as this increases your stride potential and can result in major burns.
6. If caught alone, the correct procedure is to curl up on the ground, preferably in a ditch, well away from higher objects.

It is important to note that, contrary to popular belief, lightning does strike twice or more in the same spot.

Wide-band magnetic direction finders are increasingly used to warn of incoming lightning storms.

Physics

The complexities and mysteries of lightning are the subject of major international research. Lightning can arise from any charged particles such as dust, ice or snow. A stepped leader stroke comes down from the cloud and is then met by an answering leader from earth (usually from taller structures). An arc is formed from cloud to ground with high current, a return stroke with superheating, light and thunder. There are usually several strokes at once, quicker than our perception, and they can be in both directions.

Mechanisms of strike

1. **Direct strike**
   a. Current passes through patient.
   b. Current passes over surface of patient (flashover), often via wet clothes which can explode or burn.
2. **Side flash.** The patient becomes part of the main conductor. This occurs, for example, when standing under a tree that is struck by lightning. The current can pass as in a direct strike.
3. **Direct contact.** The patient is in physical contact with the main conductor.
4. **Stride potential.** This arises when current from a lightning strike travels along the ground near the patient who has his legs separated. The current takes the path of lesser resistance up a leg, across the body and down the other leg, rather than along the high-resistance ground. This process is associated with a significant mortality.

Pathophysiology

As the injuries sustained are both multisystemic and have multiple causes from diverse sources such as electricity, heat, blunt trauma and anoxia, the clinical possibilities are vast.

The lightning patient may suffer an asystolic arrest, shocked respiratory centre with prolonged apnoea, a marked dysfunction of the autonomic nervous system with fixed dilated pupils, mottled limbs, possible vascular spasm, or possible abnormal discharge of any neuromuscular tissue.

Table 31.1 Special injuries often associated with lightning

Skin	• Burns: feathering or flowers (transient, not burns but electron showers) • Superficial (often in patterns of sweat lines, or wet exploded clothing) • Deep entry and exit wounds; imprints of metal buttons, belt clips, ignited clothing
Ear	Tympanic membrane rupture, barotrauma
Eye	Onset of cataracts, eye trauma and causing disruption of anatomy
Heart	Asystole, ventricular fibrillation, arrhythmias, infarct (rare), transient hypotension or hypertension
Limbs	Trauma: keraunoparalysis, a temporary neurovascular dysfunction in the majority of serious strikes, usually resolves in hours but permanent sequelae are possible
Central nervous system	• Seizures, mental state similar to that after electroconvulsive therapy • Amnesia (very common), psychological sequelae.

Severe burns, with their sequelae of renal failure, anaemia and tissue damage, are very uncommon.

As a generalisation, patients who survive the initial strike will usually have no major problems. Obviously clinical expertise must be used to rule out potential complications to the eyes, ears, heart and nervous system.

Clinical presentation

Pre-hospital

Rescuer safety is vital. A very special aspect of lightning victims is that they require aggressive resuscitation even in the light of asystole, apparent fixed dilated pupils or pulseless limbs. This is because, in the initial phase, these signs are caused by the electricity and may be reversed by standard life support measures.

This is also the reason for splitting up a group caught by a storm so that immediate CPR can be administered to the sickest victim. Contrary to usual disaster responses, if several people are struck by lightning at once, the care must go to the sickest (arrested) first, as the walking and talking wounded will survive whereas the arrested patient has only a brief opportunity to be salvaged.

Hospital

Patients may arrive arrested, unconscious, amnesiac, as a trauma patient or as one that has very few clinical problems.

A standard approach—e.g. advanced cardiac life support (ACLS), advanced trauma life support (ATLS)—is indicated.

The clinical picture dictates the management. It is essential that other possible causes of the clinical picture and concomitant illness be sought and excluded as part of the patient's management.

As always, the ABCs are secured. Lightning-strike patients rarely need fluid loading. Hypothermia due to exposure is very common. If there is any loss of consciousness, arrhythmia or rise in cardiac enzymes, cardiac monitoring for 24 hours is indicated. MRI scanning is useful for subtle lesions of the brain and spinal cord.

Usually the surviving victim needs mainly supportive treatment.

Appropriate follow-up is dictated by the clinical picture.

DOMESTIC CURRENT ELECTRICAL INJURIES

Epidemiology

These are a common cause of tragedy, which is nearly always preventable. The early incidence peak in 1–4-year-olds reflects young children exploring, biting cords and investigating power outlets. The next (male-dominated) peak (20–50 years) involves mainly occupational accidents, but ranges from the experienced tradesman to the foolish person.

The common hand-to-hand pathway (transthoracic) has a mortality of up to 60%. With hand-to-foot transmission (left side worse), a 20% mortality is quoted.

Physics

The type and amount of current can often be inferred from the nature of the source. However, within appliances, conversions from the more dangerous AC to DC to another voltage are very common. Usually there are clean entry and exit wounds, but the current does not travel in straight lines.

Pathophysiology

Although not totally reliable, the history can give a good guide to the possible injuries that should be excluded.

If a short circuit occurred with an explosion or a flash, it is possible that very little actual current passed through the patient, and the clinical picture is dominated by facial burns (often superficial), eye problems and sequelae of blunt trauma. If the patient was frozen to the circuit, often as a result of muscle tetany with AC, a serious, life-threatening injury has probably occurred with multiorgan and limb damage.

Domestic AC current will cause ventricular fibrillation. DC current is more likely to put the patient into asystole.

Obviously the damage to tissues can be patchy, and it may be secondary to another process such as thrombosis or oedema.

Injuries, burns, and complications are very frequently underdiagnosed and poorly documented. Because litigation often ensues, good clinical recording is mandatory.

Clinical presentation

Pre-hospital

As long as the current has been shut down, in a witnessed arrest a praecordial thump is indicated. An electrocuted patient must be treated along standard life-support guidelines. Special considerations are cardiac, major fluid losses and burn management.

Hospital

A thorough ABC reassessment, a meticulous whole-body examination, and aggressive early management must be carried out. Often fractures are present and fasciotomies of digits and limbs need to be done in the emergency department.

A good urine flow (1 mL/kg per hour) in the face of myoglobin, haemoglobin or shock is life-saving. Normal electrolyte homeostasis, especially potassium, must be ensured. A major electrical burn has facets of a crush syndrome (see Chapter 14).

In children with oral burns, delayed rupture of the labial artery in 4–5 days is well described. Tetanus prophylaxis is mandatory. Cardiac monitoring in children with no cardiac signs has not been shown to be useful. In adults it is still controversial. Cardiac enzymes, including creatine kinase isoenzyme (CKMB) and troponins, cannot be relied upon. Thus, monitoring should be done if there is any loss of consciousness or any cardiac event or signs, and in high-risk patients including those who experienced current across the thorax, or cardiac patients.

Adequate follow-up, both physical and psychological, must be arranged, as up to 70% of these patients have some long-term effects. Neurological damage has an especially poor prognosis.

Cataract formation occurs after 6–10% of electrical injuries to the head.

Special patient groups

In children and pregnant patients the relevant specialties must be involved from the onset.

Flash burns

These occur usually where a short circuit causes an explosion, e.g. switchboard, and are often seen in tradesmen. Priorities are often those of the trauma to the face, eyes, hands etc. In many cases, little current has passed through the patient, but it must be looked for.

RECOMMENDED READING

Cherington M. Lightning injuries. Ann Emerg Med 1995; 25: 517–519.
Marx JA, Hockberger RS, Walls RM, Adams J, eds. Rosen's emergency medicine: concepts and clinical practice. 5th edn. St Louis: Mosby; 2001.

32 | Hypothermia and hyperthermia

David J Lewis-Driver

Although Canadians write more about hypothermia and Saudis write more about hyperthermia, neither condition is in fact rare in Australia. Heat waves and fun runs occur every year in every Australian city. At the opposite end of the spectrum, hypothermia is a regular accompaniment to injury and disease throughout the year, and can occur in summer—for example when nursing home patients are left scantily clothed under the air-conditioner to cool them. It is important too to remember that the average multiple trauma patient in any country will become hypothermic unless specific preventative steps are taken.

PHYSIOLOGY

Temperature control requires a functioning hypothalamic centre, adequate cardiovascular function to be able to dissipate or conserve heat, adequate muscle bulk to generate heat, intact skin and sweat glands, and sufficient commonsense and mobility to escape the heat or cold. All of these may be affected by disease, trauma or environmental factors.

Cold basically slows body functions, with death in asystole unless an irritable heart is jolted into ventricular fibrillation (VF). In general, slow warming and gentle handling is appropriate. Heat eventually destroys cellular enzymes, after an initial adaptive response including heat shock proteins and acute phase reactants. Central nervous system (CNS) symptoms usually predominate, but multiorgan failure similar to overwhelming sepsis eventually occurs. Rapid cooling is necessary.

In both cases, skin circulation is a problem. Overheating cold skin induces vasodilation, which feels good but may overwhelm the pumping capacity of a cold heart, resulting in rewarming shock. Ice on hot skin induces vasoconstriction, which may limit heat transfer.

HYPOTHERMIA

This condition is defined as a core temperature <35°C. It is classified as shown in Table 32.1.

Physiology

The body responds to a fall in temperature by attempting to seek warmth and by shivering. If these efforts fail because of environmental factors, drugs, injury or disease and the temperature falls, an initial rise in respiration, pulse and blood pressure is followed by a gradual slowing of all body systems, with death due to cardiovascular failure. CNS slowing results in apathy and confusion, and cardiovascular system (CVS) slowing proceeds to death in either asystole or VF. Vigorous attempts at external rewarming can result in skin burns or death from rewarming shock, an ill-understood phenomenon that can best be considered as shunting of needed blood to the surface while the core is still too cold to cope with the demand. Core temperature lags behind surface temperature during

Table 32.1 Classification of hypothermia

Temperature	Grade	Signs
35–32°C	Mild	Shivering/apathy
32–28°C	Moderate	Confusion ↓ PR ↓ BP
<28°C	Severe	CV failure

rewarming, and healthy volunteers start to feel better when rewarmed while their core temperature is still falling due to continued cold penetration. An 'undressing phenomenon' is also well described, where failure of skin vasoconstriction as a terminal event allows return of skin circulation and leads to a sensation of warmth so that victims are found to have undressed themselves as a last act before death.

Diagnosis

If temperature is not a routine observation on every patient, ensure it is taken in those patients who are potential hypothermia candidates, as outlined in Table 32.2.

If the temp is <36°C on a standard instrument, use a low-reading thermometer. The tympanic thermometers commonly used in emergency departments will generally read down to 26°C and are thus adequate to suggest the diagnosis. However, they are not accurate enough to guide treatment. Use an electronic probe—rectal in an awake patient and oesophageal in an intubated patient.

Table 32.2 Potential hypothermia candidates

Conditions associated with accidental hypothermia
Trauma that limits protective mechanisms, e.g. neck of femur (NOF)
Overdose
Alcoholism

Conditions that may cause hypothermia
Sepsis
Myxoedema or adrenal insufficiency
Parkinsonism (failure to shiver)
Wernicke's encephalopathy
Drugs, e.g. phenothiazines; beta-blockers; clozapine; sedatives
Hypoglycaemia; diabetic ketoacidosis (affect the thermostat)
Pancreatitis
Myocardial infarction or other cause of low CO
Malnutrition/anorexia
Burns; extensive skin rashes (excessive heat loss)

Conditions for which hypothermia may be mistaken
Cerebrovascular accident
Dementia; confusion in the elderly; delirium
Hypoglycaemia
Myocardial ischaemia
Drunk and disorderly
Myxoedema

Treatment of mild hypothermia (35°–32°C)

1. **Stop further heat loss.** The most powerful way to prevent heat loss in any emergency department patient is to stem conduction and radiation loss—i.e. remove wet clothes and provide a blanket or space blanket. This is also called passive external rewarming, because prevention of heat loss allows the patient's own metabolism to raise temperature.

2. **Continuously monitor temperature.** A rise of above 0.5°C per hour is acceptable.

3. **Apply a Bair Hugger** if available. This method of active external warming using hot air is commonly available and unlikely to cause rewarming shock or burns. Active warming, however, is not vital unless the patient is incapable of generating heat because of systemic disease or a condition (e.g. cerebrovascular accident—CVA) that has reset the temperature centre. If a Bair Hugger is used, do not exceed a rise of 2°C/h. It is probably better to leave the arms exposed, because the main risk is that sequestered cold blood will be restored to the circulating pool by skin vasodilation, causing an afterdrop in the core temperature. This risk is less from the trunk than the limbs.

4. **Give O_2 and monitor O_2 saturation.** If the saturation monitor will not read because of vasoconstriction, warm the finger or even do a digital block to overcome vasospasm.

5. **Treat the underlying cause.**

6. **Set up an IV and take blood** for:

   - *Urgent blood sugar level (BSL).* Physiologically, hypothermia causes firstly a rise in BSL due to catecholamine-induced glycogenolysis, reduced insulin secretion. Finally (below 30°C) insulin stops working. But there is a high association with hypoglycaemia in alcoholics, and elderly or malnourished patients may have exhausted glycogen stores by the increased metabolism of shivering. Treat hypoglycaemia but not hyperglycaemia. If rewarming does not correct hyperglycaemia, exclude haemorrhagic pancreatitis (a complication of hypothermia) or diabetic ketoacidosis (a cause of hypothermia).

   - *Urea and electrolytes.* Fluid shifts and renal dysfunction mean that Na and K can go in either direction. Minor changes in the initial results do not require treatment and can simply be observed during rewarming. Significant changes should be treated and may be a clue to the underlying cause of the hypothermia.

   - *Lipase.* Pancreatitis is both a cause and a result of hypothermia.

   - *FBC.* Expect the haematocrit to be high (due to cold diuresis—an attempt to compensate for central fluid overload due to peripheral vasoconstriction) and the WCC and platelets to be normal or low (due to sequestration). A normal Hb/Ht may indicate anaemia and a normal WCC does not rule out infection. Thus the main reason for doing the tests is that a high WCC increases suspicion of an underlying disease process.

- *Troponin.* Patients who become hypothermic during surgery have a higher incidence of myocardial events. Subendocardial infarctions have been found at autopsy in the absence of ECG changes. In elderly patients, repeat troponin after rewarming.
- *CK.* May be a clue to rhabdomyolysis in overdose or injury.

  Note: Hypothermic patients bleed more after surgery and trauma and this is generally attributed to failure of one or more of the enzymes in the coagulation cascade and qualitative platelet dysfunction. However, coagulation screens will generally be normal because these tests are done in the laboratory at room temperature. Rewarming is the best treatment. It is not generally possible either to get the laboratory to re-do the tests at the patient's temperature or to make fresh frozen plasma (FFP) work while the patient is still cold.

7. Give 500–1000 mL **dextrose/saline or normal saline** (warmed!). Hartmann's is contraindicated because the cold liver can't metabolise the lactate. Assume that the patient is dehydrated due to third space shifts and cold diuresis. Some fluid is required to compensate for the return of skin flow during rewarming, but when the patient is warmer the third space fluid will return. Elderly patients require cautious fluid replacement but younger patients can have the full litre fairly quickly.

8. **Take an ABG** and use the result, which is uncorrected for temperature. Expect hypoxia (due to ventilation/perfusion defects plus shift in oxyhaemoglobin curve plus increased haematocrit) and a lactic acidosis due to shivering. Below 32°C a respiratory acidosis due to slowed respiration will be added. Try to keep the uncorrected pH close to normal, but only by warming and ventilation. HCO_3 is not indicated.

9. **Do an ECG.** Hypothermia increases conduction times and often causes a slow atrial fibrillation, which reverses with rewarming. The classical ECG change is the appearance of a J wave between the QRS complex and the T wave. Some computerised ECG programmes interpret this wave incorrectly as myocardial infarction.

10. **Institute cardiac monitoring.** Ventricular fibrillation is the terminal event in a significant number of hypothermia deaths, and is commonly thought to be provoked by jostling or rescue or treatment procedures. However, it is unlikely to occur above 29°C.

11. **Monitor BP.** If it drops, turn off the Bair Hugger if it is being used (rewarming shock due to skin vasodilation).

12. **Measure urine output.** Use an indwelling catheter (IDC) if required. Neither PR, BP nor urine output will be reliable indicators of hydration status, but urine output will be the best of the three.

13. **Keep nil by mouth** until 35°C is reached (poor gut motility).

14. **Consider central venous pressure (CVP).** It may be the only way to measure fluid replacement requirements in the elderly, but the risk of coagulopathy is a strong disincentive. If a CVP catheter is introduced, it should stop well above the R atrium to avoid an arrhythmia in the irritable heart.

15. **Do a chest X-ray (CXR).** Cold induces bronchorrhoea and reduces ciliary activity and resistance to infection, making bronchopneumonia more likely.

16. **Give thiamine to alcoholic or malnourished** patients, because of the association between Wernicke's encephalopathy and hypothermia.

17. Confirm that the patient can protect his/her airway, cooperate with treatment, maintain a satisfactory pO_2 on oxygen, and has a fairly stable pulse, BP and cardiac rhythm. If not, proceed to the more aggressive measures in the next section.

Treatment of moderate hypothermia (31°–28°C)

Treatment should not be based on temperature alone, particularly since core temperature may not initially reflect the rewarming that has been commenced. BP, pulse, O_2 sats and ability to protect the airway all influence treatment decisions. Because VF is a frequent complication, patients with frequent ventricular ectopic beats (VEBs) merit vigorous rewarming.

In addition to the same measures as those described above for mild hypothermia, most moderately hypothermic patients will need:

1. **Intubation.** The patient will be hypoventilating and having problems dealing with copious bronchial secretions. Use standard drugs and dosages. Pharmacokinetics and pharmacodynamics are altered by hypothermia, but there is no specific information to guide dosing. Below 30°C, most drugs do not work at all, and 'cold' intubation may be required. At higher temperatures, if the drugs work, they will generally have a longer half-life. Insert a heat-moisture-exchanger into the circuit. Seventy per cent of respiratory heat loss goes into humidifying expired air. Most emergency departments do not have mechanisms for heating inspired air, and this additional effort brings marginal benefit.

2. **Nasogastric tube (NGT).** Cold reduces gastric motility and distension is likely.

3. **Active external rewarming.** If a Bair Hugger is not available, put hands and feet in warm water or use radiant heat or hot water bottle. Be careful of burning poorly vascularised and insensitive skin.

Treatment of severe hypothermia (<28°C)

Most patients with severe hypothermia will need active core rewarming and ICU admission. Heated gastric lavage and/or bladder irrigation through the NGT and IDC are non-invasive but not as effective as peritoneal lavage (one or two catheters) or thoracic lavage (two catheters). The most effective rewarming procedure is extracorporeal rewarming using cardiopulmonary bypass or haemodialysis machines.

Give broad-spectrum antibiotic prophylaxis because of the high incidence of sepsis due to impaired resistance.

If there is no cardiac output

Death from hypothermia will be preceded by slow pulse and respirations, so more care than usual in seeking signs of life is indicated. Unfortunately, the muscular rigidity associated with severe hypothermia is similar to rigor mortis, so the clinical diagnosis of death is difficult without an ECG. But there have also been cases of cold asystolic people recovering or being resuscitated, so the axiom 'no one is dead until they are warm and dead' creates a dilemma in the emergency department, particularly if CPR has been started pre-hospital.

Some guidelines are:

1. T <15°C, or K >12 mmol/L is unsalvageable.
2. 32°C is a reasonable level to achieve. Once it has been reached, if resuscitation has not already been successful, it probably will not be.
3. <32°C, if cardiopulmonary bypass is available, use it. If it is not available, use warmed fluids through two intercostal catheters while CPR continues. VF may not respond to either drugs or defibrillation <32°C.

Spectacular reported saves in the literature involve icy immersions (rarely relevant to Australia) and cardiopulmonary bypass being readily available.

There is a tendency to persist longer in hypothermic resuscitations than normothermic, but the presence of hypothermia above 32°C in a temperate water (10°–20°C) toddler drowning does not mandate active core rewarming efforts.

HYPERTHERMIA

Hyperthermia is technically different from fever. It is a raised body temperature due to failure of the temperature regulation systems. Unlike hypothermia, it is not possible to say that the diagnosis is defined by temperature. However, it is reasonable to say that below 40°C urgent treatment is unlikely to be needed. Above 42°C, cellular damage is likely whatever the cause—fever or hyperthermia.

Definitions

In **fever**, the body's temperature regulation is reset to a new level. Resetting the temperature control with antipyretics may help.

Heat stress is a sense of discomfort in a hot environment.

Heat exhaustion is thirst, weakness, dizziness etc plus a normal or mildly elevated temperature due to water or salt depletion.

Heat stroke is a medical emergency, which is described below.

Heat stroke

This is defined as collapse plus CNS abnormalities plus T >40°C occurring once temperature regulation is overwhelmed. In athletes, it occurs despite sweating (exertional heat stroke), but in sedentary elderly or frail people (classical heat stroke) it usually occurs after sweating stops. There is a risk of multiorgan failure from the combination of hyperthermia and an exaggerated acute phase response. Once this response has started, temperature correction may not be enough to avert death. Table 32.3 shows the clinical features of heat stroke

Diagnosis

Diagnosis is easy if a patient has been exercising in hot conditions, but the presentation may be more subtle. Table 32.4 shows a list of situations that predispose to hyperthermia.

As with hypothermia, surface temperature may not reflect core temperature. Tympanic infrared thermometers are technically capable of detecting high temperatures but may be unreliable due to technique. As with hypothermia, the diagnosis, if suspected, should be confirmed with a rectal probe.

Differential diagnosis

T >40°C plus CNS dysfunction equals heat stroke, unless an alternative diagnosis is evident. The most obvious alternative diagnosis is a febrile

Table 32.3 Clinical features of heat stroke

System	Signs
CNS	Delirium; convulsions
Musculoskeletal	Rigidity; rhabdomyolysis; lactic acidosis
Skin	Dry when sweating eventually fails
Electrolytes	Hyponatraemia, hypokalaemia early Hypernatraemia, hyperkalaemia later
Gastrointestinal tract	Diarrhoea; raised hepatic transaminases; raised lipase
Endocrine	Hypoglycaemia
Haemopoietic	Coagulopathy
Renal	Oliguric renal failure
Respiratory	Hyperventilation; alkalosis/tetany

Table 32.4 Conditions predisposing to hyperthermia

Condition	Reason
Advanced age	Impaired adaptation/mobility
Infancy	Immature sweating
Cardiac disease/drugs	Unable to increase CO
Dehydration/diuretics	Less circulating fluid
Anticholinergics/skin disease	Reduced sweating
High humidity	Reduced evaporative cooling
Hyperthyroidism/stimulant drugs	Increased heat production

illness, particularly CNS infection. A more detailed list of differential diagnoses is as follows:

- Meningitis/encephalitis.
- Cerebral malaria.
- Thyroid storm.
- Anticholinergic poisoning
- Delirium tremens.
- Neuroleptic malignant syndrome.

Management

Heat stroke is a medical emergency. If the diagnosis is suspected, commence treatment immediately.

1. **Cool the patient.** Remove clothing as far as modesty permits, place a fan at each end of the bed, and continuously spray the patient with water at room temperature (or warmer) using a misting device. This evaporative cooling is the most effective cooling mechanism. If the temptation to use ice is irresistible, try to confine it to strategic areas (groin and axilla). Aim to reduce the temperature to 39°C within 30 minutes. Stop cooling when 39°C is reached.
2. **Give oxygen.** Check O_2 sats, ABGs and CXR. ABGs will show a respiratory alkalosis +/- lactic acidosis.
3. **Intubate** if hypoxic or unable to protect the airway. Remember that an intubated patient will require hyperventilating to cope with the metabolic acidosis. Convulsions are common, so the intubated patient will require electroencephalogram (EEG) telemetry and/or phenytoin.
4. **Set up an IV and take blood** for baseline:
   - *BSL.*
   - *Electrolytes, Ca, PO₄.* Electrolyte disturbances will improve with cooling, so treat only excessive derangements.
   - *Liver function tests (LFTs).*
   - *Creatine kinase* (CK—rhabdomyolysis).

- *Coagulation studies.* Use FFP and platelets if bleeding is a problem. Disseminated intravascular coagulation (DIC) may be present but treatment with heparin is controversial. Coagulation defects should correct with time and cooling.

5. Give 500–1000 mL crystalloid. The patient will have a hyperdynamic circulation with a degree of R heart failure and raised jugular venous pressure (JVP). Pulmonary oedema can occur. Yet almost by definition there will be a fluid deficit from previous sweating, so hypotension and oliguria are usually present. The best plan is to give 500 mL crystalloid stat, with a further 500 mL over the next hour. If BP and urine output are not restored, use CVP to monitor further replacement.

6. Insert an IDC. Monitor urine output. Test for myoglobinuria. If present alkalinise the urine with HCO_3 and give mannitol.

7. Consider sedation. Use a benzodiazepine to sedate the patient if agitated or confused and to control seizures.

8. Do not use aspirin or paracetamol. In theory they won't work: aspirin will exacerbate bleeding, and paracetamol will require metabolising by a deranged liver. In fact, pyrogenic cytokines have been implicated in heat stress, but there have been no controlled trials of antipyretics.

9. Consider chlorpromazine 25 mg IVI if shivering is impeding cooling, but don't use it routinely because it may lower BP and impair sweating.

If symptoms and blood abnormalities do not correct with cooling, ICU admission will be required. Heat stroke has a significant mortality rate.

MALIGNANT HYPERTHERMIA

This is a rare complication of anaesthesia that usually occurs soon after anaesthesia, but may be delayed up to 11 hours. Most anaesthetic agents (including succinylcholine) can cause it. Temperature is 41°–45°C. Treatment is similar to heat stroke but with the addition of dantrolene 2–3 mg/kg/day.

NEUROLEPTIC MALIGNANT SYNDROME

This is an idiosyncratic reaction occurring in about 0.2% of patients given neuroleptics. Haloperidol is the commonest offender. Dopamine receptor blockade leads to skeletal muscle spasticity (generating heat) and impaired hypothalamic regulation (interfering with response). The patient has T >41°C plus muscle rigidity plus altered consciousness plus autonomic instability. Treatment is as for heat stroke. Both dantrolene and bromocriptine are thought to be helpful, although there are no controlled trials.

SEROTONIN SYNDROME

See Chapter 28.

RECOMMENDED READING

Auerbach P. Field guide to wilderness medicine. 2nd edn. St Louis: Mosby; 2003.

Bouchama A, Knochel JP. Heat stroke. N Engl J Med 2002; 346(25):1978–1988.

Marx JA, Hockberger RS, Walls RM, Adams J, eds. Rosen's emergency medicine: concepts and clinical practice. 5th edn. St Louis: Mosby; 2001.

Sessler D. Complications and treatment of mild hypothermia. Anaesthesiology 2001; 95(2):531–543.

33 | Childhood emergencies

Gary Browne, Bruce Fasher, Mary McCaskill, Susan Phin

The child in the emergency department presents a challenge to the busy emergency physician, particularly in a setting where both adults and children are being treated and the general culture is not a paediatric one. Children are different in that they are dependent, developing and growing rapidly. They also differ in their spectrum of disease and response to illness.

Keep in mind that you are managing both the child and the family. Parents may often perceive their children to be sicker than staff assess them to be. In many instances they may prove to be right! It is crucial for a successful consultation to listen to the parents and get a clear understanding of their concerns. At the same time, don't be dismissive of the children; involve them in your history-taking as a prelude to examination. Parental anxiety and coping skills need to be assessed and any social disadvantage noted.

In all childhood emergencies, take a careful history and examine the whole child. A child can deteriorate rapidly. This must be anticipated. If there is any doubt about a child's condition, a paediatrician should be involved and transfer to a paediatric hospital considered.

PHYSIOLOGICAL PARAMETERS

In dealing with sick children, it is important to recognise how physiological parameters change with age and the impact this may have on the interpretation of observations and management.

Respiratory

Table 33.1 Normal respiratory values

Age	Breaths per minute
Infants	40
Preschool	30
School age	20

Endotracheal tube size = (age in years ÷ 4) + 4

Cardiovascular

Table 33.2 Normal cardiovascular values

Age	Beats per minute
Infants	160
Preschool	140
School age	120

Blood volume = 80 mL/kg
Systolic blood pressure = 80 mmHg + (age in years × 2)

Weight

In ideal circumstances, children should be weighed and the weight, height and head circumference plotted on appropriate growth charts. In emergencies, weight can be estimated using the simple formula:

$$\text{Weight} = (\text{age} + 4) \times 2.$$

IMMUNISATION IN CHILDHOOD

The emergency department offers an excellent chance to give catch-up immunisations. The recommended schedule changes frequently and is listed in the current Australian Immunisation Handbook (available from the Commonwealth Department of Health and Ageing, tel. 1800 671 811 or from the website: see 'Recommended reading'). There are few contraindications.

RESUSCITATION

In the emergency situation, a child's condition can deteriorate very rapidly. This is due to:

- The dynamic and unpredictable responses a child can have to stress.
- Physiological limitations, e.g. hypoglycaemia.

- Anatomical differences, e.g. small airways and fatigable respiratory muscles.
- Developmental differences, e.g. immune system.
- Ability or inability to communicate.
- Less characteristic illness responses, e.g. meningitis/neck stiffness.

There may also be a greater risk of acute deterioration in the following cases:

- Neonates and small infants.
- Children with congenital or genetic disorders.
- Children with chronic disease.
- Immunodeficiency or child undergoing chemotherapy.

The key to success in managing seriously ill children is early recognition. The outcome from paediatric cardiac arrest is extremely poor, as most children who arrest do so from progressive unrecognised hypoxia or through inadequate or inappropriate resuscitation.

When assessing children therefore, attention should focus on the three major systems—respiratory, cardiovascular and central nervous system (CNS)—to identify the very sick child early.

Respiratory

Increased breathing effort is a sign of increasing respiratory insufficiency and is characterised by: tachypnoea, use of accessory muscles, expiratory grunting, stridor, wheezing, nasal flare, dyspnoea or cyanosis.

Other important but often forgotten signs of impending respiratory embarrassment in children are exhaustion and apnoea.

Monitor the following closely:

1. Respiratory rate.
2. Effort of breathing.
3. Colour.
4. Oxygen saturation using pulse oximeter.

Cardiovascular

A child's haemodynamic status is assessed by examining pulses, capillary refill, blood pressure, mental status and urine output. It must be remembered that in children the ability to compensate through vasoconstriction is strong, hence blood pressure is always one of the last indicators of a decompensated haemodynamic state.

The signs of shock are:

- Tachycardia/bradycardia.
- Decreased pulse volume.
- Poor peripheral perfusion.
- Abnormal mental status.
- Oliguria.
- Hypotension.

CNS

The level of consciousness in children may be impaired for many reasons. However, invariably in the seriously ill child it is due to hypoxia. Mental state change is one of the most consistent features of shock and generally occurs when cerebral perfusion is being compromised. Neurological assessment therefore involves:

1. **Level of consciousness.**
   A—alert.
   V—responds only to vocal stimuli.
   P—responds only to painful stimuli.
   U—unresponsive.
   Children who are unresponsive to painful stimuli are very likely to have difficulty with their airway and ventilation.
2. **Pupils.** Pupillary size, reaction to light, and inequality need to be assessed. Fixed dilated pupils are a sign of severe cerebral injury.
3. **Posture.** Tone and posture need to be assessed. Decorticate (flexed arms, extended legs) or decerebrate (extended arms, extended legs) posture indicates severe cerebral injury.

The principles of resuscitation

These are similar in children and adults.

A—airway

In children the goals are to recognise and relieve obstruction, to prevent aspiration and to allow adequate oxygenation.

B—breathing

If breathing is laboured or poor in children, it should be supported with either a bag-valve-mask device or through intubation with mechanical ventilation.

C—circulation

The rate-limiting step in many resuscitative efforts in children is achieving IV access. If unsuccessful after an initial attempt, an intraosseous line should be promptly attempted. An initial fluid bolus to resuscitate a shocked child is 20 mL/kg of normal saline or Hartmann's solution. A colloid such as 4% albumin can also be used.

D—drugs

When using drugs in the resuscitation of children, it is important to be aware that their effect depends on:

- Appropriate dosage on a weight-determined basis.
- How they are delivered, e.g. diluted or undiluted.
- The route of administration, e.g. IV, endotracheal, rectal.

- How they are absorbed and metabolised, e.g. endotracheal adrenaline.
- If there are any unwanted effects in children, e.g. verapamil/asystole.

E—environment

In children it is important to consider hypothermia, hypoglycaemia and other reversible causes early in the process of resuscitation.

When CPR is performed in children, how it is performed is determined by the child's size and age (see Chapter 1).

IDENTIFYING THE SICK CHILD

Identifying the sick child can be difficult even for experienced staff. The younger the child, the more difficult it can be, particularly when trying to exclude focal bacterial infection. Following simple guidelines will help screen out those children with a greater likelihood of serious illness. Table 33.3 shows a useful approach for detecting serious illness in the child under 36 months of age. Combinations of symptoms are even more concerning. No child should be sent home from the emergency department without thorough assessment, appropriate investigations and preferably a period of observation.

Other signs of concern include fever, apnoea, convulsions, a petechial rash, cyanosis and the rapid onset of symptoms. Antibiotic use, prolonged symptoms and chronic illness are important features to note. Do not ignore the signs of bile-stained vomiting or blood in the stools alone or in the presence of abdominal pain.

AIRWAY EMERGENCIES

Croup

Croup is viral laryngotracheobronchitis characterised by a barking cough. Often several days of upper respiratory tract symptoms precede the cough. The associated respiratory distress is worse at night and with anxiety in child or parent. Spasmodic croup occurs without accompanying infective symptoms and is often recurrent. Stridor at rest is an indication of severity,

Table 33.3 The ABC of assessment of the sick child*

A	Arousal, alertness and activity	Decreased responsiveness, drowsy, floppy
B	Breathing difficulty	Grunting respirations, recession
C	Circulation	Pallor, mottling
D	Decreased input and output	Input down to half, or output less than 4 nappies in 24 hours

*See Hewson and Oberklaid

while cyanosis is a pre-arrest state. Lateral airways X-rays are not needed and are dangerous as the child is unstable.

A calming environment with the child on the mother's lap is therapeutic.

If there is moderate or severe airway obstruction, nebulised adrenaline (0.5 mL/kg of 1:1000 maximum 5 mL) can be used as a temporising measure, but rebound after 20 minutes has been well described. Oral dexamethasone (0.15 mg/kg) or prednisolone (1 mg/kg) reduce the risk of intubation and in moderate cases may allow the child to be discharged with review arranged. If this is not tolerated, IV dexamethasone or nebulised budesonide 2 mg can be given. Attention to hydration of the child is important. Humidified air has not been shown to help, and numerous burns occur from steam at home.

Epiglottitis

Epiglottitis is a severe bacterial infection of the epiglottis less commonly seen since *Haemophilus influenzae* immunisation. The disease is usually rapidly progressive over hours and the child drools, is unable to phonate, does not cough and assumes the 'sniffing the air' position to maximise the airway calibre. Cyanosis is a late, pre-arrest state. Interventions should be avoided unless the child is pre-arrest. The initial treatment is rapid transfer to the operating suite for administration of an inhalational anaesthetic and intubation. If there is doubt about the diagnosis, this can be diagnostic. If a respiratory arrest occurs before an inhalational anaesthetic is available, bag-and-mask ventilation, intubation with sedation only or needle cricothyroidotomy are needed. Muscle relaxants must not be used with the anaesthetic as the airway will be lost. Once the airway is controlled, take a swab and commence IV third-generation cephalosporins.

Bacterial tracheitis

This is a rare infection presenting similarly, with acute upper airway compromise. Usually the child appears toxic.

Foreign body inhalation

This causes an acute onset of respiratory distress, often in a child between 6 months and 2 years. If the object is in the upper airway, complete or partial obstruction may be present. If the child is moving air or coughing then removal under inhalational anaesthetic by skilled personnel is advisable. If the airway is completely obstructed, rapid back blows in an infant or the Heimlich manoeuvre in an older child should be performed. Direct visualisation and removal of the object with Magill's forceps may be possible. If this is not successful, a needle cricothyroidotomy should be performed. Cricothyroidotomy using a scalpel is not recommended for children under 5 years.

What else could it be?

- Peritonsillar or retropharyngeal abscess.
- Anaphylaxis.

RESPIRATORY EMERGENCIES

Asthma

Asthma in childhood is a common condition. Signs of respiratory distress indicating severity include tachypnoea, intercostal recession, use of accessory muscles, prolonged expiration, cyanosis and altered level of consciousness. Exacerbations are treated with salbutamol, initially with spacers or nebulised if moderately severe bronchospasm prevents adequate inspiration. In severe cases, IV salbutamol initially as a bolus, or an infusion if improvement is not maintained, speeds improvement. Except in mild cases nebulised ipratropium bromide is also given. A short course of steroids (prednisolone 1 mg/kg) for 3–5 days is given, by the IV route in severely ill patients. Ventilatory support with either continuous positive airways pressure (CPAP) or intubation, often with assistance with expiration, is needed with apnoea or altered level of consciousness. There is a high attendant risk of barotrauma. Inhalational anaesthetics can also be used as bronchodilators. Long-term preventative therapy aims to reduce the incidence and severity of exacerbations: inhaled sodium cromoglycate and, if needed, inhaled steroids.

Pneumonia

This also presents with respiratory distress. Auscultatory signs may be subtle especially in the younger child, and X-ray is needed to confirm the diagnosis. Treatment is with antibiotics, either oral or IV.

Organisms causing pneumonia are shown in Table 33.4.

Table 33.4 Organisms causing pneumonia

Common bacterial agents	
Streptococcus pneumoniae	
Staphylococcus aureus	<5 years
Mycoplasma pneumoniae	>3 years
Common viral agents	
Parainfluenza	
Influenza	
Respiratory syncytial virus (RSV)	
Epstein-Barr virus (EBV)	

Bronchiolitis

Bronchiolitis occurs particularly in 2–6-month-olds, and is caused by respiratory syncytial virus (RSV) in 75% of cases. After two days of coryza, increasing respiratory distress with tachypnoea, nasal flaring, wheezing and fever is seen and lasts several days. There may be apnoea or difficulty feeding, requiring IV hydration. Chest X-ray is normal or shows hyperinflated lungs with peribronchial cuffing in approximately 50% of cases. Treatment involves oxygen, if required, via nasal prongs, headbox or intubation and attention to hydration. Bronchodilators and steroids are of no proven benefit but a trial of bronchodilators may be warranted in the older infant. Patients who are discharged need early review by their local doctor.

Cystic fibrosis patients commonly present with respiratory decompensation related to infection. They have a chronic cough and purulent sputum, and benefit from chest physiotherapy and IV antibiotics.

Chronic lung disease occurs in premature infants and some develop respiratory failure with subsequent upper respiratory tract infection.

Pertussis is associated with spasms of coughing, an inspiratory whoop in older children and then frequently a vomit. Apnoea may be the only symptom in the infant less than 3 months old. Between coughing paroxysms the child is often asymptomatic. There is a leukocytosis of 20,000–50,000 with a predominance of lymphocytes. X-rays are usually normal. Treat with oxygen during spasms, IV rehydration if necessary, and erythromycin if the patient is in the early phase or for prophylaxis of contacts.

THE UNCONSCIOUS CHILD

Remember that the brain is more commonly the target of insult than the primary cause. Always consider and treat those conditions that are correctable, such as hypoglycaemia and hypoxia.

Always examine the whole child in the light of a thorough history.

Immediately

- Support and maintain the airway.
- If trauma is likely, take appropriate precautions to stabilise the cervical spine.
- If the airway is unmaintainable, consider repositioning and jaw thrust.
- Suction the oropharynx if this is available.
- Insert an oral airway.
- Intubation: this can be performed cold in the deeply unconscious child, or the rapid-sequence intubation technique can be used if the child is only lightly unconscious.
- Support ventilation if inadequate or impaired.
- Administer oxygen via face mask at 4–6 L/minute.

- If the circulation is compromised, establish intravenous access (intraosseous access may be necessary) and give a bolus of fluid: 20 mL/kg.
- Reassess the child regularly.

Look for

- Rashes.
- Fever or hypothermia.
- Evidence of head injury.
- High or low blood glucose.
- Blood pressure abnormalities.
- State of hydration.
- Evidence of raised intracranial pressure.
- Abnormal neurological signs.

Ask about

- Events before the child's presentation.
- Past medical history.
- Medication the child may be taking or have been exposed to.
- Specifically, accidental ingestion, diabetes, whether there has been a convulsion.

Management

- After initial stabilisation, consider the need for mechanical ventilation.
- Check a dextrose stick and if low administer 5 mL/kg 10% dextrose solution.
- Consider poisoning and antidotes, e.g. naloxone, flumazenil.
- Consider sepsis and administer antibiotics if necessary.
- Consider dexamethasone 0.6 mg/kg before antibiotics if meningitis is likely.

Investigations to be considered

- Full blood count.
- Blood culture.
- Formal blood glucose.
- Electrolytes and urea.
- Urine for glucose, ketones and drug assay.
- Lumbar puncture if meningitis is considered, no evidence of raised intracranial pressure exists and patient is not obtunded.

Monitor closely

Level of consciousness, perfusion, respiratory rate, blood pressure, heart rate, urine output, temperature—clinically.

Re-evaluate and reassess regularly.

THE FEBRILE CHILD

If the cause is still not evident, consider intussusception (may have a 'cerebral' presentation). Fever is one of the most common causes of presentation to an emergency department. Most fevers are due to viral infections, but care must be taken to exclude a bacterial infection. Diagnosis can often be difficult, particularly in the younger child, where caution is advised. The child without a clear focus presents a real challenge, with pneumococcal sepsis being the most common infective condition currently encountered. Various approaches are advised in the literature, ranging from cautious assessment and observation through to aggressive management.

A thorough clinical assessment is recommended. Appropriate investigations include a full blood count, blood culture, chest X-ray, urine microscopy and culture, and lumbar puncture in the younger child where there are associated convulsions, meningism or where the child is on antibiotics. Ensure appropriate observation, review, and if in doubt seek further consultation. The dilemma of when and where to treat and which antibiotic to use depends upon the individual and the local environment. It is better to err on the side of overinvestigating and treating.

In the acute situation, the age of the child, the highest recorded temperature (>39.5°C) and an elevated white cell count with a shift to the left are the most useful guides to underlying bacterial infection, in combination with the Hewson criteria. The higher the white cell count, the greater the risk of bacteraemia, ranging from 6% for counts greater than 10,000 to 30% and higher for counts above 20,000. Do not be lulled into a false sense of security by a temperature that responds to temperature control measures, or by a normal white cell count. Your initial assessment should set the pace for further assessment. Staging a septic work-up is only likely to delay care.

What else could it be?

Always think of underlying metabolic, cardiac and endocrine problems. The fever may be the simple harbinger of acute deterioration in these patients. One possible approach to management of the febrile child is given in Figure 33.1.

COMMON INFECTIONS

Consider:

1. Preschool children normally experience 6–8 upper respiratory tract infections (URTIs) per annum.
2. Antibiotics neither cure the URTI nor prevent complications.
3. Exclude common and dangerous causes:
   - Otitis media.
   - Tonsillitis.

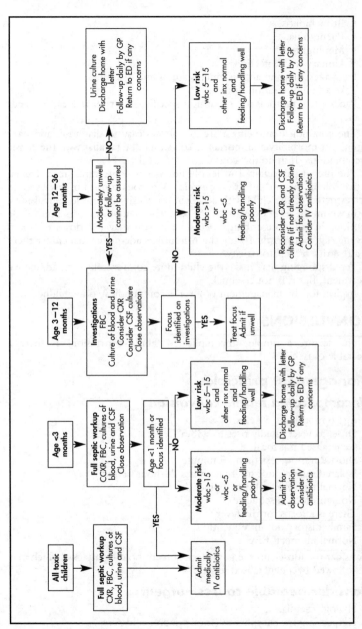

Figure 33.1 Guidelines for the management of febrile children (T 38°C) under 3 years of age without a focus of infection

- Bronchiolitis.
- Pneumonia.
- Meningitis.
- Urinary tract infection
4. Decongestants and antihistamines are of dubious value.
5. Take an immunisation history.
6. Paediatric symptoms are often non-specific—fever, diarrhoea, off feeds etc.

The common exanthemata are not always easy to diagnose, and have significant morbidity and mortality. You should be familiar with the classic presentations. If in doubt, consult.

The use of paracetamol in febrile illnesses is conjectural (fever has an active role in the anti-infection cascade). Vigorous control of fever should be restricted to the child with a known propensity to febrile convulsions, or in whom the fever exceeds 38.5°C and who is in obvious discomfort. Be cautious in your prescribing. Occasionally you may use doses of up to 15 mg/kg, but mostly 10 mg/kg 6-hourly is adequate. Remember there is a real risk of hepatotoxicity.

Tepid sponging may make the child more comfortable as an adjunctive treatment, but it is not essential.

Aspirin for the management of fever is contraindicated in childhood.

CONVULSIONS

Is the seizure a simple, uncomplicated febrile convulsion? Is there a treatable cause?

Management principles

Uncomplicated febrile convulsion

- Age 6 months to 5 years.
- Onset as fever rapidly rises to >38.5°C.
- Generalised not focal.
- Short duration, less than 15 minutes.
- Isolated seizure, not multiple over a 24-hour period.
- Normal neurological development.
- No neurological sequelae.
- There is a focus for the fever.
- Family history not infrequently.
- Normal interictal EEG.

Consider pseudoseizures, e.g. syncope, breath-holding attacks (which may be followed by a generalised seizure).

Consider treatable causes—urgent

- Hypoglycaemia.
- Herpes simplex encephalitis (focal seizure, cold sores).

- Electrolyte disturbance (especially sodium—persistent vomiting and diarrhoea).
- Meningitis.

General management

- Maintain airway.
- Oxygen.
- Diazepam IV (0.2 mg/kg)—not IM, repeat as needed. Consider midazolam (0.1 mg/kg/dose) either IV or IM, or diazepam PR undiluted 0.5 mg/kg if IV access difficult.
- If status develops, consider:
  a. Over 3 months of age: phenytoin 15–20 mg/kg IV over 20 minutes (cardiac monitor), then 3 mg/kg IV 6-hourly.
  b. Under 3 months of age: phenobarbitone 20 mg/kg (500 mg maximum) diluted in normal saline or dextrose over 20 minutes, then 5 mg/kg/day 8-hourly.

Above all, listen to parents (previous management, treatable cause etc) and recognise their distress, especially if this is the first seizure they have witnessed.

GASTROENTERITIS

Gastroenteritis is a common childhood complaint, the commonest complication of which is dehydration.

Organisms to consider are shown in Table 33.5. Most cases will be viral. Bloody diarrhoea often suggests a bacterial cause.

Signs include vomiting, diarrhoea, fever and abdominal pain. The diarrhoea with rotavirus and adenoviruses often lasts for 5–12 days, and that of bacterial diarrhoea (especially *Campylobacter*) is often bloodstained. *Giardia* infection commonly causes an epidemic and is complicated by asymptomatic carriers. Beware of attributing vomiting without diarrhoea to gastroenteritis.

Assessment

Includes the degree of dehydration. Evidence of sepsis is important, especially in the young infant. Of children under 3 months of age with

Table 33.5 Organisms causing gastroenteritis

Viruses	Bacteria	Protozoa
Rotavirus	*Salmonella*	*Giardia*
Enteroviruses	*Shigella*	Amoebae
Enteric adenovirus	*Campylobacter*	
Norwalk	*Yersinia*	
	E. coli	

Salmonella, 5–10% are bacteraemic. *Salmonella* can also cause focal infections in children with sickle cell anaemia. Abdominal X-ray commonly shows multiple fluid levels representing ileus: it is rarely helpful unless obstruction is suspected. Stool culture is advisable when bacterial or parasitic infections are suspected.

Treatment

Try oral rehydration solution in small frequent sips at a rate of 1 mL/kg every 10 minutes. If this fails, commence nasogastric tube rehydration with an oral rehydration solution. If this is not tolerated, commence IV rehydration, remembering to check the sodium level. Volumes to replace the fluid deficit and volumes for maintenance requirements should be calculated separately, added together then divided by 24 to get the hourly rate. Frequent reassessment to monitor progress is important. Antibiotics (third-generation cephalosporins) are recommended for *Salmonella* in the young septic infant, or one with a prolonged severe course of illness. Otherwise they do not convey any benefit, as they do not shorten the course or reduce the infectivity of the patient with *Salmonella*. *Campylobacter* infection should be treated with erythromycin only if the symptoms are prolonged. *Giardia* infection-causing symptoms should be treated with metronidazole.

When not to treat at home

- Dehydration.
- Diagnosis in doubt.
- Family not coping.
- Persistent vomiting.
- No consultation available.
- Deterioration.
- Anticipated deterioration.

An uncommon sequel is the haemolytic uraemic syndrome presenting usually 5–10 days after gastroenteritis, caused by enteropathic *E. coli*. It can also occur after upper respiratory tract infection. It is manifest by microangiopathic haemolysis, low platelets, raised urea, poor urine output, hypertension and renal failure.

Think again if

- Vomiting bile or blood.
- Severe abdominal pain.
- Toxic, high fever.
- Abdominal signs:
    Distension
    Tenderness, guarding
    Mass, visceromegaly
- Neonates.
- Failure to thrive.

What else could it be?

- Intussusception.
- Appendicitis.
- Urinary tract infection.
- Sepsis, otitis media.

See also below: 'Fluid therapy', 'Surgical abdominal emergencies'.

FLUID THERAPY

Children can rapidly become dehydrated because of their small size and large, insensible fluid loss (they have a high surface area to volume ratio). The aim of fluid therapy is to continue maintenance fluid intake and replace fluid in the dehydrated child. Common causes of fluid loss are gastroenteritis, fever, blood loss and poor oral intake in respiratory distress.

Maintenance fluids

Maintenance fluids can be estimated using:

- 100 mL/kg for the first 10 kg.
- 50 mL/kg for the next 10 kg.
- 20 mL/kg for every subsequent kilogram.

Maintenance fluids should be one-quarter normal saline plus 3.75% dextrose.

Potassium requirements of 2–3 mmol/kg/day should also be met.

Signs of dehydration

These can become more evident with the extent of fluid imbalance, but are altered in hypernatraemia. Percentages of fluid loss give a guide to the rate at which fluids need to be given, but frequent reassessment of the child's fluid state is vital:

- 3% dehydration manifests with reduced urine output and thirst but no clinical signs.
- 5% presents with sunken eyes, dry mucous membranes and reduced skin turgor.
- 7% manifests with a more severe presentation of the above signs as well as irritability, lethargy and tachycardia.
- 10% presents with marked lethargy, irritability and even coma, plus cardiovascular compromise with tachycardia, hypotension, coldness and sweating.

Rehydration

Acute resuscitation of the child with cardiovascular compromise should include a bolus of fluid 20 mL/kg crystalloid such as normal saline or Hartmann's solution or 5% NSA colloid. Half normal (N/2) and quarter normal (N/4) saline should not be used for resuscitation.

Volume required to replace the fluid deficit can be estimated using the fomula:

$$\% \text{ dehydration} \times \text{weight} \times 10 = \text{mL}.$$

More sodium is needed in this replacement fluid, so half normal saline plus 2.5% dextrose is used. This should be administered over 24 hours and regularly reviewed to allow for further losses to be replaced. In the case of hypernatraemia, slower rehydration over 48–72 hours is required.

Remember

- Decreased oral intake or vomiting may rapidly lead to dehydration in a child.
- Serum electrolytes, urea, creatinine should be checked if rehydrating intravenously.
- Rehydrate slowly in hypernatraemia.
- Reassess the child clinically and monitor the urine output to see if the fluid therapy is appropriate.
- If no improvement, consider repeating electrolytes and an alternative diagnosis.

DIABETIC KETOACIDOSIS AND HYPOGLYCAEMIA

These are not uncommon problems, but are best managed in a children's centre experienced in such specialised care, hence early referral is recommended.

Children with diabetic ketoacidosis at diagnosis of their diabetes have often been unwell for 4–6 weeks with progressive weight loss, dehydration and altered mental state. Because of this, mistakes in diagnosis can be made early in the acute phase.

Presentation

- Polyuria.
- Polydipsia.
- Weight loss
- Dehydration.
- Altered mental state.

Traps for young players

- Chest infection: rapid breathing due to metabolic acidosis.
- Urinary tract infection: polyuria (always check urine for glucose and ketones).
- Gastroenteritis: dehydration.
- Enuresis: polyuria (always check urine for glucose and ketones).

Always take a thorough history and completely examine the child.

Management

1. If shocked, ensure adequate airway and ventilation while administering high-flow oxygen via a face mask. Administer 20 mL/kg fluid (saline or normal serum albumin) rapidly and then reassess the child's haemodynamic status.

   Then:

2. Assess the degree of dehydration.

3. Commence replacing sodium with 0.9% saline and aim to correct over 48 hours. Be careful not to give too much fluid too soon, as children are prone to developing cerebral oedema.

4. Add potassium to fluids 5 mmol/kg/day once urine has been passed.

5. Strict fluid balance is essential.

6. Commence insulin infusion after rehydration has commenced. Commence at infusion rate of 0.05 units/kg/h, aiming to lower blood glucose 4–5 mmol/L per hour. A larger drop in the first hour is acceptable, as fluid alone would lower the blood glucose to some extent.

7. When the blood glucose falls below 12 mmol/L, change IV fluid to 0.45% saline and 5% dextrose. Maintain the blood glucose level between 5 and 10 mmol/L. If glucose falls below 5 mmol/L do not decrease the insulin infusion, but rather increase the amount of glucose in the infusion.

Investigations

1. Collect venous blood for:
   - Glucose.
   - Sodium, potassium, chloride, urea, creatinine.
   - pH, PCO_2, HCO_3, base deficit.
   - Full blood count.
2. Test all urine for glucose and ketones.

Monitor closely

- Hourly to two-hourly glucose, potassium, sodium.
- Hourly pulse rate, respiratory rate, blood pressure, blood glucose and neurological observation.
- Accurate fluid balance.
- Test all urine for ketones until clear.

Cerebral oedema/brainstem herniation

Brainstem herniation is a sudden and unpredictable complication of therapy for diabetic ketoacidosis; it occurs during the first 24 hours of treatment.

1. Monitor all patients for evidence of raised intracranial pressure with particular attention to those most at risk:
   - Severe dehydration.
   - Severe acidosis with low potassium.

- Hypernatraemia.
- Deteriorating conscious state.
- Severe hyperosmolality on presentation (>320 mOsm/L).

The onset of headache should be taken seriously.

2. Transfer to an intensive care unit and arrange neurological assessment and CT head scan. Management should be aimed at aggressively controlling any elevation in intracranial pressure.

Hypoglycaemia

Blood glucose levels <2.5 mmol/L. In diabetic children hypoglycaemic symptoms often occur at blood glucose levels under 3 mmol/L. Prolonged hypoglycaemia can cause irreversible brain damage.

In children substrate deficiency is the most common cause, either as a result of prolonged fasting or due to specific conditions such as ketotic hypoglycaemia. Other important causes include hepatic disorders, metabolic disorders and, rarely, insulin excess (Beckwith syndrome, nesidioblastosis).

Presentation

- Anxiety, flushing.
- Nausea/vomiting.
- Pallor.
- Sweating.
- Trembling, weakness.
- Tachycardia.
- Confusion, drowsiness or coma.

Investigations

- Blood glucose.
- Sodium, potassium, urea, creatinine.
- After consultation, further special tests may be necessary: alanine, cortisol, growth hormone, amino acids, free fatty acids, ammonia etc.

Management

- Resuscitate as necessary.
- Check blood glucose, draw blood for investigations.
- Administer a glucose bolus 0.5 g/kg as 5 mL/kg 10% glucose or 2 mL/kg 25% glucose IV if symptomatic and the blood glucose is <2.5 mmol/L. After recovery, if necessary continue a 10% glucose infusion at maintenance rate. If unable to secure IV access, glucagon 0.03 mg/kg IM may be used to a maximum of 1 mg (ineffective in hepatic disease). In some cases, where a child is awake and cooperative, oral glucose drinks may be satisfactory.
- Early referral to a specialist children's centre is recommended in difficult or refractory cases.
- Monitor closely.

DEVELOPMENT

Assessing normal development is a skill acquired only from constant practice and observation. Always consider seriously parents' concerns of loss of recently acquired skills or slow development of others. If you are not confident of your own skills in assessing development do not dismiss parents' concerns but rather refer appropriately. See Table 33.6 for normal developmental milestones.

FEEDING

Feeding problems are rarely emergencies. The notable exception is the parents' observation that the child is 'going off his feeds'. This can be the result of any illness from a cold to congestive cardiac failure.

History and examination are paramount:

- To elucidate a cause (infection, surgical condition, etc.) *or*
- To assess effect (weight loss, dehydration etc).

It is important to be familiar with basic feeding practices and to be able to support a breast-feeding mother through a crisis when her child is unwell. Milk allergies and intolerances are not common. Resist changing milk formulas for the lack of better inspiration. Rather than give inappropriate advice, refer the infant and mother to their local doctor, paediatrician, community health centre or in some instances an appropriate mothercraft centre.

THE INCONSOLABLE INFANT

The inconsolable infant will test the patience of all attendants. The condition is always worse in the quiet of night. Listen to the parents. Don't be dismissive—they are at the end of their tether.

Consider physical causes of pain and discomfort, especially treatable conditions such as:

- Intussusception/malrotation volvulus.
- Otitis media.
- Dental problems (rarely teething).
- Peptic ulceration (oesophagitis secondary to clinical reflux).
- Missed fractures (intentional or accidental).
- Stones—renal/gallbladder.
- Infection (paradoxically, sepsis often leads to quietening).
- Ischaemic heart disease (anomalous coronary arteries—rare).

There is a group of children (infants) for whom no physical cause can be elucidated. Their parents require immense support.

Consider admission if:

- There is a physical condition to treat.
- Children are at risk from tired, frustrated carers.

Table 33.6 Normal developmental milestones

Age	Gross motor	Vision and fine motor	Social and understanding	Hearing and speech
Newborn	Prone: pelvis high, knees under abdomen, turns face to side.	Can fix on a visual object and follow it briefly horizontally.		Variable response to sound.
1 month	Lifts head momentarily when held in a ventral suspension.	Follows visual object through 90°.	Quietens when picked up.	Soft guttural noises when content.
6 weeks	Head lag not complete when pulled to sit.	Hands often open.	Social smiling.	Quietens in response to soft sound 15 cm from ear.
3 months	Prone: lifts chest off bed taking weight on forearms. Only slight head lag when pulled to sit.	Holds rattle placed in hand. Hand regard begins.	Pleasurable response to familiar, enjoyable situations (bottle, bath).	Turns head to sound at ear level.
6 months	No head lag when pulled to sit. Prone: lifts chest on extended arms, rolls onto back.	Hand regard goes. Transfers objects between hands.	Shows fear of strangers. Can imitate (e.g. cough).	Visually locates soft sounds at 45 cm on ear level.
9 months	Crawls. Stands holding onto support. Sits unsupported for 10 minutes.	Pincer grip developing.	Looks for toy fallen out of sight. Shouts to attract attention.	Deliberate vocalisation to try to communicate. Localises soft sounds above and below ear at 1 metre.
12 months	Walks with one hand held. Can let self down from standing position.	Casts objects on floor repeatedly.	Claps hands. Knows and turns to own name.	Says 2 or 3 words with meaning.
18 months	Jumps using both feet. Walks backwards.	Spontaneous scribble. Tower of 3 or 4 cubes.	Knows 2 or 3 parts of body. Indicates toilet needs.	6–20 recognisable words. Understands many more.

Table 33.6 Normal developmental milestones (continued)

Age	Gross motor	Vision and fine motor	Social and understanding	Hearing and speech
2 years	Runs well. Kicks ball without overbalancing.	Copies vertical and circular strokes. Tower of 6 or 7 cubes.	Parallel play with other children. Mainly dry by day.	Names 4 toys. Two- and 3-word phrases.
3 years	Rides tricycle. Can stand on 1 foot momentarily.	Copies circle, 9 cube tower.	Mainly dry by night. Competent with fork and spoon.	Knows full name and sex. Uses plurals.
4 years	Hops on 1 foot for 3–5 seconds.	Copies cross. Draws men with 3 parts. Matches 4 primary colours.	Very imaginative play. Picks longer of 2 lines.	Asks many questions.
5 years	Skips on alternate feet.	Copies square. Man of 6 parts. Names primary colours.	Understands rules of play. Washes and dries face and hands.	Knows full name, address and age.

Always acknowledge carers' concerns and frustrations. This often resolves 50% of problems. Plug them into 'the system' (for ongoing support) if you intend sending the child home.

JAUNDICE

With the advent of early discharge obstetric programmes, neonatal jaundice is a concern in emergency departments.

Kernicterus (significant brain damage due to jaundice) can occur with high levels of unconjugated (indirect) bilirubin.

Be concerned by

- Jaundice in the first 24 hours of life.
- Bilirubin greater than 240 µmol/L.
- Conjugated bilirubin greater than 30 µmol/L.
- Jaundice present after day 10 of life.
- Jaundice in an unwell infant.

Consider

- Haemolysis (rhesus, spherocytes, cephalhaematomas, other).
- Infection:
    a. Intrauterine: toxoplasmosis, cytomegalovirus (CMV), rubella, other.
    b. Current sepsis, especially urinary tract infection (UTI).

- Surgical causes, some treatable (ideally early): biliary atresia, choledochal cysts.
- Genetic causes and inborn errors of metabolism:
  a. Hypothyroidism.
  b. G6pd deficiency.
  c. Galactosaemia.
  d. α_1-antitrypsin deficiency.
  e. Cystic fibrosis.
  f. Bilirubin metabolism syndromes (Gilbert's, Crigler-Najjar, Dubin-Johnson, Lucy Driscoll).

Investigations

May include:

- Bilirubin, total and direct.
- Haemoglobin, film, haematocrit, blood cultures, group, Coombs' test, reticulocytes.
- Torch titres.
- Urine microscopy, culture and sensitivity, reducing substances.
- Thyroid function (check neonatal screen).
- Galactosaemia screen.

Physiological and 'breast milk' jaundice

Physiological jaundice (slow maturation of glucuronyl transferase) and 'breast milk' jaundice (competitive use of glucuronyl transferase) are not diagnoses of convenience. Continue to monitor the child either until a cause is found or the jaundice disappears.

CHILD ABUSE

This is a common problem. It should be in the differential diagnosis of all injuries, burns, poisonings and genital injuries in both sexes.

Suspect child abuse if

1. The physical findings are inconsistent with the explanation given for the injury.
2. There is delay in seeking medical attention.
3. The explanation for the injury varies.
4. There are multiple injuries at different stages of healing.
5. There is a spiral fracture (an unusual fracture in childhood suggesting a twisting, shearing force) or metaphyseal chip fractures.
6. There are two black eyes and/or haematomas on the ears.
7. Retinal haemorrhages are present.
8. Fingerprint bruising (e.g. on upper arms, cheeks or trunk) caused by violent gripping.
9. Bruising in soft tissue areas not normally injured in play.

10. Burns on the buttocks and perineum (from dunking in boiling water) or discrete burns in other areas consistent with cigarette burns.
11. There is vaginal or anal bleeding or injury in the absence of an adequate explanation.

Management

1. Admit the child to hospital for protection and treatment.
2. Treat the injuries.
3. Do skeletal survey and radionuclide scan in children under 2 years, looking for old fractures at different stages of healing.
4. Consider CT for subdural haematoma.
5. Obtain clinical photographs.
6. Take appropriate forensic specimens for semen and check for sexually transmitted diseases (use sexual assault kit).
7. Assess child's development and behaviour.
8. Take a full social history.
9. Avoid having the child interviewed on multiple occasions. Questions must not be suggestive or leading.
10. Consult a paediatrician and social worker experienced in this area.
11. Record all findings and conversations accurately in the hospital record (they and you may be required in court later).
12. Notify the statutory authority in those places that have mandatory notification laws.

SUDDEN INFANT DEATH SYNDROME (SIDS)

By definition there is no evident cause of death. The diagnosis thus cannot be confirmed until after the autopsy. These facts affect management.

1. Resuscitation attempts are dictated by the clinical situation. Be alert for a treatable condition.
2. Parents and family, including siblings, should not be excluded from resuscitation, despite the uneasiness this may cause staff.
3. Family counselling should involve the most experienced staff available. Note the necessity of police interviews because of the coroner's involvement.
4. The family should be able to stay with the deceased infant as long as they wish, preferably in a quiet room and supported by staff.
5. Photographs and hand and foot prints are often appreciated at a later date.
6. Follow-up for the parents is important. This may need to be organised later.
7. It is often useful to involve your local SIDS association.

Prevention

- Position infants on their backs.

- Do not overheat.
- Loose-fitting clothes.
- Smoke-free environment.

SURGICAL ABDOMINAL EMERGENCIES

Abdominal pain may be difficult to assess in a young child. Examination requires warm hands and a gentle approach to gain the child's trust. The examination will be limited once pain has been elicited. Consider analgesia to aid examination.

Intussusception

This classically presents between 3 months and 5 years. It frequently follows a minor viral illness, and involves intussusception of a lymphoid follicle through the bowel, causing intermittent screaming with pallor and vomiting, usually without diarrhoea. Increasing lethargy develops between exacerbations of pain. The abdomen in usually tender and a sausage-shaped mass is often palpable in the right upper quadrant. Blood in the stools and shock are late presentations. X-ray may reveal an area of paucity of gas or obstruction; however, 30% have normal X-rays. Abdominal ultrasound can be diagnostic.

Treatment involves reduction under surgical supervision, preferably in a paediatric facility, by air enema under radiological visualisation. Cases that present late or may have perforation require reduction (and repair) in theatre. Be aware that intussusception may present masquerading as a cerebrally depressed child such that investigations pursue this avenue (CT head, cerebrospinal fluid, drug screen) until all return normal results.

Inguinal hernias

These are common in the first year of life and need early correction, as they are liable to become incarcerated. Gentle reduction is often possible in the emergency department. If they become irreducible, IV fluid therapy and urgent surgery are required.

Henoch-Schönlein purpura

This is a vasculitis that commonly occurs in the bowel causing intermittent abdominal pain in children 3–5 years. It is also associated with a purpuric rash developing on the buttocks, and arthropathy and haematuria signify renal involvement. Management is usually conservative.

Hirschsprung's disease

This is absence of intramural ganglion cells, usually in the rectosigmoid region. It is four times more common in males. It presents early in life with increasing constipation and abdominal distension from the newborn period to early childhood. Rectal examination often reveals explosive release of stool under pressure. Abdominal X-ray shows faecal loading. The complications are enterocolitis and perforation. The treatment is surgical.

Appendicitis

This can occur at any age. Under 2 years of age the appendix is an intra-abdominal organ. Appendicitis is difficult to diagnose and the appendix is often perforated at the time of surgery. The child has abdominal tenderness and sometimes fever, vomiting and diarrhoea.

Pyloric stenosis

This occurs from 1 week to 3 months of age with males four times more commonly affected than females. They present with increasing vomiting, dehydration and hypokalaemia, with a hypochloraemic metabolic alkalosis. A pyloric mass can often be felt, particularly at the end of a test feed; ultrasound or barium meal can confirm this. The child needs IV fluids and operative treatment.

What else could it be?

Urinary tract infection, mesenteric adenitis, gastroenteritis, child abuse, constipation, diabetic ketoacidosis.

ORTHOPAEDIC PROBLEMS

See also Chapter 17.

Septic arthritis

This can occur in any joint and is characterised by pain, restricted joint movement and sometimes fever, raised white cell count and erythrocyte sedimentation rate (ESR). Suspicion requires confirmation and treatment by surgical drainage in theatre, culture of the fluid, irrigation and intravenous antibiotics.

Irritable hip

This commonly occurs in children and is often (but not always) associated with a viral illness. The important differential to consider is septic arthritis. Serial examination often reveals limitation of internal rotation of the hip but preservation of some hip movement, absence of constitutional symptoms and normal blood pathology.

Limp

The child with a limp needs careful assessment to establish where the problem lies. Trauma, irritable hip, Perthes disease, slipped capital femoral epiphyses, septic arthritis or effusion in any of the joints of the limb, tumours, leukaemia, spinal problems, soft-tissue injuries and foreign bodies in the sole of the foot must all be considered. Spinal discitis may be suggested by the child refusing to walk or sit.

Pulled elbow

A pulled elbow occurs when the radial head is pulled out of the annular ligament sling with traction on the arm. It sometimes occurs recurrently in children between 1 and 4 years. Check that the story is consistent with this diagnosis, and exclude bony injury with X-ray. To relocate the annular ligament, feel over the radial head, and firmly pronate and extend the arm. Often a click is felt and the child begins using the arm within 10 minutes. If this does not occur check that nothing has been missed and arrange review the following day. The natural history is for these to spontaneously relocate over a few days.

What else could it be?

Child abuse, bony tumour.

PAIN MANAGEMENT

Pain control during procedures and with painful conditions greatly reduces the anxiety experienced by children and parents.

Anxiety reduction minimises the pain felt and should be used with all frightening or painful procedures. A confident, caring approach to the family and enlisting the parents' support for the child are vital. Clear, non-threatening and age-appropriate explanation to the child just before and during the procedure reduces the fear of the unknown.

See also Chapter 22.

Analgesics

- Paracetamol preparations in a dose of 15 mg/kg are very effective in children.
- Narcotics IV (in frequent small doses), IM or orally (morphine 0.1 mg/kg, pethidine 1 mg/kg, codeine 1 mg/kg).

Sedatives

Nitrous oxide/oxygen mixture is used with great success in experienced hands. It reduces anxiety especially when combined with verbal relaxation methods and topical cream if necessary, but consciousness is maintained. A maximum of 70% N_2O can be used. The main side effect is vomiting. This can be minimised by having the child fasted for at least 2 hours before proceeding.

Midazolam can be given orally (in juice or frozen in ice-blocks to disguise the taste) or nasally at a dose of 0.5 mg/kg or IV at 0.1–0.2 mg/kg. It is effective in about 70% of children. The main side effect is respiratory depression, especially after the noxious stimulus is withdrawn. Recovery with careful observation and oximetry for 2 hours after the procedure is important.

Ketamine, a dissociative anaesthetic given IV or IM, is very effective. Paediatric airway expertise should be present as should venous access. The airway is maintained but there is an increase in salivation. Its side effects include occasional prolonged vomiting and hallucinations. This agent is not commonly used in paediatrics but may be useful in the adolescent.

Anaesthetics

General anaesthetics should be available, especially for procedures involving intricate work and cooperation of a small child.

Topical prilocaine creams reduce the pain felt during procedures involving needles (IV cannulas, blood taking, lumbar punctures). They are safe, but should not be used under 6 months of age because of toxicity and methaemoglobinaemia. The area should be completely occluded with a dressing once the cream is applied and left for 45 minutes to ensure maximal efficacy. The cream cannot be applied to mucosal areas or areas of broken skin. Topical mixtures such as TAC (tetracaine, adrenaline and cocaine in a gel preparation) are very effective for lacerations. Toxicity from cocaine is minimised if it is not used on mucosal surfaces, where absorption is rapid.

PRESCRIBING FOR THE PAEDIATRIC PATIENT

When prescribing for the paediatric patient, oral therapy is preferred where possible. If parenteral antibiotics need to be given, avoid IM injections. Plan ahead by leaving a cannula in situ when taking blood. Dosages should be based on weight and the manufacturer's instructions carefully adhered to. There are many useful pocket guides available. Special care should be taken with newborns. Maximum dosage should be calculated based on a patient's weight not exceeding 50 kg.

Parents should be given clear written instructions on dosage and guidance on administration. Children mostly do not enjoy taking medications and will not always cooperate. When a child refuses to take medication, gentle restraint, recruiting another adult to assist or using a syringe (without needle) to instil the medication into the buccal cleft may all help.

PROCEDURES
What size tube?

Most items of equipment vary depending upon the age, weight and size of the patient. Table 33.7 provides only a guide to the size of commonly used items of equipment for use in emergency circumstances. In certain

Table 33.7 Equipment sizes for children

Age	ETT size (ID) to try first (mm)	Distance to insert ETT at lips (cm)	Chest tube (Fr)	Naso-gastric tube (Fr)	Foley's catheter (Fr)	Laryngo-scope blade
Neonate	3	10	8	6	6	1
6 months	3.5	11	8	6–8	6	1
1 year	4	12	12	8	6–8	1.5
2 years	4.5	13	12	8	6–8	2
4 years	5	15	14	10	8	2
6 years	5.5	16	20	10	8	2
8 years	6	18	20	10	8	2
10 years	6.5	19	20	12	10	2
12 years	7	20	28	12	12	3

ETT = endotracheal tube

circumstances, it may be necessary to modify the tube size (e.g. a child with croup may need a smaller tube).

Obtaining blood

It is always possible to get sufficient blood from paediatric patients for all tests—it is a matter of patience, and having the right equipment and technique. Depending on the laboratory, you may be able to use smaller samples. A superficial peripheral vein is the preferred location. If inserting an IV line, plan your investigations so that you can take blood for investigations at the same time to avoid unnecessarily hurting the child. Use topical EMLA if time allows.

Tips

- Proper reassurance distraction techniques and restraint are the secrets to success.
- Consider analgesia such as nitrous oxide.
- Be prepared and always have an assistant.
- Hand over after two failures.
- Do not overconstrict or you will prevent venous filling.
- Small veins collapse more easily—2 mL are better than 5 mL.
- Unless taking blood for cultures, free flowback often gives a better volume than aspiration.
- If not siting an IV and aspiration is difficult, use a needle with the hub removed. The hub promotes coagulation when the flow is slow.
- Do not use the femoral or neck veins as first options. It may be preferable to resort to arterial sampling instead.
- If leaving a cannula in situ, proper splinting is required, but avoid a tourniquet effect.

Urine sampling

To adequately diagnose a urinary tract infection, a sterile sample must be collected. Midstream urines are of value only in the older child. Bag urines are inadequate. Younger children require either a suprapubic aspirate or catheterisation. Over 12 months of age catheterisation is preferred.

Suprapubic aspiration

1. Ensure that the bladder is full by percussion and that the child has not passed urine for 60 minutes.
2. Use EMLA cream in anticipation.
3. Be prepared with appropriate equipment and assistant.
4. Gently restrain the child supine with legs held at the knees.
5. Prepare the site. Cleansing may lead to urination—be prepared to catch a midstream sample.
6. Insert a 23-gauge 32 mm needle on a 5 mL syringe 1 cm above the symphysis in the midline. Direct the needle caudally at a 20° angle to the vertical. Gently aspirate while advancing.
7. Repeat the procedure once only if unsuccessful, by withdrawing the needle just below the skin and advancing it with a slightly greater degree of angulation caudally.

Urinary catheterisation

Urinary catheterisation is an acceptable alternative to suprapubic aspiration. The procedure is essentially no different from the one used in adults. Use aseptic techniques, have an assistant, be prepared and most importantly be gentle. In young females, be familiar with the anatomical landmarks. If you are unable to identify the urethra do not proceed.

UTI

Criteria for the diagnosis of a urinary tract infection (UTI):

1. $>10^5$ organisms (pure growth of a single organism).
2. >100 white cells/high power field.
3. Positive leukocytes and nitrites on dipstick (should not be relied upon as a screening test).
4. Negative microscopy does not exclude UTI.
5. Up to 20% of children with UTIs have negative dipstick analysis.

Lumbar puncture

1. No child will cooperate willingly with a lumbar puncture. Use EMLA cream in anticipation but local infiltration is still preferable. Ensure adequate restraint with proper positioning.
2. Consider nitrous oxide.
3. Position the patient in the lateral decubitus position, making sure the patient is well flexed and the back is vertical to the bed.
4. Prepare the skin and drape the site.

5. Identify the L3/4 interspace (at the level of the superior edge of the iliac crest).
6. Insert spinal needle (with stylet) in interspinous space, directed slightly cephalad towards the umbilicus.
7. Advance the needle slowly. A 'give' may be felt as the dura is penetrated.
8. Remove stylet and, if no fluid is obtained, rotate the needle 90° so that the bevel is pointing in a cephalad direction.
9. If CSF does not flow freely replace the stylet and advance the needle until fluid is obtained.
10. Pressures should be measured using a manometer.
11. Collect adequate samples for testing. If bloodstained fluid is obtained use the last tube for microscopy.

Contraindications

- Obtunded patient.
- Raised intracranial pressure.
- Infection at the site.
- Bleeding diathesis including thrombocytopenia.

RECOMMENDED READING

Browne G, Choong RKC, Gaudry PL, Wilkins BH. Principles and practice of children's emergency care. Sydney: MacLennan & Petty; 1997.

Crain E, Gershel J. Clinical manual of emergency pediatrics. 4th edn. New York: McGraw-Hill; 2003.

Hewson P, Oberklaid F. Recognition of serious illness in infants. Modern Medicine of Australia 1994; 37(7):89–96.

Kilham H, Isaacs D, eds. The Children's Hospital at Westmead handbook: clinical practice guidelines for paediatrics. Sydney: McGraw-Hill; 2003.

National Health and Medical Research Council. The Australian immunisation handbook. 8th edn. NHMRC; 2003. Available from Immunisation Information Line 1800 671 811 or from the website: http://immunise.health. gov.au/handbook.htm.

Strange G, et al. Pediatric emergency medicine. 2nd edn. New York: McGraw-Hill; 2002.

34 Geriatric care

Nicholas J Brennan

This chapter is a guide to help you in assessing older patients who present to the emergency department with one of the six geriatric syndromes: confusion, depression, incontinence, falls, immobility, and dependency in activities of daily living (ADLs). Put simply, 'geriatric care' means assessment of each of these syndromes, in addition to conventional history-taking and examination. It implies detailed assessment of functional status and social context. In addition, it is important to remember to assess hearing and vision, nutritional status and dental hygiene, as well as to review all medications and the immunisation status of older patients.

The rapidly increasing population of older Australians is placing enormous pressures on all aspects of our health system. Older people come to hospitals in numbers that are approximately double their proportional representation in the community. These numbers are rapidly escalating, so we will continue to see significant increases in demand for emergency services for the elderly. Older people come to hospital more often by ambulance; wait longer in the emergency department; have a much higher rate of admission to hospital; have increased mortality; undergo more investigations and cost more money to treat. They are at increased risk of further deterioration or readmission after discharge from the emergency department. It is important that you familiarise yourself with the post-acute care services or early discharge programs that are available locally.

Geriatric medicine is not simply general medicine in old people. There are significant differences in the approach to care, diagnosis and decision-making in the frail aged. There are several important principles of practice:

1. Older patients have impaired physiological reserve, which means that diseases often present at an earlier stage. Many illnesses that present as acute emergencies are in fact minor, easily treatable and have excellent outcomes. Some older patients present late with very advanced disease. This is usually a result of abnormal illness behaviour.
2. Presentation of a new disease often depends on the weakest organ system, not the newly diseased organ system. Atypical presentation of disease is common. For example, new onset of confusion will most likely be due to infection in the urine or chest, rather than new pathology in the brain. Therefore, the first test to perform for acute confusion is a septic screen rather than a CT scan of the brain.
3. Many 'abnormal' clinical findings are common in older people and may not be responsible for a particular symptom. For example, many older

patients will have some crackles in their chest and some degree of lower limb oedema. Together, these findings are commonly overinterpreted and treated as if due to cardiac failure.

4. Occam's razor frequently does not apply in the elderly where multiple, common, coexisting pathologies combine to form a 'syndrome'. Therefore, in the emergency department, attention to detail and treatment of multiple concurrent abnormalities can result in marked overall improvement in the patient.

5. Effective treatment of older patients requires effective communication. For example, if you are prescribing medications for a patient going home, can you be certain that the patient will be able to understand the instructions and comply with your therapy? Over half of patients sent home from hospital are mal-compliant with prescribed medication, and most show inadequate medication-related knowledge.

Diagnostic information and treatment changes must be communicated directly to the local general practitioner, family and carers. It should be assumed that patients will not remember much of what they have been told during their visit to the emergency department. It is safer to take a more paternalistic approach, similar to when dealing with paediatric patients, where extra time is spent explaining the medical issues to the patient's family or carers. This is not meant to suggest that the majority of our older patients are mentally incompetent, but merely to stress the importance of good communication, especially in those situations where the older patient is dependent on a variety of coordinated community services to remain at home.

THE GERIATRIC SYNDROMES

1. Dependency in activities of daily living (ADLs)

Older people come to the emergency department for a wide variety of reasons. Their presentation will commonly be due to an acute medical illness; but equally there will often not be a 'medical' emergency, as we know it. What the older patients in emergency departments need more than anything else is for you to take a careful history, which includes speaking to family, carers, friends and local doctors.

- Always check that the patient's own account is accurate by asking someone else who knows the patient (this will save time, unnecessary investigations and costs).
- Always consider the possibility of underlying medical problems as the cause of the current presentation, especially when the initial triage suggests 'acopia'.
- You should become familiar with a brief assessment of ADLs (Figure 34.1), which should become part of your medical assessment, because dependence on basic ADLs is a powerful predictor of poor health outcomes from acute illness.

- Involvement of the emergency department social worker and discharge planning service are crucial. Patients may need temporary services at home to cope with a new disability associated with their current illness. There are significant shortages in the availability of community services, including community nursing, so do not assume that appropriate services can be arranged immediately by the social worker.
- Refer patients for physiotherapy and occupational therapy assessments.

2. Acute confusion

Presentation with acute confusion offers diagnostic and management challenges to the doctor and the staff of emergency department. A busy emergency department is the most unsatisfactory environment in which to treat an acutely confused older person, but you will be expected to do this time and time again. The family of the patient will find the situation particularly stressful. Care should be taken not to label the patient as suffering from dementia, until such time as a clear history of a dementing

Figure 34.1   Dependency in activities of daily living (ADLs)

Personal activity of daily living (tick box if patient needs help in ADL)		Instrumental activity of daily living (tick box if patient needs help in ADL)	
Bladder and bowel function	☐	Shopping	☐
Feeding	☐	Meal preparation	☐
Dressing	☐	Housekeeping	☐
Transfers	☐	Taking medications	☐
Bathing	☐	Transport	☐
Mobility	☐	Finances	☐

| ANSWER THIS QUESTION | Have you ticked any of the boxes?

YES

Referral to social worker.
Do not send home without further consultation.
Confirm the history with family, carer or GP.
Test for cognitive impairment.

NO

Can you be sure?
Is there evidence of cognitive impairment?
Have you confirmed the history with the family, carer or GP?

Being dependent in activities of daily living is strongly predictive of deterioration after being sent home from the emergency department. Patients themselves will often overestimate their level of independence. Always check the history with family or friends. Do not send the patient home with new medications unless you are sure that they will be taken correctly.

Figure 34.2 Acute confusion—why is this patient confused now?[1]

Baseline factors		Precipitating factors	
Brain disease (dementia, stroke, head injury)	☐	Trauma/injuries	☐
Use of sedatives and anticholinergics	☐	Recent introduction of new medications	☐
Visual or hearing impairment	☐	Dehydration	☐
Malnutrition	☐	Pain	☐
Severe disability	☐	Drug withdrawal	☐

illness can be obtained. Dementia is largely a diagnosis of exclusion, and you need to actively exclude delirium and psychiatric conditions such as depression before arriving at such a significant diagnosis. Dementia, depression and delirium frequently coexist, and it can be very difficult to separate them.

Diagnosis

- It is best to assume that the confused emergency department patient has some underlying acute medical problem that is contributing to the acute confusion, and to set about finding it!
- A collateral history from reliable informants must always be sought.
- Assess baseline and contributing factors (Figure 34.2).
- The Confusion Assessment Method (Figure 34.3) is a brief tool that helps to diagnose delirium. This is used in conjunction with the Mini Mental Status Examination (MMSE: Figure 34.4) that should be completed in all cases to objectively document the current level of cognitive impairment.
- Physical examination is often difficult, as the patient struggles against your valiant efforts to complete the examination.
- Routine haematology and biochemistry, urine and blood cultures, ECG and CXR should suffice as preliminary investigations in the majority of cases. Abnormal thyroid function, vitamin B_{12} and folate deficiency are uncommon causes of acute confusion which should be excluded.
- CT brain scan is a second-line investigation, unless there is evidence of objective neurological signs or a high index of suspicion for possible recent head injury, especially in those cases presenting with a 'fall and long lie'.
- Even after hospital admission and lengthy investigations, up to one-third of these patients will be discharged from hospital without a precipitant having been clearly identified.

Management

- Broad-spectrum intravenous antibiotics if there is evidence of infection (neutrophil leukocytosis, elevated temperature, cultures positive).

Figure 34.3 Confusion Assessment Method (CAM)[2]

Feature	Questions to ask	Yes = 1 No = 0
Acute onset and fluctuating course Ask a family member or carer these questions:	Is there evidence of acute change in mental status from the patient's baseline?	☐
	Did the abnormal behaviour fluctuate during the day, that is, tend to come and go, or increase or decrease in severity?	☐
Inattention This feature is shown by a positive response to the question:	Did the patient have difficulty focusing attention, for example being easily distractible, or having difficulty keeping track of what is being said?	☐
Disorganised thinking This feature is shown by a positive response to the question:	Was the patient's thinking disorganised or incoherent, such as rambling or irrelevant conversation, unclear or illogical flow of ideas, or unpredictable switching from subject to subject?	☐
Altered level of consciousness This feature is shown by any answer other than 'alert':	Alert (normal) = 0 Vigilant (hyperalert) Lethargic (drowsy, easily aroused) Stupor Coma	☐

The diagnosis of delirium by CAM requires the presence of features 1 and 2 with either 3 or 4.

Complete the MMSE (see Figure 34.4) and basic investigations

Delirium management

| ANSWER THESE QUESTIONS | Is the patient at risk from harm from falling, restlessness, wandering, AND/OR
Is there a risk of harm to others due to agitation or aggressive behaviour? |

YES	**NO**
Close supervision—use special nurse, family member or expedite admission to secure environment. Commence risperidone 0.5 mg, preferably given late afternoon, further doses of 0.5 mg.	Close supervision—remember that delirium fluctuates. The situation may be stable now, but will possibly deteriorate at night.

Figure 34.4 Folstein Mini Mental Status Examination (MMSE)[3]

Year.................................1	State...................................1
Season............................1	City 1
Date 1	Suburb...............................1
Month..............................1	Hospital 1
Day of the week 1	Floor..................................1

Registration of three items 3
Spell WORLD backwards or serial sevens.................................5
Recall of three items at one minute...3
Able to name two objects (pen and watch)..............................2
Able to repeat 'no ifs, ands, or buts' 1
Able to follow three-stage command 3
Able to read and obey 'close your eyes'..................................1
Write a sentence 1
Copy intersecting pentagons or draw a clock face 1

Total..........30

- Avoidance of iatrogenic precipitants (such as indwelling urinary catheters, addition of multiple medications, use of restraints).
- Careful use of a very low dosage of major tranquillisers such as risperidone or haloperidol.
- Individual nursing is probably the most effective 'treatment'—it prevents problems such as falls and wandering, and reduces the need for sedating medications.
- Families can play a crucial role in helping to reorientate patients to their current surroundings.
- If wandering patients cannot be safely contained within the department, there is a priority to move them to a safe environment within the hospital, rather than to restrain them.

3. Falls

One-third of all people over the age of 65 years fall every year, and half of these fall repeatedly. Falls cause pain, fear, suffering, restriction of activities and death among older people; in fact they are the leading cause of accidental death in people older than 85 years. Five per cent of falls lead to a fracture and 10% of fallers sustain other serious injuries. After a fracture, one in four will never regain previous mobility.

Elderly fallers are different from their healthy, age-matched counterparts. Although some have medical conditions that cause the fall, most have no single diagnosis, but rather a combination of risk factors for falls. The more risk factors present, the greater the likelihood of further

Figure 34.5 Falls risk assessment[4]

Baseline factors (tick box if present)		Suggested action by RMO
Postural hypotension	☐	Measure erect & supine BP
Hypnosedative agent	☐	Discuss with consultant
Use of ≥4 medications	☐	Medication review; discuss with consultant
Environmental hazards	☐	Consider occupational therapy assessment
Any impairment of gait	☐	Mobilise the patient
Any impairment of balance or transfers	☐	Observe transfers and test standing balance
Impairment of leg or arm muscle strength or range of movement	☐	Neurological examination

| ANSWER THIS QUESTION | Is the patient at risk of harm from falling over again now? |

YES

Close supervision especially if confused & falling. Physiotherapy assessment for provision of walking aid and indication of mobility status.
Daily supervised mobilisation if possible.
Do not send home without further consultation.

NO

Consider future risks; referral to community team for OT assessment; referral to outpatients for falls risk assessment and exercise programme.

About half the patients who fall will do so repeatedly. Your task is to prevent another fall; falls risk assessment coupled with appropriate interventions can reduce the risk of further falls and injury.

falls. Interventions targeted at these risk factors have been shown to reduce the rate of further falls.

- Complete a simplified falls risk assessment (Figure 34.5) on all older patients who present after having fallen.
- Exclude postural hypotension.
- Check vision.
- Perform neurological assessment.
- Perform a gait assessment, including the time to 'Up & Go' test (Figure 34.6) and review adequacy of footwear. Consult the physiotherapist in the emergency department about the gait assessment and provision of mobility aid where appropriate.
- Review all medications (in particular hypnosedative agents) and reduce medications where possible.

- A follow-up occupational therapy home visit should be organised, as 50% of falls are due to extrinsic (environmental) factors.

4. Immobility

Mobility problems are a common link in those patients who have a number of the geriatric syndromes (incontinence, falls and dependency) and are often overlooked by young doctors. It is important to determine if the immobility is an acute or chronic problem and train yourself to comment on the gait. Is it safe or unsafe? Mobility is affected by falls (pain from fractures or soft tissue injury, fear of further falling, lack of confidence), and intercurrent illness (breathlessness, muscle weakness, dizziness, fear) in the acute setting (Figure 34.7). A brief period of gait retraining is often all that is required to restore confidence and safety, and is a good reason in itself to recommend admission to hospital. Those with long-standing mobility problems may need much more intensive multidisciplinary team involvement to get home, and should be referred to the geriatric service for assessment. As in the falls assessment, the time to 'Up & Go' test is an objective measure of gait that you should perform.

5. Depression

The spectrum of depressive disorders differs in the elderly. Major depression occurs in only 1.5%, but depression of clinical significance occurs in up to 13.5%. However, depressive symptoms including anxiety symptoms, phobias and somatisation are extremely common. There is a very strong correlation between depressive symptoms and use of health services, and the rate at which old people develop depression is highly dependent on preceding disability.

- It is important to perform a full mental status examination on geriatric patients, especially when you suspect depression, self-neglect, squalor syndrome or excessive alcohol intake.
- Assess cognition using the MMSE.
- The Geriatric Depression Scale (GDS, Figure 34.8) may help you decide whether there is a likelihood of depression being present.
- Assess degree of suicidality (passive and active) and decide if you feel that either is present. Older patients will commonly tell you that they wish they were dead, especially in the setting of acute illness, pain and disability.

Figure 34.6 The time to 'Up & Go' test[5]

The time to 'Up and Go' test is a useful bedside test that correlates well with more sophisticated falls risk assessment. The patient should be able to arise from a chair, walk 6 metres and return to the seated position within 15 seconds. Failure to do so within this time limit constitutes an abnormal test and indicates a high risk of further falls.

Figure 34.7 Immobility

Why is the patient unable to mobilise? (tick box if present)	Suggested action by RMO	
Always immobile ☐	Are social supports adequate to deal with the immobility?	☐
Fear of falling ☐	Multidisciplinary team approach	☐
Pain (especially musculoskeletal) ☐	Investigate and treat	☐
General deconditioning ☐	Nutritional, cognitive and ADL assessment	☐
Acute medical illness or fracture ☐	Investigate and treat; to exclude a fracture may take time	☐

ANSWER THIS QUESTION   Can the patient mobilise independently today?

YES

Recommend daily mobilisation while in hospital to prevent deconditioning.
Perform the time to 'Up & Go' test.

NO

Referral to physiotherapist.
Do not send the patient home unless immobility is able to be managed at home.
Assume a fracture to be present if patient is not able to bear weight following a fall.

Figure 34.8 The Geriatric Depression Scale[6]

Are you basically satisfied with your life?	X	No
Have you dropped many of your interests and activities?	Yes	X
Do you feel that your life is empty?	Yes	X
Do you often get bored?	Yes	X
Are you in good spirits most of the time?	X	No
Are you afraid that something bad is going to happen to you?	Yes	X
Do you feel happy most of the time?	X	No
Do you often feel helpless?	Yes	X
Do you prefer to stay at home rather than going out and doing new things?	Yes	X
Do you feel that you have more problems with memory than most?	Yes	X
Do you feel it is wonderful to be alive now?	X	No
Do you feel pretty worthless the way you are now?	Yes	X
Do you feel full of energy?	X	No
Do you feel that your situation is pretty hopeless?	Yes	X
Do you think that most people are better off than you are?	Yes	X
Total score (one point per question answered)		**15**

- It is never appropriate to institute antidepressant therapy in the emergency department without first consulting the duty geriatrician or psychiatrist.
- The presence of passive suicidal ideation or depressed mood should prompt discussions with family and a referral to the emergency department social worker for psychological support.
- If the patient is to be sent home, involvement of social supports (both family and community) is essential to reduce the risk of self-harm.

6. Incontinence

Urinary incontinence affects up to 20–30% of community-dwelling older persons and 50–70% of those in long-term institutions. Incontinence creates embarrassment, isolation, depression and stigmatisation. It places a significant burden on caregivers and carries the risk of institutionalisation. Incontinence predisposes to skin rashes and infections, decubitus ulcers, urinary tract infections (UTIs), urosepsis, falls and fractures. For these reasons, incontinence carries very high economic costs. Despite its prevalence, morbidity and cost, however, incontinence is often neglected, poorly evaluated, often accepted as 'a normal part of ageing'.

There are numerous primary causes of incontinence in the older person. These may be primarily related to the pelvic structures or there may be various contributing factors. Frequently, the aetiology is mixed and complex. With adequate assessment and appropriate management, many patients can be cured and almost all can be significantly improved. Where cure is not possible, assistance with social continence should be achieved.

Continence requires not only the integrity of lower urinary tract function but also adequate mentation, mobility, motivation and manual dexterity (the four Ms).

Initial assessment of incontinence

See also Figure 34.9.

1. Determine whether the incontinence is a new or old problem.
2. Determine the pattern of the incontinence (urge, stress, retention with overflow, mixed).
3. Determine the contribution of the four Ms to the current presentation.
4. Exclude infection in the urine (dipstick testing; midstream urine, MSU).
5. Lower limb neurological examination.
6. Rectal examination and abdominal palpation, excluding the presence of significant post-voiding residual volume (catheter or ultrasound).

Diagnosis and management

1. Frequency–volume chart helps to accurately define the pattern of incontinence.
2. Bowel management (prescribe enemas and aperients if constipated).
3. Treat urine infection if this is present.

Figure 34.9   Incontinence—Why is this patient incontinent now?

Baseline factors	Precipitating factors	
Brain disease (dementia, stroke, head injury)	Infection in the urine or elsewhere	☐
Always has bladder or bowel problems ☐	Recent introduction of new medications, especially diuretics	☐
Pre-existing mobility problems ☐	New mobility problems	☐
Malnutrition ☐	Constipation, impaction with overflow	☐
Severe disability ☐	Severe illness	☐

ANSWER THIS QUESTION   Is the incontinence a new problem?

YES	NO
Exclude faecal impaction (PR and plain abdomen X-ray). Exclude urinary retention (examination, bladder ultrasound, residual volume). Exclude infection (MSU, CSU, in-out catheter if necessary). Discuss bladder/bowel management with nursing staff.	Discuss bladder/bowel management with nursing staff. Do not introduce IDC for management of incontinence.

Remember the four Ms (mobility, mentation, motivation and manual dexterity) when assessing incontinence in older patients. They are often the most relevant factors involved.

4. Medication review. Drugs predisposing to incontinence include diuretics (especially frusemide), calcium channel antagonists, anticholinergics (including antipsychotics, antispasmodics, anti-Parkinson's agents) and benzodiazepines.
5. Screening for prostate pathology with the prostate-specific antigen test (PSA).
6. Individualised toileting, such as prompted two-hour toileting, may improve continence in the cognitively impaired patient. This approach may fail due to apathy, ageism, inflexibility and workload.

Indwelling urinary catheters are not indicated in the routine management of incontinence. The only indications for the insertion of a urinary catheter are:

• To relieve retention with overflow incontinence.
• To monitor urinary output (as part of haemodynamic monitoring).

- An in-out catheter to collect a urine specimen and to exclude acute retention.
- When incontinence is contributing to perineal or sacral skin sepsis.

Faecal incontinence

Continence of faeces depends on sphincter function and rectal motility, as well as the four Ms of continence. Chronic constipation complicated by faecal impaction with overflow, diarrhoeal illnesses and continence problems related to dementia and acute confusion are the most common causes. Initial assessment is similar to the urinary incontinence assessment:

1. Exclusion of faecal impaction (PR and abdominal X-ray).
2. Stool culture if diarrhoea truly present.

REFERENCES

1. Creasey H. Acute confusion in the elderly. Current Therapeutics, Aug 1996; 21–27.
2. Inouye SK, van Dyck CH, Alessi CA, et al. Clarifying confusion: the Confusion Assessment Method; a new method for detection of delirium. Ann Intern Med 1990; 113:941–948.
3. Folstein MF, Folstein SE, McHugh PR. The Mini-mental State Examination: a practical method for grading the cognitive state of patients for the clinician. J Psychiatr Res 1975; 12:189–198.
4. Tinetti ME, Speechley M, Ginter SF. Risk factors for falls among elderly persons living in the community. N Engl J Med 1988; 319:1701–1707.
5. Podsialdo D, Richardson S. The time to 'Up & Go': a test of basic functional mobility for frail elderly persons. J Am Geriatr Soc 1991; 39:142–148.
6. Yesavage J, Brink T, Rose T, et al. Development and validation of a geriatric depression screening scale: a preliminary report. J Psychiat Res 1983; 17:37–49.

RECOMMENDED READING

Aminzadeh F, Dalziel W. Older adults in the emergency department: a systematic review of patterns of use, adverse outcomes, and effectiveness of interventions. Ann Emerg Med 2002; 39:238–247.

Gray L, Woodward M, Scholes R, Fonda D. Geriatric medicine: a pocket guide for doctors, health professionals and students. Port Melbourne: Ausmed Publications; 1994.

Resnick N, Marcantonio E. How should clinical care of the aged differ? Lancet 1997; 350(9085):1157–1158.

35 Emergency gynaecology

Sally McCarthy

History includes last normal menstrual period (LMP), past pregnancy history, sexual activity, contraception, pregnancy signs and symptoms, preventative health strategies (PAP smear, breast examination) as well as characteristics of presenting symptoms (commonly pain, abnormal vaginal bleeding plus or minus pregnancy, vaginal discharge, fever).

Management includes excluding pregnancy for every female of reproductive age, and early attention to vital signs, anticipating that certain conditions are associated with immediately life-threatening presentations.

Sensitivity and attention to the patient's comfort mandates conducting gynaecological history and pelvic examinations in a private area (when patient's condition is stable), using a warmed speculum, and offering analgesia early.

COMMON PRESENTATIONS

Pain

Ruptured ectopic pregnancy

- Incidence of ectopic pregnancy increasing worldwide, mainly due to the increased incidence of pelvic inflammatory disease (PID) caused by *Chlamydia trachomatis.*
- History includes abdominal pain (97%), missed period (80%), vaginal bleeding (79%), infertility (15%), use of an intrauterine contraceptive device (IUCD) (14%), previous ectopic pregnancy (11%).
- Presenting signs include abdominal tenderness (91%), adnexal tenderness (54%); less frequently, shoulder tip pain, syncope and hypovolaemic shock (5%).
- Commonly presents between the 5th and 8th week following the LMP.

Diagnosis made by positive beta human chorionic gonadotrophin (BHCG), and ultrasound (US) negative for intrauterine pregnancy. (Heterotopic pregnancy—an ectopic pregnancy together with an intrauterine pregnancy—occurs in approximately 1 in 30,000 pregnancies.)

Management

- Unstable vital signs, signs of haemoperitoneum: resuscitate with O_2, large-bore IVC and fluids, crossmatch blood, urgent obstetrics and gynaecological (O&G) consultation for operative management.

- Stable: insert IVC, perform group-and-hold (G&H), consult O&G. Management may be expectant, medical or surgical, depending on initial serum titre of BHCG and trend in titres, and local practice.

Acute salpingitis (PID)

- Often sexually acquired. Infection usually due to *Chlamydia trachomatis* or *Neisseria gonorrhoea*. Other organisms from vaginal flora may subsequently be involved.
- May result from mechanical interruption of the normal cervical barrier, e.g. postabortal, postpartum, postoperative infection, or in association with IUCDs. Infection caused by mixed pathogens including anaerobes, facultative bacteria and *Mycoplasma* species. Any IUCD or retained products must be removed as soon as possible.
- Risk factors include history of previous episode, multiple sexual partners, adolescence and IUCD.
- Long-term sequelae may include chronic pelvic pain, dyspareunia, infertility, tuboovarian abscess, increased risk of ectopic pregnancy.
- Clinical presentation includes lower abdominal pain, adnexal and cervical motion tenderness, fever, generalised malaise, purulent or mucopurulent vaginal discharge.
- Fever is usually low grade, with only one-third of patients presenting with a temperature greater than 38°C.
- No correlation between extent of disease and symptom severity.

Diagnosis is made by a combination of clinical findings and some or all of the following: positive micro from cervical secretions (swabs taken specifically for gonococcus and *Chlamydia*), leukocytosis, US documenting inflammatory adnexal mass or retained products.

Management

- Severe infection or systemically unwell or requires removal of retained products or IUCD: admit for IV antibiotics (consult local guidelines, but generally tetracyclines, metronidazole, third-generation cephalosporins while awaiting culture results).
- Milder infections may be discharged on oral therapy (antibiotics as above).
- Must treat sexual partner.

Adnexal cyst or mass complications

Ruptured ovarian cyst

- Ovarian cysts are asymptomatic until complications occur.
- Physiological cysts such as corpus luteum cysts (in pregnant or non-pregnant) and follicular cysts rupture at different points in the menstrual cycle, giving a clue to aetiology.
- Rupture of a follicular cyst with the extrusion of an ovum occurs midcycle, and gives rise to the unilateral pain of mittelschmerz.

Discomfort may last 2–3 days, may be associated with mild general malaise, and may be associated with vaginal spotting.

- Corpus luteal cyst rupture in the non-pregnant woman occurs just prior to menses, is usually associated with some intraperitoneal bleeding and may require differentiation from ectopic pregnancy.
- In pregnancy, the corpus luteum may persist until 10 weeks, so that spontaneous rupture typically occurs during the first trimester. Characteristic findings are unilateral pain and adnexal tenderness; fever and leukocytosis are uncommon (approximately 20%). Diffuse peritoneal irritation occurs with spillage of fluid into peritoneal cavity.
- Laparoscopy may be indicated.

Torsion of ovarian or tubal mass

- Usually associated with diseased ovary or fallopian tube.
- Onset of pain is sudden, sharp, intermittent, becoming increasingly severe.
- There may have been previous similar episodes.
- May be associated with nausea, vomiting, low-grade fever and leukocytosis and, infrequently, with amenorrhoea or abnormal vaginal bleeding.
- Examination findings vary from unilateral lower abdominal tenderness to peritonitis.
- Complications include ovarian necrosis and shock.

Ultrasound reveals reduced perfusion of the torted mass.

Management will include analgesia, resuscitation as appropriate and laparoscopy or laparotomy.

Other gynaecological causes of lower abdominal or pelvic pain

- Endometriosis.
- Uterine perforation: typically after intrauterine instrumentation, may present acutely due to intraperitoneal irritation secondary to intraperitoneal blood, or as delayed diffuse pain with diffuse peritonitis.
- Severe dysmenorrhoea: management is with antiprostaglandins and paracetamol.
- Denial of pregnancy and unanticipated labour: estimated at one in 2000–5000 births, the diagnosis is made when the woman presents in labour, putting both mother and fetus at risk.
- Vulvovaginitis.

BLEEDING

In early pregnancy

1. Ectopic pregnancy

See 'Ruptured ectopic pregnancy'.

2. Spontaneous abortion or miscarriage

- Common in early pregnancy.
- Several stages are recognised: threatened, bleeding occurs, cervical os closed; incomplete, products of conception in uterus, at os or in vagina; completed, when all products expelled from uterus and os closed.
- Presenting symptoms include intermittent vaginal spotting progressing to heavy bleeding with passage of clots and gestational tissue; midline, cramping abdominal discomfort occurring after bleeding has commenced.
- Signs include unremarkable abdominal examination, with possible midline suprapubic tenderness on deep palpation, uterine enlargement consistent with pregnancy.
- Shock or bradycardia may occur rarely as a result of products sitting in the cervical os. These will require urgent gentle removal.

Management involves assessment of vital signs and management of blood loss (may occasionally require IV fluids and, rarely, ergometrine or oxytocin), confirmation of pregnancy, assessment of state of cervical os (if open, uterus is unable to contract to limit bleeding adequately), ultrasound examination to confirm diagnosis, assessment of Rh status, and administration of Rh (anti-D) immunoglobulin if Rh-negative.

Miscarriages are frequently associated with grieving, and referral for counselling may be offered to the patient while she is in the emergency department.

In later pregnancy (>20 weeks)

Patients presenting with bleeding in later pregnancy should have immediate obstetric consultation, with emergency department treatment focusing on maternal stabilisation (oxygen, IVC and fluids, blood XM, FBC, coagulation status, Rh status). Vaginal examination must be left to the obstetrician.

1. Placental abruption

Placental abruption, or separation of the placenta from the uterine wall, is usually associated with characteristically dark vaginal bleeding, uterine pain and tenderness. Complications include fetal distress or death, DIC, maternal haemorrhage.

2. Placenta praevia

Placenta praevia, or implantation of the placenta over the cervical os, is usually associated with painless fresh vaginal bleeding, which may become severe with cervical probing.

Bleeding in the non-pregnant woman

Dysfunctional uterine bleeding may be associated with ovulatory or anovulatory menstrual cycles.

- Assessment of blood loss may be difficult, but menorrhagia is indicated by anaemia, use of two pads concurrently or tampon and pad, pads/ tampons changed every 1–2 hours when flow is heaviest, episodic flooding with staining of clothes or sheets, frequent clots.
- Complete history (including symptoms of clotting disorder) and physical examination is required to establish signs of endocrine dysfunction, obesity (associated with polycystic ovarian syndrome) or lifestyle or exercise contributors.
- Exclude pregnancy or pelvic infection, measure Hb if anaemia likely on history or examination findings.
- Consider clotting disorders and abnormal platelet function in women <20 years old.
- Refer for further gynaecological assessment (causes may include fibroids, malignancy).

Genital bleeding

Profuse bleeding may result from trauma. Emergency department management includes patient stabilisation, examination to discover bleeding origin and early consultation.

Vaginal foreign bodies may be associated with bleeding and/or infection.

OTHER COMPLICATIONS OF LATER PREGNANCY (>20 WEEKS)
Preeclampsia

Preeclampsia is a multisystem disorder potentially affecting the maternal liver, kidneys, brain and clotting system, as well as leading to impaired placental function.

Defined as hypertension developing after 20 weeks in a patient with normal blood pressure prior to pregnancy, associated with proteinuria or hyperuricaemia. There is no history of hypertension or renal disease, and blood pressure returns to normal within 3 months postpartum. It is more common in nulliparous women.

Hypertension in pregnancy is a systolic BP greater than or equal to 140 mmHg and/or diastolic BP greater than or equal to 90 mmHg or a rise in SBP of 25 mmHg or greater and/or a rise in DBP of 15 mmHg or greater from the patient's first-trimester BP.

Features of severe preeclampsia are BP >170/110, proteinuria >300 mg/day, hyperuricaemia, serum creatinine >0.09 mmol/L. Other features include liver pain, elevated transaminases or bilirubin, persistent headaches, visual disturbances, hyperreflexia or clonus, thrombocytopenia.

Eclampsia is the onset of convulsions in pregnancy or the postnatal period, usually preceded by preeclampsia.

Management: severe preeclampsia and eclampsia are medical and obstetric emergencies. Magnesium sulphate infusion is the agent of choice for seizure prophylaxis. Other agents may be required for BP control. Urgent obstetric consultation is obtained, and general resuscitative measures (maintenance of airway, O_2 therapy, IV access, nurse patient on side) are undertaken.

Trauma in pregnancy

The risk to the pregnancy in 'minor' trauma is significant, with pre-term labour occurring in 8%, abruption in 1%, and fetal death in 1% of pregnancies. In severe trauma, fetal death rate rises to 20% or greater.

Main determinant of fetal outcome is maternal outcome, thus ensuring maternal oxygenation and tissue perfusion is the primary goal. Positioning of the third-trimester patient with a left lateral tilt (as an entire unit to maintain cervical spine stability) is essential to displace the uterus and prevent vena caval compression.

All patients with minor trauma should be admitted to hospital for at least 24 hours. Careful fetal monitoring is essential once fetal viability has been established.

Sexual assault

Sexual assault is a common, and under-reported, violent crime. Women presenting to the emergency department following a sexual assault are preferably referred to a sexual assault service, where expertise in obtaining forensic samples, documenting the physical examination, offering pregnancy and STD prophylaxis and providing psychological support exists. Occasionally, victims require management of other injuries prior to assessment by the sexual assault service.

EMERGENCY CONTRACEPTION: MORNING-AFTER PILL

Administration of 100 µg ethinyloestradiol and 500 µg levonorgestrel to a woman within 72 hours of unprotected intercourse, with the dose repeated 12 hours later, has an efficacy of 75–98% in preventing pregnancy. Anti-emetics should always be given, and a spare dose of hormone tablets, should vomiting occur. Advice given with emergency contraception should include risk of failure and appropriate follow-up, and counselling regarding contraceptive use.

DRUGS IN PREGNANCY

Drugs should be prescribed in pregnancy only if the expected benefit to the mother is thought to be greater than the risk to the fetus, and all drugs should be avoided if possible during the first trimester. Drugs that have been extensively used in pregnancy and appear to be usually safe should be prescribed in preference to new or untried drugs; and the smallest effective dose should be used.

Few drugs have been shown conclusively to be teratogenic in man but no drug is safe beyond all doubt in early pregnancy. For information regarding specific drugs, MIMS should be consulted.

ANTI-D PROPHYLAXIS

RhD immunoglobulin (anti-D) is administered for prophylaxis against haemolytic disease of the newborn. Current indications and doses include potentially sensitising events, e.g. miscarriage, ectopic pregnancy during the first trimester (250 IU RhD immunoglobulin); potentially sensitising events during the second and third trimester (625 IU RhD immunoglobulin, plus additional doses as indicated from the assessment of the extent of feto-maternal haemorrhage).

RECOMMENDED READING

Cameron P, Jelinek G, Kelly A, et al. Textbook of adult emergency medicine. Edinburgh: Churchill Livingstone; 2000.

D'Amours SK, Sugrue M, Russell R, Nocera N, eds. Handbook of trauma care. The Liverpool Hospital trauma manual, 6th edn. Sydney: Trauma Department, Liverpool Hospital; 2002.

Mein KJJK, Palmer CM, Shand MC, et al. Management of acute adult sexual assault. Med J Aust 2003; 178(5):226–230.

National Health and Medical Research Council. Guidelines on the prophylactic use of RhD immunoglobulin (anti-D) in obstetrics. Canberra: AGPS; 1999.

36 Endocrine emergencies

Glenn Arendts and Anna Holdgate

DIABETIC KETOACIDOSIS

Diabetic ketoacidosis (DKA) is due to insulin deficiency resulting in acidosis, hyperglycaemia and fluid and electrolyte losses. It is most commonly seen in patients with preexisting insulin-dependent diabetes or as the first presentation of insulin-dependent diabetes. The principles in assessment and management of DKA are identifying and treating the precipitating cause, assessing the severity of the illness, correcting fluid and electrolyte disturbances, and administering insulin.

Assessment

Patients with DKA commonly present with vomiting, polydipsia/polyuria and abdominal pain. History and examination should be directed at identifying the precipitating event and assessing the degree of dehydration. Most commonly, DKA is precipitated in patients with Type I diabetes by intercurrent infection, although other causes should be considered (Table 36.1). It occurs infrequently in patients with non-insulin-dependent diabetes.

The diagnosis is confirmed at the bedside by the presence of urinary ketones, a blood pH <7.3 (venous or arterial blood gas) and an elevated blood sugar level (BSL) >14 mmol/L. Other important investigations include:

- Urea, electrolyte, creatinine (UEC)—potassium depletion is common and creatinine may be elevated.
- FBC—elevated white cell count (WCC) suggests infection.
- Midstream urine for microscopy and culture.
- Blood culture if febrile.
- Liver function tests and amylase if abdominal pain.
- ECG for silent myocardial infarction or arrhythmias.
- Chest X-ray (CXR) for respiratory infection.

Management

Patients with DKA are often extremely ill and should be initially observed in an area of the emergency department with continuous ECG and oximetry monitoring, and regular blood pressure measurements. If there is a depressed level of consciousness, the patient requires supportive airway management and may need intubation. Ongoing regular measurement of BSL and serum K^+ should continue throughout treatment.

Table 36.1 Precipitants of DKA

- First presentation of insulin-dependent diabetes
- Non-compliance/errors with insulin therapy
- Infection
    - Urinary tract
    - Respiratory tract
    - Gastrointestinal
    - Skin
- Other
    - Steroid medication
    - AMI
    - Pancreatitis
    - Thyroid disease/surgery/pregnancy/trauma

Fluid and electrolyte therapy

All patients with DKA are volume depleted and require rehydration with intravenous fluids. Hypotension (systolic BP <100 mmHg) should be treated with boluses of normal saline up to 2000 mL until blood pressure has improved. In the normotensive patient, 1 litre of normal saline should be given over the first hour, followed by a second litre over the next 2 hours. Subsequent fluid therapy will be guided by clinical assessment of pulse rate and hydration status, but most patients will require 5–8 litres of fluid over the first 24 hours. A dextrose-containing solution should be commenced once the BSL falls below 15 mmol/L, in addition to ongoing sodium requirements.

Potassium depletion is a feature of DKA, even in the presence of an initial elevated serum K^+. Serum potassium should be measured as soon as possible and is often available on the blood gas. If the initial K^+ is >5.5 mmol/L, the level should be rechecked every 30–60 minutes, as it will inevitably fall as a consequence of rehydration. Once the K^+ is 3.5–5.5 mmol/L, K^+ replacement should commence at 10 mmol/h, diluted in the normal saline being given for rehydration. If the K^+ is <3.5 mmol/h, K^+ replacement should be given at 20 mmol/h. Monitoring of K^+ levels every 1–2 hours is essential during the initial phase of treatment.

Phosphate and magnesium levels are commonly low in DKA, however there is no evidence to support the routine replacement of these electrolytes. Intravenous bicarbonate is of no proven benefit in patients with DKA as the acidosis usually improves with rehydration and insulin therapy. Bicarbonate should not be given without consulting a critical care specialist or endocrinologist.

Insulin therapy

Rehydration increases insulin sensitivity, and therefore insulin therapy should not precede fluid therapy. In the initial phase, insulin should be delivered via continuous intravenous infusion. A second intravenous line is usually required for this purpose. Short-acting neutral insulin should be loaded into a colloid solution to avoid binding to plastic tubing and packaging. A common regimen is 50 units of Actrapid in 500 mL Gelofusine or Haemaccel. The insulin infusion should commence at 0.05–0.1 units/kg/h (2–8 units/h), aiming for a fall in BSL of 2–4 mmol/h. The BSL should be measured hourly initially and the insulin infusion adjusted according to the rate of fall.

The insulin infusion should continue until the urine is clear of ketones. Once the BSL falls below 15 mmol/L, rehydration should continue with a dextrose-containing solution. Subcutaneous insulin can be commenced once the patient has adequate oral intake and is no longer acidotic. The first subcutaneous dose must be given before the insulin infusion is ceased.

Other therapy

- Treatment of associated infection with appropriate antibiotics.
- Subcutaneous heparin for thromboembolic prophylaxis.
- A nasogastric tube may be necessary if there is persistent vomiting.
- An indwelling catheter is often necessary to monitor urine output.

Ongoing management

The aim of treatment is to correct fluid/electrolyte disturbances and control ketosis over 12–24 hours. Strict monitoring of BSL and serum K^+ every 1–2 hours initially is vital. Other electrolytes, especially sodium, should be checked twice daily. Regular reassessment of the patient's hydration status and acidosis is necessary to determine ongoing fluid management. The patient needs to remain closely monitored with hourly observations while the insulin infusion continues.

HYPEROSMOLAR HYPERGLYCAEMIC NON-KETOTIC STATE

This condition occurs primarily in older patients with non-insulin-dependent diabetes, although it has several clinical features in common with diabetic ketoacidosis. It is characterised by relative, rather than absolute, insulin deficiency, leading to hyperglycaemia, hyperosmolarity and dehydration, with little or no acidosis. The goals of therapy are identification and treatment of the precipitating event, controlled correction of fluid and electrolyte abnormalities, and correction of hyperglycaemia.

Assessment

Hyperosmolar hyperglycaemic non-ketotic state (HHNS) is characterised by non-specific signs such as confusion, vomiting and weight loss, developing over days to weeks in elderly patients with undiagnosed or poorly controlled diabetes. Polyuria and polydipsia are not universally present. There are many possible precipitating events, which are summarised in Table 36.2. These patients often have multiple comorbidities and may be on multiple medications.

Physical examination is focused on assessing the degree of dehydration and looking for evidence of a precipitating cause. The diagnosis is confirmed by the presence of severe hyperglycaemia (often >50 mmol/L) and serum hyperosmolarity (>315 mOsm/L), with minimal acidosis (pH >7.3). Important early investigations include:

- UEC—severe dehydration may be associated with hypernatraemia. Potassium depletion and renal impairment are common.
- Septic screen—urine, blood, skin swabs +/– CSF for culture.
- Chest X-ray—for evidence of infection and to evaluate heart size and presence of cardiac failure.

- ECG—for evidence of myocardial infarction or atrial fibrillation.
- CT head—for cerebrovascular accident (CVA) or intracranial haemorrhage.

Management

These patients often have an altered level of consciousness and may have multiple comorbidities, including heart and renal disease. Therefore they must be closely observed with full cardiorespiratory monitoring.

Fluid and electrolyte therapy

In the presence of shock (hypotension or poor tissue perfusion), fluid therapy should begin with 500 mL boluses of normal saline until blood pressure and tissue perfusion are restored. After correction of shock, fluid replacement should be performed relatively slowly. Although these patients are often profoundly dehydrated, this has usually occurred over a period of days to weeks and overly rapid replacement of fluid may lead to pulmonary oedema. Most patients will have a fluid deficit of 8–12 litres and this should be replaced over a 24–48-hour period. Fluid therapy should begin with 1 litre of normal saline every 2–4 hours. Once the BSL starts to fall and the patient has an established urine output >1 mL/kg/h, normal saline can be replaced by half saline/2.5% dextrose. The patient should be regularly assessed for clinical evidence of fluid overload, and may need central venous monitoring via a central line.

Potassium levels will fall rapidly once the patient is rehydrated and receiving insulin. Potassium replacement at 5–10 mmol/h should commence if the K^+ is <5.5 mmol/L and urine output has been

Table 36.2 Precipitants of HHNS

- Poor compliance
- Newly diagnosed diabetes
- Infection
  - Urinary tract
  - Respiratory
  - CNS
  - Skin
- Cardiovascular events
  - Acute myocardial infarction (AMI)
  - CVA/intracranial haemorrhage
  - Mesenteric ischaemia
- Other
  - Gastrointestinal haemorrhage
  - Pancreatitis
  - Renal failure
  - Diuretic therapy

established. In the presence of oliguria and renal failure, K^+ replacement should be more cautious.

Insulin therapy

As for DKA, an intravenous insulin infusion should be commenced. Patients with HHNS usually require ~0.05 units/kg/h to achieve a fall in BSL of 3–5 mmol/h. As hyperglycaemia has developed over a long time period, it is appropriate to correct the BSL slowly, aiming for normalisation at 18–24 hours. This minimises the risk of cerebral oedema.

Other therapy

Precipating illnesses should be actively sought and treated. Serious diagnoses such as mesenteric ischaemia must be considered. Thromboembolic prophylaxis with subcutaneous heparin is particularly important in HHNS, due to the thrombogenic effect of profound dehydration and the presence of serious comorbidities.

HYPOGLYCAEMIA

Hypoglycaemia most commonly occurs in diabetic patients on insulin or oral hypoglycaemic therapy. It can also occur in non-diabetics secondary to diseases such as sepsis, alcohol, hepatic failure, renal failure and insulinomas.

In diabetics, hypoglycaemia may be due to excess insulin or oral hypoglycaemic treatment, missed meals, physical exertion and alcohol. It may be the first presentation of renal impairment in patients on sulphonylureas.

Clinical features

Hypoglycaemia predominantly affects the brain and the autonomic nervous system. Neurological signs can vary widely and include coma, seizures, confusion, dysarthria and focal deficits (mimicking stroke). Autonomic features include sweating, tremor, blurred vision, vomiting and anxiety. The diagnosis is confirmed by BSL <3 mmol/L on fingerprick sampling. The diagnosis should be considered in all patients presenting with confusion, seizures or an altered level of consciousness.

Therapy

Hypoglycaemia is easily reversed with oral or intravenous glucose. Prolonged, untreated hypoglycaemia can lead to permanent brain dysfunction, so early diagnosis and treatment are essential.

If the patient is still awake, oral glucose in the form of a sweet drink, biscuit or other sugary substances may be enough to restore BSL. If the patient is unable to swallow, 25 mL 50% dextrose is given as an intravenous push through a large-bore IV cannula, followed by a 2 mL saline flush (to prevent phlebitis). If the patient does not recover within 2–3 minutes, or the BSL remains <3 mmol/L, the dose can be repeated.

If intravenous access is not possible, 1 unit of intramuscular glucagon may temporarily reverse hypoglycaemia if the patient has normal hepatic function. This should be followed by oral or intravenous glucose.

Hypoglycaemia secondary to oral hypoglycaemic agents may be recurrent and prolonged, particularly in the presence of renal impairment. These patients require a 5% dextrose infusion and observation in hospital until the BSL is stable.

Once the BSL is restored, assessment and treatment of the precipitating cause is essential.

HYPOADRENAL CRISIS (ACUTE ADRENOCORTICAL INSUFFICIENCY)

Assessment

Hypoadrenal crisis develops in two clinical settings. Occasionally, the patient presents with acute haemorrhagic destruction of the adrenal glands due to sepsis, burns, trauma or anticoagulant therapy. More commonly, the crisis develops as an acute deterioration in patients with Addison's disease or other causes of chronic adrenal failure. This can be due to increased steroid requirements (infection, surgery, trauma), drug interactions that increase steroid metabolism (phenytoin, barbituates) or noncompliance with maintenance steroid therapy.

The presenting symptoms are often non-specific and include malaise, lethargy, nausea, vomiting, diarrhoea and abdominal pain. However, the patient may present with severe dehydration or haemodynamic collapse and shock requiring immediate resuscitation.

A number of investigations aid in the diagnosis and management:

- Plasma cortisol level—a low level in the setting of acute stress is highly suggestive of adrenocortical insufficiency. The short synacthen test will confirm the diagnosis if doubt exists. Adrenocorticotroph hormones (ACTH), renin and aldosterone levels may be useful in diagnosing the cause of hypoadrenalism. Treatment should not be delayed for the results of hormone assays.
- UEC—the combination of hyponatraemia and hyperkalaemia is highly suggestive of hypoadrenal crisis. Renal failure may occur.
- BSL—hypoglycaemia.
- ABG—non-anion gap metabolic acidosis.
- Ca^{2+}—hypercalcaemia.
- ECG—arrhythmias or hyperkalaemic changes.

As infection is a common precipitant, the patient often requires a septic workup as part of the initial assessment.

Management

The patient may present with haemodynamic collapse and require immediate resuscitation. Continuous ECG, blood pressure and pulse oximetry monitoring is required. High flow oxygen by mask should be applied. Hypotension should be treated initially with 1000 mL boluses of normal saline until BP or peripheral perfusion improve. Shock may be refractory to fluid resuscitation until corticosteroid therapy is commenced (see below). Even with adjuvant steroids, the patient may need inotrope support in decompensated shock. Hypoglycaemia, if present, should be treated initially with 25 mL 50% dextrose IV.

After resuscitation, further fluid requirements should be determined by assessment of the patient's hydration status. Normal saline should be used to replace any fluid deficit over the next 24–48 hours. If the patient has associated persistent hypoglycaemia, adding dextrose to the bags of normal saline is preferable to using a dextrose-containing solution with a low sodium concentration. Blood glucose, Na^+ and K^+ levels should be measured every 2–3 hours initially.

IV corticosteroids should be given promptly. A 200 mg bolus of IV hydrocortisone, followed by 100 mg every 6 hours, is an appropriate treatment. In cases where the diagnosis is in doubt and a short synacthen test is being performed, steroid treatment should not be withheld. However, as hydocortisone interferes with the integrity of this test, dexamethasone 8 mg can be used as an alternative treatment in this setting.

Other important acute management issues include the treatment of any underlying precipitant such as infection.

The majority of patients improve within 24 hours of commencing this treatment regimen. Oral combined glucocorticoid and mineralocorticoid therapy may then be commenced. After the acute treatment phase is over, patient education concerning increasing their maintenance steroid requirements at times of stress or illness is a vital part of management.

THYROTOXIC CRISIS ('THYROID STORM')

Thyrotoxic crisis is the clinical extreme of hyperthyroidism. The diagnosis is often difficult to make and this may lead to delayed treatment and a high mortality. The aims of assessment and management are to establish the diagnosis, identify precipitant causes, provide supportive care, and reduce both production and peripheral end-organ effects of thyroid hormones.

Assessment

The diagnosis of thyrotoxic crisis is entirely clinical. The clinical signs are the exaggerated features of hyperthyroidism, but three in particular help characterise thyrotoxic crisis from uncomplicated hyperthyroidism:

1. Hyperpyrexia (temperature >38°C).
2. Extreme tachycardia (HR usually 130–200 bpm).
3. Central nervous system (CNS) disturbance, ranging from restlessness and agitation to coma.

Table 36.3 Precipitants of thyrotoxic crisis

- Intercurrent illness or stress—infection, labour, major vascular events such as CVA
- Drugs—amiodarone, thyroxine overdose, cessation of antithyroid drug therapy, iodinated dyes
- Trauma—multitrauma, thyroid gland surgery, vigorous palpation of thyroid gland

Vomiting and diarrhoea are common. Potentially life-threatening cardiac complications (arrhythmias, cardiac failure) occur in more than 50% of patients.

No single test confirms the diagnosis of thyrotoxic crisis. Thyroid function tests confirm hyperthyroidism, but the levels of T_3 and T_4 in thyrotoxic crisis are usually no different from those in uncomplicated hyperthyroidism, and treatment should not be delayed for the TFT results. Hypokalaemia, hypercalcaemia, abnormal liver function and leukocytosis occur commonly. A CXR and ECG looking for specific cardiac complications should be performed.

Patients at risk of thyrotoxic crisis mostly have undiagnosed or poorly treated hyperthyroidism. The precipitants of thyrotoxic crisis that should be looked for in these patients are shown in Table 36.3.

Management

Patients with thyrotoxic crisis are usually extremely unwell and require continuous ECG, blood pressure and temperature monitoring. Unstable arrhythmias and profound cardiac failure may be evident at presentation and require urgent treatment. Early consultation with a critical care specialist or endocrinologist is important.

Good general supportive care is essential. These patients are hypermetabolic and have markedly increased oxygen, fluid, electrolyte and glucose requirements. High flow oxygen by mask should be started. The patient usually requires 5–6 litres of normal saline in the first 24 hours, although less aggressive fluid resuscitation may be necessary in the elderly or those with heart failure. Hyperpyrexia should be treated with paracetamol and external cooling methods, for example axillary and groin cold packs. Thyrotoxic crisis patients have an increased risk of thromboembolism and should receive appropriate prophylaxis.

Beta-adrenergic blockers antagonise the peripheral end-organ effects of thyroid hormones and are the mainstay of emergency therapy. Oral (or NGT) propranolol 40 mg every 6 hours is the treatment of choice, although much higher doses may be required. Intravenous propranolol is not currently commercially available in Australia and, if the patient requires intravenous beta blockade, esmolol is the best option due to its very short half-life. All beta-blockers can worsen cardiac failure and hypotension.

Oral or NGT propylthiouracil reduces the further synthesis of thyroid hormones and prevents the peripheral conversion of T_4 to the more active T_3. A loading dose of 600 mg followed by 200 mg every 6 hours should be given.

Corticosteroids improve survival in thyrotoxic crisis and are indicated in all cases. Hydrocortisone 100 mg IV every 6 hours is an appropriate choice.

The majority of patients improve within 24 hours with this management regimen, although complete recovery may take many days. In patients not responding to these standard therapies, other treatments are occasionally used. These include large doses of iodide or iodinated radiology contrast media, and plasma exchange techniques to reduce levels of circulating thyroid hormones.

HYPOTHYROID CRISIS ('MYXOEDEMA COMA')

Myxoedema coma is the clinical extreme of hypothyroidism. As with thyrotoxic crisis, the diagnosis is difficult to make and there is a high mortality rate, even with treatment.

Assessment

Myxoedema coma occurs most commonly following some precipitating event in a patient with unrecognised hypothyroidism (Table 36.4). The diagnosis is clinical and a high index of suspicion is required.

Myxoedema coma is characterised by multiorgan failure due to reduced cellular metabolism. The cardinal clinical features are:

- Decreased conscious state.
- Hypoventilation progressing to hypercarbic respiratory failure.
- Bradycardia and hypotension.
- Hypothermia.

Increased total body water is common, leading to oedema, pleural and pericardial effusions, and hyponatraemia. Paralytic ileus and urinary retention may occur.

The diagnosis of myxoedema coma is clinical, although thyroid function tests confirm hypothyroidism. A rapid thyroid-stimulating hormone (TSH) assay is often available and, if normal, excludes the diagnosis. Other important investigation abnormalities include:

- UEC—hyponatraemia, renal failure.
- BSL—hypoglycaemia.
- ABG—hypercapnia, hypoxia.
- FBC—anaemia, leukopenia.
- ECG—bradycardia, prolonged QT interval, low voltage complexes.
- CXR—pleural and pericardial effusions.

Hypothyroid crisis patients are commonly septic without exhibiting any of the usual clinical features of sepsis, and should have a septic screen as part of their initial workup.

Table 36.4 Precipitants of myxoedema coma

- Intercurrent illness—infection, GIT bleed, CVA, congestive cardiac failure (CCF)
- Drugs—CNS depressants, anaesthetic agents, beta-blockers, lithium, amiodarone, cessation of thyroxine therapy
- Environmental—cold exposure

Management

Hypothyroid crisis patients are profoundly unwell and require management in an area with full monitoring and resuscitation equipment. Intubation and ventilation is often needed but requires special precautions due to hypothermia and gastric stasis. These patients, while oedematous, usually have a reduced intravascular volume, and hypotension should initially be treated with warmed intravenous normal saline. Hypoglycaemia, if present, should be immediately corrected with 25 mL 50% dextrose IV.

Administration of thyroid hormones is the mainstay of therapy in myxoedema coma. If the diagnosis is clinically suspected, early consultation with a critical care specialist or endocrinologist is essential so that therapy is not delayed. Considerable controversy exists regarding the optimal dose, route and rate of thyroid hormone replacement. Initial intravenous therapy is preferred when ileus is present. Currently in Australia, only IV triiodothyronine (T_3) is readily commercially available, and 10–20 µg can be given as a slow bolus every 8 hours. Oral T_3 or T_4 can be commenced once the ileus has resolved. As hypothyroid crisis usually develops slowly, rapid replacement of thyroid hormones may provoke serious complications such as cardiac ischaemia or arrhythmias. Providing supportive care is adequate, giving relatively low initial doses either IV or orally, titrated to clinical response, is prudent.

IV hydrocortisone 100 mg every 6 hours should be commenced, as myxoedema coma is often associated with adrenal dysfunction.

Other important management issues include:

- Hypothermia—active core rewarming is required only in cases of refractory haemodynamic instability, but passive rewarming with warm blankets or a Bair Hugger is recommended.
- Hyponatraemia—usually corrects with water restriction but if severe and associated with altered consciousness state it may require hypertonic (3%) saline.
- Infection is common and should be covered with broad-spectrum anti-biotic therapy

Recovery time with treatment is highly variable, and improvement can occur anywhere from 24 hours to many days after commencing therapy.

RECOMMENDED READING

Bagg W, Sathu A, Streat S, Braatvedt GD. Diabetic ketoacidosis in adults at Auckland Hospital 1988–1996. Australian and New Zealand Journal of Medicine 1998; 28:604–608.

Brady WJ, Harrigan RA. Hypoglycemia. In: Tintinalli JE, Kelen GD, Stapczynski JS, eds. Emergency medicine: a comprehensive study guide. New York: McGraw-Hill; 2000:1327–1329.

Brandenburg MA, Dire DJ. Comparison of arterial and venous blood gas values in the initial emergency department evaluation of patients with diabetic ketoacidosis. Ann Emerg Med 1998; 31:459–465.

Chansky ME, Lubkin CL. Diabetic ketoacidosis. In: Tintinalli JE, Kelen GD, Stapczynski JS, eds. Emergency medicine: a comprehensive study guide. New York: McGraw-Hill; 2000:1330–1337.

Graffeo CS. Hyperosmolar hyperglycemic nonketotic syndrome. In: Tintinalli JE, Kelen GD, Stapczynski JS, eds. Emergency medicine: a comprehensive study guide. New York: McGraw-Hill; 2000:1340–1343.

Kitabchi AE, Wall BM. Diabetic ketoacidosis. Med Clin North Am 1995; 79:9–37.

Lorber D. Nonketotic hypertonicity in diabetes mellitus. Med Clin North Am 1995; 79:40–52.

Service FJ. Hypoglycemia. Med Clin North Am 1995; 79(1):7.

Young KK, Oh TE. Diabetic emergencies. In: Oh TE, ed. Intensive care manual. Oxford: Butterworth-Heinemann; 1997:443–450.

37 Metabolic disorders

Ken Hillman

ACID-BASE DISORDERS

Acid-base disorders affect the body's basic biochemistry—especially enzyme function. A primary acid-base disturbance induces a secondary response. Initial chemical buffering is followed by compensatory respiratory and/or renal adaptation. Before considering any acid-base disorder, the pH, $PaCO_2$ and bicarbonate must be determined. This is determined by arterial blood gases (Table 37.1).

Respiratory acidosis

Although the following guidelines consider metabolic and respiratory disturbances separately, many critically ill patients have combined

Table 37.1 Interpretation of arterial blood gas findings

1.	Look at PaO_2. Rapidly correct it if it is abnormal.
2.	Look at the pH value: Acidosis: pH <7.35 Alkalosis: pH >7.45
3.	Is the acidosis respiratory or metabolic? Respiratory: $PaCO_2$ >45 mmHg Metabolic: HCO_3 <22 mmHg
4.	Is the alkalosis respiratory or metabolic? Respiratory: $PaCO_2$ <35 mmHg Metabolic: HCO_3 >26 mmHg
5.	Is there any compensation? The compensation is the opposite of the original disorder (e.g. the compensation for metabolic acidosis is respiratory alkalosis). Remember, the compensation can never be greater than the original abnormality. In other words, the primary abnormality will be determined by the pH value.

disorders, which are complicated in their interpretation by artificial ventilation and drugs. It is vital to consider the underlying cause of the disorder before active treatment is commenced.

Causes

Inadequate CO_2 removal

1. Lung pathology, e.g. asthma, chronic lung disease.
2. Obstructed airway.
3. Central, nervous or neuromuscular pathology, e.g. drug-induced hypoventilation, tetanus.
4. Increased dead space ventilation.

Excess CO_2 production

For example, hypercatabolic state, rapid infusion of bicarbonate solution.

Management

1. Correct the underlying cause, e.g. obstructed airway.
2. Artificially ventilate.

It is dangerous to rapidly correct chronic hypercarbia to normal levels. Patients with chronic lung disease should have their ventilation supported to maintain adequate $PaCO_2$ levels, rather than corrected to 'normal'. Similarly, in patients with acute severe asthma who need ventilatory support, the aim should be to maintain oxygenation rather than return the $PaCO_2$ to 'normal'. This is known as permissive hypercarbia. $PaCO_2$ levels of around 100 mmHg are sometimes acceptable because of the difficulty in maintaining adequate mechanical ventilation without barotrauma—as long as oxygenation is adequate.

Respiratory alkalosis

Causes

1. Hyperventilation, e.g. acute respiratory failure and central nervous system (CNS) disorders.
2. Hypometabolism and decreased CO_2 production, e.g. brainstem death and hypothermia.
3. In response to a metabolic acidosis.

Management

1. Correct the underlying cause.
2. Decrease ventilatory minute volume or add a dead space (e.g. breathing into a bag in spontaneously breathing patients with hysterical hyperventilation).

Metabolic acidosis

Causes

1. Excessive hydrogen production, e.g. lactic acid, salicylic acid, ketoacidosis.
2. Loss of bicarbonate, e.g. diarrhoea, renal tubular acidosis, small bowel loss.
3. Failure to excrete the hydrogen ion, e.g. renal failure.

Management

1. Correct reversible causes, e.g. diabetic ketoacidosis, shock.
2. Restore circulation and oxygenation.
3. Alkali. The above measures are usually sufficient. If the acidosis is severe (pH <7.1) or resistant to supportive therapy, bicarbonate can be considered. However, bicarbonate therapy can be associated with complications such as a rebound alkalosis, paradoxical intracellular acidosis as well as large sodium and osmolar load. Previous formulae for bicarbonate have usually overestimated the amount needed and are no longer used. Commence with 1 mmol/kg and repeat as necessary. Use only in cases of severe and resistant acidosis.
4. Dialysis may be required to remove excessive hydrogen ions as a result of renal failure.

Metabolic alkalosis

Causes

1. Loss of acid, e.g. diuretics, nasogastric suction, vomiting.
2. Gain in alkali, e.g. excessive bicarbonate therapy, antacid therapy, metabolism of organic ions (e.g. lactate, citrate, acetate).

Management

1. Correct any reversible cause.

2. Correct factors which potentiate the alkalosis, such as decreased extracellular fluid and hypokalaemia.
3. Usually the alkalosis responds to addressing the underlying problem and there is only rarely a need for further treatment. Acetazolamide 500 mg IV 8-hourly. NH_4Cl and arginine monohydrochloride should be avoided, as they both require hepatic conversion and normal renal function for full activity.

ELECTROLYTE DISORDERS

Sodium

Sodium (Na) concentration variation usually reflects disorders of water rather than sodium. For example, hyponatraemia is almost always due to water excess, while hypernatraemia is due to water depletion.

Hyponatraemia

Arbitrarily defined as Na <130 mmol/L. Rarely a problem in the chronic situation unless Na <120 mmol/L.

Clinical features depend on the rapidity of onset. Rapid onset may result in confusion, seizures, central pontine myelinolysis and cerebral oedema.

Management

1. Water restriction is all that is necessary in most cases.
2. Correction should be commensurate with onset. Aim to increase the serum sodium by no more than 10 mmol/24 h if the onset has been slow (i.e over days or longer). Slowly correct to 130 mmol/L.
3. Treat the underlying cause.
4. In severe symptomatic hyponatraemia (i.e. coma or convulsions), use hypertonic saline either by itself or together with a diuretic such as mannitol (0.3 g/kg).

Hypernatraemia

This usually occurs as a result of both water and sodium loss, with relatively more water lost compared with sodium, e.g. osmotic diuresis, or gastrointestinal (GIT) loss as a result of diarrhoea or vomiting. It can cause disorders of central nervous system (CNS) function.

Management

1. Slow rehydration with 5% dextrose solution (100–300 mL/h) will correct most cases.
2. Rarely, dialysis may also be necessary.

Potassium

Compared with sodium, the body's mechanisms for retaining potassium are underdeveloped. Small shifts in serum levels can be dangerous.

Hypokalaemia

This predisposes to supraventricular and ventricular arrhythmias, coma and neuromuscular weakness. Losses are usually related to GIT (e.g. vomiting diarrhoea) or renal (diuresis) disorders.

The serum potassium level can also decrease as a result of shift into cells, e.g. after insulin or accompanying a metabolic alkalosis.

Management

Oral potassium supplements are often adequate for replacement. If severe or symptomatic, give potassium infusion via a central line (5–40 mmol/h) with frequent monitoring of serum levels and continuous ECG monitoring.

Hyperkalaemia

This predisposes to cardiac tachyarrhythmias, profound muscle weakness and eventual asystole. ECG changes include T wave elevation, widening of the QRS complex, prolongation of the PR interval and deepening of the S wave. Hyperkalaemia occurs as a result of renal failure, movement of potassium from the cells to the extracellular fluid (e.g. severe acidosis) or as a result of cellular damage (e.g. crush injury, burns, rhabdomyolysis, haemolysis).

Management

The treatment depends on the severity of the hyperkalaemia and the presence or absence of complications.

1. Calcium 10 mL 10% solution to counteract the effect of hyperkalaemia on the myocardium.
2. Glucose 100 mL 50% glucose with 20 units of short-acting insulin.
3. Sodium bicarbonate 100 mmol. Both (2) and (3) temporarily drive the potassium into the cells.
4. Ion exchange resin. Calcium resonium 30–60 g every 2–6 hours, either orally or rectally.
5. Dialysis may be required for severe or resistant hyperkalaemia.

Calcium

Almost all of the total body calcium is present in bone. Calcium is normally controlled within narrow limits and is essential for cell membrane integrity and complement activity. The ionised calcium, rather than total serum calcium, should always be measured, as the correlation between the two can be poor.

Hypocalcaemia

This can cause increased neuronal membrane irritability, tetany, seizures, heart failure and arrhythmias. It usually occurs as a result of parathyroid hormone deficiency, acute renal failure or acute deposition of calcium in soft tissues (e.g. following rhabdomyolysis).

Management

1. Correct underlying cause.
2. Correct serum phosphate and magnesium levels.
3. Oral calcium supplements or 10 mL 10% calcium solution over 10 minutes. Aim to keep plasma calcium above 1.75 mmol/L.
4. Vitamin D supplement may also be required.

Hypercalcaemia

This is usually associated with hyperparathyroidism or malignancies (e.g. disseminated cancer, myeloma, lymphoma). Symptoms do not usually occur until the serum calcium level exceeds 3 mmol/L. Clinical features include anorexia, nausea, vomiting, depression, lethargy, constipation, polyuria and polydipsia.

Management

1. May not need any specific treatment if asymptomatic.
2. Correct other fluid and electrolyte abnormalities.
3. Calciuresis with 2–3 litres isotonic saline over 4 hours together with frusemide 20 mg intravenously every 2 hours.
4. Dialysis in emergencies.
5. Long term:
   - Calcitonin 4 U/kg IV, then 4 U/kg at 12–24-hour intervals.
   - Prednisolone 60 mg/24 h.
   - Mithramycin 25 mg/kg as an IV bolus.
   - Oral phosphate supplements—to be used only as an emergency measure, as they can cause precipitation of calcium salts.
   - Biphosphates act in 24–48 hours.

Magnesium

Hypomagnesaemia

Always consider hypomagnesaemia in the presence of hypokalaemia, as it is often related to the same causes, e.g. diuretics and GIT losses. It causes tachyarrhythmias, neuromuscular excitability, as well as GIT and CNS abnormalities.

Management

Intravenous boluses of 20 mmol over 30 minutes diluted to 100 mL. Repeat as necessary.

Hypermagnesaemia

Not as common as hypomagnesaemia, this may be seen in association with renal insufficiency and is associated with impaired neuromuscular activity as well as CNS and cardiovascular depression.

Management

1. Calcium 5 mmol IV.

2. Isotonic saline with 5 mmol calcium/L over 6 hours plus frusemide 20 mg IV every 4 hours.
3. Haemodialysis if resistant and associated with symptoms.

Phosphate

Hypophosphataemia

This is commonly associated with chronic alcoholism, malnutrition and diabetic ketoacidosis and can cause severe respiratory failure and general muscle weakness as well as CNS depression.

Management

Give 20–60 mmol phosphate over 6 hours as part of an IV infusion and repeat as necessary. Phosphate usually comes in the form of potassium salt—therefore, check serum levels before administering.

Hyperphosphataemia

Usually seen in association with hypercatabolic states, chemotherapy or cell destruction.

Management

Restoring renal function and dialysis is the only reliable way of reducing serum phosphate if levels are dangerously high.

ACUTE RENAL FAILURE (ARF)

Rapid restoration of renal blood flow and blood pressure can often attenuate or prevent renal failure with its accompanying high morbidity and mortality. Most acute renal failure is related to hypotension. The elderly and those with pre-existing renal disease are particularly prone to ARF.

Investigation

The diagnosis of ARF is usually clinical—oliguria and deteriorating renal function in the presence of suggestive clinical circumstances (e.g. sepsis, hypotension). History and physical examination will usually suggest the aetiology. Nephrotoxic drugs must be excluded, e.g. aminoglycosides, tetracyclines or angiotension-converting enzyme (ACE) inhibitors in the presence of chronic renal impairment.

Investigations that should be performed include the following:

1. Biochemistry: electrolytes, urea, creatinine, blood glucose, osmolality, liver function tests.
2. Haemoglobin, full blood count, erythrocyte sedimentation rate (ESR), platelets, blood film.
3. ECG.
4. Arterial blood gases.
5. Chest X-ray.
6. Blood cultures.

7. Urine analysis for protein, blood and glucose.
8. Microscopic examination for cells and casts.

Exclude hepatitis and human immunodeficiency virus (HIV) if dialysis is contemplated. Urine culture should be on midstream or catheter specimen. Renal ultrasonography confirms the presence of both kidneys and provides information on chronicity and excludes obstruction. CT scanning may provide more detail about the site of obstruction. Radionuclide scan or angiography will help if vascular occlusion is suspected.

Renal biopsy is necessary only where the aetiology remains unclear or when glomerular disease is suspected.

Exclude obstruction.

Management

Cardiovascular system

Rapidly correct hypovolaemia with fluids. If, despite normovolaemia, the patient's normal blood pressure has not been achieved, inotropes may be necessary. The alpha-agonist effects of vasopressors will often paradoxically improve renal blood flow and urine output by improving systemic blood pressure.

It is important to maintain the patient's normal blood pressure: i.e. in a previously hypertensive patient used to autoregulating at a certain systemic pressure, that pressure must be restored.

Drugs

Avoid or closely monitor nephrotoxic drugs such as aminoglycosides.

Intraabdominal pressure (IAP)

Oliguria and renal failure result when IAP increases. If the abdomen is tense, always measure intravesical pressure, which closely correlates with IAP over a wide range. It is simply performed in a catheterised patient by running 50 mL isotonic saline into the bladder, clamping the catheter distal to the inlet and connecting the bladder to a central venous pressure (CVP) manometer measuring set. The IAP should be measured from the pubic symphysis. Pressures below 20 cmH$_2$O are safe; pressures between 20 and 30 cmH$_2$O cause an increasing deterioration in renal function and pressures above 30 cmH$_2$O significantly impair renal function. The pressure must be relieved for re-establishment of normal function.

Diuretics

Diuretics will not prevent established renal failure and may actually worsen renal function if used instead of fluid replacement, if that is required. However, there is some evidence that oliguric renal failure may be converted to non-oliguric renal failure by the use of diuretics: e.g. IV aliquots of frusemide 20 mg and higher in the presence of chronic renal impairment. Alternatively an IV infusion of frusemide 10–20 mg/h, or mannitol 0.3 g/kg over 30 minutes, repeated at 4–6 hours if successful. Cease if oliguria persists.

MANAGEMENT OF ESTABLISHED RENAL FAILURE

1. **Hyperkalaemia.** The rate of rise of serum potassium will depend on the degree of oliguria and production of potassium. For management of hyperkalaemia, see above.
2. **Acidosis.** This is not usually a problem during the early phase of renal failure. If it becomes significant (pH <7.1), bicarbonate (1 mmol/kg) can be given as a temporary measure.
3. **Serum creatinine.** The rate of rise will depend on the degree of muscle breakdown and renal impairment—usually 0.05–0.2 mmol/L/day.
4. **Water retention.** Water retention results in pulmonary and peripheral oedema. Fluid restriction is a temporary measure.
5. **Dialysis.** This is the only short-term definitive method for restoring normal fluid, electrolyte and metabolic status. Its use depends on the rate of rise of potassium, hydrogen ions, creatinine and fluid status.

RECOMMENDED READING

Adrogue HJ, Midas NE. Medical progress: management of life-threatening acid-base disorders: first of two parts. New Engl J Med 1998; 338:26–34.

Gluck SL. Acid-base. Lancet 1998; 352:474–479.

Gutierrez G, Wulf ME. Lactic acidosis in sepsis: a commentary. Intensive Care Med 1996; 22:6–16.

Kellum JA. Metabolic acidosis in the critically ill: lessons from physical chemistry. Kidney International 1998; 66:581–586.

Zaritsky, A. Unmeasure anions: déjà vu all over again? Crit Care Med 1999; 27:1672–1673.

38 Ophthalmic emergencies

Michael R Delaney

PRINCIPLES OF EXAMINATION

1. All cases of suspected eye injuries require a thorough history and examination of:
   - Visual acuity.

- Pupillary reactions.
- The fundus.
- Ocular movement.
- Fields to confrontation.
- Lids and ocular adnexae.

2. Do not put pressure on the eye to examine it (especially if there is a possible penetrating injury).
3. Do not use atropine drops to dilate the pupil. Use a short-acting mydriatic and only if essential.
4. Do not use mydriatics in cases where the ocular state and optic nerve function may need to be monitored.
5. X-ray the orbits in all cases of a suspected intraocular foreign body, especially if the patient was using a hammer on metal, e.g. a chisel. *Note:* Request X-rays with eyes in up and down gazes.

COMMON PITFALLS

1. Never use steroid drops in the emergency department in initial treatment. Refer for further assessment.
2. Eye swabs need to be plated out directly.
3. Avoid contaminated diagnostic medications. Use only sterile drop solutions.
4. Always pad an eye after instilling local anaesthetic.
5. Never give local anaesthetic drops to the patient to take away and use.
6. Use a short-acting cycloplegic, e.g. cyclopentolate 1% or homatropine 2%.
7. Do not apply ointment in cases suspected of having a penetrating injury.
8. Do not persist in trying to remove a corneal foreign body if it is not easily removed.
9. Always provide adequate systematic analgesia in cases of corneal injury.
10. When in doubt seek an ophthalmic consultation.

USE OF SLIT LAMP

These remarks apply to the Haag Streit slit lamp, but the principles apply to all slit lamps. The patient and the examining doctor must both be comfortable. In particular, the patient should not be straining to keep the chin on the chin rest, and the patient's forehead must rest comfortably against the forehead strap. The eye should be at the level of the black mark on the side of the two columns that hold the chin rest and forehead strap; this is achieved by adjusting the height of the chin rest. The slit lamp should then be adjusted so that it is in its mid-position, allowing a full range of vertical and horizontal movement. This position is adjusted by rotating the joystick, which controls the height of the slit lamp as well as its movement in all directions, thereby controlling its focus.

After the patient is positioned correctly, the eye can be examined. On the bottom of the rotating light source column of the slit lamp is a knob that controls the width of the slit beam. Further up the column, immediately under the globe housing, is a control to adjust the intensity of the light; this same control also allows the insertion of a cobalt blue filter into the light, producing the characteristic blue light used to detect corneal ulcers with fluorescein dye. Near this control is another control that adjusts the height of the slit beam.

The slit lamp can be used in many ways. The easiest of these is simply to use it as a high-powered illumination source with magnification using the broad beam; this is particularly useful to detect corneal ulceration after instilling fluorescein dye and using the cobalt blue filter. To detect and assess iritis a narrow slit beam can be shone through the anterior chamber; this will highlight any flare or cells. A slit beam can be shone directly through the pupil to retro-illuminate the iris using the red reflex; this is also a useful way of assessing the clarity of the media.

Intraocular pressures are measured using the application tonometer, which is either attached to the slit lamp on a swinging arm or is detached from the slit lamp and is placed on the platform immediately in front of the eye pieces.

TRAUMA

Foreign bodies

Conjunctiva

Carefully examine posterior lid surfaces and fornices by everting the upper lid. Remove with moist swabstick or fine forceps.

Cornea

1. Remove with a sterile swab stick or sterile 25-gauge needle. Do not attempt to remove rust ring. Apply antibiotic ointment and pad firmly.
2. Patients with a residual rust ring and foreign body remnants must be referred.

Intraocular

1. Always suspect if there has been an eye injury after using a metal hammer on metal, or if there have been high-velocity particles.
2. Often minimal signs. A CT scan or X-ray of the orbit is mandatory.
3. Treat as a penetrating injury and organise urgent ophthalmic consultation.

Corneal abrasions

1. Instil local anaesthetic drops, stain with fluorescein and examine the eye.
2. Check for subtarsal foreign body.
3. Treat with antibiotic ointment and firm pad plus adequate analgesia.

Lid lacerations

1. Inspect punctum and look for lacerations to the canaliculus, which require prompt repair.
2. Lacerations through the lid margin need meticulous repair to prevent lid notching.

Burns

Chemical: acid or alkali

1. Immediate irrigation with copious amounts of water and local anaesthetic drops if needed.
2. Lime burns and alkali burns are the most damaging of all chemical injuries. All particles of lime must be removed. Evert lids to inspect fornices. Systemic analgesia is often required.

Thermal

Instil anaesthetic drops and remove any obvious loose foreign bodies. Start antibiotic drops and pad if possible.

Flash burns

1. These are very painful. Pain can start up to 6–12 hours after injury and last for 24 hours.
2. Apply antibiotic ointment and pad. Systemic analgesia and sedation are usually needed.
3. Review in 24 hours.

Blunt ocular trauma

Severe injuries can easily be missed. The history is not always a good guide to the severity of the injuries.

Hyphaema

1. This can cause secondary glaucoma; there may be a more severe secondary haemorrhage 2–3 days after the initial bleed (especially in children).
2. Admit to hospital for bed rest and pad the eye for bed rest at home if circumstances are appropriate. Arrange for urgent consultation within 24 hours.
3. Do not give aspirin-based analgesics.

Subconjunctival haemorrhage

The appearance is alarming. No treatment is needed except reassurance. Examine the eye to exclude any other injuries.

Vitreous haemorrhage and choroidal haemorrhage

Advise bed rest at home. Needs referral within 24 hours to exclude retinal detachment.

Traumatic mydriasis and iridodialysis

1. No treatment is available. Often associated with hyphaema.
2. Remember as a cause of abnormal pupillary reactions in cases with head and eye injuries.

Lens and retinal injuries

These need referral within 24 hours.

Orbital fractures and haemorrhage

Blowout fractures

1. Often associated with fractures of malar complex and middle third of face fractures.
2. Suspect if there is restriction of movement, enophthalmos or the patient complains of double vision.
3. Admit if other injuries require treatment. Otherwise needs referral within 24 hours. Start oral antibiotics.
4. The eye must be examined during initial assessment.

Orbital haemorrhage

1. Is often associated with orbital fractures.
2. Can be sight-threatening. Needs urgent consultation if severe or the patient has reduced vision, non-reacting pupils or ophthalmoplegia and proptosis.
3. May need urgent orbital decompression.

Optic canal fractures

These often cause total visual loss.

Penetrating injuries

1. Suspect from history, especially hammering on metal.
2. Examine very gently. Do not put pressure on the eye.
3. Start systemic antibiotics and local antibiotic drops (do not use ointment). Gently pad the eye. Bed rest.
4. Order X-ray or CT scan of the orbit if there is any possibility of intraocular foreign body.
5. Admit to hospital.

THE PAINFUL RED EYE

Acute conjunctivitis

1. Red inflamed eye, less congested towards the limbus. Often gritty with copious mucopurulent discharge in bacterial infections. Serous discharge in viral infections.
2. Swab.
3. Start broad-spectrum antibiotic drops every 1–2 hours.

Acute keratitis

1. Painful eye often with blurred vision, diffuse conjunctival injection and watery discharge.
2. Stain with fluorescein, looking for branching dendritic pattern of herpes simplex ulceration.
3. If herpetic ulceration is present, start antiviral chemotherapy (e.g. acyclovir ointment 5 times a day, plus antibiotic drops 4 times a day).
4. In non-herpetic keratitis start antibiotic drops 4–6 times a day and refer.

Acute iritis

1. Heavy dull pain, with ciliary injection (more injected near the limbus); sluggish small pupil and blurred vision.
2. Intraocular pressure normal.
3. Slit lamp examination essential.
4. Dilate pupil with short-acting cycloplegic drops 3 times a day and local steroid drops 4–6 times a day.
5. Analgesia and dark glasses may be required.

Acute narrow-angle glaucoma

1. Severe pain in unilateral red eye. Poor vision and semi-dilated non-reacting pupil. Cornea usually hazy. Intraocular pressure markedly raised (including to digital assessment). The main differential diagnosis is acute iritis, which can have secondary glaucoma.
2. This condition is sight-threatening. Start miotic drops—pilocarpine 2% every 5 minutes for 1 hour, then hourly, plus timolol 0.5% twice daily plus prednisolone 0.5% 4 times a day.
3. Acetazolamide 500 mg IV, then 250 mg every 8 hours (orally if tolerated).
4. Pethidine 50–100 mg by IM injection for pain.

Orbital cellulitis

1. Oedema and swelling of eyelids and conjunctiva. Often with exophthalmos, restriction of eye movement, pyrexia and dull pain—usually secondary to trauma or sinusitis.
2. Swab any wounds, start high-dose systemic antibiotics.
3. Admit to hospital and observe the vision and the eye.

SUDDEN VISUAL LOSS IN A WHITE EYE

Retinal artery occlusion

1. Sudden painless total and partial loss of vision, more often in the elderly. Pale disc, retinal oedema, cherry red spot and narrowed arteries.
2. Look for cause to treat, e.g. temporal arteritis or emboli.

Initial treatment

If seen within 2 hours of onset of symptoms:

1. Lower intraocular pressure with digital massage and IV acetazolamide 500 mg.
2. Attempt to dilate blood vessels by breathing carbagen (95% O_2 and 5% CO_2) via mask, or re-breathing from a paper bag.
3. Continue treatment for at least 30 minutes and obtain an urgent ophthalmic consultation.
4. Do an urgent ESR to exclude temporal arteritis; if confirmed, start systemic steroids—60–100 mg prednisolone daily.
5. Admit to hospital.

Retinal vein occlusion

1. Usually incomplete but variable visual loss; painless.
2. Dilated retinal veins with multiple haemorrhages throughout the retina. Optic disc often swollen.
3. Urgent referral.
4. No treatment.

Retinal detachment

1. Initial partial field loss, after history of flashes and floaters. More common in myopic and aphakic patients; often after blunt trauma.
2. Grey elevated veil-like retina seen.
3. If macula still not detached, admit to hospital for bed rest and urgent ophthalmic assessment. If macula detached, refer for assessment within 24 hours.

Vitreous haemorrhage

1. Often preceded by large black floaters. Vision may vary up to complete visual loss.
2. Advise bed rest at home. Needs referral within 24 hours to exclude retinal detachment.

Optic neuritis

1. Variable visual loss, more frequently central field loss.
2. Afferent pupillary defect and marked loss of red saturation.
3. Urgent referral for investigation.
4. No treatment.

OPHTHALMIC CONDITIONS NEEDING REFERRAL

1. **Acute dacryocystitis.** Treat with warm compresses and massage of tear sac. Start antibiotics.

2. **Squints in children.** Need to be seen by an ophthalmologist without delay. Cover test to diagnose.
3. **Chronic glaucoma.** Patient needs full assessment and institution of therapy without delay.
4. **Meibomian gland cyst/abscess.** Treat with hot compresses plus local antibiotic drops (oral antibiotics if severe). Refer.

COMMON OPHTHALMIC MEDICATIONS

1. **Antibiotics.** Availability and use varies from country to country. A routine course of treatment would be 1 or 2 drops, 4–5 times a day for 4 days. Intensive treatment needs drops every 1 or 2 hours during waking hours with ointment at night. Antibiotic suitable for initial treatment: sulfacetamide 10%; chloramphenicol 0.5%; gentamicin 0.3%; tobramycin 0.3%.
2. **Mydriatics.** Fundal observation is best carried out using 1 drop of tropicamide 0.5% (Mydriacyl) and waiting about 15 minutes. Reverse with pilocarpine 2% drops.
3. **Cycloplegics.** Use short-acting preparations, e.g. cyclopentolate 1% or homatropine 2%, 1–3 times a day. Do not use atropine.
4. **Miotics.** Pilocarpine 2% is the most commonly used strength.
5. **Glaucoma preparations.** Timolol maleate 0.25%, 0.5%; levobunolol 0.25%, 0.5%; latanoprost; brimonidine tartrate; apraclonidine HCl; pilocarpine HCl 1%, 2%, 4%; acetazolamide 250 mg.
6. **Local anaesthetics.** Amethocaine hydrochloride 0.5% (available in minims); proxymetacaine hydrochloride 0.5%.
7. **Antiviral agents.** Acyclovir 30 mg/g ophthalmic ointment.
8. **Non-steroidal anti-inflammatory agents.** Diclofenac (Voltaren); indomethacin (Indoptol); flurbiprofen (Ocufen).
9. **Steroids.** Fluorometholone 0.1%; prednisolone 0.5%; prednisolone 1%; dexamethasone 0.1%.
10. **Frequency of use.** Remember to tell the patient to wait 5 minutes between different drops.

RECOMMENDED READING

Kranski J. Clinical ophthalmology—a systematic approach. 4th edn. Oxford: Butterworth-Heinemann; 1999.

Rhee DJ, Pyfer MF. The Wills eye manual. 3rd edn. Philadelphia: Lippincott, Williams & Wilkins; 1999.

Fraunfleder FT, Roy FM. Current ocular therapy. 5th edn. Philadelphia: WB Saunders; 2000.

EAR EMERGENCIES

➡ If no vertigo is present, ear trauma is managed conservatively.

➡ If vertigo is present, call ENT service.

Pressure injury (barotrauma)

1. Occurs because of inadequate eustachian tube function and pressure changes in air travel or diving.
2. Bruising of the eardrum and middle ear (haemotympanum) produces pain and usually a conductive hearing loss.
3. Vertigo suggests inner ear damage.

Management

1. Evaluate.
2. Analgesia.
3. Patient should avoid flying/diving.
4. If no vertigo, follow up in ENT clinic in 2 weeks.
5. If vertigo or significant hearing loss, urgent audiogram and specialist referral required.

Tympanic membrane perforations

1. Traumatic perforations most commonly occur with blows to the side of the head, or sharp objects inserted into the ear.
2. Ask about ear symptoms—hearing loss, discharge (character), vertigo, tinnitus.
3. Sharp, irregular margins of the perforation are classical.
4. Most (95%) heal with no operative intervention.

Management

1. Disturb the canal as little as possible.
2. Keep the ear dry.
3. If there is evidence of infection (mucopus) and pain, then amoxycillin for 7 days is indicated.

4. Baseline audiogram should be requested to exclude sensorineural hearing loss.
5. Refer to the ENT clinic for review in 2–3 weeks.

Temporal bone fractures

1. Occur with 5–10% of closed head injuries.
2. Are suspected with blood and/or CSF otorrhoea, Battle's sign (periauricular haematoma), hearing loss, vertigo and facial nerve dysfunction.
3. Record the patient's facial nerve function on arrival, if possible. This is important for long-term prognosis.

➡ **Check for CSF leak and check facial nerve function.**

Management

1. ABCDE (primary survey) are paramount. This injury takes low priority relative to life-threatening comorbidities.
2. Once stable, in the secondary survey record the ear examination findings, including otoscopy, hearing, vestibular and facial nerve function.
3. Diagnosis is made clinically and with CT of temporal bones (bony windows, fine cuts).
4. Referral to the ENT service is warranted.
5. If cerebrospinal fluid (CSF) otorrhoea is suspected, a sample can be tested for β_2-transferrin (1 mL fluid in a urine jar).
6. Most injuries are managed expectantly—surgery is rarely indicated to repair CSF leaks or facial nerve paralysis.

Foreign bodies in external ear canal

1. Most common in 2–5-year-olds and seen occasionally in the unfortunate adult.
2. Insects should be killed first—try topical lignocaine or oil to drown them.
3. Insects are best removed by ear alligator forceps if sharp edges are facing you.
4. Most foreign bodies, however, should be removed by sneaking behind them with a wax curette or angled hook and withdrawing the object laterally (Figure 39.1).

Equipment required

- Headlight.
- Ear speculum (sizes 5–8) for adults; children mostly do not require them.
- Ear irrigation syringe.

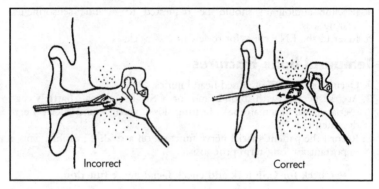

Incorrect   Correct

Figure 39.1   Incorrect and correct ways to remove a foreign body from the ear

- An angled wax curette or such instrument is invaluable.
- Ear alligator forceps.
- The parent, to calm the child and gently restrain!
- Nitrous oxide is used in some paediatric hospitals to facilitate cooperation (should be used with caution—check with your paediatric hospital emergency department staff).

> ➡ **If you lose rapport with the child, a general anaesthetic will probably be required.**

Management

1. The key to removal is establishing rapport and calming the child. Explain what you are doing in simple terms as you go.
2. Try ear syringing first. If this fails, try direct removal.
3. The safest technique is to use a blunt wax curette to move beyond the object and then gently pull the object out as you withdraw the curette, trying to minimise pressure on the ear canal as you remove it (Figure 39.1).
4. Check the ear for more foreign bodies.
5. If the canal is traumatised, Sofradex or another ototopic is suggested.
6. If you are unable to remove the object after one attempt, call the ENT service.

Otitis externa

1. Very common following water exposure.
2. Key features are pain, canal oedema, canal debris and watery discharge.
3. Irritating pruritus with cheesy discharge suggests fungal infection.

Management

1. Analgesia.
2. Ear toilet—usually cottonwool mopping of what can be seen. Avoid ear syringing in this situation.
3. Insertion of Otowick (Merocel tampon for ear)—with metal forceps—in a patent canal will help topical drop dispersion.
4. Topical antibiotics—Sofradex, Kenacomb (otic drops), Locorten-Vioform.
5. Systemic antibiotics if there is regional spread of infection (periauricular or onto neck).
6. Admission is rarely required, unless pain is not controlled by oral analgesics.

Bullous myringitis

1. Usually of *Mycoplasma pneumoniae* or viral origin.
2. Relatively normal external canal and haemorrhagic blebs on the tympanic membrane are diagnostic.
3. Produces severe pain, building to a crescendo before bloody discharge—and perhaps repetition of the cycle.
4. There may be an association with sensorineural hearing loss, so if patient complains of significant hearing loss, ENT referral and audiogram are warranted.

Management

1. Oral analgesia.
2. Amethocaine eye drops can be useful because, unlike in acute otitis media, the source of pain is superficial.
3. Keep the ear dry.
4. Antibiotics active against *Mycoplasma pneumoniae*.
5. Audiogram if hearing is clinically reduced.

Acute otitis media

1. Very common cause of ear pain in children.
2. Otoscopic features range from dilated vessels on the tympanic membrane to bulging of the tympanic membrane with a purulent effusion in the middle ear.
3. Spontaneous rupture of the eardrum heralds a relief of pain and usually heals within 3–4 weeks.
4. Most common microorganisms include *Streptococcus pneumoniae*, *Haemophilus influenzae* and *Moraxella catarrhalis*.

Management

1. Analgesia for the patient.
2. Then treat the parents—explain the condition.

3. Antibiotics—amoxycillin first line, amoxycillin and clavulanic acid for recurrent infections.
4. ENT referral if frequent infections.
5. Urgent ENT referral if suspected complications (Table 39.1).

Mastoiditis

1. Still occurs as a complication of acute otitis media.
2. Look for it in any child with ear pain.
3. Postauricular pain or oedema/fluctuance should alert you to call the ENT service.

Management

1. Analgesia.
2. FBC, UEC and blood cultures.
3. Swab of ear discharge (if present).
4. IV ceftriaxone and dicloxacillin.
5. Contact ENT service.
6. CT scan of brain/temporal bones and upper neck with IV contrast should be organised if there is cause for concern.
7. Keep the patient nil by mouth (NBM). True mastoiditis requires operative intervention.
8. If ENT consultation is not available, transfer the patient to a unit that offers the service.

➡ **Pitfalls in mastoiditis management:**
  • **Failure to suspect or diagnose.**
  • **Failure to recognise concurrent CNS complications.**
  • **Delaying ENT consultation.**

Labyrinthitis

1. Common cause of true rotatory vertigo, usually following upper respiratory tract infection.
2. Vertigo is sudden and persists for hours to days.
3. Cerebellar infarction can cause similar symptoms.
4. Admission may be required for IV rehydration.

Table 39.1 Complications of otitis media	
Local	Mastoiditis Labyrinthitis Facial nerve dysfunction
Regional	Meningitis Intracranial abscess
Systemic	Septicaemia

Management

1. Confirm the diagnosis.
2. Bed rest.
3. Try to reduce vestibular suppressant treatment (Stemetil, diazepam)—these medications prolong recovery time.
4. IV rehydration may be required if vomiting is excessive.

NOSE EMERGENCIES

Essential equipment

- Headlight.
- Nasal speculum.
- Frazier nasal sucker.
- Packing forceps.
- Metal tongue depressor.
- Wax curette.

> ➡ If you get the lighting and equipment right, most nasal emergencies can be managed satisfactorily.

Medications required

1. Drixine (oxymetazoline)—powerful nasal vasoconstrictor.
2. Cophenylcaine nasal spray—local anaesthetic and vasoconstrictor.

Epistaxis

1. Don't forget the ABC—the condition is life-threatening.
2. Many elderly patients have preexisting cardiovascular disease, so resuscitation and monitoring is paramount.
3. Detailed history may have to be delayed if there is brisk, heavy bleeding.
4. Ninety per cent of bleeding is classified as anterior, i.e. the majority of blood is exiting from the anterior nares.
5. Anterior bleeding is generally more readily treatable by the emergency physician than posterior bleeding.
6. Posterior bleeding is not readily visualised via the nose. Rather, on oral examination blood is seen streaming down the oropharynx.

Special requirements

1. Same as for the nasal examination.
2. Silver nitrate cautery sticks or hot nasal cautery wand.
3. Cottonwool for soaking with cophenylcaine and applying over the bleeding spot.
4. Vaseline packing gauze (available prepacked in 1.2 cm and 2.5 cm widths).
5. Merocel nasal tampons.

6. Epistat nasal balloon or a silicone Foley catheter (12F or 14F with a 30 mL balloon).
7. Kidney dish for the patient to evacuate blood and blood clots.
8. Don't forget your local anaesthetic and vasoconstrictor.

Management of anterior epistaxis

1. The patient should apply digital pressure over the soft external (cartilaginous) part of the nose, with head forward over a bowl or kidney dish.
2. Protect yourself first! Gowns, gloves and eye protection are mandatory.
3. Have all your equipment readily accessible—no headlight, no view.
4. Don't forget your ABC, including assessing vital signs, IV access and taking FBC, UEC, coagulation studies (coags) and group-and-hold.
5. Clear the clots (suck the nose or get the patient to blow nose).
6. Make a view for yourself and make it comfortable for the patient—cophenylcaine and/or Drixine.
7. Little's area (anteroinferior septum) is the most common site. Look for active bleeding, prominent blood vessels, small polyps or other frank pathology.
8. Are you able to see the bleeding site or potential bleeding site?
   • NO — Pack the nose with Vaseline gauze (see Figure 39.2) or insert Merocel tampons and call the ENT service.
   • YES — Place a cottonwool pledget (3–4 cm) soaked with cophenylcaine over the bleeding site for 5 minutes.
9. Silver nitrate sticks can be used directly over a slow bleed or suspiciously large vessel to cauterise—look for whitening of mucosa. (**Warning!** Don't cauterise the same site on the opposite side of the nose; there is a risk of later septal perforation.)
10. If the bleeding is controlled, observe the patient for 1 hour in the emergency department, then discharge with advice (Table 39.2), for follow-up in the ENT outpatients department.
11. If the bleeding is visible, but too brisk or heavy, pack the nose and call the ENT service.

Management of posterior epistaxis

1. Preparation and initial inspection is the same as for anterior epistaxis.
2. Generally, the bleeding site is not easily seen; blood streams from above down the oropharynx.
3. Most of these patients require urgent posterior packing using either an Epistat nasal balloon (inflating the 10 mL posterior balloon first) or a Foley catheter insufflated in the nasopharynx and Vaseline gauze packed anteriorly (Figure 39.3). **Inflate slowly** to minimise pain.
4. Call the ENT service—all posterior packed patients require high dependency/ICU monitoring to observe for cardiorespiratory disturbance.

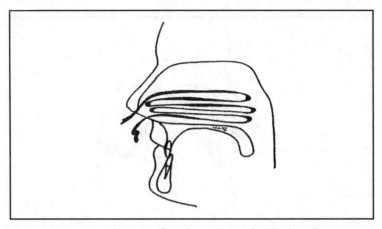

Figure 39.2   Correct placement of Vaseline gauze packing, with antibiotics commenced (possible bacteraemia in presence of nasal packing)

Table 39.2 Epistaxis discharge advice (to be followed for 5–7 days after bleeding)

- Avoid strenuous/heavy activity.
- Avoid cold/dry environments.
- Avoid caffeine and alcohol.
- Don't blow the nose hard.
- Avoid bending over/lifting/straining on the toilet.
- Expect occasional minor bleeding post-cautery.

Return to the hospital if bleeding restarts and you are unable to control it with digital pressure over the soft (cartilaginous) external nose for 10 minutes by the clock.

Trauma to the nose

1. Patients with trauma to their face should have other facial fractures excluded as well.
2. Septal haematomas occur with these injuries—look for a bilateral septal swelling.
3. Management of epistaxis is more emergent than the fracture itself.
4. X-rays (including CT of facial bones) should be considered for medico-legal reasons, if other face fractures are suspected clinically. Plain X-rays of the nose can be difficult to interpret because of the nasomaxillary suture and anterior nasal artery grooves on the bone.

Management of fractured nose

1. ABC primary survey is first.

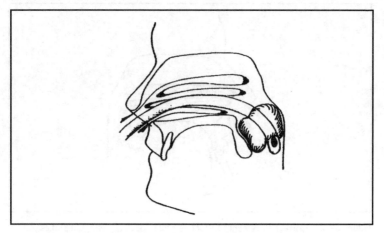

Figure 39.3 Foley's catheter used as postnasal balloon packing, with gauze anterior pack

2. In the secondary survey, manage the epistaxis, exclude other facial fractures and septal haematoma.
3. If all other conditions are satisfied, reduction of the fractured nose can occur within 2 weeks.
4. An appointment can be made with the ENT service after 3 days (to allow swelling to subside).
5. The decision to operate depends on functional (nasal obstruction) and cosmetic considerations.

Management of septal haematoma

1. If septal haematoma (i.e. bilateral septal swelling) is suspected, contact the ENT service.
2. Keep the patient fasting.
3. Drainage can be attempted under local anaesthetic (topical and direct injection).
4. Drainage and then suturing of the mucosa back down to the cartilage, with subsequent packing of the nose, is the best treatment.

Foreign bodies in the nose

1. Very common cause of unilateral nasal discharge in a 2–5-year-old child.
2. It is difficult to justify leaving a foreign body in a child's nose overnight—this situation is potentially airway-threatening.
3. The foreign body is very probably lying between the inferior turbinate and septum.
4. Developing rapport and moving slowly is essential.

5. Topical local anaesthetic 'magic mist' is useful (1–2 puffs of Cophenylcaine).
6. If unsuccessful after one attempt, call the ENT service.

➡ **Button batteries**
These are extremely **dangerous**. Any suspicion that they may be present in the ear, nose or throat is an **absolute emergency**. They require **prompt removal**.

Equipment required

1. As for nasal examination set-up.
2. An angled wax curette or such instrument is invaluable.
3. Ear alligator forceps.
4. The parent! To calm the child and gently restrain.
5. Nitrous oxide is used in some paediatric hospitals to facilitate cooperation. (It should be used with caution—check with your paediatric hospital emergency department staff.)

Management

1. Explanation, rapport and 'magic mist' are the keys to successful removal.
2. Tell the parent and child what is happening at all times—**in simple terms.**
3. Get the parent to spray the Cophenylcaine and then let the child return to play for 10 minutes.

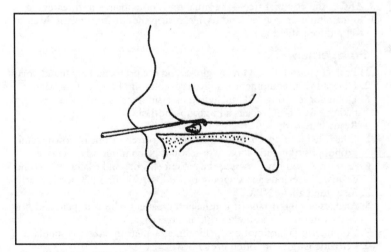

Figure 39.4   Removing a foreign body from the nose

4. No nasal speculum is required for a 2–5-year-old child. Just push the nasal tip up.
5. Suction the nose to clarify your view, and check the number of foreign bodies.
6. If foreign body is spherical or difficult to grasp, pass the angled blunt instrument gently behind the foreign body and pull the object forward out of the nose (Figure 39.4).
7. If foreign body is irregular or graspable, gently grasp and remove.
8. Recheck the nose so that you don't miss the second or third foreign body.

THROAT

Remove patient's dentures before examination.

Essential equipment

- Headlight.
- Metal tongue depressor.
- Flexible endoscope or dental mirror if concerned about laryngeal pathology.

Post-tonsillectomy bleed

1. Two to five per cent of patients will have a post-tonsillectomy bleed of some degree, and half of these patients will re-present to a doctor.
2. Most of these patients present 5–10 days postoperatively.
3. ABC is the essential step—the situation is potentially life-threatening.
4. Remaining calm yourself and trying to keep the situation relatively clean will reduce patient anxiety.

Management

1. Protect yourself first! Gowns, gloves and eye protection are mandatory.
2. Have all your equipment readily accessible—no headlight, no view.
3. Don't forget your ABC including assessing vital signs, IV access and taking FBC, UEC, coags and group-and-hold.
4. Resuscitate early.
5. If heavily bleeding, the patient should be placed in a head down (semi-prone) position and blood/clots should be continuously suctioned.
6. As soon as you have assessed the patient (history and examination) and estimated previous and ongoing blood loss, call the ENT service early.
7. Keep the patient NBM.
8. Analgesia is important (it is usually the patient who is in pain and not swallowing who is at higher risk of a bleed).
9. Commence IV antibiotics—penicillin +/– metronidazole is standard.
10. Peroxide gargles are often prescribed.
11. The ENT service determines when and if exploration is warranted.

Palatal trauma

1. More common in children, e.g. after falling face first with a pencil in the mouth.
2. Injuries can be dramatic, with full thickness mucosal and muscular tears.
3. Most tears heal without surgery, but large (>2 cm) or full-thickness injury should be looked at by the ENT service.
4. Be aware of other coincident major injury, e.g. carotid artery injuries have been reported with this mechanism of injury.

Management

1. Lateral airways X-ray to exclude retropharyngeal/parapharyngeal air.
2. Antibiotics.
3. Injuries associated with odynophagia (painful swallow) or dysphagia (difficulty swallowing) may require admission, IV antibiotics and rehydration.

Laryngeal trauma

1. Represents 1 in 20,000 emergency department admissions.
2. Usually coincident with other neck trauma.
3. Becoming less frequent because of chest restraint seatbelts.
4. Is life-threatening—patient's airway is tenuous.
5. Emergency airway access (intubating equipment, minitrach, tracheostomy tray) should always be at hand (see Chapter 2 for airway emergencies).

Management

1. Examination includes primary survey—ABC with cervical spine control, detailed secondary survey focusing on excluding concurrent neck/ chest injury.
2. Flexible endoscopy—call the ENT service to assess the endolarynx.
3. If the patient is able to lie flat, CT scan of neck bone/soft tissue with IV contrast should be organised.
4. All patients are admitted to high-dependency/ ICU for observation.
5. Keep NBM, humidified oxygen until ENT review.
6. The decision to operate depends on airway stability and degree of injury.

➡ **All suspected laryngeal injuries should be reviewed by the ENT service before discharge. Severe injury may present with minor symptoms.**

Caustic ingestion

1. Alkaline liquefactive necrosis is more damaging than acid coagulative necrosis; therefore try to determine exactly what was ingested.
2. Liquid is generally more destructive than solid ingestion (travels further).

3. In addition to ENT examination, don't forget to examine the chest and abdomen (oesophageal and gastric perforation).

Management

1. ABC is the most important first step. The child's airway is tenuous, so consult the ENT service early.
2. Admit the patient.
3. IV access, FBC, UEC and rehydration.
4. Keep the patient NBM under review by senior staff.
5. Chest and abdominal X-rays are routine, to exclude mediastinal and intraabdominal gas.
6. Antibiotics, proton pump inhibitor and steroids should be considered.
7. Most patients with caustic ingestion require an evaluation of the upper aerodigestive tract under general anaesthetic in the first 24 hours.

Pharyngeal foreign bodies

1. Ingested bones are the most common pharyngeal foreign bodies.
2. Check the tonsils, tongue base and piriform fossa—the most common sites.
3. Local anaesthetic facilitates removal, but try to get the patient to localise side and site before topicalising.

Equipment required

1. Headlight.
2. Metal tongue depressor.
3. Tilley's nasal packing forceps or Magill's anaesthetic forceps.
4. Macintosh or straight laryngoscopes can be helpful for tongue base and vallecula.
5. Topical anaesthetic (4% lignocaine).
6. Sucker.

Management

1. Get the patient to localise the foreign body, then topicalise the pharynx.
2. Wait for 5–10 minutes.
3. If the foreign body is on tonsil or tongue base, it is often easily retrievable with Tilley's or Magill's forceps.
4. If foreign body is further posterior, try putting the patient in the intubating position and use a laryngoscope in your left hand, with forceps/sucker in your right hand.
5. Two or three unsuccessful attempts justify a call to the ENT service. Keep the patient NBM.

Oesophageal foreign bodies

1. Food bolus in the adult or coins in the child are the most common oesophageal foreign bodies.

2. Complete obstruction with drooling and discomfort requires urgent endoscopic removal.
3. Beware of a sharp foreign body ingestion—if CXR shows pneumomediastinum, this is potentially life-threatening.

Management

1. Confirm the diagnosis—history, examination (drooling, complete aphagia, neck discomfort).
2. CXR helps to rule out air in the mediastinum.
3. Call the ENT service.
4. Cola gargles, glucagon and midazolam may help for partial obstruction, but rarely work for complete obstruction.

Keep NBM and workup for general anaesthetic.

Airway foreign bodies

1. If there is complete airway obstruction leading to cyanosis, back blows should be used.
2. Partial airway obstruction should never be treated with the Heimlich manoeuvre, as this may convert a serious situation into a desperate one.
3. In children a history of coughing or choking episodes followed by stridor or continuous coughing warrants admission and endoscopic evaluation.
4. Tracheobronchial foreign bodies are life-threatening—vegetable matter is especially dangerous because of irritant oils and swelling.

Management

1. History and examination is vital. Look for localised crepitus, rhonchi, decreased air entry.
2. CXR should be ordered with an inspiratory and expiratory film, looking for air trapping, hyperinflation, atelectasis or consolidation.
3. Admit the child and call ENT service.
4. Keep NBM and arrange for theatre: endoscopic assessment is always required.

Inflammation—the 'bad sore throat'

Most patients with sore throats have pharyngitis/tonsillitis, but always be aware of the two serious situations: supraglottitis and quinsy/deep neck space infections.

➡ **Beware** the patient with **sore throat and voice change**—a **tenuous airway** until proven otherwise.

Supraglottitis (or epiglottitis)

1. Previously a disease of childhood, now much more common in the adult patient not vaccinated for *Haemophilus influenzae B*.

2. In the child—toxic, stridor, patient sits upright with neck extended and drooling.
3. In the adult—toxic, sore throat, voice change, may have respiratory distress.
4. As always, ABC.

Management of paediatric epiglottitis
1. Any child suspected of this condition should not be disturbed.
2. Call senior staff/ENT service.
3. Usually the child is transported to theatre for stabilisation of airway.

➡ **Adults get epiglottitis more often than children now. The adult form involves the whole supraglottis.**

See also Chapter 33.

Management of adult supraglottitis
1. Evaluate—take history and examine.
2. The diagnosis is suspected, before endoscopic assessment, by specific localisation of pain to well below the tonsils, i.e. to the larynx.
3. Call ENT service.
4. Check ABC, including assessing vital signs, IV access and taking FBC, UEC and blood cultures if toxic.
5. IV rehydration.
6. IV antibiotics—usually ceftriaxone and dicloxacillin are empirically given after blood cultures.
7. If airway is tenuous, IV steroids can be considered.
8. Humidified oxygen.
9. Admission to high-dependency/ICU after diagnosis is endoscopically confirmed.
10. Most adult supraglottitis does not require operative intervention.

Quinsy/deep neck space infections

1. Quinsy (peritonsillar abscess) is the most common form of deep neck space infection.
2. Adolescence is the typical age group.
3. Most infections occur at the superior pole of the tonsil and manifest with severe unilateral sore throat, trismus (lock jaw) and soft palate bulging.
4. Remember that simultaneous bilateral quinsy is rare.
5. Peritonsillar abscesses can spread to other neck spaces and pose a threat to the airway.

Equipment required
- Headlight.
- Metal tongue depressor.
- Long IV cannula (>5 cm) or 20-gauge spinal needle.

- 10 mL syringe.
- Topical lignocaine
- Spit bowl/kidney dish.

Management

1. Evaluate: take history and examine. Look for 'hot potato' voice, trismus, unilateral palate oedema/pointing of an abscess.
2. IV access, FBC, UEC and blood cultures if toxic.
3. IV penicillin and metronidazole and rehydration.
4. Parenteral analgesia maybe required.
5. Topical lignocaine over the site of maximal pointing.
6. Call ENT service.

Aspiration of a quinsy

1. Patient should be sitting up with kidney dish under chin.
2. Tongue depressor in left hand to expose, needle on syringe in right hand (if right-handed).
3. Insert needle then create vacuum over maximal pointing (generally no deeper than 1–1.5 cm)—feeling for deliberate give into abscess cavity.
4. If concerned or unsuccessful, call ENT service.
5. Admission generally required for 24–48 hrs of IV antibiotics.

RECOMMENDED READING

Bull PD. Lecture notes on diseases of the ear, nose and throat. 9th edn. Oxford, Malden, MA: Blackwell Science; 2002.

Burtin M, Leighton S, Robson A, et al. Hall and Colman's diseases of the ear, nose and throat. 15th edn. Edinburgh: Churchill Livingstone; 2000.

Ludman H. ABC of otolaryngology. 4th edn. London: BMJ Publishing Group; 1997.

40 Dental emergencies

Peter Foltyn

There are many kinds of dental emergencies, some of which can be extremely subjective. Whereas a small carious lesion or infected extraction socket may cause excruciating pain for one person, a fractured jaw may be asymptomatic and discovered as an incidental finding only after routine X-rays. Emergency departments in teaching hospitals will nearly always have an accredited on-call dentist or in rural settings may refer all dental emergencies to a local dental emergency service or individual dentist. As dental emergencies are rarely life-threatening, commonsense measures such as antibiotics, sedatives and analgesics where appropriate should get the patient through the night or weekend until an appointment can be arranged for the next working day.

It would be an inappropriate use of resources to ask an on-call dentist to personally attend all cases of dental or oral pain. Many dental problems are the result of dental neglect, which would have initially presented many days or weeks earlier.

If the patient is to be admitted or there is doubt about management, contact the on-call dentist. Always have any relevant medical history at hand and try to establish a history for the dental problem. The dental history should include duration and nature of any pain or swelling and any measures taken to counter the problem by the patient or patient's own doctor or dentist.

TOOTHACHE

In the majority of instances toothache can be narrowed down to a specific tooth, which may be tender to touch, and is often a direct result of tooth decay. However, pain can be referred to adjacent teeth, the opposing jaw, facial areas or the neck, but does not generally extend across the midline except when the origin is the anterior teeth. As emergency department imaging may be limited to taking orthopantomogram (OPG) X-rays or standard views of facial bones, the source of the toothache may not immediately be evident. Clinical examination by emergency department staff may prove unrewarding without some training in oral examination. A strong light source, dental mirror and probe, and an air source are required (wall-outlet medical air or oxygen or cylinder gases and tubing are normally available in all emergency departments).

Dental caries

Dental caries may be minor or extensive and may undermine an existing dental restoration or artificial crown.

Response/advice

Provide adequate analgesia until the next working day.

Erosion or abrasion

Erosion or abrasion areas at the tooth/gum junction may produce extreme hypersensitivity.

Response/advice

Provide adequate analgesia until the next working day and suggest an anti-hypersensitivity toothpaste such as Sensodyne or Colgate Gel-Kam.

Dental pulp

Dental pulp (nerve) involvement is often an extension of decay in the body or branches of the dental pulp. Invasion by microorganisms into the dental pulp often leads to an initial acute pulpitis which may settle and return as a chronic, more diffuse pain many weeks or even months or years later. The microorganisms that invaded the dental pulp may then extend beyond the tooth apex and be responsible for dental abscess formation. (See also 'Facial swellings'.)

Response/advice

Provide adequate analgesia until the next working day. Antibiotics may also be required if there is established lymphadenopathy, pyrexia or visible dental abscess formation on X-ray. Advise the patient to see a dentist as a matter of urgency.

Fractured or split teeth

Fractured or split teeth may be the result of trauma or of a heavily filled tooth giving way. In some instances intact teeth may fracture as a result of an anatomical irregularity in their formation or as a result of an occlusal or bite discrepancy.

Response/advice

Provide adequate analgesia until the next working day. Advise the patient to see a dentist as soon as possible.

INFECTED GUMS
Gingivitis/periodontitis

Poor oral health may lead initially to marginal gingivitis, progressing over many years to moderate or severe periodontitis and associated problems with the bone surrounding the teeth. Advanced periodontal disease may lead to tooth mobility, bad breath, oral bleeding, periodontal abscess formation, extrusion, drifting or exfoliation of teeth and generalised mouth pain. Periodontal disease may be an early clinical clue for systemic diseases such as HIV infection and diabetes or following treatment in the case of graft versus host disease (GVHD) in bone marrow transplantation and radiation therapy of the head and neck.

Response/advice

Provide adequate analgesia until the next working day. Antibiotics may also be required. A chlorhexidine mouth rinse, preferably alcohol-free (Colgate—Perioguard), will reduce microorganism numbers. Advise the patient to see a dentist as soon as possible.

Acute necrotising ulcerative gingivitis (ANUG)

ANUG is a severe gingival infection often characterised by strong pain, pyrexia and bad breath with punched out and ulcerated interdental papillae. ANUG can be found in otherwise healthy mouths and is often associated with stress. ANUG is not uncommon around examination time or in times of partnership breakdown.

Response/advice

Provide adequate analgesia until the next working day and prescribe metronidazole (Flagyl) or tinidazole (Fasigyn). A chlorhexidine mouth rinse, preferably alcohol-free (Colgate—Perioguard), will reduce micro-organism numbers. Advise patient to see a dentist as soon as possible.

IMPACTED TOOTH

The usual age for eruption of wisdom teeth or third molars is between 17 and 22, but eruption can occur as early as 15. In the past, when oral health was poor and fluoridation of water supplies had not commenced, it was common for young adults to have had a number of teeth removed due to tooth decay before the end of their teenage years. Today, most young adults born and raised in communities with fluoridated water are rarely missing any teeth and have also had a minimal number of teeth restored. A consequence of having good teeth is that for many there is little room for their orderly eruption. This has now led to a significant increase in not only impaction of wisdom teeth but occasionally other teeth as well, especially when there is a discrepancy between tooth and mouth size.

Impacted teeth can cause pain for numerous reasons. In most instances the cause of pain is a result of local infection which often leads to regional lymphadenopathy. Carious breakdown with acute pulpitis and pressure on an adjacent tooth can also cause severe pain.

Response/advice

Provide adequate analgesia until the next working day. Antibiotics may also be required if there is established lymphadenopathy or pyrexia. Advise the patient to see a dentist or a specialist oral surgeon as soon as possible.

MOUTH SORES AND ULCERATION

Oral ulceration and mouth sores may be the result of a myriad of precipitating factors including stress, acidic foods and even specific foods. Sodium lauryl sulphate (SLS), a detergent commonly found in toothpastes, has also been implicated.

Random aphthous and traumatic ulceration is not uncommon, but ulceration as an oral manifestation of a systemic disease can also occur. Severe mouth sores also occur in GVHD following bone marrow transplantation and canker sores during head and neck irradiation.

Nutritional deficiencies in the aged and unwell may also lead to oral ulceration. Denture wearers who have lost more than 5 kg since the dentures were made may have experienced shrinkage of alveolar ridges and other changes inside their mouths. This shrinkage is not uniform, causing the denture to dig in.

Response/advice

Good oral hygiene and reducing stress is a starting point for limiting the recurrence of oral ulceration. Rinsing or topical application of Xylocaine viscous with a cotton bud to a specific ulcer may help. Chlorhexidine mouth rinse and topical steroids, such as Kenalog in orabase, should be prescribed until the patient can get to his/her dentist. Thalidomide has been shown to reduce pain in large intractable ulcers found in immune-compromised patients, as has nicotine-containing gum (Nicorette) in non-smokers suffering random aphthous ulceration.

NEOPLASIA

The average age of a person with an oral cancer in Australia is 64. However, young people are regularly being diagnosed with oral-based malignancies. An area of induration, leukoplakia or erythroplasia that has progressed in size or has been managed topically or systemically without resolution requires urgent attention.

Response/advice

As the consequences of delay in providing a definitive diagnosis of an oral cancer may compromise the patient in many ways, biopsy of the suspect lesion should be carried out as soon as possible. Punch biopsy or excisional biopsy can be carried out by a surgical or plastics registrar or on-call dentist.

FACIAL SWELLINGS

The most common cause of facial swellings is dental abscess formation. A dental abscess is an infection around the root of a tooth or in the gum that causes an accumulation of pus. At the early stage of infection there is often associated pain, but not necessarily swelling. If the infection is left unchecked, the accumulated pus attempts to drain and will track via the path of least resistance, accumulating as a intra- or extraoral swelling that may not necessarily be overlying the abscessed tooth. Local lymphadenopathy is common, with marked facial swellings caused by dental abscess formation.

Response/advice

Provide adequate analgesia until the next working day together with antibiotics if the swelling is slight and there is no concern about airway obstruction or progression to cellulitis. Tell the patient to rinse out the mouth with warm salty water every hour or as needed to ease the pain. If able, the patient can cover the handle of a teaspoon with cottonwool, immerse it in hot salty water and then press on the swelling. This may help to establish drainage. Using ice packs or frozen peas, 20 minutes on and 10 off, over the affected area may also help to relieve the pain. Advise the patient to return to the emergency department if:

- Swelling of the face, jaw, cheek or eye increases.
- Swelling spreads to the neck or chest.
- There are any symptoms of airway obstruction.
- The pain becomes worse.
- The patient develops pyrexia.

If the swelling is significant, has spread to the eye, neck or chest, or there is concern for potential airway obstruction (Ludwig's angina), the patient should be admitted and IV antibiotics commenced immediately (benzylpenicillin 1.2 g 6-hourly). In the more severe or unresponsive cases, add metronidazole. For patients hypersensitive to penicillin, use clindamycin 300 mg 8-hourly or lincomycin 600 mg 8-hourly. IV fluids should also be considered. Contact the on-call dentist; however, if the swelling is significant and CT X-rays are available, fine cut views in the area of the swelling will help determine if there is an accumulation of pus and if incision and drainage is required.

HEART DISEASE AND DENTAL CARE

The following recommendations from the St Vincent's Hospital Dental Department are based on guidelines and antibiotic regimens that have been endorsed by all Australian Commonwealth and all state health departments, the Cardiac Society of Australia and New Zealand and Australian Dental Association Inc.

Several heart conditions require the patient and dentist to take special precautions. These recommendations are especially important for:

1. People with artificial heart valves (aortic, mitral).
2. People with a previous history of heart-valve infection.
3. People born with or who acquire heart problems such as:
   - Most at-birth heart malformations.
   - Damaged heart valves.
   - Thickened heart muscle.

People with heart problems have three responsibilities:

1. They need to establish and maintain a clean and healthy mouth. That means practising good oral hygiene and visiting their dentist regularly.
2. They need to make sure that their dentist knows that they have a heart problem.
3. They must carefully follow both their doctor's and dentist's instructions when prescribed any medications and in particular antibiotics.

ANTIBIOTIC GUIDELINES FOR DENTAL PROCEDURES IN HIGH-RISK PATIENTS[1]

Amoxycillin 2 g (children: 50 mg/kg up to 2 g) orally as a single dose 1 hour before the procedure. (*Note*: the Australian Guidelines are now 2 g, not 3 g.)

For patients hypersensitive to penicillin, on long-term penicillin therapy or having taken penicillin or a related beta-lactam antibiotic more than once in the previous month, use: clindamycin 600 mg (children: 10 mg/kg up to 600 mg), not erythromycin or tetracycline, orally as a single dose 1 hour before the procedure commences.

POST-EXTRACTION INSTRUCTIONS

Often teeth need to be removed because of excessive dental decay or formation of a dental abscess. Immediately following a tooth extraction, the patient should be advised to keep biting on the rolled gauze, which has been placed in their mouth for at least 20–30 minutes. If the patient is still bleeding provide extra gauze.

General advice to patient

- Do not smoke.
- Do not rinse mouth vigorously.
- Do not spit or continually wipe away blood.
- Do not drink through a straw for 24 hours.
- Do not suck on the extraction site.

These activities may disturb the healing blood clot.

Immediately after a tooth is extracted, the patient may experience discomfort and notice some swelling. This is normal. The initial healing period typically takes 1–2 weeks, and some swelling and residual bleeding should be expected in the 24 hours following an extraction. It is important not to dislodge the blood clot that forms on the wound. Occasionally, this clot can break down, leaving what is known as a dry socket. This can cause temporary pain and discomfort that will subside as the socket heals through a secondary healing process.

Response/advice

To limit swelling:

- Place ice packs or frozen peas on the area of the face overlying the extraction site, 20 minutes on and 10 minutes off for 2–3 hours.
- Should there still be bleeding after 2–3 hours, place a teabag on the extraction site and bite down on it firmly but without rupturing the bag.
- Avoid strenuous activity for 24 hours.
- Drink plenty of fluids and maintain as normal a diet as possible, which may be limited to soft foods for the first few days.

- Avoid alcoholic beverages and hot liquids.
- Brush and floss normally, being extra careful around the extraction area.
- On the day following the extraction, gently rinse the mouth with warm salt water (half a teaspoonful in one glass of water).
- Medication may be prescribed to help control pain and infection.

DRY SOCKET

Alveolar osteitis, or dry socket, is a severe pain that often follows a recent extraction. It is the result of disintegration of the blood clot formed in the socket after the extraction and may not be relieved by over-the-counter analgesics. The pain may radiate to the ear and is often accompanied by fetor oris, or bad breath. When the usual process of healing is disturbed, the blood clot may be dislodged, leaving bone within the socket exposed to saliva, food and other mouth debris rather than surrounded by an organising blood clot. If a dry socket occurs, it usually does so immediately following the extraction, although breakdown of the blood clot occasionally occurs after several days of uneventful healing.

Response/advice

Provide adequate analgesia, which may include the addition of an non-steroidal anti-inflammatory drug (NSAID), until the next working day; however, antibiotics may also be required if there is established lymphadenopathy or pyrexia. Advise the patient to attend a dentist as soon as possible to have the dry socket irrigated and dressed.

ORAL BLEEDING

Generally warfarin or antiplatelet medications need not be stopped prior to dental extractions or deep cleaning. However, appropriate local measures should be adopted in addition to checking with the patient's cardiologist, in the case of an underlying cardiovascular disease, or haematologist if the concern is due to a blood dyscrasia. Most patients can be managed in a general dental practice setting and do not need to be admitted to hospital. St Vincent's Hospital has adopted dental recommendations from the United Kingdom as the basis for new prescribing and formulary guidelines.[2]

Patients being treated with oral anticoagulant medication who have an International Normalised Ratio (INR) below 4.0 may have dental extractions without interruption to their treatment. Local measures, which include suturing and packing the extraction site with absorbable gelatine sponge, are generally sufficient to prevent post-extraction bleeding. However, excessive post-extraction or oral bleeding for other reasons may still occur. The most common cause of post-extraction bleeding for the patient with no known systemic problems is failure to follow instructions from the dentist.

Response/advice

If bleeding persists despite repetition of local measures as described in the above section, or if a bleeding disorder or dyscrasia is suspected, follow the St Vincent's Hospital Dental Department Protocol for local anti-fibrinolytic treatment, as follows:

- Dilute IV Amicar (aminocaproic acid) 5 mL in 10 mL sterile water and ask patient to rinse.
- Wet but do not saturate a sterile gauze square in undiluted Amicar.
- Fold or roll the gauze so that it can be placed on the extraction site and press firmly.
- Repeat after half an hour or as required.
- If patient is being discharged, provide the remaining Amicar and additional bite pads to repeat at home if required.
- Tell the patient to use an alcohol/phenol-free mouthwash twice daily, commencing after 24 hours.

TRAUMATIC INJURIES TO TEETH

Fracture

Tooth fractures can be divided into five categories:

Grade 1: Involves minor chipping of the incisal edge limited to enamel.
Grade 2: Involves fracture through to dentine without pulpal or nerve exposure.
Grade 3: Fracture with pulpal or nerve exposure.
Grade 4: Root fracture.
Grade 5: Complex.

Response/advice

If the traumatic injury is the result of a minor accident, provide analgesia if required until the next working day. If, however, the injury is the result of a motor vehicle accident, assault or other significant incident, an OPG X-ray should be taken, if available. Often, undisplaced and asymptomatic fractures of the body of the mandible, ramus, condylar head or coracoid process may be detected with an OPG. With grade 3–5 fractures where there are no bodily injuries present other than minor local lacerations, provide analgesia until the next working day. Should the patient be admitted or require observation in the emergency department for any length of time, contact the on-call dentist.

Luxation

A tooth is considered luxated when it has been moved, often occupying a position other than its original one. Luxated teeth can be divided into five categories:

Grade 1: Tooth loosened but still in its original position (subluxation).

Grade 2: Loosened and out of position.
Grade 3: Significantly out of position.
Grade 4: Pushed into upper or lower jaw.
Grade 5: Complex (out of its original position with a grade 2–5 tooth fracture).

Response/advice

Except for a grade 1 luxation, always contact the on-call dentist as soon as possible. If there are no other bodily injuries precluding dental management, repositioning and splinting of the loosened teeth will generally be required.

Avulsion

Evidence suggests that avulsed or knocked out teeth that are reimplanted within 30–45 minutes have a reasonable chance of long-term retention. However, after 2 hours out of the mouth, the prospects are diminished. Correct handling, transportation and storage of the knocked-out tooth is critical.

Response/advice

Ideally the patient should be encouraged to push the tooth back into the socket, even if it is out of alignment and loose. If this is too painful or not possible, holding the tooth in the floor of the mouth will keep the root bathed in the patient's own saliva. Should other injuries or the patient's mental state preclude the above, immediate storage in UHT milk is preferred to whole milk or water. Handle avulsed teeth only by the enamel and do not rinse in any disinfectant solution. Always contact the on-call dentist as soon as possible, as implantation, repositioning and splinting of an avulsed tooth will be required. Should the dentist be unavailable immediately, small rectangular strips of Stomahesive Wafer by Convatec can be used to hold the tooth provisionally.

TRISMUS AND TEMPOROMANDIBULAR JOINT (TMJ) DYSFUNCTION

Many people have pain or discomfort in and around the TMJ at some time during their lives. The symptoms may include pain, tenderness, spasm, clicking or crepitus as well as direct or referred pain in the muscles of the face, neck, shoulder and ears. TMJ dysfunction may lead to loss of jaw function, with the pain ranging from a mild discomfort in the morning to a chronic debilitating pain rendering a patient unable to open the mouth by the afternoon.

Conservative treatment (NSAIDs plus alternating hot and cold packs or compresses and rest) may prove effective following acute trauma to the jaw after a motor vehicle accident, fall or bashing. Direct trauma to the TMJ area or either jaw may also cause chronic or latent damage which may eventually contribute to a TMJ problem, often years later.

Bruxism is a non-functional clenching or grinding of the teeth. Some people brux during waking hours, but bruxing is generally carried out subconsciously while asleep. Although bruxing while asleep is extremely common and can lead to enamel wear, pathological bruxing can lead to significant TMJ damage over time especially when the dentition is less than optimal in the first place. Dentists can fabricate a variety of splints which the patient generally wears at night and help in either alleviating the symptoms of TMJ dysfunction or in the retraining of the facial musculature.

DENTAL NOMENCLATURE

The international numbering system of teeth (Fédération Dentaire Internationale—FDI) should be used in any written or verbal communication. The mouth can be divided into four quadrants. In the adult dentition (Figure 40.1) the maxillary right is quadrant 1; the maxillary left, quadrant 2; the mandibular left, quadrant 3; and the mandibular right, quadrant 4. The individual teeth are numbered from the central incisor outwards to the third molar. This provides an easy-to-use two-digit code to indicate the tooth or region of concern. Deciduous or baby teeth follow a similar pattern. The maxillary right is quadrant 5; the maxillary left, quadrant 6; the mandibular left, quadrant 7; and the mandibular right, quadrant 8. The complete deciduous dentition has only five teeth in each quadrant, as opposed to eight teeth in each quadrant in the adult dentition.

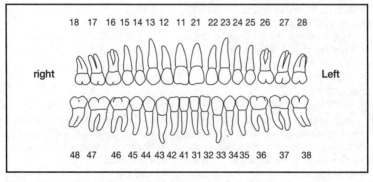

Figure 40.1 The international numbering system for adult dentition

REFERENCES

1. Therapeutic guideline: antibiotics. 11th edn. Melbourne: Therapeutic Guidelines; 2003. Also online. Available: http://www.tg.com.au.
2. Online. Available: http://www.ukmi.nhs.uk/med_info/documents/Dental_Patient_on_Warfarin.pdf; http://www.ukmi.nhs.uk/med_info/documents/Dental_Patient_on_Antiplatelet_Medication.pdf

Copies of information sheets referred to in this chapter are available from pfoltyn@stvincents.com.au.

Psychiatric presentations

Beaver Hudson and Neil Ballard

MANAGEMENT OF PSYCHIATRIC PATIENTS
(Beaver Hudson)

This chapter is not intended to replace a comprehensive psychiatric assessment; rather it is to help you in the effective and efficient gathering of relevant information, which will enable an appropriate psychiatric referral/consultation to be made and assist in the development of an immediate/interim management strategy.

Mental health type presentations can be many and varied. The most common of these are:

• Self-harm with suicidal intent.
• Self-harm without suicidal intent.
• Suicidal thinking.
• Aggressive or threatening behaviour.
• Depressed and withdrawn behaviour.
• Bizarre behaviour.
• Anxiety.
• Psychosis.
• Combinations of the above.

Before the assessment takes place, issues of safety must be taken into consideration. Physical environments must be assessed for potential hazards to either patient or clinician. Assessment rooms specifically set up for this kind of examination are highly recommended.

If a friend or relative has accompanied the patient, this may help or hinder the assessment process. The best suggestion is that the patient be asked, in private, if they would prefer to have the friend or relative present during the assessment process. Many people in psychosocial distress will feel more willing to share personal information when given this option.

Before any intervention, an assessment of the current physical and mental state will need to be performed. Psychiatric assessment must include investigation of physical cause. In the first instance, it is critical to rule out an organic cause for the presenting problem. Medical and psychiatric practitioners are less likely to medically examine a patient meticulously when the presenting symptoms fit into a well-defined psychiatric syndrome or the patient is known to have an established psychiatric diagnosis.

There are many medical conditions that can superficially give the appearance of mental illness. Should any of the symptoms below be evident, a medical assessment must take precedence:

- Pyrexia.
- Impaired, clouded or depressed levels of consciousness.
- Recent and abrupt onset of confusion, disorientation and impaired memory.
- Visual and tactile hallucinations.
- Periods of complete inactivity during which time there is a loss of awareness of surroundings for short periods.
- Known to be a diabetic.
- 24-hour history of seizure, head injury or history of recent head injury.

Use of a Mini Mental State Examination (see Figure 34.4, p 384) will identify cognitive deficits or a possible delirium. This will also help you decide whether the patient is too sedated, sleepy or disorientated to provide a valid history.

In the emergency department the following questions will help you to rapidly assess psychosocial distress for potential mental health problems, establish the degree of urgency for psychiatric referral and identify any need for safety and/or security measures to be instituted.

1. **First establish the nature of the problem.** Is it:
   - Suicidal ideation?*
   - Anxiety/panic?
   - Depression?
   - Thought disordered?
   - Bizarre behaviour?
   - Hallucinating?*
   - Aggression?*
   - Stress?
   - Alcohol or other drug withdrawal?
   - Delusional?
   - Agitation?*
2. **Establish why this problem requires attention now:**
   - Self-referral.

These problems may require immediate action to prevent the patient from self-discharging or failing to wait for a thorough psychiatric assessment.

- General practitioner referral.
- Police referral.
- Concern from others.
- Deliberate self-harm.
- Uncommunicative patient.
- Personal crisis.
- Involuntary—mental health legislation.

The triage sister should prioritise these patients using the mental health triage system (Table 41.1).

History

To give meaning to any mental health presentation it must be understood in a context: why here and why now? Preliminary information gathering can significantly expedite the assessment process. In some instances there may well be a 'management plan' for such occasions, which might be found in the patient's file. Early enquiries and review of previous presentations or an existing mental health record can reveal important and valuable information regarding the involvement of other healthcare providers or provide an established working diagnosis. If there is a working diagnosis, take note of any current medications.

Corroborative history from others is especially valuable, but you will need to seek the patient's consent if not under a mental health act.

People/places to approach

- Family, friends or significant others.
- General practitioner.
- Community health centre.
- Voluntary or non-government agencies.
- Case managers, psychiatrists, counsellors and psychologists.
- In the waiting room (enquire about children, and where they are now).

What does the patient want?

Most patients who present in distress will have an idea of what they feel they need or want. Determine what this might be at the outset. Once again, this will further assist you in getting to the core of the problem and possible solution quickly. It will be helpful to Psychiatry if you are able to tell them what the patient wants. Is it:

- Medication?
- Accommodation?
- Someone to talk to?
- Psychiatric treatment as an inpatient or an outpatient?
- Detoxification from alcohol or other drugs?
- They have no idea?

Now would be a good time to start compiling a problem list.

Table 41.1 Mental Health Triage Scale (From: South-eastern Sydney Area Health Service: Mental Health Triage Guidelines for Emergency Departments)

Triage code	Description	Treatment acuity	Typical presentation	General principles of management
1	Definite danger to life (self or others)	Immediate	**OBSERVED** • Violent behaviour • Possession of weapon • Self-destructive behaviour in emergency department	**SUPERVISION** • Continuous visual surveillance* **ACTION** • Provide safe environment for patient and others • Ensure adequate personnel to provide restraint/detention **Consider** • 1:1 observation • Alert mental health team • Consult mental health specialist
2	Probable risk of danger to self or others Severe behavioural disturbance	Emergency Within 10 min	**OBSERVED** • Extreme agitation/restlessness • Physically/verbally aggressive • Confused/unable to cooperate • Requires restraint **REPORTED** • Attempt at self-harm/threat of self-harm • Threat of harm to others	**SUPERVISION** • Continuous visual surveillance* **ACTION** • Provide safe environment for patient and others • Ensure adequate personnel to provide restraint/detention **Consider** • 1:1 observation • Alert mental health team • Consult mental health specialist

Continued p 454

Table 41.1 (continued)

Triage code	Description	Treatment acuity	Typical presentation	General principles of management
3	Possible danger to self or others Moderate behaviour disturbance Severe distress	Urgent Within 30 min	**OBSERVED** • Agitation/restlessness • Intrusive behaviour • Bizarre/disorganised behaviour • Confusion • Withdrawn and uncommunicative • Ambivalance about treatment **REPORTED** • Suicidal ideation Presence of psychotic symptoms: • Hallucinations • Delusions • Paranoid ideas • Thought disorder • Bizarre/agitated behaviour Presence of affective disturbance: • Severe symptoms of depression/anxiety • Elevated or irritable mood	**SUPERVISION** • Close observation* **ACTION** Consider • Consult mental health specialist • Re-triage if evidence of increasing behavioural disturbance: – restlessness – intrusiveness – agitation – aggressiveness – increasing distress
4	Moderate distress	Semi-urgent Within 60 min	**OBSERVED** • No agitation/restlessness • Irritability without aggression • Cooperative • Gives coherent history	**SUPERVISION** • Intermittent observation* **ACTION** Consider • Re-triage if evidence of increasing behavioural disturbance

Continued p 455

Table 41.1 (continued)

Triage code	Description	Treatment acuity	Typical presentation	General principles of management
4 (cont.)			**REPORTED** • Symptoms of anxiety or depression without suicidal ideation	– restlessness – intrusiveness – agitation – aggressiveness – increasing distress
5	No danger to self or others No acute distress No behavioural disturbance	Non-urgent Within 120 min	**OBSERVED** • Cooperative • Communicative • Compliant with instructions **REPORTED** • Known patient with chronic psychotic symptoms • Known patient with chronic unexplained somatic complaints • Request for medication • Minor adverse effect of medication • Financial/social/accommodation/relationship problems	**SUPERVISION** • General observation* **ACTION** Consider • Referral to mental health specialist/social worker • Mobilise or establish support network—community team/LMO/family

FACTORS TO CONSIDER

Consideration should be given to assigning a *higher* triage category where the following factors apply:

- Unaccompanied by a responsible adult
- Brought in by police under Section 24 of Mental Health Act
- Age: under 18 or over 65
- Concurrent physical conditions
- Recent history of self-harm
- Recent history of aggression or violence
- Past history of absconding
- Concurrent drug and/or alcohol intoxication
- Adult accompanied by baby/young child

Establish the degree of urgency

This will depend on:

- The immediate needs of the patient.
- Whether the patient requires psychiatric consultation immediately.
- Whether the information you have is accurate and sufficient to refer to psychiatry.
- Whether the patient can be discharged safely.
- Who will follow up the patient and how.

Good follow-up is essential for ongoing care: it may be necessary for you to notify other health care providers right away; can you fax/message them?

THE INTERVIEW

Ensure risk to yourself or others is minimised. Tell others where you will be and who you are with. If you are interviewing in a single-exit room, don't place yourself between the door and the patient. Consider whether the patient is safe to be left alone or requires observation. If there is a 'personal duress system', make sure you know how to activate it.

It is important to maintain a professional but empathetic attitude in your attempt to develop a rapport with the patient. Questions should be conversational, yet direct. Asking about suicidal thoughts or plans will often elicit a sense of relief from the person who has been thinking about such acts.

Risk of self-harm

Some of the questions that will determine risk of harm to self are:

- Have you been thinking life is not worth living?
- Have you thought about harming yourself?
- Are you thinking of killing yourself?
- Have you thought about how you would do it?
- Have you already done anything to harm yourself?
- Have you tried to harm yourself before?
- How many times have you tried before?
- When was the most recent time?

Other relevant questions are:

- How often are you getting these thoughts?
- Do you have the means of taking your life and are they easily accessible?
- When would you intend to take your life?
- Is there anything that would stop you from taking your own life?
- Do you know anyone who has died by suicide?
- Do you have access to a firearm or other weapon? *Note:* If you suspect the patient to be in possession of any weapon(s) the interview should be terminated and security called immediately!

Suicide attempt

If a suicide attempt has already be made:

- Does the patient still have access to the method used?
- Did the patient use alcohol or other drugs before the attempt?

Degree of risk to patient

Some factors to be aware of when determining the increased degree of risk are:

- Definite plan.
- Hopelessness.
- Severe depression.
- Psychotic symptoms (command hallucinations).
- Recent discharge from a psychiatric facility.
- Use of alcohol and/or other drugs (especially if recent escalation in use).
- Recent suicide attempt.
- Single men who are young, elderly or homeless.
- Medical illness.
- History of sexual/physical abuse.
- Recent suicide of friend or family member.
- Temporary effects of alcohol and or other drugs.

Degree of risk to others

Questions to determine the degree of risk to others:

- Have you been thinking of hurting anyone else?
- Have you ever acted on these thoughts?
- Have you been involved in any fights recently?
- Were you using alcohol or other drugs at that time?
- Were you ever assaulted as a child or adult?
- Have the police ever charged you with assault?

Predictors of violence

These may include:

- History of violence.
- History of impulsivity.
- Alcohol and other drug use.
- Violent father.
- Criminal charges for violence.
- Antisocial behaviour.

Psychotic symptoms

Some questions to elicit psychotic symptoms are:

- Do you feel safe at the moment? (This question may elicit paranoid thoughts.)
- Do you hear a voice(s) that others do not hear? (Auditory hallucinations)
- Does this voice(s) tell you what you must do? (Command hallucinations)

- Has your relationship to religion changed recently? (Religious delusions)
- What are your energy levels like? (Psychomotor excitation/retardation)
- Do you feel you or your thoughts are being controlled? (Ideas of passivity)
- Do you receive communications from the TV, radio etc? (Ideas of reference)

If the responses are garbled or illogical, it is likely the patient is experiencing thought disorder. It is important try to keep the patient on the subject if possible and give time for him/her to respond to questions. This may also uncover possible thought blocking—another form of thought disorder.

Summary: key points

- Consider physical safety: first your own, then that of your patient and of others!
- Is there a physical explanation for the behaviour?
- Preliminary information gathering and corroborative history is essential.
- Will the patient be safe if left alone?
- Most patients will have an idea of what they feel they need or want.
- Conduct a Mental State Examination.
- Questions should be conversational, yet direct.
- The patient who has been having suicidal thoughts or plans will often have a sense of relief when asked directly.
- If you suspect the patient to be in possession of any weapon(s), the interview should be terminated and security called immediately!

THE VIOLENT PATIENT (Neil Ballard)

There are many causes of aggressive behaviour, varying from psychosis and antisocial/borderline personality traits to organic causes such as head injury, delirium and a post-ictal state. Other common causes include drug or alcohol intoxication, and anxiety. There are also concerns that are particularly relevant to the emergency environment, such as the stress resulting from grief or helplessness that may be experienced by family members/friends of patients. Stress may also be due to concern that patients and others seem not to merit appropriate consideration by staff who are dealing with several issues at once.

Violence is usually prefaced by warning signs of aggressive or frustrated behaviour. The subject may be loud and threatening, or may become withdrawn. He/she may report violent thoughts/urges or hallucinations/delusions with violent content.

Interviewing the violent patient

The potentially violent or violent patient needs to be interviewed in a manner that minimises the chances of escalation, while maintaining your safety and that of the patient. This is best done in an environment with at least two exits (one for the clinician and one for the patient) that can be observed by other staff (this may need to be done discreetly out of respect for the patient's privacy).

The presence of potential dangers should be considered and appropriate steps taken. Furniture should be too heavy to throw and anything that could be used as a weapon (e.g. IV poles) should be removed. Also consider removing ties, necklaces, stethoscopes, pens etc from your person. If available, a duress alarm may prove invaluable.

Security personnel should be alerted and present nearby, especially if the patient has committed an act of violence before arriving in the emergency department.

Consider that the patient may have a concealed weapon—a search of their person or belongings may be appropriate. This is a potentially difficult step that may be made easier by having it clearly signposted as departmental policy that a safe working environment is a right of the staff and that a condition of entry is that searches may be instituted.

History, assessment and treatment

The aim of initial contact is to defuse the situation, but this will often depend on elucidating and treating the underlying cause, so history taking, assessment of mental state, and looking for other diagnostic clues should proceed simultaneously. Your approach should be empathetic and non-confrontational—avoid making the patient feel threatened either verbally (e.g. by using ultimatums) or physically (e.g. by standing over a seated patient or blocking their exit).

Get as much information as possible before approaching the patient (e.g. medical records, family, other involved clinicians), always bearing in mind the possibility that a delay may exacerbate the situation. From these sources and from the patient, establish what the current concerns and precipitants are. Are there specific threats? A history of violence is the best predictor of future violence. Other relevant history includes that of substance abuse, impulsive or reckless behaviour in the past, and details of previous medical or psychiatric conditions. An understanding of the patient's social circumstances and supports is vital.

As is the case with many presentations in emergency medicine, assessment may need to proceed concurrently with treatment. Indeed thorough history taking, mental state and physical examination may need to be deferred until the acute situation is under control.

On mental state examination you should look for evidence of intoxication from drugs or alcohol, confusion (which may suggest the presence of delirium), psychosis (is the patient reporting or responding to hallucinations or delusions?), or mania (pressured speech, grandiose ideas, elevated mood). A thorough physical examination should be performed when it is safe to do so, focusing particularly on vital signs (pulse rate, blood pressure, temperature, pulse oximetry and blood sugar level), nervous system examination as well as looking for signs of drug or alcohol abuse, and evidence of other conditions that may cause behavioural change (e.g. head injury, febrile illness, metabolic disturbance).

There are no routine investigations for the violent patient. Choice of investigations should be guided by information obtained during history taking and physical examination, and may include basic blood tests, drug levels, urinalysis, and appropriate imaging (e.g. computed tomography of the head).

Controlling aggression

There are a number of different ways of controlling aggression, ranging from verbal de-escalation to pharmacological and/or physical restraint. Often a number of strategies will need to be employed. The underlying cause, especially if it is organic in nature, needs to be identified and treated.

Verbal de-escalation

Verbal de-escalation and distraction is almost invariably the initial means of approaching the aggressive patient. This needs to be done in a non-judgemental and non-confrontational manner. Allow the patient to talk about her/his concerns while stating your desire to sort things out in the manner most appropriate for everyone. Although there is often a role for the setting of limits of acceptable behaviour, issuing ultimatums will frequently result in escalation of the situation. Avoid getting drawn into long-term grievances or issues beyond your control.

Simple courtesies, such as offering something to eat or drink (this should be avoided if sedation is possible) or somewhere to sit, may assist you in establishing a rapport with the patient, which is vital to successful resolution of the situation. If appropriate, try to get the patient to accept help such as psychiatric assessment, or to voluntarily take oral sedative/antipsychotic medication.

'Show of force'

Should this approach fail a 'show of force' may be necessary. This is where an obvious presence of security/police officers backs up the clinician, with the aim of convincing the patient that further escalation is unwise and in the hope that the patient will then agree or take medication. One person (usually the clinician involved) should lead the staff and interact with the patient. A fallback plan should always be in place at this stage: if the violence/aggression appears due to a medical or psychiatric condition and physical/pharmacological restraint is legally justifiable, it should be the next step; if not, the patient/subject should be escorted from the department by security or police.

Physical restraint

Physical restraint should be used in an emergency situation only in the treatment of a delirious or psychiatrically unwell patient. In these cases, it must be done in a manner aimed at minimising the chance of injury to patient or staff, and should always be followed by pharmacological sedation. There must be sufficient staff with well-defined roles. Usually seven staff are required: one to immobilise each limb, one for the head and neck, one to administer medication, and a runner/scribe. One person should be in charge, will nominate when immobilisation will take place (it will often have to immediately follow a failed negotiation or 'show of force'), and will be responsible for talking to the patient. Throughout, extreme care must be taken to avoid injury to staff (e.g. punching, biting, spitting by patient) or patient (e.g. asphyxia, broken limbs during restraint).

Sedation

If physical restraint is required, sedation will have to be by parenteral route. Beware of needlestick injury. Intravenous injection is preferred because of quicker onset of action; the best choice here is diazepam. An initial dose of 10 mg should be given, with further increments of 2.5–5 mg every 3–5 minutes. Beware of using too small a dose initially, as it is important to achieve sedation rapidly.

If intravenous access is not available, midazolam is the benzodiazepine of choice for intramuscular sedation, as it is more reliably absorbed via this route than diazepam. The initial dose should be 10 mg which can be repeated at 15–20 minutes, and intravenous access should be gained as soon as possible.

The major side effect of benzodiazepine is respiratory depression, so the sedated patient should be closely observed, given supplemental oxygen, and have pulse oximetry, +/− non-invasive blood pressure (NIBP) and ECG monitoring in place. If possible, the patient should be nursed in the left lateral position.

If control is not achieved with repeated benzodiazepine doses (reasonable limits are 60 mg diazepam IV or 20 mg midazolam IM per sedation event), an antipsychotic should be added. Haloperidol or droperidol may be given IM or IV in 5–10 mg increments (up to 20 mg over 24 hours). These agents may lead to dystonic reactions (which may be treated with benztropine 2 mg IV/IM), hypotension, and QT prolongation, so the patient must be closely observed and monitored. Antipsychotics should be avoided in the elderly if possible, and smaller doses of benzodiazepines used.

Occasionally parenteral sedation will be used in a situation where the patient agrees to take medication; usually oral medication will be used in this case. The first-choice agent would be oral diazepam, 10–20 mg, with olanzapine, 10–30 mg, an alternative for the clearly psychotic patient. Be aware that the desired effect may take 20–30 minutes. Once sedated, the patient again needs to be closely observed and monitored, and may require supplemental oxygen.

Documentation should clearly explain the reasons that sedation and/or restraint were required, and the doses, routes of administration and timing of any medications used. At the earliest possible time fill out the legal forms (schedules).

RECOMMENDED READING

Centre for Mental Health. Mental health for emergency departments—a reference guide (amended May 2002). Sydney: NSW Health Department; 2002.

Slaby AE. Handbook of psychiatric emergencies. 4th edn. Norwalk, CT: Appleton & Lange; 1994.

Treatment Protocol Project. Management of mental disorders. 2nd edn. Sydney: World Health Organization Collaborating Centre for Mental Health and Substance Abuse; 1997.

42 Dermatological emergencies

Frank Isaacs

Emergencies in dermatology mainly arise from:

1. Extensive acute skin disease causing disruption of normal skin function, e.g. toxic epidermal necrolysis, pustular psoriasis.
2. Dermatological manifestations of severe systemic disease, e.g. meningococcaemia.

The skin's most important functions are:

1. Prevention of body fluid and electrolyte loss to environment.
2. Temperature regulation.
3. Prevention of infection.

In most dermatological emergencies, monitoring the above parameters is thus essential to correct management.

ERYTHRODERMA

For acute and chronic forms of erythroderma, or generalised exfoliative dermatitis, see Figure 42.1.

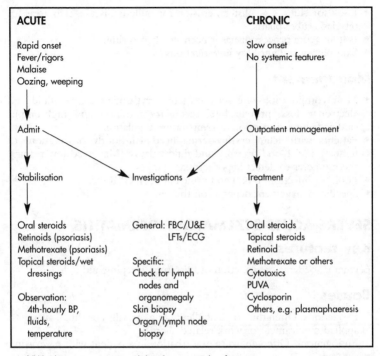

ACUTE		CHRONIC
Rapid onset Fever/rigors Malaise Oozing, weeping		Slow onset No systemic features
↓		↓
Admit		Outpatient management
↓		↓
Stabilisation	→ Investigations ←	Treatment
↓		↓

Oral steroids
Retinoids (psoriasis)
Methotrexate (psoriasis)
Topical steroids/wet
   dressings
 	
Observation:
   4th-hourly BP,
   fluids,
   temperature
	General: FBC/U&E
	         LFTs/ECG
	
	Specific:
	Check for lymph
	   nodes and
	   organomegaly
	Skin biopsy
	Organ/lymph node
	   biopsy
		Oral steroids
		Topical steroids
		Retinoid
		Methotrexate or others
		Cytotoxics
		PUVA
		Cyclosporin
		Others, e.g. plasmaphaeresis

FBC full blood count   U&E urea and electrolytes   LFTs liver function tests
PUVA psoralen ultraviolet A therapy   BP blood pressure

Figure 42.1   Erythroderma (generalised exfoliative dermatitis)

Key features

Generalised erythema and scaling of skin (red man). This is a general term for inflammation of the entire skin.

Causes

These include eczema • psoriasis • drug eruptions • pemphigus • pityriasis rubra pilaris • sarcoid • lymphoma/leukaemia • idiopathic • graft-versus-host disease • others. The condition may be acute or chronic. Acute forms need admission to hospital.

Assessment

- History of recent medication ingestion.
- Past history of skin or other systemic disease.

- Look for clues, e.g. blisters/erosion for bullous disease, skip areas for pityriasis rubra pilaris.
- Is it an acute process or has it been slowly evolving?
- Skin biopsy and ancillary investigations.

Management

- Most complications are seen in acute erythrodermas, i.e. fluid and electrolyte loss, protein loss, secondary infection and high-output cardiac failure, disruption of temperature regulation.
- Patients with acute erythroderma need 4th-hourly observations of temperature, blood pressure and fluid balance. May need low-reading thermometer to detect hypothermia.
- Look for infection: blood and urine cultures, CXR etc.
- Specific management depends on the cause.

SEVERE ACUTE ECZEMATOUS DERMATITIS

Key features

Erythema, oedema, vesiculation or blistering, weeping and itch.

Causes

1. Exogenous. Often due to plant allergy (e.g. grevillea or rhus), allergy to applied medicament or work-related allergen.
2. Endogenous. Often an acute exacerbation in a patient with preexisting eczema.

Assessment

Exogenous

- History of contact with allergen.
- Rash localised to area of contact.
- Linear or unusually shaped lesions.
- Patch testing can be done once the rash has settled in order to confirm contact allergy.

Endogenous

- Preexisting atopic diathesis/eczema.
- No history of contact with allergen.
- Involves areas normally affected by endogenous eczema, e.g. cubital fossa.

Note that it is not uncommon for a patient with dermatitis to be misdiagnosed as cellulitis. Swelling and erythema is common to both. Infection is usually accompanied by fever, pain and lymphadenopathy. Dermatitis is accompanied by itch.

Management

See Figure 42.2.

- The acute weeping/oozing stage is best treated with cool wet dressings until the weeping ceases. Solutions commonly used for wet dressings include saline, Condy's solution (a few crystals in bowl of water to make a light pink-coloured solution), Burrow's solution (diluted by 1 part in 20 parts of water) and chlorhexidine solution (1:50).
- Follow with application of corticosteroid creams as weeping decreases.
- Once weeping/oozing has ceased the corticosteroid creams can be continued without wet dressings.
- Oral corticosteroids are indicated in severe cases, especially if exogenous in aetiology.
- Look for secondary infection: bacterial • herpes simplex • fungal. Treat accordingly.

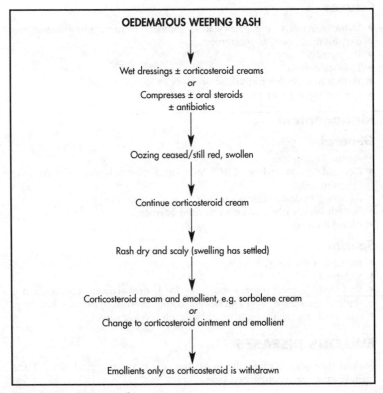

OEDEMATOUS WEEPING RASH

↓

Wet dressings ± corticosteroid creams
or
Compresses ± oral steroids
± antibiotics

↓

Oozing ceased/still red, swollen

↓

Continue corticosteroid cream

↓

Rash dry and scaly (swelling has settled)

↓

Corticosteroid cream and emollient, e.g. sorbolene cream
or
Change to corticosteroid ointment and emollient

↓

Emollients only as corticosteroid is withdrawn

Figure 42.2 Treatment of acute eczema

GENERALISED PUSTULAR PSORIASIS

Key features

Sterile pustular lesions of varying extent, fever and prostration if severe. In pregnancy this is known as impetigo herpetiformis.

Pustules in psoriasis may be seen in the following circumstances:

1. As a localised eruption on palms and/or soles—not associated with risk of generalisation.
2. Within the more usual scaly plaques—may generalise with injudicious treatment.
3. Generalised pustular psoriasis
   - Waves of small pustules.
   - Fever, malaise, toxicity, prostration.
   - Significant mortality.

Causes

- Drug reactions, e.g. salicylates, iodine, lithium, phenylbutazone, oxyphenbutazone, progesterone.
- Pregnancy.
- Hypocalcaemia.
- Withdrawal of systemic corticosteroids.
- Irritant topical therapy, e.g. tar, dithranol.

Management

General

- Admit to hospital.
- General investigation, FBC, urea and electrolytes, calcium/liver function tests.
- General physical examination.
- Fourth-hourly observations and fluid balance.
- Blood cultures.

Specific

- Bland wet dressings.
- Sedatives.
- Very mild topical application, e.g. 1% hydrocortisone cream. If not settling or severe fever/metabolic complications, systemic therapy is indicated, e.g. acitretin, systemic steroids, cyclosporin.

BULLOUS DISEASES

Bullous diseases are often the most dramatic dermatological cases. Their main features are summarised below.

Neonatal/childhood

Epidermolysis bullosa

- A genetically inherited group of mechano-bullous diseases due to defective attachment of epidermis, resulting in easy separation of part or whole epidermis.
- Often fatal. Various patterns of inheritance. Needs urgent referral. Presents as blisters/erosions, often at birth.

Incontinentia pigmenti

- X-linked dominant.
- Males are more severely affected (usually incompatible with life) than females.
- Self-limiting blisters at or soon after birth. Associated with other malformations, e.g. brain, eye, bone, teeth.

Staphylococcal scalded skin syndrome (SSSS)

Due to a toxin elaborated by *Staphylococcus aureus*. Circulation of this toxin causes a generalised erythema of the skin, followed by peeling in sheets. Superficial loss of stratum corneum. Has low mortality with appropriate treatment. Treatment is with antibiotics (usually flucloxacillin) and attention to fluid and electrolyte balance.

Bullous impetigo

Localised bullae due to the same toxin as SSSS. Treatment is with flucloxacillin (orally) and mupirocin (topically).

Chronic bullous dermatosis of childhood

Bullae often around lower trunk and pelvic region but tend to become generalised. Associated with IgA deposition at dermo-epidermal junction. Responds to dapsone.

Adult/childhood

Erythema multiforme minor/major (Stevens-Johnson syndrome)

Key features

Erythema multiforme minor usually involves the extremities and is more common on extensor surfaces. Erythema multiforme major includes the above but is often more extensive and there is prominent mucous membrane involvement (especially ocular) and fever. Upper airway involvement and pneumonia may occur. Renal changes have been described. Mortality rates of 3–19% reported.

As the name suggests the morphology of the lesions in this disease may be quite variable and includes:

- Macules, papules and urticarial lesions.

- Plaques with purpuric centres and red rims (target lesions).
- Plaques which become vesicular or bullous.
- Erosions on mucous membranes.

Causes
- Infections, especially viruses (herpes simplex most common), *Mycoplasma*.
- Drugs.
- Others, e.g. neoplasms, vaccinations, X-ray therapy.
- Idiopathic.

Assessment
- Clinical.
- Skin biopsy.

Treatment
- If possible, identify and eliminate cause.
- Topical steroids on non-eroded lesions.
- Silver sulfadiazine (SSD) cream (or similar) on eroded lesions.
- Antiseptic/anaesthetic applications/washes for mucous membranes.
- Antibiotics/eye consultation for ocular involvement.
- Antihistamines for itch and sedation.
- May need hospitalisation if severe.
- Systemic antibiotics often given.
- Other systemic medications that may be considered for severe cases include corticosteroids, cyclosporin and intravenous immunoglobulin. These medications are likely to be of most help if used early in the disease.

Toxic epidermal necrolysis

Key features
Severe disease is characterised by generalised erythema and swelling of skin, followed by separation and lifting off of full-thickness epidermis. Mucous membrane involvement may be severe. The disease is associated with severe pain, fever and often other organ involvement, e.g. gastrointestinal and respiratory tracts, liver and kidney.

Causes
- Largely as for erythema multiforme.
- Drugs are the most common cause, especially sulfonamides, anticonvulsants, NSAIDs.

Assessment
- Clinical picture and skin biopsy to confirm diagnosis.
- History of infection or drug ingestion.
- Extent of involvement.
- Check for infection, fluid and electrolyte problems.

Treatment

- Admission to hospital (usually to ICU or burns unit) for supportive care until skin re-epithelialises.
- High doses of corticosteroids are usually given.
- Other systemic agents that have been used with success include cyclophosphamide, cyclosporin and intravenous IgG.

Prognosis

- Mortality approaches 25%—mainly from infection.
- High incidence of scarring, especially mucosal surfaces.

Pemphigus

Key features

A blistering disease, usually involving skin and mucous membranes. The blisters are thin-walled and often present as erosions on inflamed or non-inflamed skin. There is little tendency for lesions to heal, and thus patients develop widespread loss of epidermis. It usually occurs during the fourth and fifth decades of life. Mortality is high when the disease is untreated and significant even with treatment. The condition can be drug-induced.

Causes

This is an autoimmune disease characterised by attachment of immunoglobulin to the epidermal intercellular adhesion molecules.

- Idiopathic.
- Drug-induced—captopril • penicillamine • gold salts (exacerbation) • rifampicin.
- Paraneoplastic—severe mucosal involvement and polymorphic cutaneous lesions.
- Endemic (Brazil).

Assessment

- Mucosal erosions are the most common presenting feature.
- Presence of cutaneous blisters.
- Skin biopsy for histology and immunofluorescence.
- Blood for circulating intercellular cement antibodies.

Treatment

- Extensive, progressive disease often needs hospitalisation.
- Corticosteroids (often 100 mg/d prednisolone or higher) or IV pulse therapy.
- Immunosuppressives used in addition to oral corticosteroids include azathioprine, cyclophosphamide, cyclosporin.
- Other treatments include plasmaphaeresis, intravenous IgG, dapsone, gold.
- Infection is a common complication.

Prognosis
Mortality of 5–15%.

Bullous pemphigoid

Key features
A blistering disorder characterised by erythematous oedematous plaques, which then develop tense blisters. It is usually generalised and occurs mainly during the seventh decade. Variants include:

- Localised pemphigoid.
- Herpes gestationis (pemphigoid of pregnancy).
- Cicatricial pemphigoid (mainly mucous membranes).
- Pemphigoid nodularis.

Causes
- Idiopathic autoimmune disorder characterised by circulating antibodies to the basement membrane zone. Antigens are the hemidesmosome-associated antigens BP230 and BP180.
- Occasionally drug-induced—frusemide • nalidixic acid • psoralens • sulphasalazine • captopril • penicillamine.

Assessment
- Itchy eruption with urticarial plaques and blisters.
- Occasional mucosal involvement.
- Biopsy shows subepidermal blister and immunofluorescence shows IgG and/or C3 along the epidermal basement membrane.
- Blood shows circulating antibasement membrane antibodies in 75% of cases.

Management
- Admission to hospital is usually not needed.
- Oral steroids (medium dose—30 mg/day prednisolone is usually sufficient).
- Other drugs that may be of use include minocycline, nicotinamide and immunosuppressives such as azathioprine, cyclosporin, cyclophosphamide.

Prognosis
- Usually remits in 3–6 years.
- Can be fatal, especially in the infirm.

Dermatitis herpetiformis

- A chronic disorder characterised by intensely itchy vesicles/blisters mainly on extensor surfaces, and associated with gluten-sensitive enteropathy.
- It responds best to dapsone and gluten exclusion.
- Biopsy of skin shows subepidermal blister and IgA deposition in the dermal papillae.

Fixed drug eruption

- A drug reaction characterised by single or multiple oedematous plaques that often blister.
- It often heals with post-inflammatory hyperpigmentation.
- Genital lesions are common.
- The most common offending drugs are—tetracycline • sulfonamides • phenolphthalein • pyrazalone derivatives, e.g. phenylbutazone • barbiturates.

Urticaria/angio-oedema

Key features

See Figure 42.3.

- Intensely itchy.

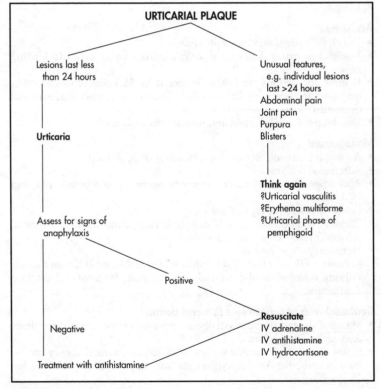

Figure 42.3 Urticaria

- Plaques with pale centres and red rim having a circular, serpiginous or polycyclic shape.
- Individual lesions come and go rapidly (in less than 24 hours).
- More diffuse swellings are known as angio-oedema.

Causes

Some common causes include:

- Foods—shellfish, nuts, chocolate, artificial colours, preservatives, naturally occurring salicylates.
- Drugs:
  - Histamine releasers—opiates, polymyxin, radiocontrast, curare.
  - Allergic reactions to drugs—usually IgE-mediated.
  - Agents altering arachidonic acid metabolism, e.g. salicylates, non-steroidal anti-inflammatory drugs (NSAIDs).
- May be seen in a large variety of other disease states, e.g. after infections, tumour-associated, thyrotoxicosis, autoimmune disorders.
- Idiopathic.

Assessment

- Check for early stages of anaphylaxis.
- Evanescent nature helps to distinguish from other urticarial-looking rashes.
- If individual lesions are lasting longer than 24 hours, consider other diagnoses including erythema multiforme, urticarial vasculitis, urticarial dermatitis.
- Skin biopsy for H&E stain and immunofluorescence.

Management

- Avoid precipitating factors, e.g. offending drug or food.
- Adrenaline if severe.
- Antihistamines—maximal doses may be necessary/combination H_1 and H_2 blockade.
- Corticosteroids (rarely necessary).
- Dietary changes to avoid ingested triggering factors (artificial colours/preservatives and salicylates).
- Hereditary angio-oedema:
  - Acute—C1 isoniazid (INH) infusion if available, fresh frozen plasma.
  - Long-term—anabolic steroids to increase level of C1-esterase inhibitor.

Treatment with antihistamines (general points)

- Maximal doses may be needed, e.g. cyproheptadine 4 mg three times daily up to 32 mg/day.
- If not responding, antihistamines of different chemical classes can be used in combination, e.g. cyproheptadine 4 mg tds plus promethazine 25 mg bd.

- Non-sedating antihistamines are often preferred, e.g. loratadine, cetirizine, fexofenadine.
- The addition of a H_2 blocker may be helpful.

INFESTATIONS

Scabies

Caused by *Sarcoptes scabiei* var. *hominis*. Incubation of approximately 4 weeks before itch starts.

Symptoms and signs

- Generalised itch, worse at night (spares head and face).
- Vesicles/burrows mainly on fingers but burrows may be seen on other areas, e.g. hands, wrists, elbows, nipples, axillary margin, genitalia, feet.
- Non-specific, papular, erythematous rash affecting body and limbs but not face/head.

Diagnosis

- Typical symptoms and signs.
- Scraping burrow or vesicle to demonstrate mite under microscope.

Management

- Permethrin applied all over body except face/head. Leave for 12 hours, then wash off. Repeat in 1 week. (Alternatives are 25% benzyl benzoate; 8% precipitated sulfur in white soft paraffin.)
- All contacts need to be treated simultaneously.
- Clothing and bedclothes need to be washed in hot water or dried in a dryer or packed away for 1 week.
- Babies' heads may be affected (use sulfur ointment for babies).
- Norwegian scabies (crusted scabies) is the term for scabies in patients with decreased resistance to infection. These patients are teeming with mites and are highly infectious. Look for hyperkeratotic crusted eruption on the hands in particular.

Complications

- Scabetic nodules—usually in the genital region and buttocks. These are very slow to resolve but do not necessarily indicate persistent active infection in adequately treated patients. They may respond to corticosteroids (topical or intralesional) or topical tar preparations.
- Post-scabetic itch—persistent itch in adequately treated patients. Responds gradually to emollients, e.g. sorbolene cream and mild steroid cream, e.g. betamethasone 0.02% valerate.
- Persistent symptoms may be due to wrong diagnosis, failure of treatment or reinfection. Check method of application of scabecide, length of treatment, treatment of contacts, decontamination of clothing and bedding.

Lice

Head lice

- Usually occur on the occipital scalp. Look for eggs (nits) cemented to hair shafts, as lice are hard to find.
- Itchy.
- Infected excoriations are common.

Treatment

- Kill lice with malathion shampoo. Use with caution in young children and pregnant women because of percutaneous absorption. Or use pyrethrins, e.g. Pyrifoam Shampoo/Lyban Foam.
- Remove nits with a fine-tooth comb (nit comb).
- All contacts should be treated simultaneously.
- Sharing of hats, towels, pillows etc should be avoided.

Pubic lice

- Look in pubic hair for lice (may need magnifying glass) and nits.
- Treatment is as for head lice.
- The lice are often spread by sexual contact, therefore sexual partners need treatment, even if asymptomatic.

VIRAL INFECTIONS

Herpes simplex

Most cases of recurrent herpes simplex are minor in nature.

Emergencies due to herpes simplex are seen in:

1. Primary herpes simplex infection, which may be severe and present as a gingivostomatitis or vulvovaginitis. In both cases hospitalisation may be needed for support (IV fluids/catheterisation), pain relief and acyclovir/famciclovir.
2. Corneal infection.
3. Disseminated herpes simplex infection.

Disseminated herpes simplex infection

This may be seen in:

- Immunocompromised patients.
- Patients with preexisting skin disorders, most commonly eczema (eczema herpeticum).
- Neonatal disseminated herpes simplex, which may be seen as a result of ascending infection in women about to give birth who have active genital infection (usually primary). May need caesarean section to prevent ascending infection.

In all the above situations therapy with acyclovir/famciclovir is usually indicated.

Table 42.1 Common viral infections

	Measles	German measles	Chickenpox
Duration			
Incubation	10–11 days	14–21 days	14 days
Spread	Droplet, via infectious secretions	Droplet, via nasopharynx	Mainly respiratory via droplets
Infective period	Viraemia and pharyngeal shedding ceases by second day of rash.	Greatest at the end of the incubation period and rapidly falls during the 4 days after appearance of the rash.	Infective for 1 to 2 days before the exanthem and for 4 to 5 days after (until the last vesicle has crusted—crusts are non-infectious.
Clinical features			
Prodrome	High fever, cough, coryza, Conjunctivitis. Last 3–4 days. Persist as rash appears.	Rare in young children. Others: low fever, headache, conjunctivitis, sore throat, rhinitis, cough. Disappear as rash appears. Lymphadenopathy, especially cervical (begins 5–7 days before the rash).	Often absent in young children. Others: 2–3 days of fever, headache, anorexia, ± sore throat, dry cough.
Enanthem	Koplik spots appear 24–48 hours before onset of rash.	Forschheimer's sign in up to 20% during prodrome or on first day, dull red macules or petechie on soft palate.	Vesicles common in mouth and other mucous membranes (at same time as rash).
Exanthem	Generalised maculopapular. Head to neck to trunk to extremities. Lasts up to 5–6 days.	Pink macules face to neck, arms, trunk, legs. Last 2–3 days.	Macules to papules to vesicles to crusts. Develop in successive crops for up to 1 week. Mainly trunk and proximal limbs.
Complications	Encephalitis. Purpura (platelets). Bacterial infection • Otitis media • Pneumonia. Subacute sclerosing panencephalitis.	Arthritis. Encephalitis. Purpura (platelets). Peripheral neuritis. Congenital rubella.	Secondary bacterial infection of lesions. Varicella pneumonia (adults). Encephalitis. Systemic dissemination (immunity). Purpura (various causes). Others rare.

Herpes zoster

This usually does not cause major problems, but some patients may develop complications as follows:

- Post-herpetic neuralgia.
- Severe cutaneous involvement with haemorrhage/severe blistering/scarring.
- Dissemination of infection.
- Severe ocular involvement. All patients with facial involvement should be referred to an ophthalmologist for urgent assessment.

Treatment

- Systemic antiviral, e.g. acyclovir (800 mg 5 times per day) or famciclovir (250 mg 3 times per day), if started <72 hours after the onset of the rash.
- Oral steroids (beginning at 60 mg prednisone/day) may decrease the risk of post-herpetic neuralgia in at-risk individuals (usually elderly people with trigeminal nerve involvement) if started early. Check for contraindications.
- Topical therapy is mainly to prevent secondary bacterial infection, dry lesions and relieve symptoms. Calamine lotion is suitable.

BACTERIAL INFECTIONS

Staphylococcus aureus

Common infections are folliculitis, boils, impetigo and wound infections. Other less common infections include ecthyma, cellulitis. Note that impetigo and ecthyma may be due to *Streptococcus pyogenes, S. aureus,* or both.

Management

- Infections are best treated with a penicillinase-resistant penicillin or other antibiotic depending on sensitivities.
- Mupirocin is an effective topical antibiotic that does not cross-react with currently available systemic antibiotics.
- Most cutaneous infections require systemic antibiotics.

Complications

Besides direct infection of the skin, patients may present with toxin- or allergen-mediated reactions to staphylococcal infections. These include:

- Staphylococcal scalded skin syndrome due to epidermolytic exotoxin produced by phage group 2 *S. aureus.* Primarily seen in children.
  Staphylococcal scarlet fever due to staphylococcal erythrogenic toxin.
- Toxic shock syndrome due to toxic shock syndrome toxin-1 (TSST-1) or enterotoxin B. These superantigens can trigger massive inflammatory reactions.
- Staphylococcal toxins can also cause food poisoning.

Streptococcus pyogenes

- Common infections include wound infection, impetigo, cellulitis and erysipelas.
- Less common are ecthyma, necrotising fasciitis.

Management

Treatment of pure *Streptococcus pyogenes* infection is with penicillin V.

Complications

Streptococcus pyogenes may secrete a number or enzymes, toxins and erythrogenic toxins, causing a variety of diseases:

- Scarlet fever due to release of erythrogenic toxin.
- Erythema marginatum rheumaticum (of rheumatic fever).
- Erythema nodosum.
- Various forms of vasculitis, including Henoch-Schönlein purpura.

Table 42.2 Bacterial infections

Infection	Clinical features	Treatment	Organism
Folliculitis	Superficial pustule around hair follicle	Antiseptic cream	*Staphylococcus aureus*
Abscess	Red, nodular and painful	Antibiotic (flucloxacillin) ± drainage	*Staphylococcus aureus*
Carbuncle	Large area of subcutaneous infection draining to surface via multiple sinuses	As above, plus attention to any predisposing illness, e.g. diabetes	*Staphylococcus aureus*
Impetigo	Erosions and crusting (*Streptococcus*) or vesicular/bullous (*Staphylococcus*)	Systemic antibiotics. Bathing off crusts with antiseptic soaks. Topical mupirocin	*Staphylococcus aureus* ± *Streptococcus pyogenes*
Erysipelas	Well-defined area of erythema. Pain, fever and rigors	Penicillin (high dose)	*Streptococcus pyogenes*
Cellulitis	Diffuse erythema and oedema. Less well defined than erysipelas. Lymphangitis	Penicillin (high dose) ± flucloxacillin ± ampicillin	*Streptococcus pyogenes*. Occasionally *Staphylococcus aureus* and gram-negative rod or other organism, especially in immuno-compromised patient

- Streptococcal toxic shock syndrome isolate is usually M Type 1; less common are Types 3, 12, 28. Pyrogenic exotoxin A and/or B.

FEBRILE PATIENT WITH RASH

Faced with a febrile, unwell patient (child or adult) with a rash, +/− mucous membrane involvement, a large number of differential diagnoses have to be considered. These include:

- Drug reactions.
- Exfoliative dermatitis.
- Bullous/erosive diseases.
- Erythema multiforme.
- Toxic epidermal necrolysis.
- Mononucleosis.
- Erythema infectiosum/fifth disease parvovirus B19.
- Rubella.
- Other viral exanthems.
- Kawasaki disease in children: fever, cardiac abnormalities, oropharyngeal lesions, cervical lymphadenopathy, erythema, oedema or desquamation on hands/feet; erythematous rash. Treatment with aspirin/intravenous IgG.
- Staphylococcal scalded skin syndrome.
- Toxic shock syndrome (staphylococcal).
- Streptococcal toxic shock syndrome.
- *Arcanobacterium haemolyticum* infection—pharyngitis +/− membrane formation, cervical lymphadenopathy, morbilliform or scarlatiniform rash in 25% of cases. Treat with erythromycin.
- Severe sunburn.

VASCULITIS

This may be purely cutaneous or have systemic involvement (renal, GIT, musculoskeletal, pulmonary, cardiac etc).

Key features

- Purpura (usually palpable) in acral/dependent areas.
- Necrosis leading to ulceration.
- Nodules.
- Livedo reticularis.
- Pustular purpura.

Causes

These are numerous, but include drug reactions, infections and collagen vascular diseases.

Diagnosis

- Typical clinical appearance.
- Biopsy is usually taken: for H&E stain and immunofluorescence • frozen section for cholesterol embolisation.

Other investigations

- To determine extent of disease.
- To find cause.

Treatment

- If possible, identify and eliminate causes.
- If purely cutaneous vasculitis is localised to the legs, bed rest is often all that is necessary, ± oral corticosteroids if not settling.
- Systemic organ involvement may dictate need for specific therapy.

DRUG REACTIONS TO SYSTEMIC OR TOPICAL MEDICATIONS

Most commonly these are maculopapular or urticarial/angio-oedema, but drug reactions may mimic almost any skin disease.

Other types of drug reactions include: vesiculo-bullous • erythema multiforme • lichenoid • phototoxic • photoallergic • fixed drug reaction • erythroderma • toxic epidermal necrolysis • nail changes/loss • hair increase/loss, texture and colour change • pigmentary changes • mucous membrane disorders • eczematous • psoriatic • vascular reactions/ vasculitis • purpura • acneiform • lupus erythematosis • carcinogenesis • pruritus.

As patients are often receiving many medications it may be very difficult to pick which is to blame. In general, the most recently started drug should be the most suspect.

In substituting drugs, be aware of cross-reactions: e.g. cross-reaction between sulfonamide nucleus-based drugs, including oral hypoglycaemics, phenothiazines and diuretics (thiazides and frusemide).

In critically ill patients where a drug cannot be suspended, it may be possible to continue treatment despite the rash as long as the reaction is not urticarial (risk of anaphylaxis) or of a severe nature, e.g. erythema multiforme/toxic epidermal necrolysis.

HAIR LOSS

Acute hair loss may occasionally be seen and may need urgent treatment/ referral. Causes may include:

- Drugs including cytotoxics.
- Alopecia areata.

- Disruption of hair follicle cycle—telogen and anagen effluvium.
- Breakage of hairs, e.g. too much perm/dyeing, hair-pulling tics.
- Systemic diseases, e.g. systemic lupus erythematosus (SLE)/syphilis.

ACNE

See Table 42.3.

MELANOMA

- 70% are superficial-spreading—surface-spreading lesions usually with irregular shape and variable colour.
- 20% are nodular melanoma—black nodule (may be amelanotic, i.e. reddish or reddish/black).
- 10% are acral-lentiginous—flat lesions in acral areas (may be subungual) or lentigo maligna melanoma—usually on the face of elderly.

Note: Melanoma may be a rapidly evolving tumour and any suspicious lesion should be referred urgently for assessment. The most common sites are: males—back, then leg; females—leg, then back.

Key early features of malignant melanoma

- Growth—usually with a horizontal spreading appearance.
- Irregular shape.
- Variegated colour.

Of these features, growth is the most important. All varieties of melanoma may be amelanotic.

Table 42.3 General treatment of acne

Symptom	Treatment
Comedones (blackheads and whiteheads)	Topical therapy e.g. Benzoyl peroxide Tretinoin/isotretinoin Sulfur lotion Topical antibiotics (clindamycin, erythromycin)
Inflammatory lesions + comedones	Often need systemic antibiotics and topical therapy Hormonal therapies often helpful in women
Cystic acne	Systemic antibiotics ± oral steroids ± intralesional steroids Isotretinoin if response unsatisfactory

TINEA

Tinea may occasionally present in the emergency room as a severe vesicular or even bullous eruption on the feet. This may be associated with a sympathetic, similar vesicular or bullous eruption on the hands ('id reaction'). Treatment is usually with a systemic antifungal and Condy's crystal soaks (diluted to a light pink colour).

RECOMMENDED READING

Rook Arthur, Wilkinson DS, Ebling FJG, Champion Robert. Textbook of dermatology. 6th edn. Oxford, Malden, MA: Blackwell Science; 1998.
Reeves John RT, Mailbach Howard I. Clinical dermatology illustrated: a regional approach. 3rd edn. Philadelphia: FA Davis; 1998.

43 | Infectious diseases

John L Harkness

SEPTICAEMIA

Patients with suspected septicaemia require a minimum of two and a maximum of three blood cultures taken aseptically as soon as possible before institution of antibiotic therapy. Treatment will be guided by the most likely focus of infection. Suggested antibiotics are shown in Table 43.1.

Patients with suspected penicillin allergy require a detailed history to be taken. Frequently evidence of genuine allergy is lacking. If hypersensitivity has occurred previously, cephalosporins may be used with a 5–8% chance of cross-reactivity.

Erythromycin, clindamycin and vancomycin are used for gram-positive infections in patients with documented significant penicillin allergy.

MENINGITIS

A patient with headache, neck stiffness and photophobia must be investigated for meningitis. The usual causes are viruses, *Streptococcus pneumoniae*, *Haemophilus influenzae* or *Neisseria meningitidis*. *Cryptococcus neoformans* is the most common cause of meningitis in patients infected with human immunodeficiency virus (HIV).

Lumbar puncture and blood cultures should be performed urgently. If there is to be any delay before lumbar puncture, a statim dose of 1.8 g

Table 43.1 Suggested antibiotics for use in septicaemia

Likely focus	Antibiotics
No focus apparent	Di(flu)cloxacillin 2 g IV 6-hourly *plus* Gentamicin 4–6 mg/kg IV daily
Urinary tract	Gentamicin 4–6 mg/kg IV as a single daily dose *plus* (Amoxycillin) ampicillin 2 g IV 6-hourly
Gastrointestinal tract	(Amoxycillin) ampicillin 2 g IV 6-hourly *plus* Gentamicin 4–6 mg/kg IV as a single daily dose *plus* Metronidazole 500 mg IV 12-hourly If gentamicin is contraindicated, substitute ceftriaxone 1 g IV daily *or* cefotaxine 1 g IV 8-hourly
Staphylococcal infection	Di(flu)cloxacillin *or* cephalothin 2 g IV 6-hourly
Suspected methicillin-resistant *S. aureus* (MRSA) infection	Vancomycin 1 g IV 12-hourly

benzylpencillin should be given IV: 2 g ceftriaxone may be given to patients allergic to penicillin. Treatment, guided by cerebrospinal fluid (CSF) results, is outlined in Table 43.2.

ACUTE HEPATITIS

Presentation

Clinical expression ranges from a mild anicteric illness to fulminant hepatitis. The main viral causes of hepatitis are not distinguishable clinically.

Symptoms

Fever, malaise, myalgia, nausea, vomiting and pruritus.

Signs

Clinical jaundice, dark urine, hepatomegaly, pain under right costal margin. The presence of maculopapular or urticarial rash, arthralgias and polyarthritis make hepatitis B more likely.

Table 43.2 Treatment of meningitis

Likely organism	Antibiotics
Not known	Cefotaxime 2 g IV 6-hourly *or* Ceftriaxone 2 g IV 12-hourly *plus* Penicillin 1.8 g IV 4-hourly
Pneumococcus	Benzylpenicillin 1.8 g IV 4-hourly Vancomycin 1 g IV 12-hourly if penicillin resistance is suspected or proven
Meningococcus	Benzylpenicillin 1.8 g IV 4-hourly
H. influenzae	Cefotaxime *or* ceftriaxone as above If the organism is susceptible (amoxy)ampicillin 2 g IV 6-hourly Close contacts of a patient with meningococcal or *H. influenzae* meningitis should be treated with rifampicin 600 mg orally once daily for 4 days, *or* ciprofloxacin 500 mg orally as a single dose
Cryptococcus neoformans	Amphotericin B 0.7 mg/kg IV *or* Fluconazole 800 mg orally daily initially Specialist advice should be sought

Aetiological agents

Hepatitis A virus (HAV), hepatitis B virus (HBV), hepatitis C virus (HCV), hepatitis delta agent (HDV), hepatitis E virus (HEV), hepatitis G virus (HGV). Less common causes are cytomegalovirus (CMV), Epstein-Barr virus, rubella virus, herpes simplex virus (HSV), yellow fever virus and enteroviruses.

Epidemiology

Hepatitis A is seen in children and adults and may be acquired locally or during recent travel in developing countries.

Hepatitis B is common among injecting drug users (IDUs), homosexuals and the sexually promiscuous. Hepatitis C was the usual cause of hepatitis following blood transfusion before the introduction of routine screening. Acquisition of hepatitis C now is most commonly found in IDUs, associated with contaminated needles. Hepatitis caused by the delta agent in association with hepatitis B leads to a more severe hepatitis and a greater likelihood of developing chronic hepatitis. Hepatitis G virus may be transmitted via blood transfusion or contaminated intravenous needles. Hepatitis E may be acquired overseas and causes hepatitis that may be fatal in pregnant women.

See also Table 43.3.

Investigations

Liver function tests (LFTs)

Raised transaminases are the usual biochemical abnormalities found in viral hepatitis.

Serology

1. Acute hepatitis A
   a. IgM antibodies to HAV present.
   b. IgG antibodies indicate previous infection with HAV.
2. Acute hepatitis B
   a. Surface antigen (HBsAg) positive.
   b. IgM core antibody (anti-HBc) positive.
3. Presence of anti-HBs or anti-HBc indicates immunity.
4. Hepatitis C is diagnosed by finding specific antibodies present (anti-HCV). Polymerase chain reaction (PCR) for HCV and ribonucleic acid (RNA) to detect HCV in blood may be indicated in some circumstances.
5. A test for delta antigen is available.
6. A test for hepatitis E antibodies is available (anti-HEV).
7. No diagnostic test is yet readily available for hepatitis G.

Infectivity

Hepatitis A

1. By the time symptoms occur, most patients with hepatitis A are excreting very little virus and are relatively non-infectious.
2. Peak infectivity is before symptoms occur.
3. Patients are advised to practise thorough hand washing to prevent faecal-oral spread.
4. Close family members should be given gamma globulin and hepatitis A vaccine. There is no chronic carrier state.

Hepatitis B and hepatitis C

1. Meticulous care must be taken in handling blood and secretions from these patients. All specimens must be treated as an infectious risk.
2. Some 5–10% of patients will become hepatitis B chronic carriers (much higher for hepatitis C).
3. Close contacts (sexual contacts, family members) should be given hyperimmune gamma globulin and hepatitis B vaccine. No vaccine is yet available for hepatitis C, but interferon and ribaviron therapy is effective in prevention post-exposure.

Table 43.3 Epidemiology of acute hepatitis

Feature	HAV	HBV	HCV
Incubation period	2–7 weeks	4–20 weeks	2–20 weeks
Route of infection	Faecal/oral	Parenteral and sexual contact	Parenteral
Occurrence of virus in blood	2 weeks before until 1 week after jaundice	Months/years	Months/years
Occurrence of virus in faeces	2 weeks before until 2 weeks after jaundice	Absent	Probably absent

FOOD POISONING AND GASTROENTERITIS

Patients with vomiting and diarrhoea may have an infective cause for their symptoms. A history of the food eaten is important, particularly if an outbreak has occurred. Appropriate specimens for culture include food, faeces and vomitus. Microscopy of faeces may give the most rapid indication of the causative organism.

Sudden onset of symptoms within 1–4 hours of eating is usually due to *Staphylococcus aureus* or *Bacillus cereus*. *Salmonella*, *Shigella*, *Campylobacter*, *Clostridium perfringens*, *Vibrio parahaemolyticus* etc. all have an incubation period of 12–36 hours. Viral causes such as Norwalk agent or rotavirus have an incubation period of 1–3 days.

In most patients the attack is self-limiting and antibiotics are not required (see Table 43.4 for appropriate antibiotics if treatment is required). Drugs that decrease intestinal motility are contraindicated as they lead to retention of enterotoxins. Electrolyte and fluid replacement is most conveniently achieved by administering rehydration therapy (Electrolade). IV rehydration is required for patients who are severely dehydrated.

Amoebic dysentery

This is a possibility in any patient with severe colitis. It is more likely in people who have travelled overseas, although the organism is endemic in Australia. It is the only organism for which a warm stool is required to enable motile trophozoites to be seen. Treatment is with tinidazole or metronidazole.

TYPHOID FEVER

Patients with typhoid present with a febrile illness, general malaise and a dry cough and are often constipated.

Diarrhoea is not usual with typhoid fever. A history of travel is important in making a diagnosis. On examination there may be hepatosplenomegaly, and rose spots should be sought on the abdomen. Bradycardia despite a high fever is characteristic.

Table 43.4 Appropriate antibiotics for gastrointestinal pathogens (if treatment is indicated)

Organism	Antibiotics
Salmonella	Ciprofloxacin 500 mg orally 12-hourly. If oral therapy cannot be tolerated, ciprofloxacin 200 mg IV 12-hourly
Shigella	Norfloxacin 400 mg orally twice daily
Campylobacter	Erythromycin 500 mg orally twice daily *or* Norfloxacin 400 mg orally 12-hourly
Clostridium difficile	Metronidazole 200–400 mg orally 8-hourly *or* Vancomycin 125 mg orally 6-hourly
Giardia lamblia	Metronidazole 400 mg orally 8-hourly *or* Tinidazole 2 g orally as a single dose

Diagnosis is made from blood cultures, and later in the illness from faecal and urine cultures. Treatment is with ciprofloxacin 500 mg orally 12-hourly for 14 days. If oral therapy cannot be tolerated, IV ciprofloxacin 200 mg 12-hourly should be given.

Ceftriaxone IV is an alternative in children. Amoxycillin, chloramphenicol or co-trimoxazole may be given orally once the susceptibilities are known.

SEXUALLY TRANSMITTED DISEASES

Gonococcal infections

There is an increasing incidence of *Neisseria gonorrhoeae* infections resistant to penicillin. Choice of treatment will vary according to local sensitivity patterns. Chlamydial infections often coexist, thereby necessitating therapy for both organisms.

Specimens

Swabs and smears should be taken from the urethra, endocervix and rectum, and a specimen of urine should be sent without delay to the laboratory. *Gonococcus* and *Chlamydia* can be identified using PCR or SDA technology on urine and swabs.

Chlamydial infections

Appropriate swabs should be collected for *Chlamydia* antigen detection by direct fluorescent antibody (DFA) or enzyme immunoassay (EIA). Urine should be collected for *Chlamydia* nucleic acid detection using PCR or SDA technology.

Genital herpes simplex

Responsible for ulceration of penis, vagina and cervix. Culture or antigen detection by direct fluorescent antibody provides confirmation. Treatment is with oral aciclovir, famciclovir or valaciclovir.

Syphilis

Primary

If a chance is present, a specimen of exudate should be collected for dark ground examination, and serological tests are also done.

Secondary

This is diagnosed by the rash that is often present on the palms and soles. All serological tests are strongly positive.

Late syphilis

Later manifestations of syphilis are protean and suspected on clinical grounds. Diagnosis is made serologically and a lumbar puncture should also be done for cell count, biochemistry and serology.

Treatment

Gonorrhoea

Penicillinase-producing *Neisseria gonorrhoeae* (PPNG) is commonly isolated from patients in Victoria and New South Wales and from those who have recently visited South-East Asia. To cover this organism the treatment of choice is ceftriaxone 250 mg IM as a single dose, or spectinomycin 2 g IM as a single dose, or ciprofloxacin 250 mg orally as a single dose. Each of these should be used with either azithromycin 1 g orally as a single dose or doxycycline 100 mg orally for 10 days.

In other areas, or if penicillin-sensitive *Neisseria gonorrhoeae* is known to be present, use amoxycillin 3 g orally with probenecid 1 g orally as a single dose, together with either azithromycin or doxycycline as above.

Syphilis

In primary, secondary or early latent syphilis, treat with procaine penicillin 1 g IM once daily for 10 days or benzathine penicillin 1.8 g IM as a single dose. In patients allergic to penicillin, doxycycline or erythromycin may be used, but advice should be sought.

Late latent syphilis is syphilis of more than 1 year's duration. Treatment is with benzathine penicillin 1.8 g IM once weekly for 3 weeks or procaine penicillin 1 g once daily for 15 days.

Neurosyphilis

Specialist advice for treatment should be sought. Recommended regimens are procaine penicillin 2 g IM daily together with probenecid 500 mg orally every 6 hours for 20 days, or benzyl penicillin 1.8–2.4 g IV every 4 hours for 15 days. For penicillin-allergic patients use doxycyline 100 mg orally every 8 hours for 20–30 days.

MALARIA

Malaria is caused by four species of *Plasmodium*, *P. falciparum*, *P. vivax*, *P. malariae* and *P. ovale*. It should be suspected in any febrile patient who has recently travelled to a malarious area overseas or who has recently ceased taking prophylactic antimalarials. Travel and medication history are thus very important. The exact area of travel is important as it may indicate the likely presence of chloroquine-resistant *P. falciparum*.

Clinical symptoms

The hallmark of acute malaria is a high fever, chills and rigors. Headaches, chest pain, abdominal pain, nausea, vomiting and arthralgia may also be present. Paroxysms may occur regularly every 48 hours as with *P. vivax*, with the patient being well in between, or they may occur irregularly.

Signs

Moderate hepatomegaly and splenomegaly are frequently present and, less frequently, jaundice, urticaria and conjunctival suffusion. The abdomen may be tender.

Diagnosis

The diagnosis is made by examining thick and thin peripheral blood films for malarial parasites. Thick films allow a volume of approximately 10 times that of thin films to be examined. Different *Plasmodium* species are distinguished morphologically in the blood film. This is extremely important, as therapy is determined by the presence or absence of *P. falciparum*.

Therapy

Uncomplicated malaria

(*P. vivax*, *P. ovale*, *P. malariae*, chloroquine-susceptible *P. falciparum*.) Chloroquine phosphate 600 mg (4 tabs) orally statim, 300 mg (2 tabs) at 6 hours, 24 hours and 48 hours (total dose 1500 mg).

Primaquine 15 mg orally daily for 2 weeks will be required to eliminate the hepatic phase.

Chloroquine-resistant P. falciparum infection

Quinine sulphate 600 mg orally every 8 hours for 7 days or quinine dihydrochloride IV 20 mg/kg (up to 1.4 g) given over 4 hours, followed by 10 mg/kg IV (up to 700 mg) every 8 hours until the patient is able to tolerate oral quinine.

Doxycycline 100 mg once daily for 7 days is administered concurrently.
Alternatively as a single agent mefloquine 750 mg orally statim followed by 500 mg in 6–8 hours.

INFECTIONS IN TRAVELLERS

Pre-travel advice

Prospective travellers should discuss their itinerary with a doctor familiar with the infectious diseases found in overseas countries. Appropriate prophylaxis against malaria requires up-to-date information, as resistance patterns change. Advice on avoiding mosquito bites is of paramount importance in a discussion of general principles regarding safe food and water consumption in overseas countries. Vaccination for diphtheria, tetanus, hepatitis A, polio, typhoid, tuberculosis and possibly meningococcus, yellow fever or Japanese encephalitis may be advised. Cholera vaccine, although available, is frequently omitted due to poor efficacy.

Travellers with fevers

A good travel history is essential, documenting countries visited, food eaten (particularly uncooked), water drunk, freshwater swimming, mosquito and tick bites, whether other members of travelling group are also unwell, risky sexual activity and prophylaxis used.

The usual investigations include haematology, basic biochemistry, liver function tests, CXR, thick and thin films for malaria, blood cultures for typhoid and other bacteria, urine culture and serological tests for dengue, hepatitis viruses, EBV, HIV and possibly *Rickettsia*, Q fever, brucellosis and leptospirosis. Mycobacterial disease should be excluded. Viral infections with haemorrhagic manifestations are potentially lethal and are highly contagious. Specialised units exist for the management of these patients and they should be contacted immediately.

Repeated blood films may be required to diagnose malaria. Advice from a clinical microbiologist or infectious diseases physician may be prudent.

TETANUS

1. Must always be thought of with any wound.
2. Debridement and good wound care are essential.
3. Any penetrating contaminated wound, especially if foreign matter or devitalised tissue is involved, is particularly tetanus-prone.
4. Table 43.5 summarises the Australian Immunisation Handbook's guidelines for management of tetanus-prone wounds.

Tetanus may occur without an obvious wound being found, or several weeks after the injury. Hence be suspicious in patients with muscle stiffness

Table 43.5 General measures for treatment of tetanus-prone wounds

History of tetanus vaccination	Time since last dose	Type of wound	DTP, DT, Td or tetanus toxoid as appropriate	Tetanus immuno-globulin*
≥3 doses	<5 years	All wounds	NO	NO
≥3 doses	5–10 years	Clean minor wounds	NO	NO
≥3 doses	5–10 years	All other wounds	YES	NO
≥3 doses	>10 years	All wounds	YES	NO
<3 doses, or uncertain	—	Clean minor wounds	YES	NO
<3 doses, or uncertain	—	All other wounds	YES	YES

* The recommended dose for TIG is 250 IU, to be given as soon as practicable after the injury, unless >24 hours has elapsed, in which case 500 IU should be given.

or spasms. It is part of the differential diagnosis of meningitis and extrapyramidal drug reactions.

NEEDLE-STICK INJURY

Following a needle-stick injury or other injury due to sharps potentially contaminated with blood, or the splashing of mucosal surfaces with blood or secretions infected with hepatitis B or HIV, the affected areas should be well washed under a running tap. An antiseptic solution such as alcohol 70%, or chlorhexidine 0.5% should then be applied to skin wounds (not mucosal surfaces).

If the donor is known to be HBsAg (surface antigen) positive and/or HIV-positive, no further blood tests from the donor need be taken. If, however, the HBV or HIV status of the donor is unknown, blood should be taken, clearly marked 'donor of needle-stick injury' and forwarded for HBV, HCV and HIV serology after consent is obtained. One tube of clotted blood is to be collected from the recipient of the sharps injury. This, together with a request clearly stating vaccination history and 'recipient of needle-stick injury', should have tests for anti-HBc (core antibody) or anti-HBs (surface antibody) performed. Recent literature has shown more than 90% eradication of hepatitis C virus after needle-stick injury with interferon-alfa monotherapy. Hospital will be producing protocols as the evidence becomes available.

The needle or sharp can be tested for HIV at certain laboratories. If the injured person has not been vaccinated against hepatitis B and the sharps injury donor is known to be hepatitis B antigen-positive, the first dose of hepatitis B vaccine should be given immediately, while serological investigations are being performed. Even if the donor is found to be hepatitis B surface antigen-negative, routine vaccination should be commenced for future protection.

In addition, hepatitis B hyperimmune globulin is available for recipients known to have no immunity to hepatitis B who suffer a sharps injury from a known or strongly suspected hepatitis B carrier. It should be administered within 1 week, preferably within 72 hours of the injury, and is given concurrently with, but in a different site from, the first dose of hepatitis B vaccine.

A tetanus booster should also be given if 10 years have elapsed since immunisation.

Needle-stick medication

Where the contact is known to be HIV-infected, it is recommended that triple therapy should be initiated immediately following a needle-stick injury, using at least two agents to which the source has not been exposed. The standard regimen is stavudine (d4T) 40 mg bd, lamivudine (3TC) 150 mg bd and tenofovir (TFV) 300 mg daily all administered for 4 weeks. Combination therapy with other antiretroviral agents may be indicated, according to the donor's therapeutic history. Following any injury or splash with infected blood, the healthcare worker should contact a microbiologist, infectious diseases physician or specialist in HIV medicine for advice regarding appropriate management.

RECOMMENDED READING

Therapeutic guidelines: antibiotic. Version 11. Melbourne: Victorian Postgraduate Foundation Committee; 2000. Available: http://www.tg.com.au.

Mandell G, Douglas RG, Bennett J. Principles and practice of infectious diseases. 5th edn. New York: Churchill Livingstone; 2000.

The Australian Immunisation Handbook. 8th edn. Canberra: NHMRC; 2003. Available: http://immunise.health.gov.au/handbook.htm.

Yung AP, McDonald MI, Spelman D, Street AC, Johnson PDR, eds. Infectious diseases: a clinical approach. Mount Waverley, Victoria: Cherry Print; 2001.

44 Patients with HIV infection

David A Brown, Ronald Penny, Sarah Pett
and Christopher Weatherall

Since infection with the human immunodeficiency virus (HIV) was first identified as the cause of the acquired immunodeficiency syndrome (AIDS) in 1981, the pandemic has had a dramatic impact on medical practice. Reported estimates of the total number of people in the world infected with the virus, at the end of 2001, were in the order of 40 million, and of these 17.6 million are women. Five million people were infected worldwide in the year ending December 2001. In the same year three million died of AIDS. In Australia, by the end of December 2001 there had been 6124 deaths and 18,854 patients infected with HIV.

Patients with HIV present to emergency centres with HIV-related disease such as seroconversion illness, opportunistic infection and malignancy, and other clinical conditions with coincidental HIV infection. Highly active antiretroviral treatment (HAART) has had a significant impact on the course and prognosis of HIV, but the complexity and potency of some treatment regimens can also lead to presentations with adverse drug reactions or syndromes of immune reconstitution.

INDIVIDUALS AT RISK

1. The sexually active, particularly men who have sex with men and individuals with partners from HIV-endemic areas (Asia, sub-Saharan Africa, South America).
2. Injecting drug users, particularly if unsafe injecting use was overseas.
3. Recipients of blood and blood components (mass screening of blood commenced in 1985 in Australia), particularly if exposure to blood products has been overseas in countries where the safety of these products is doubtful.
4. Infants and children of HIV-infected or at-risk mothers.

A careful history should be taken from such patients, with particular emphasis on sexual and drug-injecting practices, receipt of blood products, risk behaviours in endemic areas and previous testing for HIV. All patients at risk of HIV infection should have HIV antibody testing done with informed consent and emphasis on the important social and medicolegal aspects of a positive test.

Patients found to be HIV antibody-positive should, in addition, have plasma HIV viral load and T cell subset testing (CD4+, CD8+ T cells and their ratio), as these parameters substantially influence the clinical assessment. In addition, all patients found to be HIV-1/2-positive should be screened for the presence of other sexually transmitted infections (STIs) including gonorrhoea, non-specific urethritis (NSU), syphilis and hepatitis A, B and C. Other risk factors for opportunistic infection should be assessed, including travel history (includes remote history), occupational and tuberculosis risk. All HIV antibody-positive patients should receive professional counselling with consideration given to referral to an expert service. This should include the issue of contact tracing.

ACUTE HIV INFECTION

Within 1–6 weeks (occasionally as long as 12 weeks) of HIV exposure, an acute illness (seroconversion illness) resembling infectious mononucleosis develops in 50–70% of individuals. The most common features (see also Table 44.1) are fever, myalgia, arthralgia, pharyngitis, lymphadenopathy, an erythematous maculopapular (face, trunk, occasionally palms and soles) rash and lethargy. There may also be dermatological, neuropsychological (including aseptic meningitis), gastrointestinal and respiratory features—*Pneumocystis carinii* pneumonia has been reported in primary infection, albeit extremely rarely. The differential diagnosis includes acute Epstein-Barr virus (EBV) infection, cytomegalovirus (CMV) or viral hepatitis, toxoplasmosis, secondary syphilis, rubella, primary HSV (rare in adults), cat scratch disease, drug reaction, opportunistic infection on a background of chronic HIV, and acute presentations of leukaemias/lymphomas.

Initial laboratory assessment

This should include full blood count and film for atypical mononuclear cells, biochemical profile (including liver function and bone screen),

Table 44.1 Clinical manifestations of primary HIV-1 infection

General	Dermatological
Fever (95%)	Erythematous maculopapular rash
Lymphadenopathy (70%)	Roseola-like rash
Pharyngitis (70%)	Cutaneous urticaria
Arthralgia/myalgia	Desquamation
Lethargy	Hair loss
Anorexia, weight loss	Cutaneous and mucosal ulceration
Neuropsychological	**Gastrointestinal**
Headache and retro-orbital pain	Oropharyngeal candidiasis
Meningoencephalitis	Nausea and vomiting
Neuropathy (can be part of a mononeuritis multiplex)	Diarrhoea
Radiculopathy	**Respiratory**
Ascending polyradiculopathy (Guillain-Barré)	Cough (rarely PCP can occur
Cognitive or affective changes	at seroconversion)

serology (IgM and IgG) for EBV, CMV, hepatitis viruses, toxoplasmosis, syphilis and relevant cultures, e.g. oral lesions (for fungi and viruses), blood (if sepsis cannot be excluded) and genital secretions if there are symptoms suggestive of an STI, as well as HIV antibody testing.

If acute seroconversion is suspected, HIV antibody tests may initially be negative, although the p24 antigen and HIV pro-viral DNA test would be positive in a symptomatic patient. These tests are always included in a 'seroconversion screen', which should be requested if there is a high index of suspicion. Arrangements for confirmatory repeat antibody testing within 2–4 weeks of presentation should be made at the time of initial testing. In the interim appropriate counselling about potential transmission risks should be given. Specialist advice should be sought immediately and appropriate referral made, as HAART may be offered in symptomatic primary HIV infection in many centres.

PERSISTENT GENERALISED LYMPHADENOPATHY

Patients with persistent generalised lymphadenopathy (PGL) are likely to present to emergency centres with unrelated illnesses. The detection on routine examination of generalised asymptomatic enlargement of extra-inguinal lymph nodes, especially axillary, anterior and posterior cervical, occipital and epitrochlear nodes, should trigger a search for further historical or examination findings of HIV. In addition, other causes of PGL +/– HIV should be excluded. Identification allows the opportunity for timely HIV assessment, including the introduction of HAART and counselling with respect to transmission risks and disease prognosis.

Laboratory assessment

This is as for acute HIV infection, except that a more detailed clinical assessment looking for opportunistic infections and malignancy (e.g. tuberculosis, Kaposi's sarcoma) should be undertaken. Pro-viral DNA and p24 antigen testing will not be necessary, but assessment should include estimation of T-cell subset (which includes CD4+) cells and plasma HIV viral load. Investigations relevant to the current clinical problem should be performed.

SPECIFIC PROBLEMS IN HIV

A recent CD4+ count and HIV viral load estimate are useful in narrowing the differential diagnosis, bearing in mind that estimates performed by a GP or HIV physician in the past 1–2 months will often be a more accurate reflection of true disease state. Acute intercurrent infections impact negatively on CD4+ cell count and HIV virus load; this effect is usually transient. (See Table 44.2.)

Table 44.2 Condition versus CD4+ T-cell (cells/L) count in HIV infection

	>400	300	200	100	0
Bacterial pneumonia					
Tuberculosis					
Lymphoma					
Kaposi's sarcoma					
Pneumocystis pneumonia (PCP)					
Cryptococcal infection					
Toxoplasmosis					
Cytomegalovirus infection					
Cerebral lymphoma					
Mycobacterium avium complex					

CD4+ T-cells/µL

Pulmonary syndromes

Presentation

The most common serious causes of respiratory disease in HIV are bacterial pneumonias caused in particular by *Streptococcus pneumoniae*. These occur at any CD4+ cell count, including those above 500 cells/mL. Ninety-five per cent of pneumococcal pneumonia is accompanied by bacteraemia (which may precede radiographic changes); pneumococcal sinusitis is also common and can be very severe.

At lower CD4+ cell counts (<200 cells/µL), particularly in those not previously known to have HIV infection or in those with low CD4 who are poorly compliant with co-trimoxazole prophylaxis, *Pneumocystis carinii* pneumonia (PCP) must be excluded. Characteristic symptoms include cough +/− sputum, progressive dyspnoea, fever and night sweats, chest pain (rare), pneumothorax, debilitation and other signs of immuno-compromise (oral candidiasis, oral hairy leukoplakia, wasting, seborrhoeic dermatitis, herpes simplex and PGL). This diagnosis is less likely in patients compliant with Bactrim prophylaxis, but in those using inhaled pentamidine prophylaxis upper lobe PCP is well described.

In addition to PCP, the differential diagnosis of a dry cough should include pulmonary TB, especially in a patient from an area with both endemic TB and HIV, atypical pneumonias (e.g. *Mycoplasma*, *Legionella*, fungi including *Cryptococcus*), CMV, Kaposi's sarcoma of the lung, lymphoid interstitial pneumonitis (usually manifests in children), pulmonary embolism, and other pulmonary neoplasms. The relative risk of these diagnoses will depend very much on current CD4+ cell count and HIV viral load (see Table 44.2). The risk of opportunistic infections (OIs) has declined substantially in the era of HAART, even in those with CD4+ cell count <200 cells/µL if HIV plasma viral load is well suppressed and OI prophylaxis is appropriate. Purulent sputum is more suggestive of bacterial pneumonia (e.g. *Streptococcus pneumoniae, Haemophilus influenzae*).

Bacterial pneumonia

There is an increased incidence of bacterial pneumonia in HIV infection concomitant with T and B cell dysfunction. These episodes are often associated with the usual organisms, e.g. *S. pneumoniae, H. influenzae* and *S. aureus*.

The X-ray features are generally the same as in an immunocompetent patient, although it should be noted that in the case of neutropenia there might be a delay between the clinical onset and radiological changes. The response to therapy is approximately the same as with a non-HIV-infected patient. Co-infection with PCP is unusual.

Pneumocystis carinii *pneumonia*

Pneumocystis carinii pneumonia (PCP) is one of the most common AIDS-defining illnesses in patients with a CD4+ count less than $200/mm^3$ who are not taking prophylaxis. Presentation is often after a prolonged (2–3 weeks) prodrome of flu-like symptoms, commonly fever, weight loss and fatigue. The development of progressive dyspnoea, non-productive cough and high fevers usually precipitates presentation. A new (or newly altered) antiretroviral regimen can also unmask subclinical infection as the recovering immune system begins to clear organisms, resulting in PCP at unexpectedly high CD4+ levels. However, immune-restoration PCP is still rare.

The most important factor in the history besides the low T-cell count is the type of primary/secondary prophylaxis and the level of compliance. Co-trimoxazole prophylaxis is superior to other forms, such as pentamidine (inhaled or IV), dapsone and trimethoprim, where breakthrough is more common.

Clinical examination is often unremarkable, and when signs are present they are usually confined to tachypnoea, decreased expansion and fine crepitations. In long-standing or repeat infections, signs of pneumothorax may be present. Extrapulmonary infection is rare.

The X-ray findings may be normal in 5–10% of patients (check for desaturation of oxygen on exertion), but usually show a diffuse interstitial pattern extending initially from the hila, which may be asymmetrical but is more commonly symmetrical. Later in the disease, alveolar filling may be present and all other patterns of radiological lung involvement have been reported. Pleural effusions are rare in PCP and are more typically seen in Kaposi's sarcoma of the lung and occasionally with lymphomas of the thoracic cavity.

Low PaO_2 is an important prognostic factor and an indication for treatment with steroids (see below). Definitive diagnosis is obtained from induced sputum or bronchoalveolar lavage. The most effective treatment for PCP is co-trimoxazole at a dose of 20 mg/kg/d trimethoprim combined with 100 mg/kg/d sulfamethoxazole in 3–4 divided doses IV for 21 days.

Investigations

CXR, blood gases, sputum for routine microbiology, cytology and auramine/Ziehl-Neelsen staining, induced sputum (using hypertonic saline) for *Pneumocystis*. If induced sputum is unsatisfactory, patient may require bronchoscopy with brushings, washings and/or transbronchial biopsy. Neither induced sputum nor bronchoscopy is safe in patients with severe hypoxia and the patient should be treated presumptively for PCP.

Initial management

If sputum is purulent, initiate antibiotic therapy to cover community-acquired pneumonia.

If *Pneumocystis* is suspected clinically, empirical treatment may be initiated with co-trimoxazole orally (20 mg/kg/day of the trimethoprim component, in four divided doses) or IV (if nauseated, vomiting or significantly ill). Sulphonamide-sensitive individuals can be managed with IV pentamidine (4 mg/kg/day for 21 days) but must be admitted for careful monitoring of blood pressure (fatal hypotension reported), blood glucose (hypo- and hyperglycaemia), renal (including calcium), liver function, pancreatic lipase and FBC. Corticosteroids are routinely used in hypoxic (PaO_2 <70 mmHg) patients with PCP and significantly improve prognosis in this setting. Prednisone 40 mg bd or equivalent (methylprednisolone) should be commenced in conjunction with the specific antimicrobial. Initiation of treatment does not interfere with subsequent confirmation of *Pneumocystis*, and should not be delayed. In extremely hypoxic patients, ventilatory support (i.e. continuous positive airway pressure—CPAP or mechanical ventilation) must be considered, particularly as the prognosis from first-episode PCP is extremely good and more so in the era of HAART.

Tuberculosis

Tuberculosis (TB) is less prevalent in the Australian HIV population than it is in the United States HIV population. It is more common to have reactivation or primary infection with T-cell counts that are greater than 400 cells/μL. TB can therefore be the first manifestation of HIV and all patients with TB, regardless of assessed risk, should be tested for HIV. TB should be considered in the diagnosis of respiratory disease presenting with cough, haemoptysis, fever and dyspnoea, especially on a background of weight loss, night sweats and generalised debility. In early HIV disease the radiological appearance of TB is similar to that of an HIV-negative individual, with upper lobe cavitatory disease being the most common finding. With more advanced disease (CD4+ cell count <400 cells/μL), reactivation or progressive primary disease is common. In addition, extrapulmonary manifestations occur in 50% of cases and include lymph node, gastrointestinal tract (GIT) and bone marrow involvement. CXR changes are less typical and while hilar lymphadenopathy is the most common finding, this may progress to diffuse, coarse interstitial densities or localised infiltrates, especially in the mid to lower lung zones; 10–20% have pleural effusion. Frank 'miliary' changes are uncommon in advanced HIV, as patients are so immunocompromised they are unable to form granulomata properly.

Treatment is with multidrug regimens as in the immunocompetent, but with dose adjustments and monitoring to take into account interactions with other medications, particularly protease inhibitors (PI). Specialist advice should be sought, in particular with respect to respiratory isolation procedures and obtaining respiratory specimens for diagnosis.

Pulmonary thromboembolism

There is an increased incidence of pulmonary thromboembolism in patients with HIV, primarily due to an increase in anticardiolipin antibody and decreased levels of proteins C and S. This should be considered in the differential diagnosis of dyspnoea. The presentation is that of pulmonary thromboembolism in HIV-negative patients and the treatment is the same.

Neurological syndromes

Presentation

Patients may present with a variety of neurological symptoms including focal cortical epilepsy, headache, fever, neck stiffness and organic brain syndrome.

Assessment

This involves full neurological examination, computerised tomography (CT), followed by lumbar puncture if the CT is normal and provided there are no focal neurological signs (see Table 44.3). Cerebrospinal fluid (CSF) opening pressure should be recorded, and a relatively large volume (8 mL), if feasible, collected. Initial testing includes routine microscopy, Indian ink staining, cultures, biochemistry (protein, albumin and glucose), cryptococcal antigen (CRAG) titres, TB polymerase chain reaction (PCR) and VDRL if either TB or syphilis are suspected, beta$_2$-microglobulin and neopterin (matched CSF and serum samples). In many centres it is also common to assess CSF HIV viral load, although perhaps not in the acute setting. A moderate pleocytosis and elevated protein is characteristic of HIV and therefore not specific. Nucleic acid testing for CMV, HSV and other viruses can be requested where diagnosis remains problematic or where clinically indicated.

Blood should be drawn at the same time as CSF for full blood count, electrolytes including magnesium, calcium and phosphate, cryptococcal antigen, syphilis serology and a drug screen (+/– urine drug screen). Magnetic resonance imaging can be useful in further characterisation of focal lesions identified on CT.

Table 44.3 Diagnosis based on cerebral CT appearance (with contrast)

CT-negative	Cryptococcal meningitis
	HIV-related seizure
	Multifocal leukoencephalopathy
	Syphilis
	Drug-related delirium
	Metabolic delirium
	AIDS dementia complex
	Cytomegalovirus infection
Mass lesion on CT	*Toxoplasma* can be CT-negative
	TB meningitis
	Toxoplasmosis
	1° cerebral lymphoma
	Cryptococcoma and tuberculoma (very rarely seen)
	Multifocal leukoencephalopathy
	Abscess

Cryptococcal infection

Cryptococcus neoformans causes disease, most commonly meningitis, in about 10% of patients with HIV. It is the first AIDS-defining illness in as many as 40% of patients. CD4+ counts are usually less than $100/\text{mm}^3$.

The onset of meningitis is often insidious and the mean time from onset of symptoms to diagnosis is of the order of 1 month. The most common features are fever, headache, nausea and malaise. Photophobia and neck stiffness may not be prominent features (only one in four); one in five will have focal neurological findings, including cranial nerve palsies. A depressed level of consciousness is the most important predictor of poor outcome, necessitating intensive treatment. There may be sites involved outside the central nervous system (CNS) including skin (a molluscum-like rash in 3–10%), joints and genitourinary tract (especially the prostate as a reservoir site) and lungs.

A contrast-enhanced CT brain scan should **always** be performed to exclude a space-occupying lesion before lumbar puncture (LP). *Cryptococcus* rarely causes focal brain lesions in HIV (in contrast to immunocompetent hosts), although cryptococcomas can be a manifestation of immune restoration disease. An elevated CSF opening pressure is very suggestive of cryptococcal meningitis, and fluid should be removed to halve the opening pressure. Some patients require daily lumbar punctures to maintain levels of less than 250 mm H_2O. Indian ink staining/CRAG can provide rapid confirmation of the diagnosis. Cryptococcal antigen should be measured in blood and CSF (positive in up to 99% of cases); blood cultures may be positive for *Cryptococcus*.

Treatment should be initiated with fluconazole 400 mg bd unless there is suspicion of a resistant organism. This may occur in the setting of prolonged treatment of oral candidiasis or relapse of meningitis while on fluconazole. If organism resistance is suspected, and when the level of consciousness is decreased, amphotericin B (0.7–1.0 mg/kg/d infused centrally over 4–6 hours) (with or without flucytosine 25 mg/kg po q6h) should be used.

An urgent HIV neurology and ophthalmology opinion must be sought in patients with very high CSF pressure. Aggressive CSF pressure management in the form of repeated LP with CSF drainage, ventriculoperitoneal (VP) shunting and lumbar drains may be life-saving; fenestration of the ocular nerve may protect against pressure-induced visual damage; acetazolamide has been used in some cases.

It is important that any patient diagnosed with *Cryptococcus* at a site other than the CNS has a lumbar puncture to exclude cryptococcal meningitis, even if asymptomatic.

Toxoplasmosis

The domestic cat is the definitive host of this protozoon, and a significant proportion of the population is seropositive. The most common route of infection is the consumption of undercooked meat. Up to 45% of untreated HIV patients who are seropositive will develop *T. gondii* encephalitis. Co-trimoxazole prophylaxis has been shown to reduce the frequency of cerebral toxoplasmosis and in a compliant patient infection is unusual.

Encephalitis usually presents with a focal neurological picture in a patient with a T-cell count below $50-100/\text{mm}^3$: 70% present with altered mental state, 60% with hemiparesis or other focal signs, 50% with headache, 30% with seizures. Fever, confusion and coma are also seen. Ring-enhancing lesions, particularly in the cortex/basal ganglia, and mass effect are the classical findings on a CT scan. The major differential diagnosis is cerebral lymphoma, which can present with multiple irregular lesions on CT, although solitary lesions are also common. It is very unlikely that a patient with negative *T. gondii* serology has cerebral toxoplasmosis.

After contrast-enhanced cerebral CT scanning the patient should have blood collected for routine tests including *T. gondii* serology, that is if their serostatus is unknown. Treatment with sulphadiazine (1–1.5 g q6h po), pyrimethamine (200 mg od loading dose reducing to 75–100 mg od), folinic acid (15–25 mg od po) and anti-epileptic prophylaxis should be commenced where the clinical, serology and imaging studies are consistent. Sulpha-allergic individuals should commence a regimen of pyrimethamine and folinic acid, with clindamycin (600 mg po/IV q6h) or azithromycin 1–1.5 g od or clarithromycin 1 g bid as the third agent. Steroids (dexamethasone) can be used if there is significant mass effect, but should be avoided if possible as they may mask the true diagnosis, i.e. lymphomas will shrink with steroids. The use of steroids in suspected

Toxoplasma encephalitis should be discussed with an HIV neurologist. A poor response (within 7–10 days) to treatment or inconsistent findings may prompt further assessment, particularly for lymphoma. Definitive diagnosis is by brain biopsy.

Seizures

Seizures affect 10% of HIV patients, typically those with severe immunosuppression. A third of these will have an underlying mass lesion, and a number will have cryptococcal infection, metabolic disturbance or AIDS dementia complex. After history and investigation, including imaging, EEG and CSF analysis, up to 46% have no cause other than HIV. Recurrence rate is 70%, so prophylaxis is suggested, usually with sodium valproate or clonazepam (caution if patient on PI and/or efavirenz), which have the best side-effect profile in HIV.

Progressive multifocal leukoencephalopathy (PML)

PML is caused by JC virus, a polyomavirus. It presents in advanced HIV (CD4+ <100 cells/µL) with focal neurology ranging from seizures (20%) to cranial neuropathies, pyramidal (limb weakness in 33%), cerebellar signs (13%), visual defects (33%), altered mental status (33%). CT may be normal or show focal hypodensities. Increased T2 signal intensity within white matter tracts on MRI is more sensitive but still often less severe than the clinical signs; there is usually no mass effect. HAART is indicated to improve an otherwise poor outlook. Signs may worsen temporarily 10–14 days after commencement of antiretrovirals. CSF can be screened for JC PCR, definitive diagnosis is by brain biopsy but not required if the MRI findings are characteristic.

AIDS dementia complex (ADC)

ADC usually occurs at CD4+ cell counts <200 cells/µL. The median onset pre-HAART was CD4+ 70 cells/µL, and paradoxically in the era of HAART the median CD4+ at onset is higher at 170 cells/µL. ADC is characterised by poor memory, psychomotor slowing, myoclonic jerks and ataxia, and on examination by dysdiadochokinesia, brisk symmetrical reflexes and primitive reflexes. Diagnosis of less florid disease may require neuropsychometric evaluation. It may present initially to the emergency department when unmasked by one of the above neurological conditions or by acute drug-induced or metabolic derangement, and all of these need to be ruled out. Both CT and MRI will show cortical atrophy, but MRI is more useful for detecting confounding pathology. It is potentially reversible with HAART.

Psychiatric manifestations

Presentation

Patients may present with an acute or severe depressive, psychotic or anxiety state. It is important to distinguish organic neurological syndromes due to opportunistic infection or tumours, adverse drug reactions (e.g. efavirenz) or substance abuse (illicit/alcohol). It is important to note that ritonavir substantially increases the half-life of ecstasy, amphetamines and their metabolites.

Assessment

Careful clinical neurological evaluation, a CT brain scan, lumbar puncture, metabolic investigations including a drug screen, and psychiatric/neurological consultation are required.

Malignancy in HIV

Kaposi's sarcoma

Kaposi's sarcoma (KS) is the most common neoplasm affecting HIV patients and is predominant in homosexual patients because of the co-infection with human herpesvirus 8. The skin is usually the first site of involvement with painless, violaceous, hyperpigmented nodules of 0.5–2 cm, which may coalesce to larger lesions. Lesions are often symmetrical along skin tension lines, and the head and neck are favoured sites. Oral lesions (palate/gums) may precede other skin lesions; 40% of those with skin lesions will have GI involvement. It is uncommon for KS to occur with T-cell counts greater than 200–300 cells/μL, although immune restoration KS has been reported with HAART and the use of immunotherapeutic agents such as interleukin-2 (IL-2).

KS can affect any organ in the body other than the brain. It most commonly affects the gut and the lung, and should be considered in the differential diagnosis of lung pathology (especially if pleural effusion is present) and fever of unknown origin. KS of the gut can cause pain, acute GIT bleeding, obstruction and perforation, although this is unusual.

In KS involvement of the lung there can be confusion with a diagnosis of PCP and TB. In the CXR, pleural effusions are common and 50% of patients have hilar lymphadenopathy. There may be a reticulonodular or diffuse interstitial pattern on X-ray. It should be noted that pleural effusions are rare in the case of isolated PCP.

The best treatment for KS is effective HIV therapy. Isolated KS lesions can be treated with cryotherapy or intralesional vinblastine. Widespread and visceral disease responds to systemic chemotherapy.

Non-Hodgkin's lymphoma

There is an increased incidence of non-Hodgkin's lymphoma (NHL) and Hodgkin's lymphoma in patients with HIV. These are usually high-grade lymphomas, and can occur over a wide range of T-cell counts; however, those patients presenting with primary cerebral NHL almost always have T-cell counts <50/μL.

NHL can present in any organ. Extranodal presentation is common, with GIT, CNS, bone marrow and liver the most common. Fifteen per cent of patients will have skin involvement—the lesions are nodular. The differential diagnosis includes *Mycobacterium avium* complex and CMV. It is important to note that the presentation of NHL in the era of HAART is becoming more like that in an HIV-negative individual with more focal disease.

Primary cerebral lymphoma may be indistinguishable from cerebral toxoplasmosis, even with nuclear magnetic resonance scanning. Presentation is usually with mass effect, 60% have altered mental state and 15% have seizures. In most cases empirical treatment for *T. gondii* should be instituted before brain biopsy is undertaken.

Systemic opportunistic infections

Mycobacterium avium-intracellulare *complex (MAC)*

MAC occurs almost exclusively in advanced HIV infection with T-cell counts <50/μL and occurs in about 20% of HIV patients at some stage. The incidence of MAC has declined substantially in the era of HAART and primary prophylaxis with azithromycin. It is a ubiquitous soil and water saprophyte. It may be isolated from blood with specific culture or from samples of affected tissues including bone marrow. PCR may establish the diagnosis.

MAC usually presents with disseminated infection manifesting with fever, weight loss, anaemia, night sweats and neutropenia (Table 44.4). Diagnosis is made by blood cultures and/or aspiration and culture of bone marrow and mesenteric lymph node; the latter are usually enlarged on CT scan. The lungs can be involved, and CXR shows interstitial infiltrates. MAC and TB can coexist. The finding of MAC in stool or respiratory secretions is not sufficient to make the diagnosis, but colonisation of these sites can precede systemic disease.

The usual initial therapy for MAC is rifabutin (300 mg/d), ethambutol (20 mg/kg/d) and clarithromycin (500 mg bd). At least two drugs should be used at all times, preferably including clarithromycin. Rifabutin has several interactions with protease inhibitors, and dose adjustment is necessary. Single-drug prophylaxis for MAC using rifabutin or

Table 44.4 Clinical syndromes associated with disseminated MAC infection in AIDS

Systemic
Fever, malaise, weight loss, often associated with anaemia and neutropenia

Gastrointestinal
Chronic diarrhoea and abdominal pain
Chronic malabsorption
Extrabiliary obstructive jaundice secondary to periportal lymphadenopathy

azithromycin is used with T-cell counts less than $100/\mu L$; azithromycin has in addition some prophylactic value against PCP.

HAART may lead to immune restoration, leading to worsening symptoms due to MAC. This can present with painful generalised lymphadenopathy, scrofula, massive hilar and mesenteric adenopathy, fever, leukocytosis, lung infiltrates, and cutaneous nodules. Expert advice should be sought in this situation.

Cytomegalovirus disease

Cytomegalovirus (CMV) infection is very common in advanced-stage HIV and virtually all patients have T-cell counts $<50/\mu L$. Autopsy studies show that upward of 90% of patients have evidence of CMV infection even if asymptomatic/undiagnosed. Retinitis occurs in about 25% and GIT disease occurs in 5–10%. Presence of CMV does not always indicate active disease. The patient with retinitis usually presents with the complaint of floaters, visual field loss or decreased visual acuity. Fundoscopy reveals the typical 'cheese and tomato sauce' appearance, initially in the periphery, which should be differentiated from cottonwool spots, which are usually benign. Fulminant vitreitis may occur as part of a HAART-induced immune restoration and requires an urgent ophthalmological opinion.

In other sites in the CNS, CMV infection causes a subacute encephalopathy, characterised by headache, fever, poor concentration, personality change and polyradiculopathy. CMV polyradiculopathy occurs as a spinal cord syndrome with paraesthesiae, spasticity, weakness, areflexia and urinary retention. Lumbar puncture should be performed; a pleomorphic neutrophilia suggests CMV involvement. CMV PCR on CSF should be obtained as well as an MRI of the lumbar-sacral spine. An urgent HIV neurology opinion should be sought before initiating dual therapy of IV foscarnet with IV ganciclovir. CMV colitis occurs in 5–10% of patients presenting with diarrhoea, weight loss, anorexia, fever and GIT haemorrhage. All areas of the gastrointestinal tract can be affected.

When CMV causes pulmonary disease (rare in HIV), it is usually an interstitial pneumonia that is very difficult to differentiate from PCP. Hypoxia is almost always present and empirical treatment for PCP should be commenced. CMV pneumonias may be precipitated following the use of high-dose corticosteroids for PCP treatment.

An addisonian picture of hyponatraemia and hypotension can point to CMV adrenalitis. Clinical diagnosis in any of these sites is aided by the finding of CMV inclusions or antigens in biopsies, and isolation of CMV nucleic acid from blood (or CSF). Ophthalmic review is necessary when systemic CMV is diagnosed because there is a 20% rate of retinal co-infection.

Treatment with ganciclovir, an analogue of acyclovir, at a dose of 5 mg/kg twice daily for 2–3 weeks, is usually first-line. Newer agents such as oral valganciclovir (900 mg bid for 21 days followed by 900 mg od maintenance) are now licensed for use in CMV retinitis. If there is significant bone marrow depression or a history of resistant disease, foscarnet (90 mg/kg bid IV for 14–21 days) is used. The dose of both drugs should be reduced in renal impairment. CMV in the CNS is life-threatening and dual therapy with GCV and foscarnet is usual—expert advice should be sought.

Diarrhoea in HIV

Diarrhoea occurs in over 50% of patients at some time during their disease, and is a major cause of morbidity (Table 44.5).

In the patient presenting with diarrhoea, investigation should include multiple stool cultures and microscopy for ova, cysts and parasites, *Clostridium difficile* toxin, electrolytes and full blood count analysis. The treatment is initially symptomatic and, when the cause is identified, specific. Adjustment of antiretroviral treatment may be necessary either to remove a poorly tolerated medication or to improve immune function and hence clearance of pathogens. Investigation should include colonoscopy and biopsy if initial investigations are negative.

Summary

In patients presenting with advanced HIV (treated and failing therapy or untreated), it is important to appreciate that multiple diagnoses may coexist as a manifestation of severe immunodeficiency. It is therefore important to perform a full clinical examination and screen for other serious OIs, even when the main diagnosis has been made. The tests chosen should be based on the most likely other OIs for the level of immunodeficiency even if the patient is asymptomatic. For this reason, in patients with CD4 <100 cells/µL it is crucial to perform a CXR, ECG,

Table 44.5 Causes of diarrhoea in HIV

Viral	Parasitic
Cytomegalovirus	*Giardia lamblia*
Adenovirus	*Isospora belli*
Rotavirus. Seasonal small round viruses (Norwalk etc)	*Strongyloides* (rare in Australia)
	Cryptosporidium
Herpes simplex virus	Microsporidium
Bacterial	**Tumour**
Campylobacter jejuni	Kaposi's sarcoma
Salmonella spp.	Lymphoma
Shigella spp.	**Drugs**
Clostridium difficile	Protease inhibitors (very common)
Escherichia coli	
Mycobacterium avium complex	

MAC and blood cultures and a serum cryptococcal antigen as well as the routine haematology and biochemical tests.

ADVERSE DRUG REACTIONS

Forty per cent of Australian HIV patients are on antiretroviral treatment (Table 44.6). HAART has had a profound influence on the prognosis of HIV infection. Its long-term success in any one patient is strongly tied to medication compliance, which is, in part, dictated by side effects and tolerability. Adverse drug reactions are more common in HIV patients than in the general population, and this is exacerbated by the complicated multidrug treatment (see Tables 44.7 and 44.8). Some of the important and common reactions for emergency department practice are summarised below.

Hypersensitivity reactions, most commonly maculopapular or morbilliform rashes, are 100 times more common in the HIV population. The rash may be pruritic, prominent on the arms and trunk, and is frequently accompanied by myalgias, fatigue and fever. Common culprits include:

- All antibiotics including co-trimoxazole.
- All of the non-nucleoside reverse-transcriptase inhibitors.
- Amprenavir.
- Abacavir.

Most reactions occur within 1–3 weeks, and are rare after 8 weeks. Up to 50% of hypersensitivity reactions will resolve spontaneously, despite continued therapy (except in the case of abacavir—see below). Indications for cessation of a drug are: blistering or exfoliation, mucosal involvement, fever >39°C, intolerability to the patient, or a rise in transaminase levels to >5 times normal. Stevens-Johnson syndrome is described in 0.5% of cases.

Abacavir hypersensitivity occurs in 5%. Certain human leukocyte antigen (HLA) types are predisposed to this allergic reaction. The test for human leukocyte antigen is in development as a possible screening tool. The hypersensitivity is characterised by a flu-like syndrome consisting of myalgia, fever >39°C, headache, dizziness, shortness of breath and cough, rash and diarrhoea. It can also result in respiratory difficulty and labile blood pressure—deaths have been reported and, once the drug is withdrawn, the patient should never be rechallenged. Expert advice should be sought.

Pancreatitis is associated with didanosine (ddI) (1 in 1000 patient-years) and less commonly with stavudine (d4T), zalcitabine (ddC), lamivudine (3TC) and hydroxyurea. Hypertriglyceridaemia from protease inhibitor use may also contribute. The drug should be ceased and pancreatitis managed supportively.

Renal colic as well as vague abdominal pain and painless haematuria can be related to indinavir crystals in urine. Indinavir should be withdrawn and urolithiasis managed as usual.

Table 44.6 Antiretroviral medications

Generic name	Abbreviation	Proprietary name	Size of tablet/ capsule	Usual dose	Brief description
Nucleoside analogues (NRTIs)					
zidovudine	ZDV = AZT	Retrovir	250 mg	250 mg bd; occ 200 or 300 mg bid used	blue/white banded capsule
stavudine	d4T	Zerit	30 or 40 mg	30 mg bd in <60 kg; usual dose is 40 mg bd	orange capsule
didanosine	ddI	Videx-EC	250 mg or 400 mg enteric coated capsule	250 mg in <60 kg or on tenofovir 400 mg/d	white capsule, red lettering
lamivudine	3TC	Epivir	150 mg	150 mg bd	white rhomboid tablet
abacavir	ABV	Ziagen	300 mg	300 mg bd (600 mg bd used in ADC)	gold ovoid tablet
deoxycytidine	ddC	Hivid	0.75 mg	0.75 mg td	light blue ovoid tablet
tenofovir	TFV	Viread	300 mg	300 mg/d	grey-white kite-shaped tablet
zidovudine + lamivudine	ZDV/3TC	Combivir	one	300/150 mg bd	white ovoid tablet
abacavir + lamivudine + zidovudine	ABV/3TC/ZDV	Trizivir	one	300/150/300 mg bd	green ovoid tablet
Non-nucleoside reverse-transcriptase inhibitors (NNRTIs)					
nevirapine	NVP	Viramune	200 mg	200 mg bd (200 mg od for two weeks at commencement)	grey-white ovoid tablet
delavirdine	DLV	Rescriptor	100 mg	600 mg tds	white ovoid tablet
efavirenz	EFV	Stocrin/Sustiva	200 mg, soon to be released as a 600 mg capsule	600 mg/d	yellow capsule

Table 44.6 Antiretroviral medications (continued)

Generic name	Abbreviation	Proprietary name	Size of tablet/capsule	Usual dose	Brief description
Protease inhibitors (PIs)					
saquinavir (soft gel capsule)	SQV (SGC)	Fortovase	200 mg	1200 mg tds 1200 mg bd when given with TV boost, occ 1600 mg od used	brown capsule
saquinavir (hard gel capsule)	SQV (HGC)	Invirase	200 mg	600 mg tds 1200 mg bd when given with RTV boost, occ 1600 mg od used	black/yellow capsule
indinavir	IDV	Crixivan	400 mg	800 mg tds (400–800 mg bd when given with a RTV boost)	white capsule
nelfinavir	NFV	Viracept	250 mg	750 mg tds or 1250 mg bd when used with SQV	blue ovoid tablet
ritonavir ('baby dose' with other PI)	RTV	Norvir	100 mg	100 mg–200 mg bd	white capsule
amprenavir	APV	Agenerase	150 mg	1200 mg bd	brown capsule, 2 lines longitudinally
lopinavir + ritonavir	LPV/RTV	Kaletra	133 mg LPV and 33 mg RTV per capsule	400/100 mg bd or 533/133 mg bd if given with nevirapine or efavirenz	orange capsule

Lactic acidaemia is related to the long-term mitochondrial toxicity of nucleoside reverse-transcriptase inhibitors, particularly d4T and ddI, but has been reported with zidovudine (AZT) and ddC. It often presents insidiously with fever, nausea, vomiting, dyspnoea, weight loss and abdominal pain; myopathy has been reported and CPK may be elevated. Hepatomegaly may be detected due to hepatic steatosis. Respiratory failure and death may ensue. Anion gap is elevated and serum lactate levels elevated. Levels >5 mmol/L (normal range <2.2 mmol/L) mandate cessation of the drug; levels >10 mmol/L have 80% mortality. Treatment is supportive. Thiamine, riboflavin and haemodialysis have been used with mixed success. Expert advice from an HIV specialist and nephrologist must be sought. Once the drug is ceased, lactate levels take up to 10 weeks to return to normal.

Abnormal liver function tests can be related to virtually any antiretroviral as well as to antifungals, antimycobacterials and other antibiotics including co-trimoxazole. Ritonavir in particular is a potent inhibitor of cytochrome P450 metabolism and therefore prone to interaction with multiple drugs.

Immune reconstitution syndrome describes a clinical deterioration or flare-up of HIV-related diseases, which may have been quiescent or even subclinical, following the introduction of effective HAART. The increasingly competent immune system begins to recognise/eliminate the infection (or malignancy) with resultant inflammatory cascades. Well-recognised immune restoration syndromes include those seen with TB, MAC, CMV, *Cryptococcus*, PML, hepatitis B/C and less commonly PCP. The timing is usually from 10 days to several weeks after commencement

Table 44.7 Drugs that should not be co-administered with HIV protease inhibitors because of demonstrated or predicted interactions with the potential for serious events or loss of efficacy

Drug class	Drug names
Antiarrhythmics	amiodarone, lignocaine (systemic), bepridil, quinidine
Antihistamines	astemizole (withdrawn), terfenadine (withdrawn)
Ergot derivatives	dihydroergotamine, ergotamine, ergonovine
GI motility agents	cisapride (withdrawn)
Neuroleptic	pimozide
Sedative/hypnotics	midazolam, triazolam, diazepam
Antimycobacterials	rifampin (rifampicin in several countries)
HMG-CoA reductase inhibitors	lovastatin, simvastatin
Phosphodiesterase type 5 inhibitors	sildenafil
Herbal products	St John's wort

Table 44.8 Drugs that may require dose modification when administered with HIV protease inhibitors based upon demonstrated or predicted interactions with the potential for serious events or loss of efficacy

Drug class	Drug name
Anticoagulant	warfarin
Antimycobacterial	rifabutin
Antibacterial	erythromycin, dapsone
Antifungal	itraconazole, fluconazole
Immunosuppressants	cyclosporin, tacrolimus, rapamycin
Anticonvulsants	carbamazepine, phenobarbital, phenytoin
Narcotic analgesic	methadone
antidepressants	all SSRIs (cipramil requires no adjustment of HAART)

of effective therapy. Where anticipated, the syndrome is minimised by treating the opportunistic infection with specific therapy to reduce the pathogen load prior to HAART. Occasionally steroids and/or temporary cessation of HAART are required to dampen the overenthusiastic immune response, but these strategies should be undertaken only in consultation with an HIV specialist.

It is critical that HAART not be commenced in a patient with an active opportunistic infection. There is considerable debate as to when HAART should be introduced in this situation; most experts would agree that an interval of at least 1 month or more is appropriate. This is to minimise the risk not only of immune restoration disease but also of difficulties in attributing side effects such as rash either to the drugs used to treat the OI or the antiretrovirals.

In Australia, the HIV-infected population is approaching middle age and it is important to appreciate that not all presentations to the emergency department will be HIV- or HAART-related.

COUNSELLING AND SUPPORT

HIV-positive patients need support to manage the emotional crises created by HIV infection and related illnesses, especially when presenting for the first time. Early intervention with skilled counsellors, social workers, nursing and other support staff, including voluntary organisations, is important. Patients must receive appropriate information and education about prevention of HIV transmission and the need to contact/trace at-risk partners for HIV testing.

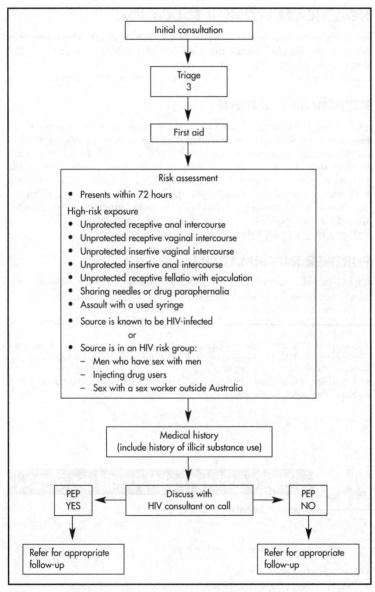

Figure 44.1   Outline of post-exposure prophylaxis (PEP) (adapted from St Vincent's Hospital guidelines)

HEALTHCARE WORKER EDUCATION

All institutions and hospital departments, but especially the emergency department, should direct education towards relevant aspects of HIV disease, modes of transmission, avoidance of discrimination towards HIV-infected patients, and adherence to infection control procedures.

INFECTION CONTROL

The adoption of universal blood and body fluid precautions, whereby all blood and body fluids are considered potential sources of infection, is recommended, and direct exposure should be avoided. All healthcare workers should refer to national, state or institutional policies for specific recommendations regarding infection control guidelines. In addition, HIV-infected healthcare workers should conduct their clinical activities in accordance with approved policies. All directors of emergency departments should ensure vigorous adherence to all recommendations.

Post-exposure prophylaxis is summarised in Figure 44.1.

FURTHER INFORMATION

Up-to-date online information can be obtained from the following websites:

1. AIDsinfo: a service of the US Department of Health and Human Services. Treatment guidelines. Available: http://www.aidsinfo.nih.gov.
2. Johns Hopkins AIDS Service. Textbook and guidelines. Available: http://www. Hopkins-aids.edu.
3. Liverpool HIV Pharmacology Group, Department of Pharmacology, University of Liverpool, UK. Information on HIV drug interactions. Available http://www.hiv-druginteractions.org.
4. University of California San Francisco. HIV InSite knowledge base. Available: http://www.hivinsite.ucsf.edu.

45 The cancer or neutropenic patient

John B Roberts

Oncologic emergencies may be due to:

1. Direct effects of the malignancy.
2. Side effects and complications of treatment.
3. Comorbid conditions.

Patients rarely present to an emergency department with the primary presentation of a previously undiagnosed malignancy.

Primary presentations include:

- Fever, fatigue, malaise, anaemia.
- Stridor, cough, haemoptysis, pneumonia.
- Headache, behaviour change, seizures.
- Abdominal pain.
- Constipation.
- Gastrointestinal bleeding.
- Unremitting pain.
- Abnormal FBC.

When malignancy is diagnosed or suspected, care should be taken to ensure that communication is clear and unambiguous and, if admission is not required on first presentation, that the follow-up arranged is timely and appropriate. Owing to the nature of modern oncological treatment, patients commonly attend the emergency department because of complications or side effects of therapy. Patients may also attend the emergency department through inability of palliative care services to meet their needs, symptoms related to progression of the underlying disease or as a result of catastrophic terminal events.

Oncology patients presenting to emergency department are often dehydrated and in a poor state of general nutrition. Patients are generally treated in oncology units by specialised staff in a controlled environment and they have high expectations of their emergency department visit. Oncology units often offer 'fast-track' or 'drop-in' services and these can be very effective. Cure rates for paediatric cancers are in the order of 60–70%, and oncologists are also able to offer improved cure rates or life expectancy to many of their adult patients.

The history should focus on the patient's cancer history and the patient's wishes and expectations regarding treatment. Information from the treating oncologist and the patients' treating doctors can be vital in determining the appropriate course of action.

Medical staff treating oncological emergencies should be aware of the legal and ethical issues surrounding these patients concerning living wills, 'Do not resuscitate' orders, power of attorney and the rights of next of kin, particularly when patients are unable to communicate their own wishes.

Pain, nausea and vomiting are common presenting complaints. Cancer patients are often acutely hypersensitive to simple procedures causing discomfort and pain, and extra care should be taken to minimise such stimuli. Narcotic analgesics should be used liberally to treat pain and titrated according to the patient's level of discomfort rather than a rigid dose schedule. Admission for pain control alone is often appropriate.

THE FEBRILE NEUTROPENIC PATIENT

Fever in the neutropenic patient is presumed to be due to infection until proved otherwise. The lack of other clinical findings is often remarkable. Patients who present looking well may die within hours of presentation. Untreated, there is a 50% mortality within 48 hours.

Management of the febrile neutropenic patient should be expedited by development of local protocols which ensure appropriate early treatment and early consultation with the treating oncology team.

Fever is defined as a temperature >38.3°C on any one occasion or temperature >38.0°C persisting for more than 1 hour in the absence of obvious environmental causes. Patients are often advised to keep a temperature chart and attend hospital if they have an oral temperature of 38°C or greater.

Neutropenia is defined as a neutrophil count of less than 0.5×10^9/L. Patients with a count less than 1.0×10^9/L, particularly if falling fast or expected to fall further rapidly, are also at increased risk.

A rapid, focused history and examination to identify treatment priorities and possible sources of infection should be performed. Digital rectal examination should not be performed. However, a careful inspection of the anus and perineum may reveal a focus of infection. Blood cultures should be taken from each lumen of an indwelling IV catheter and also from a peripheral vein if possible. A full septic work-up is conducted promptly.

Broad-spectrum antibiotics should be administered through an indwelling IV catheter if present or via a peripheral vein. Selected low-risk patients may be treated with oral antibiotics according to specific protocols. Selection of antibiotics should be based on protocols developed with regard to local patterns of resistance and aimed at broad coverage of potential pathogens. For example: Timentin 3.1 g qid plus gentamycin 5 mg/kg daily; or if the patient has penicillin allergy, cefepime 2 g bd plus gentamycin 5 mg/kg daily. For suspected IV catheter infection or severe mucositis, add vancomycin 1 g bd. For suspected GIT or perineal focus of infection, add Flagyl 500 mg bd.

There is increasing prevalence of gram-positive organisms due to the increasing incidence of mucositis associated with cancer treatment regimens, the use of long-term IV catheters and the use of prophylactic antibiotics to reduce the incidence of gram-negative sepsis. There is also an increasing incidence of fungal pathogens, particularly in patients with prolonged and profound (less than 0.1×10^9/L) neutropenia.

SPINAL CORD COMPRESSION

Most patients will complain of spinal pain before the onset of neurological symptoms.

The best chance of avoiding permanent paralysis is to investigate and treat before the development of neurological signs. More than 70% of lesions are in the thoracic spine and occur most commonly in patients with prostate, lung and breast carcinoma, although almost any malignancy may be associated with this condition.

Once weakness, sensory loss or incontinence has developed, treatment must be commenced within hours to give the patient any chance of regaining these functions. The initial symptoms and signs of weakness and/or paraesthesiae may be very subtle. Despite early treatment the prognosis remains poor.

Treatment is commenced with intravenous steroid, e.g. dexamethasone 20 mg stat, then 4 mg qid. MRI scan of the spine to localise the lesion should be followed by commencement of localised radiotherapy within hours. Surgical treatment is an option for selected cases.

HYPERCALCAEMIA

Hypercalcaemia of malignancy is common and occurs as a result of increased mobilisation of calcium from bone, often combined with impaired renal excretion. It is a marker of poor prognosis, the median survival being as short as 30–90 days.

Patients present with non-specific symptoms, including fatigue and muscle weakness, lethargy, anorexia and altered mental status, which may proceed to coma. Diagnosis is made using the corrected calcium level to measure ionised calcium. Corrected calcium = serum calcium + (0.02 × 40-serum albumin).

Initial treatment is focused on rehydration with isotonic saline IVb. When rehydrated, diuretics may be added to promote renal excretion of calcium. Biphosphonates (e.g. pamidronate) by infusion and calcitonin may be used to further reduce the calcium level.

CEREBRAL HERNIATION

Headache, usually of gradually increasing severity combined with signs of raised intracranial pressure (ICP) or localising neurological signs, requires rapid investigation and treatment. IV dexamethasone 20 mg and IV mannitol should be given. Consideration should be given to intubation and hyperventilation if rapid reduction of ICP and/or sedation for urgent head CT is required.

SUPERIOR VENA CAVA (SVC) OBSTRUCTION

SVC obstruction may be a primary presentation of lymphoma, lung or breast cancer. Symptoms include dyspnoea, chest pain, cough, headache and dysphagia. Signs include swelling of the neck, face and upper extremities, distension of neck and upper limb veins, and cyanosis of the face and upper extremities. While seldom immediately life-threatening, the condition requires prompt investigation and treatment.

CARDIAC TAMPONADE

Often a terminal event diagnosed at autopsy, but can occasionally occur in patients with treatable lesions or with a relatively good short-term prognosis. Breast and lung cancer are responsible for 75% of malignant pericardial effusions. Emergency treatment is with a pericardial drain if the patient is moribund and referral to a cardiothoracic surgeon for pericardiotomy.

TUMOUR LYSIS SYNDROME (TLS)

While this syndrome usually occurs after treatment has commenced, it may occur spontaneously. TLS most commonly occurs 72 hours after commencement of chemotherapy for leukaemia and lymphoma.

The cause of TLS is the breakdown of tumour cells and the accumulation of products of cell breakdown in the bloodstream. TLS is characterised by the rapid development of high serum nitrate, uric acid and phosphate levels and acute renal failure. Profound metabolic acidosis may occur, in excess of the degree of renal failure.

The syndrome may be prevented and treated by maintaining hydration and high urine output, use of allopurinol and keeping urinary pH >7.0 by addition of 50–100 mg sodium bicarbonate to each litre of IV fluids.

HYPERLEUKOCYTOSIS

This is defined as an extreme elevation of the WCC count $>100 \times 10^9/L$. Patients with acute myelocytic leukaemia (AML) have a significantly increased risk of early death if the WCC count is $>100 \times 10^9/L$. Patients with chronic lymphocytic leukaemia (CLL) tolerate such extreme cell counts better. Patients are at risk of tumour lysis syndrome (TLS) and leukostasis, particularly when the WCC is $>200 \times 10^9/L$.

Leukostasis is caused by an increased blood viscosity, which affects predominantly the cerebral and pulmonary circulations, causing headaches, dizziness, confusion, visual symptoms, acute coronary syndromes and changes in mental status, shortness of breath and right heart failure.

Initial treatment is to maintain hydration and treatment to prevent TLS as above and referral for exchange transfusion and/or leukaphaeresis.

RECOMMENDED READING

Kelly KM, Lange B. Oncologic emergencies. Pediatric Clinics of North America 1997; 44(4):809–830.

Schiff D, Batchelor T, Wen PY. Neurologic emergencies in cancer patients. Neurologic Clinics of North America 1998; 16(2):449–483.

Ducharme J. Acute pain and pain control: state of the art. Ann Emerg Med 2000; 35(6):592–602.

Krimsky WS, Behrens RJ, Kerkvliet GJ. Oncologic emergencies for the internist. Cleveland Clinic Journal of Medicine 2002; 69(3):209–222.

Flombaum CD. Metabolic emergencies in the cancer patient. Seminars in Oncology 2000; 27(3):322–334.

Yeung SJ, Escalante CP, Holland JF, Frei E. Holland-Frei oncologic emergencies. Hamilton, Ont: BC Decker; 2002.

46 Emergency presentations of drugs and alcohol

Alex Wodak

Alcohol and drugs share the common property of affecting mood or thought (i.e. are psychoactive) in a pleasurable manner and thus tend to be used repeatedly.

Problems resulting from alcohol and drug use can be classified as:

1. Acute—overdose, withdrawal.
2. Chronic—organ damage, dependence.

After dealing with the presenting complaint, some attempt must always be made by the emergency medical officer to intervene effectively with the underlying cause of the presentation, i.e. the alcohol or drug use. An effective intervention could be as simple as an explanation or a referral.

ALCOHOL

1. Use of >60 g/day (males) or >40 g/day (females) is considered hazardous. (Remember: one standard drink, e.g. one glass of wine, = 10 g alcohol.)
2. Over 5% of Australian men and 1% of Australian women drink hazardous quantities of alcohol.
3. One in six medical admissions to Australian hospitals is directly attributable to alcohol, and another one in six patients drinks hazardously but admission is required for reasons unrelated to alcohol.
4. Alcohol contributes to a substantial proportion of accident and emergency presentations.
5. Studies show emergency department staff grossly underestimate the proportion of intoxicated patients and, where recent alcohol use has been detected, the extent of intoxication is usually underestimated.

6. Alcohol can easily be measured in blood, breath or urine. Inexpensive portable machines are now available which will improve the rate and accuracy of diagnosis.
7. The presence of high blood alcohol concentrations in an individual who appears to have no psychomotor impairment suggests the presence of tolerance to alcohol and thus regular consumption of large quantities.
8. The most important aid to diagnosis is a high level of awareness.

Acute presentations
Overdose

1. The signs of alcohol intoxication are well known, e.g. slurred speech, ataxia, clouded judgment, disinhibited behaviour.
2. Alcohol intoxication can be fatal. The risk correlates roughly with the blood alcohol concentration (BAC). Any patient with a BAC >0.40 mg/100 mL should be regarded as high risk.
3. Alcohol intoxication results in respiratory depression. Inhalation of vomitus is a serious potential hazard.
4. Severely intoxicated individuals should be managed like other drug-overdosed patients, i.e. carefully observed and nursed lying on the side. Emetics are dangerous and cathartics are unnecessary as alcohol is absorbed rapidly.
5. The severity of central nervous system (CNS) depression is increased by other sedatives such as benzodiazepines, barbiturates, antihistamines and opiates.

Alcohol withdrawal scale (AWS)

The alcohol withdrawal scale (Figure 46.1) is a widely used, simple instrument for measuring the signs of alcohol withdrawal. It has several virtues: the fact that it is a standardised instrument encourages a better quality of care. The simplicity of the AWS makes it easy to use and encourages an earlier response. However, like all other instruments used in medicine, the AWS must be applied critically. The signs of alcohol withdrawal can be produced in many other conditions. Therefore, the diagnosis of alcohol withdrawal should always be reviewed in patients who do not respond to treatment.

Alcohol withdrawal

1. Alcohol withdrawal usually starts within 48 hours of abrupt cessation or decreased consumption of drinking.
2. In individuals who are used to high BACs and tolerant to alcohol, withdrawal symptoms may appear when the BAC has fallen but not yet reached zero.
3. Withdrawal is usually manifested by agitation, tremor and sweating. Confusion, anxiety and hallucinations are often present to a minor degree but the patient can usually be 'brought back to reality'.

4. Hallucinations are usually tactile, and less commonly visual. Auditory hallucinations can occur but usually suggest other diagnoses.
5. The presence of severe confusion, tremulousness, anxiety and hallucinations, where the patient cannot be 'brought back to reality', constitutes delirium tremens (DTs). This is relatively uncommon.
6. The risk of developing symptoms of alcohol withdrawal is poorly correlated with previous exposure to alcohol. Withdrawal symptoms following abrupt abstinence may not recur on future occasions.
7. Alcohol withdrawal is exacerbated by physical illness, injury or surgery.
8. People withdrawing from alcohol are very sensitive to their environment. An uncaring or hostile reception by medical and nursing staff in a crowded and noisy emergency department often rapidly results in an aggressive and violent patient.
9. The key to management is manipulation of the environment. Emphasise peace and quiet, even lighting without sharp shadows, and most of all a caring attitude from staff. It is often difficult to obtain these conditions in emergency departments.
10. Special detoxification centres are available in some hospitals for the management of intoxicated people or those going through alcohol withdrawal. If such a centre is not available or the patient has a medical or surgical problem requiring admission to hospital, the withdrawal can be attenuated by using a (cross-tolerant) sedative.

Diazepam

This long-acting benzodiazepine is ideal for the management of withdrawal. The therapeutic index is high. The aim of management is to achieve patient comfort. Doses of 10–20 mg are given orally and repeated every 1–2 hours until the patient has been comfortably sedated.

Frequent review is mandatory when the medication is being given every 2 hours. The diazepam is stopped once the patient is reasonably comfortable. Diazepam can be given by slow IV injection under careful supervision if the patient is fasting. The anticonvulsant properties of diazepam are also helpful. Avoid discharging patients who are still receiving benzodiazepines. Review the diagnosis if the patient has not responded to 80 mg diazepam.

Haloperidol (Serenace)

If alcohol withdrawal is severe (and not responding to benzodiazepines) or if delirium tremens is present, haloperidol is preferred. Doses of 2.5–5 mg can be given orally and repeated every 2–4 hours, provided the patient is being closely supervised. Haloperidol can also be given parenterally. Doses can be increased if the patient is exceedingly restless.

Phenothiazines

These are not recommended for use in alcohol withdrawal (or delirium tremens) as they lower the seizure threshold.

ALCOHOL WITHDRAWAL SCALE

MRN		SURNAME		
OTHER NAMES				
DOB		SEX	AMO	WARD/CLINIC

Please enter patient information or affix patient information label

Record AWS hourly for 4 hours, then at least 4/24 for 48 hours.

If total score is >5 increase observations to hourly. If total score is >6 notify medical officer.

DATE: / /	Time	Time	Time	Time	Time	Time	Time	Time	Time
Item 1 Perspiration									
Item 2 Tremor									
Item 3 Anxiety									
Item 4 Agitation									
Item 5 Temperature									
Item 6 Hallucinations									
Item 7 Orientation									
TOTAL SCORE									
Sedation/Type/Dose									

DATE: / /	Time	Time	Time	Time	Time	Time	Time	Time	Time
Item 1 Perspiration									
Item 2 Tremor									
Item 3 Anxiety									
Item 4 Agitation									
Item 5 Temperature									
Item 6 Hallucinations									
Item 7 Orientation									
TOTAL SCORE									
Sedation/Type/Dose									

See over for explanations of items and scoring guide

Figure 46.1 Alcohol withdrawal scale

ITEM 1
PERSPIRATION

No abnormal sweating	0
Moist skin	1
Localised beads of sweat on face, chest etc	2
Whole body wet from perspiration	3
Profuse maximal sweating—clothes and linen are wet	4

ITEM 2
TREMOR

No tremor	0
Slight intentional tremor	1
Constant marked tremor of upper extremities	2
Constant marked tremor of extremities	3

ITEM 3
ANXIETY

No apprehension or anxiety	0
Slight apprehension	1
Apprehension or understandable fear, e.g. of withdrawal symptoms	2
Anxiety occasionally accentuated to state of panic	3
Constant panic-like anxiety	4

ITEM 4
AGITATION

No sign of agitation—resting normally	0
Slight restlessness, unable to sit or lie still, awake when others are asleep	1
Moves constantly, looks tense, wants to get out of bed	2
Constantly restless, getting out of bed for no obvious reason, returns to bed if taken	3
Maximal restlessness, aggressive, ignores requests to stay in bed	4

ITEM 5
TEMPERATURE

Temperature of 37°C or less	0
Temperature of 37.1°C to 37.5°C	1
Temperature of 37.6° to 38°C	2
Temperature of 38.1°C to 38.5°C	3
Temperature greater than 38.5°C	4

ITEM 6
HALLUCINATIONS

(Spontaneous sense of perceptions of sight, sound, taste or touch for which there is no external basis)

No evidence of hallucinations	0
Distortions of real objects—aware these are not real if they are pointed out	1
Reports appearance of totally new objects or perception—aware these are not real if pointed out	2
Believes hallucination is real—remains orientated to place and person	3
Believes being in total non-existent environment, is preoccupied, unable to be reassured	4

ITEM 7
ORIENTATION

Fully oriented in person, place and time	0
Oriented in person, unsure of place and time	1
Oriented in person, disorientated in place and time	2
Doubtful of personal orientation, disoriented in place and time, short periods of lucidity	3
Disoriented in place/time and person. No meaningful contact can be made	4

Alcohol withdrawal may be a life-threatening condition that requires medical intervention in clinical settings.
The alcohol withdrawal scale is designed to alert medical staff to the possibility that the patient may be developing alcohol withdrawal and may be in need of appropriate sedation.

Figure 46.1 (continued)

Chronic presentations

Organ damage

Gastrointestinal bleeding is an emergency presentation frequently associated with excessive alcohol consumption.

Central nervous system (CNS)

Fitting

1. Occurs in 1–2% of episodes of alcohol withdrawal or delirium tremens.
2. Caused by metabolic changes secondary to rebound hyperventilation following removal of CNS depressant.
3. It is difficult to achieve therapeutic blood levels of phenytoin in patients who have suddenly stopped consuming alcohol.
4. Diazepam is the best agent to control fitting in the emergency department.
5. The first episode of fitting in an individual should always be investigated. Subsequent fits are investigated only if unusual features are present or if the seizure has occurred more than 48 hours after alcohol cessation.
6. Long-term anticonvulsants to control fitting in patients who have uncontrollable alcohol consumption is often problematic. Phenytoin compliance is variable and patients will often fluctuate between phenytoin intoxication and zero blood levels.
7. Subdural haematomas occur more frequently in patients drinking large quantities of alcohol because head injury, impaired coagulation and cerebral atrophy are common. They can present as epilepsy or as a space-occupying lesion.

Wernicke-Korsakoff syndrome

1. These two conditions are now considered to be one entity.
2. Episodes of Wernicke's encephalopathy manifest by confusion, ophthalmoplegia, nystagmus and ataxia. Patients frequently present with only one or two of these signs. Treatment with parenteral thiamine is strongly recommended in all such cases. Thiamine is a cheap and safe preparation, and should be administered generously to patients at risk of developing the Wernicke-Korsakoff syndrome. If untreated, this condition results in severe and irreversible brain damage requiring permanent institutionalisation. Prophylactic use of thiamine in at-risk patients is recommended. Alcohol-related brain injury is common, rarely diagnosed and usually manifests as subtle impairment of decision making.

Subdural haematoma

Early diagnosis is important, so a high degree of awareness is essential. Presentations are diverse but any unexplained drowsiness or lateralising signs should be investigated promptly.

Metabolic problems

1. Hypokalaemia is frequent and usually due to poor nutrition, vomiting or diarrhoea.
2. Rarer metabolic problems resulting from alcohol include lactic acidosis, hypoglycaemia and renal failure secondary to myoglobinuria.

Trauma

Patients presenting with multiple injuries (including head injuries) are often severely intoxicated.

Alcohol dependence

This manifests by:

1. Narrowing of drinking repertoire—inability to vary type of beverage or quantity consumed according to the social occasion.
2. Tolerance—increasing amounts of alcohol required to achieve the same degree of intoxication.
3. Salience—alcohol seen to dominate the priorities in a patient's life.
4. Compulsion to drink—patient plans the day so that a steady supply of alcohol, often covert, is always available.
5. Withdrawal symptoms—tremulousness, dysphoria, anorexia, nausea, vomiting, sweating (or some of these) usually occurring in the morning soon after waking.
6. Relief of withdrawal symptoms—the patient learns that withdrawal symptoms can be ameliorated by consuming alcohol and thus commences drinking earlier in the day as time passes.
7. Reinstatement after abstinence—rapid development of dependence following prolonged abstinence and then relapse.

Management of drinking problems

Diagnosis

1. To achieve a high diagnostic rate, a high level of awareness of particular risk groups is essential.
2. Males are more at risk than females, but this difference is diminishing.
3. High-risk occupations include: employment in beverage industry, police force, armed forces, administrators, businessmen, employment away from family.
4. The diagnostic rate will be improved by estimating BAC (or breath alcohol) as a routine, especially in conditions such as trauma.
5. A sound knowledge of alcohol-related medical conditions will increase the possibility of a correct diagnosis.
6. Be alert for subtle signs, e.g. conjunctival injection, facial telangiectasia, Dupuytren's contracture, spider naevi.

Assessment

1. Remember to ask every patient in a non-judgmental manner about alcohol consumption. Do not ask: 'Do you drink a lot?' Find out how many days a week a patient usually drinks and how much on each occasion.
2. Assess the severity of alcohol dependence by asking about the presence of early-morning alcohol withdrawal symptoms (see above) or other indicators of alcohol dependence.
3. Enquire systematically about medical or non-medical alcohol-related problems, including marital, employment, legal, financial and driving.
4. Recent research indicates that brief interventions by practitioners can be very effective, especially with individuals who have yet to develop well-established alcohol dependence or organ damage but are drinking hazardously.
5. Establish a 'contract' with the patient and help to advise whether alcohol consumption should be reduced (and, if so, how much) or whether abstinence is the desired goal.
6. Discuss ways of achieving these ends.
7. When a management plan has been established, arrange for long-term follow-up by the general practitioner, social work department, community health centre, hospital clinic or Alcoholics Anonymous. A telephone service available in each state provides advice and contact details about specialist agencies and services available throughout Australia.

TOBACCO

Minimal intervention with smokers presenting to emergency departments for conditions unrelated to tobacco can achieve a modest but none the less significant reduction in smoking prevalence. All smokers should therefore receive advice to stop immediately, and to consult a general practitioner or specialist agency if help is required in ceasing smoking. Smokers should be advised that mere reduction in tobacco consumption is pointless.

Wherever possible patients, relatives, visitors and staff must be discouraged from smoking for the comfort of the majority of the population who are non-smokers and, more importantly, because of the (now appreciated) hazards of passive smoking.

OPIOIDS

1. Injecting drug users (IDUs) are a heterogeneous population. The conventional stereotype represents only one segment of this population.
2. It is important to recognise that psychological as well as pharmacological factors maintain drug dependence.
3. IDUs increasingly use a wide variety of psychoactive drugs. Cannabis, barbiturates, hallucinogens, cocaine, amphetamines, benzodiazepines, tobacco and alcohol are used as substitutes or adjuncts to opioids.

4. Overdose is the major adverse pharmacological effect of opioids. Other problems result from microbiological (bacterial, viral, fungal and parasitic) and chemical contamination.

5. The death rate is lower than generally recognised (approximately 2% per annum) while spontaneous remission is commoner than generally believed (approximately 40% per 10 years).

Acute presentations
Overdose

As in other self-poisoning presentations, the patient is nursed on his/her side if the airway is endangered and careful observations are maintained. Charcoal and mannitol may be used if (as frequently occurs) the overdose includes other ingested drugs.

Renal failure associated with myoglobinuria may sometimes develop if the patient has been unconscious for some period and has developed muscle necrosis from pressure. The urine is stained intensely brown. Laboratory confirmation of this diagnosis should be arranged promptly.

Naloxone (0.4 mg/mL), a specific antagonist, is given first IM and then IV up to a maximum of 3 ampoules because the half-life of 30–90 minutes is much shorter than that of heroin. IM doses are absorbed more slowly. If only given IV, patients may wake up at the end of the injection and leave the emergency department (often against advice), and then collapse later from the same overdose.

Withdrawal

Opioid withdrawal is objectively milder than alcohol withdrawal and has been likened to a 'bad cold'. However, many experiencing heroin withdrawal complain about distressing symptoms. Withdrawal can be recognised in patients who are often restless, have a tachycardia and sweat profusely. They may complain of diarrhoea, abdominal cramps or a curious nasal snuffling. The pupils are widely dilated. The most helpful objective signs are mydriasis and gooseflesh, which can be seen fleetingly across the trunk and abdomen. Patients in opioid withdrawal should be referred to specialist detoxification centres (when available) unless a medical or surgical condition requires hospital admission.

Opiate withdrawal can be readily managed with sedation. Benzodiazepine is effective, and more recently clonidine at a dose of 15 mg/kg/24 hours (in divided doses) has been introduced for this purpose. The medication is slowly reduced over 3–4 days. Alternatively, methadone can be given. Usually 15–20 mg twice daily is sufficient but slightly higher doses may sometimes be necessary. It is best to give methadone in divided doses for the first 1–2 days until the patient's opioid tolerance is known. In addition to the above, symptomatic treatment can be given for diarrhoea (e.g. loperamide), abdominal pain (paracetamol) or muscle cramps (quinine). Sublingual buprenorphine is now regarded as the most effective drug for managing heroin withdrawal but assessment of the dose requires some experience.

Organ damage

Local infections

Phlebitis, cellulitis or deep abscesses may develop from local injection sites. These can usually be treated adequately with antibiotics, but surgical intervention is sometimes required.

Systemic infections

Septicaemia, endocarditis, lung abscesses and brain abscesses are some of the serious and well-recognised systemic infections. The endocarditis is often right-sided and difficult to diagnose. Lung abscesses are often associated with endocarditis. The complications of HIV infections should also be considered in the differential diagnosis.

Hepatitis

This may be due to hepatitis B, hepatitis C, D or sometimes hepatitis A. Admission to hospital may be required if the hepatitis is severe. Patients should be advised about the risk of spreading infection to others by needle or sexual contact. Advice should be given about alcohol consumption, diet and physical exercise, as the symptoms of hepatitis may recur following overindulgence or participation in active physical exercise before the liver has recovered.

Patients with hepatitis B or C should be referred for long-term follow-up. Patients without evidence of hepatitis B should be encouraged to be vaccinated.

Dependence

This is assessed by enquiring about drug use (number of injections per day, duration of drug use, expenditure on drug use) and psychological factors (which will be indicated by the damage to social development, e.g. relationships, employment).

Management

Diagnosis

The medical officer should be alert for drug-seeking behaviour, needle track marks or unexplained inconsistencies in the patient's history.

Assessment

A history of the patient's drug use and drug dependence should be obtained and specific enquiry made about medical and non-medical opioid-related problems.

Management plan

All patients should be advised that help is readily available. The risks of needle sharing (hepatitis, HIV) should be discussed. A number of specialised agencies are available in major cities. Information about resources available for treatment can be obtained by contacting telephone information services (e.g. Australian Drug Information Service in NSW). Several larger hospitals have clinics for referral, and community health centres usually have an alcohol or drug counsellor who can provide assistance.

Infection control procedures should be followed scrupulously because of the hazards of occupational exposure to agents such as HIV, hepatitis B or hepatitis C.

BARBITURATES

Acute problems

Medical indications are limited. These drugs are now rarely obtained by street drug users in Australia.

A range of barbiturates exist with widely differing durations of action. Overdose and withdrawal fits are the major pharmacological problems associated with barbiturates.

Overdose

1. Barbiturates were commonly included in the cocktail of drugs taken for self-poisoning episodes by street drug users.
2. 'Barbiturate blisters' containing clear fluid are seen on pressure areas.
3. Coma and respiratory depression following barbiturate overdose are often prolonged. Neurological pressure palsies or renal failure subsequent to myoglobinuria are very common.

Withdrawal

1. This may extend up to 2 weeks with longer-acting barbiturates.
2. Fitting is relatively uncommon.
3. The withdrawal can be managed with cross-tolerant benzodiazepines.

Management

The same principles are followed as with opiates.

BENZODIAZEPINES

A range of benzodiazepines are available with markedly different durations of action and some pharmacokinetic differences.

This group of drugs is relatively safe when used sparingly. Indiscriminate use is relatively rare. Some elderly patients are very sensitive to even small doses.

Benzodiazepine antagonists such as flumazenil are now readily available and their ability to rapidly and selectively reverse the inhibitory effects of benzodiazepines has been well demonstrated. Regimens involving bolus doses and in some cases infusions of flumazenil are rarely used because of the risk of inducing refractory fitting.

Overdose

Death from an overdose of benzodiazepines alone is unlikely. Usually benzodiazepines are taken with a mixture of other CNS depressants.

Withdrawal

1. The symptoms of benzodiazepine withdrawal may be somewhat similar to the original presenting complaint, e.g. insomnia, anxiety. Perceptual distortions are often present.
2. Fitting can occur as part of benzodiazepine withdrawal.
3. Benzodiazepine withdrawal begins 5–7 days after stopping the medication. Onset may be earlier with shorter-acting drugs or later with longer-acting medication.
4. Management is achieved by slowly reducing the dose of a longer-acting benzodiazepine (e.g. diazepam) over a fortnight.
5. Patients undergoing benzodiazepine withdrawal should always be referred for follow-up.

Organ damage

There is no significant organ damage associated with benzodiazepine use.

Dependence

To reduce benzodiazepine dependence, the dose and duration of treatment should be the minimum required to achieve the desired therapeutic effect. It should be noted that benzodiazepine users (when no clinical indication is seen to exist) should be referred for management. Usually it is possible to slowly reduce the dose over several weeks (with the agreement of the patient).

PRESCRIBED DRUGS

Emergency physicians should always be cautious about prescribing parenteral opioids to patients not known to the hospital, especially if the patient presents just before closing time, appears very familiar with drug names which are often slightly misspelt or mispronounced. Characteristic presentations are renal colic, backache, migraine or pancreatitis. Wherever possible, some objective evidence of the condition should be obtained, e.g. inspect freshly voided urine (passed under supervision) for the presence of microscopic haematuria in renal colic. Take-away doses of parenteral opioids should not be provided unless there is a good indication, e.g. disseminated malignancy or authentic letter from a medical practitioner. Avoid prescribing pethidine, which is responsible for most difficult cases of iatrogenic dependence.

COCAINE

Cocaine use has been increasing in Australia for some years but is still mainly confined to Sydney and is still much lower than in most other Western countries.

Overdose

1. Psychosis is a common presentation. This should be treated with benzodiazepines. Aggressive behaviour is common.
2. Fitting. Again the benzodiazepines are recommended. Caution should be used when intubating as cocaine causes sensitisation of the bronchial tree.
3. Arrhythmias, myocardial ischaemia, cerebral ischaemia occur.

Withdrawal

Some individuals report a rebound self-limiting period of mild depression following cessation of cocaine use. It is uncertain whether this represents a true withdrawal phenomenon.

Chronic use

Organ damage

1. Snorting of cocaine is associated with the development of nasal septal necrosis.
2. 'Free-basing' of cocaine is a method of inhaling cocaine following treatment of the salt (cocaine hydrochloride) with volatile solvents. Pulmonary damage can occur following inhalation of cocaine (as free base).
3. IV administration is associated with problems similar to the complications of heroin IV self-administration.

Management

Cocaine users who present with psychosis should be encouraged to remain and be reassured until they have returned to their normal state. Drug and alcohol counsellors are of assistance. Telephone information and counselling services provide information on specialised agencies.

ECSTACY

MDMA is a drug which has both amphetamine and mild hallucinogenic properties. Use of MDMA increased rapidly in many countries around the world in the 1990s, although the drug had been first synthesised many decades earlier. Side effects are uncommon but deaths have been attributed to MDMA. There is controversy about the degree of risk, but deaths are rare compared to the very large estimated number of episodes of use. There is also concern based on animal studies of possible nerve and brain damage. However, it is often difficult to ascertain the extent of risk of illicit drugs because of the uncertainty about the nature of the drugs actually taken. The short-term risks of MDMA may be reduced by ensuring that people taking the drug do not become dehydrated.

GHB

In the last few years, GHB (gammahydroxybutyrate) has become popular in many Western countries. GHB releases dopamine in the brain, causing effects ranging from relaxation to sleep at low doses.

Disorientation, nausea, muscle spasms, vomiting, convulsions and deep coma have been described following use of the drug. As with other illegal drugs, the dose taken is always uncertain. Deaths following the use of GHB have been reported, and admission to intensive care is not uncommon among those who require treatment from emergency departments of major hospitals.

TRENDS

The use of legal and illegal drugs is volatile. Overall, alcohol consumption has been declining in Australia since the early 1980s, although binge drinking among young people is increasing. Tobacco consumption has been declining slowly for some decades. Cannabis consumption has been increasing for decades in Australia but consumption has fluctuated somewhat in recent years. Amphetamine consumption has been increasing in Australia for more than a decade. The number of people injecting heroin in Australia has been increasing rapidly for decades but declined during the heroin shortage that began in late 2000 and continued during 2001. Cocaine and amphetamine use increased as heroin availability declined. During 2002, these trends reversed.

Other modern recreational drugs are discussed in Chapter 28.

RECOMMENDED READING

Australian Drug Information Network. Website. http://www.adin.com.au.

Cami, Jordi, Farre, Magi. Mechanisms of disease: drug addiction (review article). N Engl J Med 4 September; 349(10):975–986.

General toxic poisoning and drug overdose clinical resources. Online. Available: http://fsumed-dl.slis.ua.edu/clinical/emergency/conditions/toxicities/over-dose.htm.

Goldfrank LR, et al. Goldfrank's toxicologic emergencies. 7th edn. New York: McGraw-Hill; 2002.

Harrison's On Line. Biology of addiction. Available: http://harrisons.accessmedicine.com/server-java/Arknoid/amed/harrisons/co_chapters/ch386_p01.html.

Harrison's On Line. Cocaine and other commonly used drugs. Available: http://harrisons.accessmedicine.com/server-java/Arknoid/amed/harrisons/co_chapters/ch389_p01.html#.

Ward J, Mattick R, Hall W, eds. Methadone maintenance treatment and other opioid replacement therapies. Amsterdam: Harwood; 1998.

47 Emergency department haematology

Anthony J Dodds

THE ANAEMIC PATIENT

Anaemia is defined as a reduced haemoglobin (Hb) concentration in the blood. The red cell mass and the plasma volume can affect this value, so both these factors must be considered when interpreting a single value.

The symptoms and signs of anaemia (pallor, faintness, lethargy and anorexia) are unreliable. Anaemia may be asymptomatic and detected only on a routine blood count. The cause of anaemia can be ascertained by a logical sequence of investigation as follows. (This is based on the mean corpuscular volume—MCV.)

Microcytic

Low MCV

Causes

1. Iron deficiency serum: ferritin ↓.
2. Thalassaemia:
   • Hb studies.
3. Anaemia of chronic disease (may also be normocytic—see below):
   • Serum ferritin normal or ↑.
   • Serum iron ↓.
   • Serum transferrin normal or ↓.

Normocytic

Normal MCV

Causes

1. Secondary anaemia:
   e.g. chronic disease, renal failure.
2. Bone marrow disease:
   e.g. aplastic anaemia, marrow infiltration, malignancy.

3. Acute blood loss—reticulocyte count ↑.
4. Haemolysis—reticulocyte count ↑.

Macrocytic

Raised MCV

Causes

1. Megaloblastosis—low serum B_{12} or folate levels, marrow biopsy may be indicated.
2. Secondary macrocytic anaemia, e.g. alcohol, liver disease, hypothyroidism, some marrow disorders, marked reticulocytosis.

Principles of therapy

1. Establish the cause and treat.
2. Blood transfusion indicated only for acute anaemia with hypovolaemia
   • refractory anaemias (marrow failure) • severe symptoms, e.g. angina.
3. Most anaemias do not need blood transfusion. Transfusion can be risky with severe compensated anaemia, especially in the elderly and with cardiac disease.

THE PATIENT WITH ABNORMAL BLEEDING

Screening haemostasis tests are not warranted or cost-effective in the absence of clinical signs or history to suggest a bleeding diathesis.

The following are suggestive of a haemostatic disorder:

1. Family history of bleeding disorder.
2. Past history of excessive bleeding with minor haemostatic insults, e.g. tooth extraction, minor surgery, minor trauma, childbirth.
3. Excessive local bleeding without an obvious cause.
4. Generalised bleeding or bruising.

The usual screening tests are:

1. Vascular or platelet disorder: platelet count (PC) • platelet function.
2. Coagulation disorder: prothrombin time (PT) • activated partial thromboplastin time (APTT) • thrombin time (TT).

The following is a guide to the interpretation of these tests.

Platelet and vascular defects

PC↓

1. Marrow failure: e.g. aplastic anaemia, malignancy. Marrow biopsy abnormal.
   or
2. Peripheral destruction or sequestration: e.g. idiopathic thrombocytopenic purpura (ITP), hypersplenism (clinical splenomegaly), disseminated intravascular coagulation (DIC).

Table 47.1 Summary of the abnormalities seen in the commonly encountered acute conditions

N = normal

Condition	PT	APTT	TT	PC	SBT	XL-FDP
Liver disease	↑	↑	N or ↑	N	N	N or ↑
Heparin therapy	↑	↑ ↑	↑	N	N	N
Oral anticoagulant therapy	↑ ↑	↑	N	N	N	N
DIC	↑	↑	↑	↓	↑	↑ ↑
Massive blood transfusions	↑	↑	N or ↑	↓	↑	N or ↑

PC normal

1. Primary platelet dysfunction.
2. Secondary platelet dysfunction, e.g. aspirin, uraemia.

Coagulation defects

PT↑, APTT↑, TT↑

1. Heparin therapy.
2. DIC.
3. Hypofibrinogenaemia (rarely).

PT↑; APTT↑; TT normal

1. Oral anticoagulant therapy.
2. Vitamin K deficiency.
3. Liver disease.
4. Factor X, V or II deficiency (rarely).

PT↑, APTT normal, TT normal

1. Mild liver disease.
2. Early oral anticoagulant therapy.
3. Factor VII deficiency (rarely).

PT normal; APTT↑; TT normal

1. Lupus inhibitor.
2. Haemophilia (factor VIII or IX deficiency).

Figure 47.1 is a simplified version of the coagulation system to illustrate what the various coagulation screening tests are testing.

Therapy

Specific therapy is usually required only if the patient is bleeding or an operative procedure is contemplated.

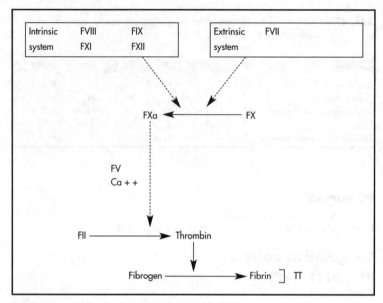

Figure 47.1 The coagulation system (simplified)

Components available include:

1. Fresh frozen plasma (FFP)—DIC, massive transfusion, liver disease, oral anticoagulant reversal.
2. Platelet concentrates—thrombocytopenia due to marrow failure.
3. Factor concentrates—specific deficiency.

See also Table 47.2.

ANTICOAGULANT THERAPY

Unfractionated heparin

Heparin inhibits coagulation at a number of sites, mainly via antithrombin-III. Administration is usually via constant IV infusion. Can also be given subcutaneously (SC), usually as prophylaxis.

Monitoring

APTT is the usual method. A baseline APTT should be established, then repeated at 4 hours and then daily. The APTT should be 2–3 times the baseline.

Table 47.2 Blood components

Product	Storage	Indications
Fresh whole blood	4°C	Massive blood loss
Red cell concentrate	4°C	Anaemia Moderate blood loss
Platelet concentrate	22°C	Thrombocytopenia bleeding Platelet dysfunctional bleeding
Fresh frozen plasma	-20°C	Massive transfusion DIC Liver disease Reversal of vitamin K antagonists
Factor concentrates	4°C	Specific factor deficiency

Reversal

For an overdose or serious bleeding, stop the heparin and give protamine sulphate IV slowly (1 mg/100 u heparin).

Side effects

1. Bleeding.
2. Thrombocytopenia—thrombosis (HITTS).

Low molecular weight heparins

These are mainly used for prophylaxis but can also be given for ambulatory full-dose therapy. They are usually given SC. They have a much longer half-life than unfractionated heparin. They cannot be monitored by APTT testing and cannot be reversed by protamine sulphate. They may cause less bleeding and less thrombocytopenia.

Vitamin K antagonists/oral anticoagulants e.g. warfarin

These inhibit synthesis of vitamin K-dependent clotting factors (II, VII, IX, X plus protein C and protein S).

Monitoring therapy

International normalised ratio (INR) is used. This is a standardised prothrombin ratio. The usual therapeutic range is 2.0–3.5.

Side effects

1. Bleeding.
2. Rash.
3. Teratogenesis.

Surgery in patients receiving vitamin K antagonists

What to do will depend on the type of surgery and the reason for administering anticoagulants. For minor procedures (e.g. tooth extraction), stop therapy 2 days before and recommence on the evening of surgery. For major procedures, it may be necessary to change to heparin, if continuing anticoagulation is required (e.g. artificial heart valve).

Changing from heparin to vitamin K antagonists

When commencing these drugs, the INR begins to fall within 36 hours, but this reflects only factor VII levels. It is necessary to continue heparin at lower doses for at least a 3-day overlap when commencing oral anticoagulants.

Reversal

FFP will acutely reverse the effect in bleeding patients. Vitamin K will act more slowly and permanently reverse the effect, but it may be more difficult to anticoagulate the patient again.

BLOOD TRANSFUSION

Transfusion reactions

Haemolytic

1. Immediate (haemolysis of donor cells usually due to ABO incompatibility).
   a. Flushing, backache, chest pain, rigors, haemoglobinuria.
   b. Treatment: stop blood. Take urine and blood sample. Watch urine output and give frusemide or 20% mannitol depending on the intravascular volume. If oliguria persists, treat as acute renal failure.
   c. Watch for shock and DIC. Differential diagnosis: already haemolysed blood from freezing or heating.
2. Delayed (1–2 weeks after transfusion). Due to secondary antibody response. Often no incompatibility at initial crossmatch.
   a. Fall in haemoglobin or late jaundice.
   b. Recheck Coombs' test and antibody screen.

Note: It is recognised that the majority of haemolytic reactions to red cells are due to clerical errors in transfusion practice.

Reactions to white cell antibodies

These occur after previous transfusion or pregnancy. 'Febrile reactions':

1. Are delayed from 0.5–3 hours after start of transfusion.
2. Brisk rise in temperature to 38–40°C with chills and headache.
3. Diagnosis by presence of white cell antibodies.
4. Give paracetamol orally or antihistamine IV and slow rate of transfusion.
5. Leukocyte-poor blood may also be used with a leukocyte blood filter.

Urticarial and anaphylactic reactions

1. Anaphylaxis (rare—due to allergy to donor plasma):
   a. Occasionally in IgA-deficient individuals.
   b. Shock—bronchospasm, laryngeal oedema, severe urticaria.
   c. Stop blood, treat with adrenaline, antihistamines and occasionally corticosteroids.
2. Urticarial reaction (occasionally accompanied by asthma):
   a. Usually a response to antihistamines.
   b. Washed red cells may be used.

Reactions to bacterial pyrogens and bacteria

1. Pyrogenic reaction:
   a. Extremely rare.
   b. Clinical picture resembles leukocyte and platelet antibody reaction.
2. Infected blood. Causes shock, fever, coma, convulsions, sudden death. Beware blood removed prematurely from blood bank or heavily haemolysed supernatant or previously punctured top.
   a. Take blood for cultures.
   b. Treat shock and give large doses of appropriate antibiotics.

Circulatory overload

Slow or stop transfusion. Treat as for cardiac or pulmonary oedema. May need venesection.

Air embolism

1. Raised JVP, cyanosis, hypotension, praecordial murmur.
2. Treat with head down, feet up and patient on left side.
3. Administer 100% oxygen.

Citrate intoxication

Only in neonate, impaired liver function and massive blood transfusion.

1. Muscles twitching, hypotension, ECG changes, bleeding.
2. Give calcium gluconate 10 mL 10% by IV injection.

Massive transfusion

1. Hypothermia (use blood warming).
2. Deficiency of coagulation factors. Check coagulation profile (use FFP).
3. Thrombocytopenia (use platelet transfusion).
4. Acidosis.
5. Hypocalcaemia.

Infectious complications—possible risk with nucleic acid testing (NAT)

1. HIV (<1:920,000).
2. Hepatitis B (<1:100,000).
3. Hepatitis C (<1:10,000).

4. HTLV-I (<1:100,000).
5. Others, e.g. syphilis, malaria, cytomegalovirus (CMV). CMV has the highest incidence but lowest risk to patients unless they are immunocompromised.

INAPPROPRIATE USE

There is considerable evidence of inappropriate use of blood components. Various strategies have been developed to reduce this inappropriate use, including guidelines, consensus conferences, monitoring, education and self-audit by clinicians.

RECOMMENDED READING

Provan A, Amos A, Smith A. Clinical haematology: a postgraduate exam companion. Oxford University Press: Butterworth-Heinemann; 1997.
Hoffbrand AV, et al. Essential haematology. 4th edn. Oxford: Blackwell Scientific Publications; 2001.
Clinical practice guidelines on the use of blood components. Commonwealth of Australia; 2002.

48 Diagnostic imaging in emergency patients

E S Seelan

The aim of this chapter is to explain briefly the need for and usefulness of diagnostic imaging services in emergency situations. Many of these emergencies arise 'after hours' and most emergency departments have no immediate access to radiologists. The chapter also outlines the various diagnostic imaging modalities available, the basic principles involved in each modality and some clues to interpreting some of the most obvious lesions.

IMAGING MODALITIES
Plain X-rays

- Commonly used modality.
- X-ray beam is passed through the body.

Different tissues of the body absorb different amount of X-rays. Unabsorbed X-rays are recorded on a film placed on the opposite side. Bone absorbs the most, hence it looks white on film. Air absorbs almost none, hence it looks black on film. Other tissues are demonstrated in shades between black and white.

Plain X-rays are performed as the first line of emergency investigations in many instances, as in fractures, abdominal or chest pain.

Ultrasound

Transducers used in this examination pass ultrasound into the body and also receive the echoes. Intensity of echoes depends on the degree of absorption of sound waves by various tissues. On the image, echogenic areas appear white and sonolucent areas (that transmit sound, e.g. fluid) appear black.

Immediate and instant demonstration of organs by real-time ultrasound imaging plus the fact that it is non-invasive and harmless (no radiation) have made this tool very popular. It is used in the following:

1. To find out whether a lesion or lump is solid or cystic.
2. Abdominal and pelvic organs: liver, gallbladder, bile ducts, pancreas, spleen, kidneys, aorta, inferior vena cava (IVC), bladder, prostate, uterus and ovaries, renal stones, gallstones, aortic aneurysm, traumatic and other haematomas, abscess and abnormal fluid collections can be demonstrated.
3. Small parts (thyroid, testes and breast) and neonatal heads for ventricular size etc.
4. Obstetrical workup including study of fetus for early detection of abnormalities. For emergencies like ectopic pregnancy, vaginal ultrasound is extremely useful.
5. Ultrasound-guided biopsy and interventional procedures.
6. Musculoskeletal investigations, e.g. shoulder, knee, muscles and tendon injuries, acute tenosynovitis.
7. Duplex and colour doppler ultrasound:
   - With the advent of duplex and colour-flow Doppler, it is now easy to identify arteries and veins non-invasively. This modality should be the first line of imaging for the detection of deep vein thrombosis (DVT) in the limbs. (This study can be difficult in extremely swollen, oedematous lower legs.) In difficult cases, venography can be performed. It should be remembered that ultrasound is non-invasive and can be performed repeatedly even in pregnant patients with suspected DVT.
   - Duplex ultrasound is useful in identifying superficial thrombophlebitis.
   - While excluding thrombosis, ultrasound study can also diagnose other causes of a swollen, tender calf such as ruptured Baker's cyst, haematoma in calf muscle, e.g. a gastrocnemius tear, mass in groin, axilla.

- Doppler ultrasound is useful in detecting and localising acute arterial occlusion in the limbs and in the investigation of peripheral vascular disease and carotid arterial disease.
- It is also useful in assessing renal artery stenosis and renal parenchymal vascular disease in the investigation of hypertension.

Computerised tomography (CT)

The same principles as in plain X-rays are applied in CT, but there are two main modifications:

1. The X-ray tube is rotated around the body in an axial plane.
2. Instead of an X-ray film, detectors are used on the opposite side. Multiple fixed detectors are placed around the body to pick up the signals as the X-ray tube rotates around the body. Signals from the detectors are digitalised and the computer builds up an image, which can be seen on a TV monitor or recorded on a film.

The resulting images are transverse sections of the part examined. Using the stored information of consecutive thin transverse sections, the images can be reconstructed in sagittal, coronal and oblique planes. CT is now a proven diagnostic tool which delivers valuable information to help the early diagnosis of many lesions and disease. Its use is greatly appreciated in many emergencies such as head injuries and some chest and abdominal emergencies. It is also useful in demonstrating fractures that are not shown by plain X-rays.

Helical CT scanning

Helical or spiral CT scanning is an improvement that allows very quick scanning of a patient (shorter scanning time than conventional CT) with increased accuracy of lesion detection resulting from volumetric data acquisition. In conventional CT, X-ray exposure and patient movement through the gantry alternate, whereas in helical CT, X-ray exposure and patient movement take place simultaneously, giving a 'spiral impression'.

Advantages
1. Greater length of patient's body can be scanned with one 'breath-hold' thus producing contiguous images without interruption, e.g. a 30-second scan can cover most of the chest.
2. Eliminates respiratory artefacts and reduces partial volume effect, peristaltic and other movement artefacts.
3. Produces overlapping images without extra radiation exposures.
4. Using a window workstation, the acquired images can be reconstructed in multiplanar and three-dimensional images with excellent clarity.

Multislice CT scans

This is a recent advancement whereby the speed of scanning and resolutions are considerably improved by using more efficient detectors and obtaining thinner slices per rotation of the X-ray tube as the patient passes through the gantry.

Scanners are available to obtain 4, 8 or 16 slices (per rotation) of about 0.3–0.5 mm thickness.

Advantages and uses

1. Speed—some scanners can complete a body scan in 20 seconds. This is useful in ICU, paediatric, elderly, trauma and postoperative patients, where a shorter breath-hold and quick scanning is required.
2. High resolution and fewer artefacts.
3. Low radiation.
4. Less IV contrast usage by allowing the scanning to start when the contrast reaches the area of interest (contrast detection system).
5. Multi-planer reconstruction without loss of resolution.
6. 3D reconstruction is useful for surgical planning.
7. CT angiography (including pulmonary angiography to detect pulmonary embolism) and cholangiography.
8. CT fluoroscopy—useful in interventional work, e.g. placement of needle for biopsy, facet joint injection.
9. Virtual endoscopy—enables a bronchoscopic view or colonoscopic view to be obtained.
10. Coronary angio—introduction of 16-slice CT will be useful for cardiac and coronary assessment without the need for catheterisation.

Magnetic resonance imaging (MRI)

In the past 20 years MRI has gradually become the technique of first choice in the investigation of many diseases. The physics involved in MRI is more complex than for any other radiological technique. However, the basic principle is indicated in the original terminology, nuclear magnetic resonance (NMR).

Nuclear

1. Unlike X-ray images, which are produced by attenuation of X-ray photons by the outer orbital electrons in the atoms of the elements in the body tissue, the MRI signal arises from the centre of the atom— the nucleus. The nuclei used in MRI are those of hydrogen atoms.
2. Hydrogen is selected because:
   - It makes up about 80% of the human body.
   - Its nucleus has only one proton and has magnetic property.
   - Solitary protons give it a larger magnetic field (or moment).

Magnetic

1. The hydrogen proton is a small, positively charged particle with associated angular momentum or spin. This situation represents a current loop and results in the formation of a magnetic field with north and south poles (dipoles). In other words, the protons behave as a tiny

magnet within the tissues. All nuclei used in MRI must have this property.

2. In the absence of influence from any external magnetic fields, the protons tend to orientate randomly in all directions. However, when a strong static external magnetic field is applied, these dipolar protons tend to align parallel to the direction of the external magnetic field (longitudinal plane).

3. The strong external magnetic field must be homogeneous over a volume large enough to contain the human body. This explains why the magnet tunnel is much longer than the CT gantry.

Resonance

1. This is a phenomenon whereby an object is exposed to an external oscillating disturbance that has a frequency similar to its own frequency of oscillation. Therefore, when the hydrogen proton is exposed to an external disturbance with a similar frequency to its own, the proton gains energy from the external disturbance. This is called resonance. This can happen only if the external disturbance is applied at 90° to the magnetic field of the proton. The oscillation frequency of the hydrogen proton in a static magnetic field strength used in clinical MRI corresponds to radio-frequency band (RF) in the electromagnetic spectrum.

2. Therefore, for resonance of hydrogen to take place, an RF pulse at the same frequency as the hydrogen proton must be applied at 90° to the magnetic field of the proton. The application of RF pulse that causes resonance is called excitation, as it results in the nuclei gaining energy. This energy causes the magnetic field of the protons to change direction. Enough RF pulse energy is given to the proton to change the direction from longitudinal to transverse plane (flip angle of 90°). Now the protons are rotating in the transverse plane. According to the laws of electromagnetism, if a receiver coil is placed in the transverse plane, the transverse magnetisation produces a voltage in the coil. This voltage constitutes the MR signal.

3. When the RF pulse is turned off, the hydrogen protons return to their original positions in the longitudinal plane. This is called relaxation. There are two main types of relaxations (T1 and T2). T1 is the return of net magnetisation to the longitudinal plane. T2 is the decay of magnetisation in the transverse plane. These two relaxations and their time variances are used to create imaging sequences. All relaxation times are based on fat and water. This is where most of the body's hydrogen protons are.

4. T1 images are known for their anatomical details. In T1 images, fluid appears black and fat appears white.

5. T2 images are known for their contrast. In these images, the fluid appears white and fat appears grey.

6. Proton density images are a combination of T1 and T2. These images specifically look at the concentration of hydrogen protons.

The above is a simple explanation of the basics, but the more complex physics involved in the formation of MR images is beyond the scope of this chapter.

Summary

MRI involves the use of:

1. Large magnet to produce static magnetic field.
2. RF generator to produce RF pulses.
3. Hydrogen nuclei—different tissues have characteristic differences in hydrogen protons concentration. Therefore, the MR signal and hence the image obtained basically represent the different distribution of hydrogen protons in the body.
4. Computer to convert the signals into images in various anatomical planes.

Advantages and uses

1. No ionising radiation.
2. Free of artefacts from adjacent bones and gas. Therefore it is excellent to demonstrate soft tissues adjacent to bones, e.g. base of brain and spinal cord.
3. Excellent resolution—even without contrast enhancement, MR is much more sensitive in detecting contrast differences between various tissues. This is due to the intrinsic differences in hydrogen proton density as well as T1 and T2 relaxation, magnetic susceptibility and motion in various tissues.
4. Uses:
   - **Brain**—very early infarction, occlusion of major intracranial vessels, haematoma (parenchymal and subdural), dural sinus thrombosis, aneurysm. Demyelination, congenital abnormality, meningeal disease, investigation of epilepsy. Tumours, posterior fossa lesions including acoustic neuroma, pituitary and parasellar lesions.
   - **Spine**—cord compression, trauma, cord infarction, tumour, myelopathy, radiculopathy, brachial plexus avulsion etc.
   - **Musculoskeletal**—musculotendinous injury and pathology, joint injury and pathology (e.g. rotator cuff injury in shoulder, meniscal and ligamentus injury in knee), fractures not detected by X-ray (e.g. fracture of neck of femur), bone infection, avascular necrosis, marrow disorders, bone and soft tissue tumours.
   - **Chest**—constrictive pericarditis, aortic and great vessel dissection, congenital cardiac and great vessel abnormality, lung cancers closer to the chest wall and apex (e.g. Pancoast's tumour).
   - **Abdomen**—adrenal mass using chemical shift imaging, cholangiography etc.
   - **Pelvis**—uterine and cervical tumours and abnormalities, differentiation of adenomyosis from fibroids, endometriosis assessment, bladder tumour etc.

Contrast-enhanced MRI

In spite of the excellent tissue contrast definition without intravenous contrast, the contrast-enhanced MRI (gadolinium) provides even better imaging sensitivity and specificity.

The enhanced contrast shows subtle parenchymal as well as leptomeningeal lesions not otherwise visible, e.g. very small metastatic lesions, acoustic neuromas of 2–3 mm, pituitary microadenomas, differentiation of the actual size of tumour from the surrounding oedema and differentiation of more malignant areas from less malignant areas. These are helpful for the purpose of treatment and to select the exact site for biopsy.

Ongoing research into the development of new contrast agents targeted at specific organs, disease processes, cells or gene type is likely to result in considerable expansion of the use of MRI.

MR angiography (MRA)

Protons in flowing blood (moving protons) produce a high signal against the background of little or no signal from the surrounding stationary tissues—hence the development of the MR angiogram without display of the background soft tissue.

Contraindications

Cardiac pacemakers, ferromagnetic intracranial aneurysm clips (except where MR-compatible clips have been used), cochlear implants, intravascular stainless steel stents inserted less than 6 weeks previously, surgical clips in chest and abdomen inserted less than 1 week previously, metal workers with metallic foreign body in the eye.

Disadvantages

Because of the length of the magnet (tunnel), some patients may experience claustrophobia. This can mostly be overcome by sedation.

Contrast study

The main limitation in the use of plain X-rays is the superimposition of the shadows of various organs. In many instances this can be overcome by introducing contrast.

1. Barium to demonstrate the gastrointestinal tract (GIT).
2. Intravenous pyelogram (IVP)—IV contrast demonstrates kidneys, collecting system and bladder. Helpful to assess function (excretion) and to detect stones, obstruction, space-occupying lesion, deformities of renal tract etc.
3. Micturating cystourethrogram (MCU)—to demonstrate urethra, bladder and vesicoureteral reflux.
4. Arthrography—e.g. shoulder, to detect rotator cuff tears. Sometimes this is combined with a CT scan, which helps to identify glenoid labral

injury etc (arthrograms may not be required if there is access to high-resolution ultrasound and MRI scan).

5. Herniography—contrast injected into the peritoneal cavity to detect clinically undetectable inguinal or femoral hernia that is producing symptoms.

6. Myelography—contrast injected via lumbar puncture demonstrates the subarachnoid space around the spinal cord and nerve roots. With the advent of CT and MRI the need for this examination is almost nil.

7. Cholangiography—in the past, oral cholangiograms were performed, but this is now replaced by CT cholangiography. This examination requires slow infusion of contrast (which is excreted by bile) followed by helical CT scan and 3D reconstruction of the biliary tree.

8. Sialography—contrast injected into the salivary ducts (parotid or submandibular) to identify stones, strictures, sialectasis and lesions in the glands.

9. Hysterosalpingogram—contrast is injected into the uterine cavity to demonstrate the uterine cavity, fallopian tubes and to detect patency of the tube in the investigation of infertility.

10. Sinogram and fistulogram—contrast injection shows the cavities and communications.

11. Venography—could detect clots, incompetent perforators and varicose veins (current trend is to do Doppler and colour Doppler ultrasound examination).

12. Arteriography—contrast injected into various arteries using catheters demonstrates the arteries in various organs. It is used to demonstrate occlusions, narrowing of arteries, aneurysms, bleeding points, AV malformation and tumours. Digital subtraction angiography (DSA) has replaced conventional angiograms. In this technique, the X-ray images are digitalised, and stored and manipulated by computer. The image signal of an area or organ obtained before the injection of contrast is subtracted from the image signal obtained after injection of contrast into the vessels. This is done by the computer.

Advantages

1. The resulting image will demonstrate the vessels and branches without superimposition of bones and other soft tissue shadows.

2. Owing to the fact that the image signals can be intensified by the computer, contrast of low concentration and volume can be used with thinner catheters.

Interventional radiology

Radiologists are able to perform certain therapeutic and interventional diagnostic procedures using various imaging equipment (fluoroscopy, ultrasound, CT and MR), needles, catheters and guide wires.

1. Dilation of narrowed arteries—transluminal angioplasty, insertion of vascular stents.
2. Embolisation—of bleeding vessels, preoperative tumour embolisation to assist surgery by reducing blood loss and reducing the duration of surgery, palliative embolisation of tumours, embolisation of some vascular abnormalities.
3. Thrombolysis—using local low-dose intraarterial injection of thrombolytic agents to relieve thromboembolism in certain vessels such as coronary artery and peripheral arteries.
4. Inferior vena cava filter insertion to prevent pulmonary embolism caused by clots arising from pelvis and lower limbs.
5. Percutaneous insertion of stents to relieve biliary or ureteral obstruction.
6. Percutaneous drainage of cysts, abscesses, pleural effusion etc.
7. Percutaneous removal of renal or biliary stones when other methods are contraindicated.
8. Biopsy of deep and superficial lesions—lesions in liver, pancreas, kidneys, other abdominal masses, chest lesions, breast, thyroid, lymph node and other superficial and deep lesions.

Intravenous contrast reaction

Even though the incidence of fatality is much less than in street accidents, it is a great worry to doctors. Some statistics show that about 1 in 80,000 patients developed severe or fatal reaction when ionic contrast was used. Incidence of mild reaction is probably about 5–15%, moderate reaction about 1–2% and severe reaction is probably about 0.2%. However, with the use of non-ionic contrast and taking good precautions, the incidence of reaction is said to have reduced to about one-third to one-quarter of the frequency.

Usually patients who develop a severe reaction have some other aggravating disease as well.

The exact pathogenesis of the reaction is not very clear. However, the following are possible mechanisms:

1. Chemotoxic effect.
2. Hyperosmolar reactions causing erythrocyte or endothelial damage, blood–brain barrier damage and vasodilation.
3. Vasomotor reactions with release of vasoactive substances such as histamine, serotonin and bradykinin.
4. Vaso-vagal reaction with inhibition of enzymes such as cholinesterase.

Symptoms and signs

Most reactions occur within minutes of injection. However, delayed reactions have also been reported.

Mild reactions—hot flush, burning sensation, arm pain, dizziness, nausea, vomiting, headache and urticaria—are thought to be due to systemic effects as a result of histamine liberation. Usually reassurance and restoration of the patient's confidence is all that is required, but sometimes oral antihistamine for urticaria, mild analgesics and sometimes tranquillisers for anxiety (5 mg benzodiazepine) may also be helpful.

Moderate reactions involve a slightly more serious manifestation of the above symptoms, with or without a moderate degree of hypotension and bronchospasm. They usually respond to reassurance and antihistamine (IM or IV), benzodiazepine 5 mg, salbutamol inhalation for bronchospasm, hydrocortisone (100–500 mg IM or IV) and occasionally adrenaline 0.3–1 mL of 1/1000 IM.

Severe reactions can be life-threatening and involve a severe form of the above reactions plus convulsion, unconsciousness, laryngeal oedema, bronchospasm, pulmonary oedema, arrhythmia, hypotension, cardiac arrest, anaphylactic shock. Severe reactions require urgent treatment (see treatment of anaphylaxis, Chapters 12 and 13).

Predisposing factors—in the presence of these, the incidence of reaction can be about 2–10 times as severe:

1. Previous adverse reaction to contrast.
2. Significant allergic history including iodides.
3. Asthma.
4. Cardiac disease.
5. Dehydration—all patients should be adequately hydrated as dehydration is dangerous, especially in patients with diabetes, renal impairment and multiple myeloma.
6. Haematological and metabolic conditions such as sickle cell anaemia, patients with known phaeochromocytoma.
7. Renal disease—patients with preexisting renal disease, especially patients with diabetes, have an increased risk of reaction as well as of renal failure. Metformin drugs used for diabetic treatment are excreted by the kidneys and in patients with renal impairment this has been known to cause lactic acidosis and lead to acute alteration of renal function. In view of this, all diabetic patients treated with metformin drugs must have serum urea and creatinine levels reviewed before the intravascular contrast injection (serum urea must be less than 6.7 mmol/L and serum creatinine must be less than 0.10 mmol/L). The metformin drugs should be discontinued from 48 hours before until 48 hours after the injection and should be recommenced only after checking the serum urea and creatinine. If required, another hypoglycaemic agent may be used during this period.

Prevention and precautions

1. Always try to use non-ionic contrast.
2. Like other drugs, contrast agents should be used only if indicated and should be used in the smallest possible dose and concentration that will result in adequate imaging.
3. Weigh the possible advantages of using contrast against the possible risk. In patients with a strong history, contrast should be avoided. In many

cases the contrast study may be replaced by another examination such as ultrasound, CT or MRI.

4. A test dose may not help. However, some authors advise a small test dose of about 1 mL IV in high-risk patients who definitely require contrast for diagnosis.

5. In some patients (e.g. asthmatic and allergic patients) premedication with oral corticosteroid and possibly antihistamines could be given during the 24 hours preceding the test. The patients should also be adequately hydrated.

IMAGING OF THE HEAD

Common emergencies are: trauma, severe headaches, collapse, syncope, seizures and stroke.

Trauma

Plain X-ray of skull

Indications

1. History of unconsciousness.
2. Palpable or visible depression on skull.
3. Laceration or penetrating wound.
4. Cerebrospinal fluid (CSF) or blood discharge from ear or nose.
5. Fits.
6. Presence of neurological signs.

Views

1. Anteroposterior, lateral, Towne's and basal views.
2. 'Shoot through' lateral (patient in supine position and X-ray beam horizontal) is useful to demonstrate air–fluid levels, especially in sinuses.

Interpretation

1. Every doctor working in the accident and emergency department should try to be familiar with the appearance of normal skull X-rays. The best way to detect abnormality is to know the normal. (This applies to every modality of imaging.)

2. One should be familiar with the skull sutures, vascular markings, venous lakes along the inner table of the skull vault, appearance of normal sinuses and normal intracranial calcifications (e.g. pineal body, choroid plexus).

3. Fracture of the skull can be an undepressed crack fracture or a depressed fracture.

4. Do not misinterpret sutures and vascular markings as fractures. You can avoid this by knowing the normal positions of sutures and vascular markings. Sutures are usually serrated. Fracture lines are usually 'blacker' than the vascular markings.

5. Beware of metopic sutures—in some patients such a suture may persist throughout life and may look like a fracture.

In depressed fractures, one or more fragments may be depressed. In some cases, oblique or tangential views may be needed to demonstrate depression.

If pineal calcification is present, look for shift. This indicates a space-occupying lesion such as a haematoma. (Towne's view is ideal for this.)

Look for air–fluid level in sinuses or air in ventricles in the horizontal beam lateral view.

Plain X-rays of the face

Most facial injuries can be evaluated clinically. However, X-rays are performed for:

1. Confirmation.
2. Assessment of the degree of displacement or depression of fragments.
3. Detecting fractures in the presence of extreme facial swelling that makes palpation difficult.

In some cases facial fractures are associated with other serious emergencies such as intracranial, neck or chest injuries, which may require emergency management such as maintenance of airway. In these patients, X-rays of the face can be postponed to the latter part of the management and may even be deferred for a few days.

Views

- Routine facial views—posteroanterior (PA), occipitomental (OM) and lateral.
- Special views—nose (AP, lateral and axial), zygoma (Towne's or modified basal view for the arch), orbital, mandible (PA, lateral, oblique and sometimes pantomogram—OPG—and occlusal view for symphysis menti).

Classification

For convenience, facial fractures can be divided into three types: upper third, middle third and lower third.

1. **Upper third.** The upper third, which is above the superior orbital margin, includes the superior orbital margin, the frontal sinuses and the adjacent frontal bone:
   - Fracture of superior orbital margin appears as interrupted cortical margin with or without depression, either craniocaudally or posteriorly.
   - Fracture of the frontal sinuses may involve the anterior wall or both anterior and posterior walls.
   - Fracture may be linear or comminuted, depressed or undisplaced.
   - Fracture of sinus may extend into orbit—therefore look for orbital emphysema.
   - Fractures causing laceration of mucosa in sinus or fractures communicating with skin laceration are compound fractures.

2. Middle third. This includes the nose, zygoma, orbit (floor, lateral and medial walls) and maxillae (midfacial bones).

- *Nose.* Nasal fracture and deviations are easily detectable clinically, but X-rays are needed in patients with severe swelling or for confirmation of the degree of damage. Fractures of nasal bones are better seen in lateral view (soft tissue exposure). Deviation is seen in axial view. PA view may demonstrate fracture of frontal process of maxilla and also deviation of fracture of the bony part of nasal septum. Associated fractures in severe cases are: bony nasal septum, cribriform plate, frontal process of maxilla, anterior nasal spine of maxilla.

- *Zygoma.* Fracture of the arch usually involves three sites causing depression of the arch. A commonly seen severe form of fracture is of the zygomaticomaxillary complex. One fracture line extends from the zygomaticofrontal suture across the orbital process of zygoma (lateral wall of orbit) up to the lateral aspect of the inferior orbital fissure. Another fracture extends from the lateral wall of maxilla to the inferior orbital margin (near the inferior orbital foramen) and extends along the floor of the orbit to the lateral aspect of the inferior orbital fissure, thus completing a circle. This fracture can cause separation of the zygomatic bone from the maxilla and orbit. (This fracture can be well understood if the reader takes a dry skull and follows the line of the fracture described above.)

- *Orbit*—blowout fracture. The orbital margin is stronger than the floor and medial wall of the orbit. The posterior half of the orbital floor is formed by the thin orbital plate of the maxilla. The medial wall is formed by the orbital plate of the ethmoid. These two orbital plates are very weak. Sometimes the orbital margin can be intact and the force of injury can be transmitted to the floor and medial walls of the orbit, causing blowout fractures into the adjacent sinuses. Therefore, in the presence of orbital emphysema, a blowout fracture should be suspected.

- *Maxilla*—fractures of midfacial bones. These fractures tend to follow a certain pattern. There are three common patterns, which are named after the person who described them—Le Fort I, II and III fractures.

  a. Le Fort I is the lowest and an almost horizontal fracture through the maxilla, causing separation of the lower part of the maxilla. The fracture line extends from the inferolateral aspect of the nasal aperture horizontally across the lower part of the anterolateral and posterolateral walls of the maxilla. It then passes almost horizontally across the lower part of the medial and lateral pterygoid plates, reaches the medial wall of the maxillary antrum and extends to the inferolateral aspect of the nasal aperture, thus completing a circle.

  b. Le Fort II fracture separates the midfacial bones from the cranium and the lateral aspect of the face. The medial part of the fracture line is across the nasal bone, nasal septum, frontal process of the maxilla, lacrimal bone and runs posteriorly along the ethmoidal bone. Laterally the fracture runs obliquely downwards from the inferior orbital margin (near the zygomaticomaxillary suture) along the anterolateral wall of the maxilla and then slightly ascends up the posterolateral wall of the maxilla to the inferior orbital fissure.

  c. Le Fort III is the highest of the fractures and is bilateral, causing complete separation of the midfacial bone from the base of the skull. The fracture line passes across the nasofrontal region to the ethmoid and runs posteriorly to the inferior orbital fissure. It also involves the pterygoid plates. Laterally the fracture involves the lateral wall of the orbit and the zygomatic arch.

The Le Fort fractures may occur in combination. The above description is useful for surgical planning.

3. **Lower third.** This includes the mandible. Common sites of fractures are the alveola (weakest part), condyles, angle of the mandible, body (usually the fracture is around the canine tooth because of maximum convexity). Bilateral fractures are common. Fractures of the body on one side and the angle on the other side are also common.

CT findings in head injury

If CT is available it is the quickest way of detecting intracranial trauma. It has been reported that about 10–15% of patients with head injury with no neurological signs were found to have abnormal CT findings. In contrast, about 75% of patients with neurological signs demonstrated abnormal CT findings.

The following lesions may be seen in CT.

Haematomas and contusion (acute and delayed)

Haematomas appear as high-density areas (white) on CT without contrast. Haematomas are fairly homogeneous, but contusion shows patchy dense and low-density areas. Low-density areas are due to oedema. Fresh blood appears as dense areas due to haemoglobin. (In anaemic patients it may be isodense with the rest of the brain or even hypodense if the haemoglobin level is low.)

Most haematomas become isodense in 1–3 weeks and in some cases get even smaller and hypodense. The isodense haematomas may be missed unless other signs of mass effect are looked for.

Delayed haematomas may appear 2–7 days after trauma. Haematomas and associated oedema usually cause space-occupying effects—midline shift, compression on ventricles, cisterns etc.

Subdural haematomas

These usually appear as dense areas and follow the brain surface with a concave inner border and convex outer border. They tend to be diffuse and extend along the subdural space. Thin haematomas (e.g. less than 5 mm) and haematomas near the vertex may be difficult to identify. However, indirect evidence such as midline shift may help. Beware of bilateral subdural haematomas, which may not cause any shift.

Acute haematomas (occurring 0–1 weeks after trauma) are usually dense.

Subacute haematomas (occurring 1–3 weeks after trauma) may be isodense.

Chronic haematomas (more than 3 weeks after trauma) are usually hypodense.

Acute-on-chronic haematomas show mixed density.

Epidural haematomas

These are caused by traumatic separation of the dura from the inner table causing damage to the middle meningeal arterial branches, venous branches or diploic veins. An epidural haematoma is usually seen as a biconvex density under the inner table of the skull. The biconvex appearance is due to firm adhesion of the dura to the inner table. For this reason the epidural haematomas are demarcated by sutures.

Oedema

Oedematous areas appear as low-density areas in the CT. They may be focal, patchy or diffuse. Due to the oedema there may be space-occupying effects, such as compression on the adjacent ventricles and midline shift.

Note: Oedema may have other causes such as infarction. Therefore it should be differentiated. A history of trauma and the site of involvement may be helpful.

Intraventricular and subarachnoid haemorrhage

These may occur with some head injuries and appear as dense areas within the ventricles, basal cistern, sylvian fissures, interhemispheric fissures or cerebral sulci. Resolution of the haemorrhage within the ventricular system and subarachnoid space is fairly quick and may disappear within a week.

Fractures and displaced or depressed bony fragments

These can be seen in CT when viewed with bone windows. The CT is useful to identify soft tissue contusion and foreign bodies in the scalp or in the intracranial region. It is also useful to identify any traumatic pneumocephalus.

Post-traumatic changes

Acute or delayed hydrocephalus is caused by blood in the subarachnoid space causing some obstruction to the CSF pathways.

Ischaemic infarction appears as low-density areas.

Post-traumatic atrophy is seen in almost one-third of patients with severe head injury. Due to the atrophy there may be compensatory dilation of the ventricles usually adjacent to the site of atrophy.

Post-traumatic abscess—this may be seen in penetrating injury or fracture, or as a complication following surgery. It appears as a low-density area with ring enhancement after contrast injection. This ring enhancement is usually surrounded by a large area of oedema. The lesion will also produce a space-occupying effect.

The use of CT in facial trauma

In some cases plain tomography is performed to demonstrate facial fractures, but CT of facial bones in coronal and axial planes is very useful, not only to demonstrate the fractures but also to show the extent, degree of depression of fragments and associated haematomas, especially in the adjacent sinuses, orbits etc.

Angiography in cerebral trauma

This has been almost eliminated by CT scanners. However, it is indicated if there is suspicion of vascular damage such as occlusion of an artery or injury to an AV malformation.

MRI in head injury

Even though MRI is superior to CT in detecting small haematomas, especially near the bones, CT is preferable as the initial investigation not only because the examination time is shorter but also because sometimes haematomas that are less than 1–2 days old may not be shown by MRI. CT shows acute haemorrhages well.

Head injury in children—CT appearance

Appearance of haematoma is almost the same as in adults. However, haemorrhagic contusions are less common than in adults due to greater pliability of the skull.

The paediatric brain may demonstrate acute generalised oedema causing narrowing of ventricles and subarachnoid space. Oedema is less marked in adults.

Acute severe headache and collapse

Sudden onset of severe headache or sudden collapse may be caused by intracranial haemorrhage. The haemorrhage could be from: aneurysm, AV malformation, capillary bleed in hypertension, bleeding disorders or bleeding from a tumour.

The haemorrhage may be intracerebral, subarachnoid or intra-ventricular.

In these cases CT is rewarding. Blood appears as dense areas. Valuable clues about the site of bleeding and the cause may be provided by CT. However, in most cases angiograms (CT or DSA) will be required to show the exact site and cause of bleeding. Multiple vessel studies are necessary as there may be multiple aneurysms. An angiogram will also show the site of the lesion and, in cases of AV malformation, the feeding vessels to the malformation. Angiograms are not necessary in cerebral parenchymal haemorrhage.

In suspected subarachnoid haemorrhage, CT scan is performed before lumbar puncture. If haemorrhage is marked, or hydrocephalus or space-occupying effect is detected, lumbar puncture is avoided. However, in cases where no haemorrhage is detected, lumbar puncture can be performed. This is because very small haemorrhages may not be shown by CT. Small amounts of blood are not enough to change the CSF density, or in some (anaemic) patients the haemoglobin content may not be enough to change the CSF density.

Syncope and seizures

Of the many causes of syncope only a few need radiological assistance for diagnosis or confirmation.

1. Syncope caused by reduced cardiac output may need echocardiography, cardiac catheterisation and angiography.
2. Syncope is rarely caused by cerebrovascular disease, e.g. transient ischaemic attacks, subclavian steal, vertebrobasilar insufficiency. In these cases Doppler ultrasound or angiography will be useful.
3. In cases of seizures, CT of the head may be required to exclude any underlying pathology.

Stroke

Transient ischaemic attacks (TIAs) may represent an early warning sign of impending stroke. Therefore arteriography (DSA) of the neck vessels and cerebral arteries is performed in cases of TIA.

Even though arteriography gives a more definite answer, ultrasound examination of the neck vessels (Duplex and colour Doppler studies) could be performed initially.

In all patients with stroke, CT should be the initial radiological examination. However, if MRI is available it is preferred to CT, as MRI is better at detecting early infarction (within a few hours of vascular occlusion). CT sometimes gives negative results within the first 24–48 hours.

EMERGENCIES IN THE NECK

Major emergencies are trauma, foreign bodies, and croup and laryngeal inflammation in children.

Trauma

Cervical spine injuries are common and can be life-threatening. They range from nerve root compression and paralysis to death. Therefore, X-ray evaluation of the cervical spine is important in trauma.

Plain X-ray views

1. The first film to obtain is a 'brow up—shoot through' lateral view. (Patient in supine position; movement of neck should be avoided.) Film should be well penetrated. All the cervical vertebrae and possibly the

upper thoracic vertebrae should be demonstrated. Demonstration of the lower cervical and upper thoracic spine may be difficult in most patients. Swimmer's lateral projection or a lateral film with shoulder traction could be useful. Sometimes the patient's condition may not permit this. Alternative ways to demonstrate this area are tomography in lateral projection or CT scan if available.

2. If no abnormality is seen in the first film, do an open-mouth AP view of 'peg' to exclude any fracture of the 'peg'. In suspicious cases the rest of the views are done only after expert examination of the films: a radiologist should be consulted if available.

3. If no abnormality is seen in the above two views, do the rest of the views, i.e. AP and two obliques. Patients must move the neck themselves.

4. Lastly, if there are no neurological signs, a flexion and extension view (functional view) could be done. Do not force the neck—the patient must move the neck. In suspicious cases the oblique and functional views should be done under the supervision of the attending doctor.

5. If no abnormality is seen in the above and the symptoms are still suspicious of fracture, tomography of selected areas could be done. If CT is available, it will be useful to show the vertebrae in transverse plane and to detect haematomas. If a helical or multiple-slice scanner is available, high-resolution images could be obtained in sagittal and coronal planes as well as 3D images.

Clues for interpretation of X-rays

1. For proper interpretation one should be familiar with the normal appearance of the vertebrae, facetal joints, disc spaces and the soft tissues around the spine.

2. Lateral and peg views should be inspected first.

3. Look for fracture lines or deformities in each vertebral body, neural arch and the facets. Look for dislocation or subluxation of facetal joints and any malalignment of vertebrae.

4. Loss of lordosis and scoliosis may indicate bony injury or soft tissue injury.

5. If the disc is damaged the space may be narrow.

6. Soft tissues anterior to the spine (prevertebral soft tissue) should be inspected for swelling (haematomas). Normal AP distance of the prevertebral soft tissue in the retropharyngeal region (at the anteroinferior angle of C2) is about 6–7 mm in adults and children. Retrotracheal soft tissue at the level of the anteroinferior angle of C6 is about 14–15 mm in children and about 15–20 mm in adults (these measurements are the upper limit of normal). Haematoma may be due to fracture or rupture of the anterior spinal ligament.

7. To identify upper cervical subluxation in the lateral view, draw a line along the anterior cortical margin of the spinous processes from C1 to C3 (posterior cervical line). If there is more than 2 mm displacement,

it is diagnostic. This is usually seen in odontoid fracture or Hangman's fracture.

Note: In children slight anterior subluxation of the body of C2 on C3, especially in the flexion view, is normal. In these cases note the posterior cervical line, which will be normal.

8. Look for common fractures. Fractures are common at the C1–C2 articulation, 'peg', and from C5 to C7.
9. Pitfalls: in the AP view of the peg, watch for superimposed shadow of an incisor tooth which will look like a fracture. Also look for a separate ossification centre of the peg. (In some cases tomography of the peg may be needed to identify the fracture.)
10. CT can be performed to determine the state of soft tissue structures around the spine.
11. It is also useful in cases of suspected instability at the fracture and to identify suspected bony fragments within the vertebral canal.
12. CT (in bone windows) will demonstrate the neural arches and facetal joints. This will be useful to identify fractures or dislocation at the joints. Modern CT scanners can image the spine in various anatomical planes.
13. MRI is more sensitive than CT in demonstrating the spinal cord.

Classification of cervical spine injury

Cervical spine injuries can be classified according to the type of injury—flexion injury or extension injury. However, in many instances the patient is unconscious or cannot describe the injury. As far as the treatment is concerned, it is important to decide whether the fracture is stable or unstable. The X-ray findings are useful in making this decision.

Flexion injury

The various kinds of flexion injury are described in order of severity:

1. **Hyperflexion sprain.** Partial damage to posterior ligaments including interspinous ligaments. Flexion lateral view may demonstrate widening or fanning of the space between adjacent spinous processes.
2. **Unilateral or bilateral facetal dislocation.**
   - In lateral view, look for anterior displacement of one vertebral body on the other by less than 50%.
   - In AP view look for malalignment of spinous processes (especially in unilateral dislocation). Facets may be locked, i.e. inferior articular facet of the vertebra above is locked in front of the superior facet of the vertebra below.
3. **Anterior wedging of vertebral bodies or compression fractures.** If the neural arches are not fractured this may be a stable fracture.
4. **Comminuted fracture of vertebral body ('teardrop' fractures).** In these fractures, look for any fragments in the vertebral canal. These fragments could cause damage to the spinal cord. CT scan would be useful in these cases to identify any fragments in the canal.

Extension injury

The various kinds of extension injury are described in order of severity:

1. **Hyperextension sprain.** This causes damage to the anterior longitudinal ligament. Due to hyperextension, there may be protrusion or bulging of the disc posteriorly. There may also be some haematoma and swelling from the ligamentum flava. The disc bulging and the swelling from the ligamentum flava can cause compression on the spinal cord. In these cases the X-ray may be normal. CT scan or MRI would be useful in these patients.
   - Sometimes lateral plain X-ray may show soft tissue swelling (haematoma) within prevertebral tissue.
   - Extension injuries may be associated with fractures of the anterior angles of the vertebral bodies.
   - Extension injuries may not be stable in extended positions of the neck but are stable in flexion.
2. **Hangman's fracture.** Fracture of both pedicles of axis with displacement of the body of C2 anteriorly and posterior displacement of neural arch of C2. This is well seen in the lateral view.
3. **Jefferson bursting fracture.** This fracture is unusual and occurs mainly when vertical compression injury causes bilateral fractures of anterior and posterior arches of C1. In the open-mouth AP view there will be lateral displacement—both lateral masses of C1.
4. **Fracture of peg.** Look for fracture line (not to be confused with superimposed shadows and separate ossification centres). Also look for alignment in lateral view—posterior cervical line.

Stable fractures

1. Unilateral fracture of lamina pedicle or lateral mass.
2. Unilateral facetal fracture or dislocation.
3. Wedge fracture.
4. Burst fracture—disc forced into fractured end plates of body.
5. Fracture of spinous process.

Unstable fractures

1. Bilateral fracture of lamina.
2. Bilateral dislocation of facets.
3. Comminuted fracture body (any fracture dislocation).
4. Hangman's fracture.
5. Peg fracture.

Foreign body in neck—pharynx and upper oesophagus

Most swallowed foreign bodies lodge at the level of the cricopharyngeal muscle or in the upper oesophagus. The most common foreign bodies are fish bones, meat or chicken bones, large pieces of meat, and coins.

Lateral film of the neck is the most useful view. Film of soft tissue exposure may be necessary to identify faintly calcified bones. Radiopaque materials are fairly easy to detect. Superimposition of calcified hyoid, thyroid, cricoid and laryngeal cartilages will be a problem. However, an understanding of their normal expected anatomical position will help to distinguish a foreign body. Pattern of calcification of cartilages (irregular) will also help. Swallowed bone may have a linear cortex. In difficult cases a barium swallow may help to identify the foreign body. Swallowing cottonwool soaked in barium (usually under fluoroscopic control) will occasionally help. This may get caught on the foreign body.

CT is also useful to locate smaller foreign bodies not shown by X-ray.

Epiglottitis and croup

Young children may develop severe acute inflammation of the epiglottis and larynx. In most cases, if the condition is severe, radiological examination is postponed until the patient's condition is stable.

1. A lateral view of the neck (soft tissue exposure) is the best view. Rarely, a single midline tomogram in lateral projection may be necessary.
   - A swollen epiglottis will look like a thumb—the swollen aryepiglottis may also be seen.
   - In croup usually the subglottic region from the vocal cord to the level of the inferior border of the thyroid cartilage shows mucosal swelling which causes narrowing of the airway. Vocal cords will also be affected. The need for radiology is debatable. However, if the patient's condition permits, it will be useful to perform an AP and lateral view of the neck. Swollen vocal cords, obliteration of laryngeal ventricles and narrowing of the subglottic airway by swelling can easily be seen.
2. Helical CT scan of larynx and trachea with sagittal and coronal reconstruction would be useful if time permits.

EMERGENCIES IN THORACIC AND LUMBAR SPINE

Injury and acute disc prolapse or rupture

Views

1. If the patient is immobilised, a 'shoot through' lateral view is initially performed.
2. Lateral film of the thoracic spine is obtained while the patient is breathing. This is to 'blur' the superimposed ribs.
3. Swimmer's lateral or lateral tomography may be required for demonstration of the upper 3–4 thoracic vertebrae.
4. AP view is fairly easy to obtain.
5. In cases of suspected ligamentous rupture, flexion and extension views in lateral projection are obtained.
6. In lumbar spine, if the condition of the patient permits, oblique views are also performed. These demonstrate the laminae and facetal joints well.

7. CT scan is useful to demonstrate the integrity of disc and bony elements. They are also useful to detect facetal dislocation, subluxation and any posterior dislodgment or bony fragments into the vertebral canal. It is also useful to demonstrate the soft tissues around the spine.

Interpretation of X-rays

Look for:

1. Reduction in the height of vertebral body and disc spaces (compression or wedge fractures).
2. Fracture lines or displaced fragments in the vertebrae, including transverse process and spinous process (also look for posterior rib fracture in thoracic region).
3. Paravertebral haematoma (loss of psoas shadow in lumbar region, displacement of pleural lining in thoracic region etc.).
4. Subluxation, kyphosis, gibbus and scoliosis.
5. Look for any underlying causes of fracture such as secondary deposits, Paget's disease and osteoporosis.
6. Beware of limbus vertebra non-united secondary ossification centre, butterfly vertebra and narrowing of vertebral bodies caused by long-standing scoliosis and kyphosis.

Unstable injury

1. Transverse fractures through vertebral bodies and neural arches.
2. Fracture dislocation.
3. Rupture of ligaments (in the lateral view, the interspinous distance is wide, especially in flexion view).

Disc prolapse

1. Plain X-ray may show disc narrowing—this is not always seen. Therefore, if symptoms persist, CT scan of the disc would be useful to show disc prolapse.
2. High-resolution scanners can differentiate disc material, nerve roots etc.
3. MRI scan is superior in demonstrating spinal cord, nerve roots, discs, ligaments and bone oedema from trauma.

CHEST EMERGENCIES

Routine views

1. PA and lateral—obtained in erect position, both with full inspiration.
2. If patient cannot stand erect, PA or AP and lateral in sitting position (in full inspiration) are obtained.
3. If patient cannot sit or stand, supine AP is obtained. This is unsatisfactory because the patient may not be able to take a full inspiration and the diaphragm appears elevated. It also causes magnification, especially of the mediastinum.

Additional views

1. Oblique views for ribs.
2. Apical lordotic view to demonstrate lung apices (to get the superimposed clavicle out of the way).
3. Inspiration and expiration films to demonstrate pneumothorax.
4. Penetrated film to see mediastinum or lung bases.
5. Lateral decubitus (patient lying down on one side—right or left, and film obtained with horizontal beam). This demonstrates mobility of pleural fluid on the dependent side.

Interpretation

There are two ways to interpret:

1. An experienced person will use a problem-oriented approach, depending on the clinical information.
2. An inexperienced person should look at a chest film in a routine, systematic manner.
   a. Start looking at the mediastinal shadows. Cast your eyes along the:
      • Anterior mediastinal structures: thymus (enlargement in infants; tumour in adults), thyroid (retrosternal), lymph nodes (if enlarged).
      • Middle mediastinum: heart, aortic arch and branches, pulmonary artery, superior and inferior vena cavae.
      • Posterior mediastinal structures: trachea, bronchi, oesophagus, descending thoracic aorta, lymph nodes, (abnormal) neural tissues, look for hiatus hernia, spine.
   b. Look at the hilar shadows.
   c. Look at the lung parenchyma and other lung markings (pulmonary vasculature and bronchi).
   d. Pleura.
   e. Chest wall (including ribs).
   f. Cast your eyes along the periphery of the film, e.g. the shoulder, under the diaphragm.

Trauma

Rib fractures

First, second and third rib fractures are seen only in severe trauma. Commonest are from fourth to ninth ribs. Flail chest is seen when three or more ribs are fractured at two points. These are usually seen from the fourth to eighth ribs. A common site of fracture is the lateral angle. Because of this, oblique views are essential. Rib fractures can cause pneumothorax and haemothorax. Fracture of the tenth, eleventh and twelfth ribs can cause damage to the liver, spleen and kidneys.

Lung contusion

Appears as an area of consolidation. It is not always associated with rib fracture. It may not appear immediately (sometimes a day later) and begins to resolve 2–3 days after injury. It usually resolves completely in about 10–15 days.

Rupture of thoracic aorta

Seen in motor vehicle accidents—usually the ligamentum arteriosum. In this region the aorta is relatively fixed. Sudden deceleration and compression injury causes laceration at this relatively fixed portion of the aorta.

In chest X-rays there will be evidence of superior mediastinal widening, shift of the trachea to the right with obscuring of the aortic arch, and there may be haemothorax on the left. CT scan and aortography are the other radiological investigations in these patients.

Rupture of trachea or bronchus

Common findings in chest X-rays are pneumomediastinum, pneumothorax and surgical emphysema. Occlusion of fractured bronchus can cause collapse of the corresponding lung, lobe or segment.

Rupture of diaphragm

Seen in direct blunt trauma and penetrating injury. Sometimes not diagnosed immediately. In an X-ray the outline of the dome may not be normal. It may be elevated, there may be haemothorax or segmental lung collapse. On the left side, the bowel may herniate into the thorax and on the right side the liver may herniate. Rupture in blunt trauma is common on the left side.

CT in chest trauma. If helical or multislice scanner is available, it will be useful for better demonstration of chest in sagittal and coronal planes as well as in 3D format. CT angiogram could be performed to demonstrate aorta and great vessels.

Breathlessness

Asthma and acute-on-chronic CAL

In chronic airflow limitation (CAL), chest X-ray shows overinflated lung, flattened domes of diaphragm, widened retrosternal space, hyper-radiolucency, a barrel-shaped chest, a relatively small and elongated heart shadow, prominent main pulmonary arteries and pruning of peripheral pulmonary arteries (associated pulmonary artery hypertension), and thickened bronchial walls (end-on ring shadows and tramline shadows).

In asthma, overinflation of lungs and bronchial wall thickenings may be seen. Other findings may include atelectasis caused by mucous plugging or consolidation.

High-resolution CT of 1 mm thickness is useful for investigation of CAL, especially to identify bronchiectasis, emphysematous bullae and interstitial fibrosis.

Radiological appearance in acute heart failure

Heart failure may be divided into left and right heart failure.

X-ray findings in left heart failure

1. Distension of upper lobe veins (normally the upper lobe veins are smaller in calibre than the lower lobe veins).
2. Interstitial pulmonary oedema. In the early stages the oedema forms around the hilar region, causing blurring of the hilar markings. Septal lines are due to accumulation of fluid along the lymphatics: 'A' lines are long and radiate from the hilar region to the periphery; 'B' lines are short and are seen in the region of the costophrenic angles.
3. Alveolar pulmonary oedema. This is due to filling of the alveolar spaces with exudates. It is seen as haziness radiating from the hilar region and produces a butterfly-wing appearance. In the severe form, the alveolar oedema produces a patchy or cottonwool appearance.

X-ray appearances in right ventricular failure

1. Prominence of superior vena cava (SVC) and azygos vein.
2. Pleural effusion. In heart failure often more fluid is seen on the right side. In the early stages, small pleural effusions are seen in the costophrenic angles as a homogeneous density demonstrating a 'meniscus sign'. The meniscus sign is seen in the erect position. The fluid in the base changes to a haziness in the supine films. This indicates mobility of the fluid. Small fluid collections are first detected in the lateral view—in the posterior costophrenic angles. In the average chest, the posterior costophrenic angle can accumulate about 150–200 mL of fluid without being seen in the PA view. In the early stages fluid can also accumulate in the fissures between the lobes. This appears as thick oblique fissures.

Pleural effusion

Pleural effusion may have various other causes, e.g. tumour. Large pleural effusions can obscure the underlying cause. If the fluid is mobile a lateral decubitus view would be useful to demonstrate the lung bases. (Alternatively, CT scan could be performed to identify any mass in the lung base.)

Lung collapse

There are two major radiological signs:

1. Density—collapsed portion of the lung appears dense.
2. Signs of loss of volume:
   - Shift of fissures—fissures are shifted towards the opacity.

- Diaphragmatic elevation.
- Mediastinal shift towards the side of collapse.
- Splaying out of lung markings on the side of collapse due to compensatory overexpansion of the remaining lung.

Chest pain

Only the causes where radiology plays a part are included in this section.

Myocardial infarction

Chest X-rays are performed to look at the heart size and shape, and also to look for evidence of heart failure. Upper limit of normal cardiothoracic ratio (CTR) is 50% (CTR = transverse diameter of the heart divided by transverse diameter of the chest).

Pericardial effusion

Chest X-ray is also useful to identify pericardial effusion. In the supine position the heart appears globular in shape and in the erect position it produces a 'tent shape'. The angle between the right atrium and the right diaphragm is lost. On fluoroscopic examination, poor pulsation may be demonstrated in cases of pericardial effusion. (For proper demonstration of pericardial effusion, echocardiography or CT scan is more useful.)

Pulmonary embolism

1. Within 24–48 hours there may not be any radiological change. However, if large pulmonary arterial branches are blocked, there may be a cut-off sign (i.e. abrupt ending of an arterial branch).
2. Raised hemidiaphragm—on the side of infarction.
3. After about 24–48 hours, an almost triangular density with its base towards the periphery of the chest may appear.
4. There may be a small associated pleural effusion.
5. Sometimes the main pulmonary artery on the affected side may enlarge.
6. Later in the process, in the area of infarction there may be atelectasis or scar formation.
7. Nuclear isotope ventilation perfusion scans are usually performed for diagnosis, but sometimes this is not confirmatory. However, a normal chest X-ray and abnormal isotope scan could be indicative of pulmonary embolism.
8. Pulmonary arteriography is the best means of establishing or excluding pulmonary embolism. This is rarely performed because of adverse reactions and the cost. However, recently, with the introduction of the multislice scanner, CT pulmonary angiogram could be performed. This would be sensitive to detect emboli in pulmonary arteries up to about the fourth or fifth level of branching.
9. Doppler study or venogram of the lower limb veins may show the origin of the clot.

Dissecting aneurysm

1. In the PA view there may be widening of the superior mediastinum with the ascending aorta bulging to the right.
2. The lateral view may show bulging of the ascending aorta anteriorly. A long-standing aneurysm of the ascending aorta can cause erosion of the posterior aspect of the sternum.
3. Leak from the aneurysm into the pericardium causes a large globular heart.
4. When the dissection extends into the arch and descending thoracic aorta, the diameter widens towards the left. Sometimes a double aortic knuckle shadow can be seen. Some aneurysms leak into the pleural cavity and appear as a pleural effusion. In some patients uniform haziness can be seen in the left lung, due to blood spread along the bronchi and pulmonary arterial planes.
5. CT scan can demonstrate a dissecting aneurysm and its extent.
6. In order to demonstrate the exact site of rupture some surgeons prefer an aortogram.

Pneumothorax

1. Usually PA films in expiratory and inspiratory phases are obtained in the erect position.
2. A large pneumothorax is well seen in a normal PA film. A small pneumothorax is usually demonstrated in the expiratory film.
3. In order to identify the pneumothorax, follow the lung markings towards the periphery. The markings stop well short of the chest wall. A white visceral pleural line can be seen at this level.
4. Do not confuse the accompanying shadow caused by intercostal muscles along the ribs with visceral pleura.
5. Look for an associated pneumomediastinum (air can leak from bronchi in asthmatics) and subcutaneous emphysema along the chest wall and neck.

Fever, cough and pain

Pleurisy

1. Early stages—no radiological findings.
2. Later stages—small amounts of pleural fluid may be seen; there may be associated lung consolidation.

Pneumonia

1. Bronchopneumonia—patchy shadows.
2. Lobar or segmental pneumonia:
   - Homogeneous localised shadows.
   - Air bronchogram may be seen.
   - Usually no loss of volume of lungs (this helps to differentiate from lung collapse).

Haemoptysis

Pulmonary infarction

See 'Pulmonary embolism', above.

Tumour

A mass, either solitary or multiple, can be seen in the hilar region or elsewhere in the lung. If there is any doubt about the diagnosis, CT would be useful. CT may also demonstrate any enlarged lymph nodes.

Other accidents

Drowning

Pulmonary oedema is seen in cases of near-drowning in both fresh and sea water. Pulmonary oedema may not develop for up to two days. Therefore, negative findings in immediate CXRs do not exclude later development of oedema.

Inhalation of toxic gases/smoke

1. In toxic gas inhalation, pulmonary oedema develops quickly—in about 4–24 hours.
2. In smoke inhalation, the oedema may not develop for up to 2–4 days.
3. In CXRs oedema appears as patchy infiltrates. There may be segmental atelectasis. These changes usually resolve faster.

Ingestion of hydrocarbons (e.g. petroleum)

May develop patchy pneumonic consolidation in lung bases, usually within 1–2 hours. Severity depends on the amount ingested. Takes up to 2 weeks to resolve.

Foreign body

1. Radio-opaque foreign bodies in bronchi are easily seen in CXRs. Foreign bodies like nuts, seeds and plastics may be difficult to see.
2. Radiological signs are usually indirect, i.e. signs of obstruction.
3. In children obstruction is usually ball-valve type, causing air trapping.

PA films are obtained in inspiration and expiration. The inspiratory film may be normal but in the expiratory film there will be hyperradiolucency and signs of increased volume on the affected side (flat diaphragm and shift of mediastinum to the opposite side).

Chest screening is very useful to detect air trapping. Normal lungs show normal density and change of volume during breathing in comparison with the affected lung, which shows fixed volume and density.

In adults, obstruction usually causes collapse of the lung or lobes.

RADIOLOGY IN ABDOMINAL EMERGENCIES

Almost all modalities of imaging (plain X-ray, contrast study, CT and ultrasound) are used in abdominal emergencies. Of these, plain X-rays are the most commonly used.

Views

1. Routine views—AP in supine and erect position.
2. Additional views—lateral decubitus in patients who cannot stand up, to look for fluid levels or free peritoneal gas.
3. In some cases an erect chest X-ray is also performed to look for gas under the diaphragm or any pleural fluid in the lung bases.

Interpretation

An inexperienced person finds it difficult to interpret an abdominal X-ray owing to superimposition of various organs. This difficulty can be greatly reduced if the film is looked at in a routine manner, for example as follows:

1. Look at the bowel shadows—these are easily identifiable because of gas and faeces. Stomach, small and large bowel can be differentiated by their anatomical sites and their pattern of mucosal folds and wall—valvulae conniventes in jejunal loops and haustral pattern in large bowel. Note any fluid levels and bowel dilation.
2. Look at the four major organs: liver, spleen, kidneys and bladder, for their size, position, outline and density.
3. Look at the psoas shadows and fat planes in the flank and along the pelvic walls.
4. Look for radio-opaque stones (gall and renal) and abnormal calcification (pancreatic, hepatic and abdominal aortic).
5. Look above and below the diaphragm for abnormal gas, fluid or air collections.
6. Any abnormal mass causing displacement of adjacent structures.
7. Look at the bony elements (lower ribs, lumbar spine and pelvis).

Acute abdomen

In the plain X-ray of the abdomen, the main aim is to identify obstruction, perforation or ileus in the bowel shadows.

Radiological signs of bowel obstruction

1. There may be gaseous distension of the bowel up to the site of obstruction. In complete or almost complete obstruction, very little gas is seen in the bowel distal to the obstruction.
2. Multiple fluid levels are seen in erect films.
3. A step-ladder pattern of air–fluid levels is seen in small bowel obstruction. In large bowel obstruction fluid levels are seen around the

periphery. In complete obstruction of large bowel there may be fluid levels in the small bowel as well.

4. In gastric outlet or duodenal obstruction, a distended stomach with a large air–fluid level is seen.

5. Volvulus. In sigmoid volvulus look for a dilated loop of bowel in the form of an inverted U in the left hypochondrium. In caecal volvulus the base of the dilated caecum usually points to the right iliac fossa. The volvulus can be confirmed by performing a limited dilute barium or gastrograffin enema.

6. Intussusception. A sharp cut-off of bowel gas pattern is seen. Common intussusception is at the ileocaecal junction. There may be a dilated small bowel with multiple fluid levels. Limited barium enema examination may show a coil-spring appearance. In children the barium enema can be therapeutic and in most cases will be able to reduce the intussusception.

Radiological signs of ileus

1. **Generalised.** Slight to moderate gaseous distension of small and large bowel with multiple small fluid levels can be seen. Generalised ileus is usually seen in postoperative patients, peritonitis and retroperitoneal conditions.

2. **Localised.** The bowel loops in close proximity to an inflammatory area may show slight dilation and some fluid levels. One or two loops may be involved. This is called sentinel loop, e.g. jejunal loops and transverse colon are involved in pancreatitis and acute deep gastric ulcers. Terminal ileum is involved in conditions such as appendicitis. Hepatic flexure and some small bowel in the right hypochondrium may show fluid levels in cholecystitis. In renal colic there may be sentinel loops on the affected side.

Radiological signs in perforation

1. Free peritoneal gas is usually seen under the diaphragm in the erect position. In a lateral decubitus film, free gas may be seen along the flank. The free gas is sometimes seen only after 24 hours.

2. Loculated peritoneal gas, e.g. in perforation of a duodenal ulcer there may be loculated gas along the inferior liver margin. If there is a collection of gas in the lesser sac, in the plain X-ray there may be a double gas shadow projected over the fundus of the stomach.

3. Retroperitoneal gas from perforation of the retroperitoneal portion of the large bowel.

4. In order to identify the site of perforation, gastrograffin contrast may be used (extravasated contrast is absorbed by the bloodstream and excreted by the kidney). In cases of suspected upper GIT perforation the contrast may be given orally. In cases of colonic perforation it may be given rectally. Not all perforations can be demonstrated by this technique.

GIT bleeding and ischaemia

It is difficult to demonstrate bleeding points by barium study. However, this examination may be useful in demonstrating the presence of oesophageal varices, peptic ulcers, diverticula or tumours.

Highly selective coeliac, superior or inferior mesenteric arteriograms may demonstrate bleeding points. Angiography is also useful to demonstrate occluded arteries causing mesenteric ischaemia. A bleeding rate of 1 mL/min is usually required.

Pancreatitis

1. Plain X-rays may show only indirect evidence such as sentinel loops or calcification in the region of the pancreas.
2. Barium meal may show a widened loop of duodenum due to enlargement of the pancreas.
3. Ultrasound is able to demonstrate the size and texture of the pancreas. It may also demonstrate oedematous change or any pseudocyst formation. However, sometimes it is difficult to demonstrate the pancreas by ultrasound due to obesity of the patient and presence of excessive gas.
4. A CT scan is the ideal examination to demonstrate the pancreas, especially in the obese patient. The sensitivity is such that it can demonstrate inflammatory changes, a small amount of calcification, a mass, a pseudocyst and also the state of surrounding tissues. It is also useful for follow-up study.
5. Skinny needle biopsy under CT or ultrasound control has greatly improved the diagnostic ability.
6. Endoscopic retrograde cholangiopancreatography (ERCP) demonstrates the state of the pancreatic ducts.

Cholecystitis

1. Plain X-ray may demonstrate radio-opaque gallstones and sometimes demonstrates sentinel loops (localised ileus).
2. Ultrasound is the diagnostic tool of choice. It can demonstrate stones, thickness of the wall of the gallbladder and any oedematous change. It can also demonstrate the size of the bile ducts or any stones in the duct. However, demonstration of the lower common bile duct may be difficult.
3. In a post-cholecystectomy patient with symptoms of biliary colic, CT cholangiography could be useful to exclude any retained stones in the bile duct, strictures etc.

Aortic aneurysm

1. The majority of aneurysms are asymptomatic. However, these patients usually present to emergency departments when there is a rupture or

leak. Severe rupture is fatal. If a slow leak is suspected radiological investigation is carried out.

2. Plain X-ray (AP and lateral) shows a soft tissue mass, especially in the posterior abdominal wall. This is usually on the left side of the lumbar spine and is better seen in the lateral view. Fifty per cent of aortic aneurysms may have some calcification in the wall of the artery, which is very useful for identification of an aneurysm.

3. Ultrasound or CT scans are non-invasive, easy and quicker methods of diagnosing aneurysms. A CT scan is superior to ultrasound. It can demonstrate the site and length of the aneurysm. It can also demonstrate the diameter of the aneurysm and the presence of clot. CT is the study of choice in many patients, especially in obese patients. With the modern scanners CT aortography gives excellent results which also show the relationship of renal arteries to the neck of the aneurysm. This is useful for surgical planning.

4. Digital angiography is still used by surgeons to demonstrate the aneurysm and the branches of the abdominal aorta. However, this would show only the lumen and not the actual diameter of aneurysm or the intraluminal clot.

Renal colic

1. Plain X-rays may show radio-opaque calculi and may demonstrate localised ileus.
2. An IVP may demonstrate: • obstruction (partial or complete) • radio-lucent stones • state of kidneys and collecting system.
3. If there is a non-functioning kidney and there are no radio-opaque stones, retrograde pyelography would be warranted.
4. Ultrasound may not detect all the stones in the kidney. It would demonstrate hydronephrosis in the case of ureteric obstruction.

Haematuria

Severe cases of haematuria may present to the emergency department.

1. An IVP may reveal tumour in the kidneys, ureters or bladder.
2. CT is used to demonstrate renal and bladder tumours as well as any extension of the tumour.
3. Ultrasound can be used if CT scan is not available or if the patient is allergic to contrast medium.

Abdominal trauma

Blunt trauma is more common. Radiological investigations depend on the patient's condition. The investigations include: plain abdominal X-ray, IVP, arteriograms, ultrasound and CT.

Renal contusion and laceration

1. Plain X-ray may show: loss of renal outline, loss of psoas shadow, scoliosis with concavity towards the side of injury, localised ileus on the side of injury, fracture of lower ribs, vertebrae (including transverse processes) and pelvic bones.
2. IVP may show: non-functioning kidney or delayed nephrogram; extravasation of contrast from ruptured kidney, ureter or bladder; clots, seen as filling defects within the pelvicalyceal system, ureter or bladder.
3. Arteriogram. If an IVP shows non-function and renal laceration is suspected, an emergency renal arteriogram is performed to assess the state of the renal arteries. (Renal vessel repair should be performed within a few hours.)
4. Ultrasound and CT, if available, are useful. They can demonstrate rupture, contusion and haematoma. CT is superior to ultrasound.

Renal vein thrombosis

1. An IVP shows an enlarged kidney, prolonged nephrographic phase and reduced excretion.
2. Ultrasound with Doppler may assist but helical CT in rapid sequential imaging after contrast injection has about 90% success in detecting renal vein thrombosis. Other findings include prolonged parenchymal enhancement and delayed excretion.
3. MR imaging is also an excellent method of demonstrating renal vein thrombosis.

Bladder trauma

1. May be contusion or rupture (either intraperitoneal or extraperitoneal).
2. In these cases a cystogram will be useful to demonstrate the site of the rupture.

Urethral rupture

1. Usually seen in males.
2. Site of rupture can be demonstrated by a retrograde urethrogram.

Spleen and liver injury

Splenic injury is more common than liver. Sometimes the plain X-ray signs may be non-specific. If there are some signs, further investigations may be necessary to confirm the diagnosis. Radiological signs depend on whether there is capsular damage or not.

Plain X-ray of abdomen and chest

1. Elevation of left diaphragm in splenic injury and right in liver injury.
2. Left or right effusion in spleen or liver injury respectively.
3. There may be atelectasis at the left or right base.
4. There may be fracture of the lower ribs.

5. Blurred liver or splenic outline.
6. In splenic haematoma, the stomach may be displaced medially and the splenic flexure of colon downwards. In liver injury the hepatic flexure may be displaced.
7. In cases of rupture there may be loss of flank stripes, separation of walls of bowel loops by peritoneal fluid, obliteration of splenic or hepatic outline and general haziness of abdomen.

Ultrasound

1. May show fluid (haemoperitoneum). Blood (fluid) is seen in the lateral gutters and pelvic recesses.
2. May show contused areas of the organ.

CT

This is the best examination. If CT is not available, ultrasound is performed. CT can demonstrate intracapsular haematomas, laceration and haemoperitoneum.

Angiogram

Selective arteriograms would be useful to study the state of the arteries and also to demonstrate rupture.

Hollow viscus

Rupture or perforation rarely occurs with blunt trauma, but may be seen in penetrating injury. When it occurs, there may be gas collections in the peritoneal cavity. Sometimes retroperitoneal and mediastinal gas can be seen. This can be detected in plain abdominal and chest X-rays. Gastrograffin study may be useful to demonstrate the site of perforation but this is not usually required.

CT is useful to identify free peritoneal air and any other injury to the adjacent organs.

SOME OBSTETRIC EMERGENCIES

Bleeding in pregnancy

This can be due to: abortion—threatened, incomplete, complete or missed; ectopic pregnancy; placenta praevia; hydatidiform mole; placental separation (abruptio placentae).

All the above causes can be assessed by ultrasound (using transabdominal and transvaginal probes), which is the examination of choice. The fetal viability can also be assessed.

Intrauterine fetal death

This can be confirmed by ultrasound.

Intrauterine trauma

Ultrasound is also used to assess the fetus after abdominal trauma.

FRACTURES OF PELVIS AND LIMBS

1. Most fractures are easy to recognise on X-rays. However, some are difficult, e.g. hairline undisplaced fractures. In suspicious cases repeat examination in 10–14 days should be performed (e.g. scaphoid fracture).

2. In about 10–14 days some bone absorption occurs adjacent to the fracture line, which makes the fracture visible. In addition periosteal reaction (callus) may begin to form.

3. Undisplaced fractures through the epiphyseal plates are also difficult to recognise. These fractures will also demonstrate bone resorption and callus in about 2 weeks' time.

4. In minor fractures, look at the cortical bone for any discontinuity or dents. Also look for any irregularity in the trabecular pattern.

5. In some areas, e.g. femoral neck and scaphoid, tomogram, CT or nuclear scan may be required to demonstrate an undisplaced crack fracture.

6. If suspicious areas are encountered, oblique views should be done (thin fracture lines are visible only when the X-rays pass perpendicular to the fracture line).

7. In oblique fractures of the metaphysis, always look at the depth of the epiphyseal plates, as the fracture might extend along the plate causing widening of the growth plate.

8. In the forearm and leg, if one of the bones is shortened or dislocated, usually the other bone will have a fracture or dislocation. Therefore, in the distal limbs have a good look at the entire length of the bones, especially the proximal and distal ends and the adjacent joints.

9. In young patients look at the location of ossification centres around the joints to identify any dislocation of the epiphysis, e.g. elbow. If in doubt consult a radiologist or do a comparative view of the opposite joint.

10. In the wrist, do not miss dislocation of carpal bones, e.g. lunate. Try to identify the position of carpal bones in the lateral view.

11. In the joints, look for indirect signs of haemarthrosis, i.e. displacement of adjacent fat pad. If there is haemarthrosis, always look hard to identify any hairline fracture or epiphyseal displacement. If in doubt, X-ray again in 10–14 days.

12. Look for soft tissue swelling in the X-ray (sometimes the X-ray has to be viewed under bright light). If found, concentrate on this area to identify any fracture.

13. The pelvis is like a ring—in compression injuries it might break in two or more places. Fracture of pelvic bones may be associated with dislocation or subluxation at the sacroiliac joints or pubic symphysis.

EDITOR'S COMMENT

Although long, this chapter contains a wealth of practical information. Very few emergency patients escape diagnostic tests. Always, if there is any doubt, talk to radiographers/radiologist about any study. Always arrange for follow-up of the formal report as emergency physicians are not radiologists and are simply giving the patients an impression.

RECOMMENDED READING

Grainger RG, Allison DJ. Grainger and Allison's diagnostic radiology: a textbook of medical imaging. 4th edn. London: Churchill Livingstone; 2001.

Lau LS, James P, Acton CM, et al. Imaging guidelines. 4th edn. Royal Sydney: Royal Australian and New Zealand College of Radiologists; 2001.

Radiologic Clinics of North America. Advances in emergency radiology. I: May 1999; II: September 1999. Philadelphia: WB Saunders; 1999.

49 | The general practitioner

Salie Greengarten and Gordian W O Fulde

The general practitioner (GP) is a vital link in the healthcare chain. Many patients are referred to the emergency department for specialised care by their own doctors, who know them well and are able to give relevant history and treatment details promptly. This can be especially valuable, for example, when patients are old, sick, confused or unfamiliar with English. Obtaining accurate patient data will expedite safe patient care: most GPs are only a phone call away and contacting them can be very time-efficient for busy emergency doctors. Technology such as mobile phones, fax machines and email makes the exchange of information even easier, with many GPs now online.

Most GPs wish to be involved with and informed of their patients' problems, whether during or after normal hours. Each emergency department should have a list of local GPs with their phone numbers (including home or mobiles). The divisions of general practice enhance the communication process, with some divisions having uniform referral forms that ensure relevant information is provided concisely in hard copy or electronically.

Patients sent in by a general practitioner should be assessed by a senior doctor before being discharged. Ideally a quick phone call from the emergency department to the GP before discharge will ensure continuity of care, but obviously the local doctors are not available 24 hours, seven days a week, like an emergency department. A note providing the relevant information is now expected to be given to the patient for the nominated local doctor (legally the norm, but increasingly electronically and automatically sent directly to the doctor). This obviates many serious complaints, unnecessary tests and investigations, and unscheduled returns ('bounces') caused by lack of follow-up.

Several surveys and published material underscore that GPs require only basic information. Now, the data at hospitals is in digital, compatible common computer language that can easily be collated into a discharge letter format by the electronic emergency department information system. The discharge information must be sent out, after the patient has signed permission as required by privacy laws.

The minimum of information required includes the following:

- Patient's name (and date of birth).
- Date, time of arrival and discharge.
- Presenting symptom.
- Tests ordered.
- Test results.
- Provisional diagnosis.
- Disposal (especially if patient dies).
- Medication given.
- Prescription details.

It should be noted that at law, where follow-up of abnormal test results is required to be organised by the GP, or other events have taken place in the emergency department which vitally affect the patient's ongoing management, it is the responsibility of the emergency department doctor to ensure the GP receives the relevant information. A patient may not deliver the letter and so a copy should always be sent by email, mail or fax. If important, a phone call is also made and documented.

With the pressure on hospital services and reduced bulk billing by GPs, more patients are using emergency departments as their primary doctor, especially out of hours. However, making full use of GPs can free resources for those patients who really need them. Many patients attending an emergency department are frightened and intimidated, and do not comprehend or retain what has happened to them. Inevitably they return to their GP for a proper explanation.

It behoves all emergency departments to advise those patients without a GP to seek one, as it is inappropriate for them to continually return to the hospital with obviously non-urgent complaints. Simply stated, it is better for patients to see a trained GP whom they know and trust rather than a different (and often junior, inexperienced and overtaxed) resident each time they visit the hospital.

As GP–hospital interaction has traditionally been neglected, it may be fruitful initially to set up a formal liaison, e.g. a joint committee to put in place the mechanisms to enable the communication.

It is desirable that GPs be accredited and encouraged to visit their patients in hospital, including the emergency department, as this allows for a smooth transition back to their care. To encourage this to happen, make GPs feel welcome when they come to the emergency department. An improved two-way relationship and understanding will get rid of a lot of unnecessary hassles.

50 Medicolegal issues and assuring quality in emergency care

S Lesley Forster and Sally McCarthy

THE LAW AND EMERGENCY MEDICINE
(S Lesley Forster)

There have been a number of recent changes in society and in the law that greatly affect the practice of medicine in general, and emergency medicine in particular. Those practising emergency medicine need to be aware of these changes and to ensure that their practice conforms to the legal requirements. In court, ignorance of the law is no excuse.

This chapter also considers ways of decreasing the likelihood of legal action, and what to do if you are sued.

Confidentiality

The overriding ethical maxim in the treatment of patients is that doctors must keep secret anything they hear about the patient. There are, of course, exceptions: for example, where a patient consents to the disclosure of information, or when giving evidence in court.

When police officers request information about a patient's condition, the doctor should ideally first obtain the written consent of the patient. It is the doctor's duty to ensure that information is given only to those who are entitled to it.

It is accepted that in some instances public interest can override a doctor's duty of confidentiality. If, for example, a patient confides to a doctor an intention to commit a serious criminal offence such as homicide or sexual assault, it would be in order for the doctor to provide a relevant third party with that information.

There are other circumstances where the situation is not quite so clear, and judgment must be made according to the circumstances at the time as to what constitutes a serious criminal offence. It seems to be fairly well accepted among the medical profession, for example, that a doctor should not notify police of a patient's involvement in minor criminal activities such as personal use of illicit drugs or property offences.

Some occasions arise where there is no absolute answer to the problem: for example, if a patient known to be involved in drug trafficking presents to the emergency department. In such a case, where doubt may exist, the

---

Table 50.1 St Vincent's Hospital policy and procedure for management of patients with internally concealed drugs (Reproduced with permission)

These patients may present of their own accord or may be brought in by the police.

1. Heroin and cocaine may cause death if leakage occurs. This is much less likely with hashish. Mechanical problems such as obstruction may occur with any ingested packets.
2. Medical management should proceed as appropriate. Drug screens and other investigations are performed if medically indicated. Abdominal and chest X-rays may be required. Close observation and supportive therapy are indicated. Specific antidotes such as naloxone may be required. Decontamination may be needed if packet rupture and toxicity have occurred (toxicity may occur by diffusion without packet rupture). Glycoprep (or similar) may be used to hasten transit. Laparotomy may be indicated to relieve mechanical obstruction or to urgently remove leaking packets which cannot be otherwise retrieved.
3. If in the judgment of the treating doctor the amount of substance is small, i.e. unlikely to be intended for large scale trafficking but rather intended for individual use, and the patient was not brought in by the police, then it is not mandatory that the police be contacted. Where large quantities are involved then the following steps should be taken:

- Contact the Emergency Department Director.
- Contact Medical Administration.
- A decision will then be taken regarding the need to contact police. The police will be contacted where the patient has obviously been involved in drug trafficking.
- Medical management should never be impeded and remains first priority.
- Patients should not be forcibly restrained.
- Consent issues for medical procedures and treatment apply in the same way as with all patients.
- The safety of St Vincent's Hospital staff should not be compromised.
- Packets recovered are the responsibility of the police if they are present. If the police are not present, recovered packets should be placed in a signed, sealed bag, labelled and locked in the S.8 cupboard (checked in by two RNs). A check should be made between shifts to ensure that the seals remain unbroken. This must be documented in the S.8 book and in the patient's medical record. The packets should then be passed on to the police when they arrive.
- Ensure that the documentation in the medical record is comprehensive and precise as the history may be called in evidence.

---

advice of colleagues and, even better, the advice of a medical defence organisation should be sought in order to assist the doctor in deciding whether to override the duty of confidentiality.

For guidance, the St Vincent's Hospital policy regarding internally concealed drugs is shown in Table 50.1.

Telephone calls

Whether to give information about a patient over the telephone is a decision that frequently has to be made in the emergency department.

As a general rule, unless the patient has given consent, specific information about that patient should not be given over the telephone if it is impossible to be sure of the identity of the caller.

Whenever possible, relatives of very ill patients should be asked to come to the hospital, where any information can be thoughtfully and sympathetically given. As a general rule, the results of tests (e.g. pregnancy, human immunodeficiency virus—HIV, sexually transmitted diseases) that have been performed in the department should not be released by phone. The patient should return to the emergency department or receive the results from the local doctor. In this way, mistakes and even medicolegal complications can be avoided (see also Chapter 44).

Legal issues in HIV medicine

The emergence of HIV has led to a number of legal issues for the emergency physician. These include notification, obligations and confidentiality.

Notification

This is mandatory and requires coded reporting by medical practitioners of all HIV-positive test results by laboratories, and of clinical acquired immunodeficiency syndrome (AIDS) diagnoses and deaths.

Obligations

Some states impose specific additional obligations on doctors in regard to HIV/AIDS patients. In NSW, for example, medical practitioners who believe a patient may be suffering from a sexually transmitted condition are required to do the following:

- Advise the patient of his/her obligation under the Public Health Act, 1991, to disclose his/her medical condition to any partners before any further acts of sexual intercourse take place ('informed intercourse'). The patient's penalty for failure to do this is $5000.
- Advise on the means of minimising the risk of infecting others.
- Provide diagnosis and prognosis of the patient's condition.
- Advise on treatment options.

Failure to comply with these obligations can result in a maximum penalty of $5000 for the doctor concerned.

Confidentiality

In addition to the general duty of confidentiality, most states specifically protect HIV/AIDS sufferers by statute from revelation of their condition. For example, in formal notifications and in test request forms, only initials can be used and no addresses.

There are, however, a number of exceptions to the confidentiality clause. A person's HIV or AIDS status may be disclosed in the following circumstances:

- In connection with administration of the Public Health Act.
- Where a court orders it.
- Where the recipient of the information is involved in the provision of care to the patient.
- In NSW, if a person has reasonable grounds to believe that failure to provide the information could 'place the health of the public at risk', then such information can be provided direct to the Director-General of Health. This means that in NSW a doctor can inform the Director-General of Health when he/she believes that the patient will, unless restrained, infect others with HIV or 'place the health of the public at risk'.

HIV- and hepatitis-infected healthcare workers

The likelihood of transmission of HIV or hepatitis B (HBV) from a doctor to a patient in the healthcare setting is very low. There are, however, a number of legal issues.

1. Is there a duty to test for HIV/HBV?

All doctors should assess their risks and undergo testing if appropriate. Where it is likely that they will be exposed to HBV, they should undergo a course of immunisation and appropriate boosters. Regular testing is not essential. There is no statutory duty to test, but failure to do so could result in a successful legal suit if a patient were to become infected.

2. Exposure-prone procedures

The NSW Department of Health strongly recommends that exposure-prone procedures (i.e. where there is potential for direct contact of the skin of the doctor and sharp surgical instruments, needles, or sharp lesions such as bone spicules in body cavities or in poorly visualised or confined body sites, including the mouth) should not be performed by healthcare workers who are hepatitis Be antigen, HBV-positive or HIV antibody-positive, because injury to the worker could result in blood contamination of a patient's tissues.

If an infected doctor performs an exposure-prone procedure on a patient that results in that patient being infected, the doctor may be liable in court.

3. Is there a duty to inform your patient of your HIV/HBV status?

As a general rule, the answer is no, nor do you have to tell your employer or co-workers.

However, it is advisable to tell the employer in order to take reasonable steps to protect patients. The employer is required to keep the information confidential.

It could be argued that if doctors know their HIV/HBV status, or suspect it, and know that there is a material risk that they might expose patients to infection by performing particular procedures, then failure to tell might constitute a breach of the duty of care.

On the other hand, if doctors do tell patients, they may be 'telling the world', as there is no duty of confidentiality on the part of the patients. A possible solution is to use a consent form for the procedure which includes an undertaking by the patient not to disclose the doctor's status.

More legal obligations

Blood alcohol

In Australia, as in many countries, the treating doctor in an emergency department must perform a venipuncture and obtain a blood alcohol sample (refer to your own state legislation), basically within 12 hours of an accident, if the patient was on a public road and could have directly contributed to that accident, i.e. pedestrian, driver, skateboarder.

These tests must be done with supplied police kits. Also there is a special kit for public transport accident victims (e.g. passenger in a bus who fell).

Drug tests

At times the police may bring someone to the emergency department for drug testing, for which each state has special kits, guidelines and strict conditions, such as supervision of the passing of urine. Sometimes the test (e.g. DNA sampling) should be done by police doctors instead of the emergency department.

Forensic tests

Sexual assault forensic tests should be done at sexual assault crisis units with trained staff and protocols.

How do you avoid a law suit?

The usual assumption is that good doctors are not sued. Sadly, this is not true. Good doctors are sued even when they do everything right, and if we are honest, even good doctors have bad days.

In a recent study, the most common reasons given for beginning a malpractice suit against a doctor were:

- Advice from a knowledgable friend (comment: be careful what you say about your colleague's work).
- Anger at being manipulated by medical personnel.
- Belief that a 'cover up' was taking place.
- Outcome failed to meet expectations.
- Was not told what was happening.

Think about these reasons carefully—they show that the remedy is in your own hands, but it has very little to do with your medical knowledge.

If you do not want to be sued, treat your patients and their relatives the way you would want to be treated in the same circumstances. Be open, friendly and concerned, and above all talk to them and tell them what is happening. The attitude of your other staff (nurses, clerks etc.) is equally important: if the department is rude and uncommunicative, the hospital and the doctor will be sued.

'Make your patients and their relatives feel you value them as people and that you will spend the time and thought needed to make them well. Patients do not expect to be cured, but they do expect that everyone will treat them courteously.' (Stubbs G, personal communication)

Consent

There has been a change in the legal definition of informed consent following the recent *Rogers v Whittaker* decision. Courts now believe that in giving informed consent, a patient must be informed of all material risks. A risk becomes 'material' if the judge believes that a reasonable person in the patient's position would be likely to attach significant importance to it in deciding whether or not to have treatment.

As a general rule, emergency physicians who do not plan to perform a patient's definitive surgical or medical procedure should **not** accept the responsibility of 'getting a consent'. The emergency physician may not even know exactly what the procedure involves, and cannot possibly be aware of all the material risks. In such a situation, it is impossible to obtain an 'informed consent' from the patient. However, for any invasive procedure—e.g. lumbar puncture, central line insertion, chest tube—a consent, if possible, should be obtained and signed by the patient and a witness.

Reports and records

Comprehensive records written when you saw the patient are the keystone of your defence if you are sued. The better the records, the better your chance of a successful defence.

It does not matter what you did; if you didn't write it down, you didn't do it! Conversely, if you did write it down, you did do it!

Whenever you are asked for a report by the police or by a lawyer acting for a patient, you should immediately make several copies of all the hospital records pertaining to that period. This includes your notes, inpatient notes, test and X-ray results. **Do not alter the records:** this is the surest way to ensure you are found guilty.

Read your notes and for your own information expand them—explaining them and adding extra information that you remember (it may be years before you get to court, and your memory will decline with time).

When you are asked for a report, make sure that the person asking is entitled to have one and has gone through the correct hospital procedures. Make sure that the patient has signed the relevant release.

Make your report factual, comprehensive and comprehensible and you may avoid going to court. Remember, you can report only on what you learned first-hand. Do not draw conclusions, just report the facts (e.g. you can say 'the patient smelt of alcohol' or 'was unsteady of gait', but you cannot say 'he was drunk').

Going to court

The important rules in court appearances are: talk to a senior colleague before you go, stay calm, pause before you answer, keep it simple.

1. The best answers are yes or no. Do not attempt to expand answers or to explain.
2. Do not 'second guess' where the questioner is heading. If you do not understand a question, ask for an explanation.
3. Do not try to beat the barrister at his own game—you can't, any more than he can intubate someone.
4. Do not get angry—if you do, you will look bad and the lawyer has won.
5. Tell the truth, but say no more than you have to.

Out-of-hours/away from workplace

The well publicised law case *Woods v Procopis and Anor* has potentially radically changed the practice of medicine. While the eventual legal principles will be established in future cases, the implications for emergency doctors include:

- If a doctor in hospital is about to leave at the end of his shift, he/she has a common law duty to attend to an emergency.
- If a doctor is at a theatre or sports event or similar, not as a doctor, and a call is made 'Is there a doctor here?', the doctor may or may not have a duty of care towards the patient (we are not discussing moral duty here, just legal duty).
- If a doctor is not working, but is somewhere where he is known to be a doctor (such as a favourite restaurant or in an aeroplane) or can be identified as a doctor (e.g. by the badge on his car), it is not clear whether the doctor is under a legal duty of care, but probably he/she is. The obvious solution is not to let people know you are a doctor, even in simple activities like booking airline seats, unless you are prepared to act in a case of emergency.

Duty of care

Patients who refuse treatment

The practice of emergency medicine has been based on the principle that it is always desirable to preserve life, and that all individuals want their lives to be preserved.

This tenet is now being challenged. The Northern Territory's euthanasia law, for example, demonstrates clearly that there are individuals who do not wish to preserve their lives at all costs. This raises questions for doctors in an emergency setting, who must balance their own obligation to treat versus the patient's 'right' to decline.

Where a patient who is believed to need life-saving medical intervention refuses treatment, the future legal questions would possibly focus on the patient's competence, at that time, to make such a decision. Unless there is previously written and witnessed evidence of a preexisting refusal by the patient, it is necessary for the doctor to be convinced that the patient is capable of making such a momentous decision (the patient's mind may be clouded by drugs, pain, or the nature of the illness). While the outcome of a legal challenge would be by no means certain, the truth is that unless the doctor is absolutely certain (and can prove it) that a patient is mentally competent when refusing life-saving treatment, then the doctor should err on the side of active management.

QUALITY (Sally McCarthy)

Clinical quality

Much of the recent discussion concerning quality in health has arisen from reports such as the *Quality in Australian Healthcare Study* (1995) and similar international studies, which found unacceptably high rates of adverse events in hospitalised patients, resulting in significant morbidity and mortality. Subsequent attention has been focused on clinical quality, with one definition of quality in health being: doing the right thing, the first time, in the right way, and at the right time. Clinical care and services must be safe, effective, appropriate, customer-focused, accessible and efficient.

Customer-defined quality

More broadly, quality is defined with reference to the customer: that is, there may be a difference between what a customer wants from the emergency department service and the perception of the actual performance of the service.

A customer is anyone who comes into contact with the work of an emergency department (ED). Customers may include internal customers—those within the organisation who will be affected by the work of the ED (e.g. diagnostic services, inpatient team registrars, ward nursing staff) and external customers—those outside the organisation who are affected by the work of the ED (e.g. patients and their families, ambulance service, GPs, taxpayers, politicians).

Organisation-wide quality

Quality management in an organisation is an organisation-wide effort to achieve sustained, ongoing improvements in quality, based on a study of organisational processes, and with decisions and results based on, and measured by, data. The management style is emphasised as a key to success—a management style that is proactive and leading, rather than reactive and authoritarian. Management recognises that employees care about their work and will take initiatives to improve it; and that employees are empowered to perform to their full potential when supported with appropriate tools and training. Management also recognises that quality is ultimately the responsibility of top management.

Clinical governance, with its concept of managerial legal responsibility for patient mishap, and clinical quality as an equal partner to fiscal control at board level are consistent with a quality management approach.

Patient satisfaction

In emergency medicine, the available body of knowledge suggests that most ED patients want the same things: promptness, courtesy, compassion, privacy and information. Providing quality ED care hinges on our ability to empathise and communicate—to understand and be sensitive to the feelings, thoughts and experiences of our patients.

Communication with patients

Introduce yourself by title and name. Establish eye contact at the beginning of the consultation and maintain it at reasonable intervals to show interest. Apologise for the wait if appropriate, and indicate by your manner that you are ready to give the patient your full attention.

Key tasks to be covered in your communication with patients:

- Eliciting the patients' main problems, their perceptions of these problems, and the physical, emotional and social impact on themselves and their families.
- Tailoring information to what patients want to know; and checking their understanding.
- Eliciting patients' reactions to the information given and concerns raised.
- Determining how much patients want to participate in decision making (when treatment options are available).
- Discussing treatment options so that patients understand the implications.
- Maximising the chance that patients will follow agreed decisions and advice.

583

Patients' expectations

Management of patients' expectations is fundamental to satisfaction. Studies suggest that dissatisfaction increases as patients' triage acuity decreases. The actual wait time to be seen by a physician and total length of stay in the ED are not significant predictors of patients' satisfaction. Managing the perception of waiting time, by communicating an expected wait time to patients, seems to be more important to satisfaction than the actual wait time.

Complaints

Avoidance of complaints is facilitated by good communication with patients. A review of reasons patients complained or litigated demonstrated the main reasons for patient dissatisfaction: patients felt their opinions were 'devalued'; information was poorly delivered; their viewpoints were not understood by doctors; their complaints were not acknowledged, or they felt that honest explanations of adverse outcomes were not given. Criticism of treatment by a second doctor also made patients more likely to take legal action.

Dealing with complaints successfully involves apologising and 'owning' the problem, doing it quickly, giving a factual explanation of what happened and what is being changed to prevent a recurrence, and thanking the person for bringing the problem to your attention. It is advisable to involve a senior staff member in this process.

Risk management

Risk is the exposure to the possibility of such things as economic or financial loss, physical damage, injury or delay, as a consequence of pursuing or not pursuing a particular course of action. Risks and their consequences in the ED include:

- An adverse event during the care process.
- A failure of equipment or computer systems.
- Dissatisfaction of patient or family.
- A threat to physical safety.
- A breach of legal or contractual responsibility.
- Unfavourable publicity.
- A breach of a patient's privacy.
- Fraud.
- Loss of a patient's valuables.

Human factors engineering (or ergonomics) is the study of how human beings interact with their environment, or the study of factors that make work easy or hard. Managing risk requires proactive attention to predictable risk areas and moving away from the traditional approach to error in medicine, with its emphasis on personal responsibility, autonomy and accountability.

A 'human factors' approach emphasises:

- Systems rather than people: e.g. rosters to be according to 'safe hours' practices (nights shifts preferably 8 hours or less, no more than three consecutive nights, no shift exceeding 16 hours, avoid on-call shifts with frequent night calls followed by normal working days, roster adequate time off after nights) to prevent fatigue-induced poor performance.
- Non-punitive approach to adverse events—viewing error or near misses as a chance to learn about the system
- Emphasis on the multifactorial nature of errors.
- Assumption that errors will occur so that systems of work should be designed to make it difficult for clinicians to act erroneously; errors should be obvious before they cause harm; and there should be multiple buffers to minimise the effect of errors.
- Emphasis on team interactions.
- Sharp end, blunt end: considering not only the point where the actual error occurred but the organisational policies and resource allocation decisions that created the system.

Occupational health and safety obligations of employers include maintaining a safe workplace for all employees through reducing the risk of occupational illness and injury. Specific examples in the ED include infection control measures, minimisation of aggression and violence in the ED through staff training, and provision of environmental controls (controlled access points to the ED, video surveillance, security personnel, personal duress alarms, safe observation rooms for potentially violent patients).

Quality assurance

Ongoing monitoring of aspects of clinical care, human resource management, adverse events, complaints, and staff wellbeing occurs to demonstrate compliance with basic standards.

Indicators assess compliance across the dimensions of:

- Access—for example, waiting times; access block.
- Safety—for example, staff absence due to work-related injury, needlestick injury, patient falls, aggressive or violent incidents towards staff.
- Acceptability/customer focus—for example, complaint rate, appreciation letters.
- Effectiveness—for example, admission by triage category, time to thrombolysis or analgesia.
- Efficiency—for example, waiting time by triage category, total treatment time.
- Appropriateness—rate of unnecessary testing, antibiotic choice.

EDITOR'S COMMENT

Although these topics are not the first in the hearts of health carers, they are ignored at your peril as they are essential parts of what we do.

RECOMMENDED READING

Australian Council for Safety and Quality in Health Care. Website. Available: http://www.safetyandquality.org.

Bronstein DA. Law for the expert witness. Florida: Lewis; 1993.

Dix A, Errington M, et al. Law for the medical profession in Australia. 2nd edn. Port Melbourne: Butterworth-Heinemann; 1996.

Forrester K. Essentials of law for health professionals. Sydney: Harcourt; 2001.

Garvin DA. Building a learning organization. Harvard Business Review 1993: 71(4):78–91.

Standards Australia International. Guidelines for managing risk in healthcare. Sydney: Australia/New Zealand Handbook HB 228; 2001.

Maguire P, Pitceathly C. Key communication skills and how to acquire them. BMJ 2002; 325(7366):697–700.

Sun B, Adams J. Determinants of patient satisfaction and willingness to return with emergency care. Ann Emerg Med 2000; 35(5):426–434.

Vincent C, Taylor-Adams S, Stanhope N. Framework for analysing risk and safety in clinical medicine. BMJ 1998; 316(7138):1154–1157.

Acknowledgment: Thanks are due to Dr G Stubbs, orthopaedic surgeon, who kindly provided assistance with the medicolegal issues section of this chapter.

Compiled by Fiona Chow

APPENDIX A
Adult emergency drugs

A1 DRUGS FOR CARDIAC ARREST	
Drug	**Dose and route of administration**
Adrenaline	1 mg 1:10,000 IV
Amiodarone	5 mg/kg IV
Atropine	0.5 mg IV (maximum total dose 3 mg)
Lignocaine	1–1.5 mg/kg IV (cardiac arrest)
Magnesium	1–2 g IV over 1–2 minutes
Sodium bicarbonate 8.4%	1 mEq/kg IV

Drugs able to be given via ETT (mnemonic—LEAN):
    Lignocaine
    Epinephrine
    Adrenaline
    Naloxone	

A2 OTHER DRUGS

Drug	Dose and route of administration
Adrenaline	1 mg 1:10,000 IV (cardiac arrest) 0.3–0.5 mg 1:10,000 IV (anaphylaxis) 0.3–0.5 mg 1:1000 IM (allergic reaction)
Adenosine	6 mg IV—if necessary 12 mg then 12 mg (maximum total dose 30 mg)
Atropine	0.5 mg IV (maximum total dose 3 mg)
Amiodarone	5 mg/kg IV
Benztropine	2 mg IV/IM/PO
Clonazepam	0.5–1 mg IV
Diazepam	2.5–5 mg IV
Haloperidol	2.5–5 mg IV
Lignocaine Lignocaine (local anaesthetic, LA) Lignocaine + adrenaline (LA)	1–1.5 mg/kg IV (cardiac arrest) 3–4 mg/kg SC (maximum) 7 mg/kg SC (maximum)
Bupivicaine (LA) Bupivicaine + adrenaline	2 mg/kg SC 3 mg/kg SC
Fentanyl	1–2 µg/kg IV
Flumazenil	0.2 mg IV (max. total dose 2 mg)
Glucagon	1 mg IV/IM
Hydrocortisone	100–200 mg IV
Ketamine	0.5–1 mg/kg IV (analgesia) 1–2 mg/kg IV (anaesthesia)
Magnesium	1–2 g IV over 1–2 minutes
Mannitol	0.5–1 g/kg IV
Midazolam	1–2 mg IV
Morphine	2.5–5 mg IV 5–10 mg IM/SC
N-acetylcysteine	Initially 150 mg/kg IV over 15 min; then 50 mg/kg IV over 4 hours; then 100 mg/kg IV over 16 hours
Neostigmine	2.5 mg IV for reversal of neuromuscular blockade (administer with 0.6 mg IV atropine)
Phenytoin	15–20 mg/kg IV loading dose infusion rate <50 mg/min
Propofol	1–2 mg/kg IV (induction dose) 1–3 mg/kg/h IV (maintenance infusion)
Rocuronium	0.6–1.2 mg/kg IV for induction 0.15 mg/kg IV (maintenance of paralysis)
Suxamethonium	1–1.5 mg/kg IV
Thiopentone	3–5 mg/kg IV
Vecuronium	0.1 mg/kg IV

APPENDIX B
Cardiology

B1 CAUSES OF PULSELESS ELECTRICAL ACTIVITY (PEA)

Hypoxia
Hypovolaemia
Hyper/hypokalaemia and metabolic disturbances
Hypothermia
Tension pneumothorax
Tamponade (cardiac)
Toxic/therapeutic disturbances
Thromboembolism (pulmonary embolism)
Massive myocardial dysfunction (AMI, myocarditis, toxic myocardial depressants)

B2 CARDIAC MARKERS: TIME SEQUENCE FROM ONSET OF SYMPTOMS

Cardiac marker	Earliest rise (hours)	Peak rise (hours)	Normalise (day)
CK	3–8	12–24	3–4
CK MB	3–12	12–24	2–3
Troponin I	3–12	12–18	5–10
Troponin T	3–12	12	5–14

B3   THROMBOLYSIS

Indications for reperfusion therapy

Ischaemic/infarction symptoms >20 min
This would include not only chest pain but other symptoms of myocardial infarction, such as chest discomfort or pressure, shortness of breath, pulmonary oedema, sweating, dizziness and light-headedness.

Patient's symptoms commenced within 12 hours.

- ST elevation ≥1 mm in 2 or more contiguous limb leads *OR*
- ST elevation ≥2 mm in 2 or more contiguous chest leads *OR*
- new LBBB on ECG

No contraindications to reperfusion therapy.

Absolute contraindications

1. Risk of bleeding
- Active bleeding
- Recent (<1 month) major trauma or surgery

2. Risk of intracranial bleeding
- History of haemorrhagic stroke ever *OR* ischaemic stroke within a year
- Anatomical abnormalities, intracerebral neoplasm, AV malformation

Relative contraindications

1. Risk of bleeding
- Prior use of anticoagulants, INR >2.0
- Non-compressible vascular punctures
- Prolonged CPR (>10 minutes)

2. Risk of intracranial haemorrhage
- Previous stroke at any time
- Previous TIA
- Severe hypertension that cannot be controlled, systolic BP >180 mmHg and/or diastolic BP >110 mmHg

3. Other
- Pregnancy

Adapted from Heart Foundation Guidelines

APPENDIX C
Respiratory

C1	OXYGEN DISSOCIATION CURVE (APPROXIMATIONS)			
pO_2 (mmHg)	30	40	50	60
% oxygen saturation	60	70	80	90

95% oxygen saturation = 80 mmHg

C2 CORRELATION BETWEEN FiO₂ AND EXPECTED pO₂ ('FACTOR OF 5' RULE)

Examples

21% FiO_2 = pO_2 ~ 100 mmHg

100% FiO_2 = pO_2 ~ 500 mmHg

C3 APPROXIMATE OXYGEN CONCENTRATION RELATED TO FLOW RATES OF SEMI-RIGID MASKS

O_2 flow rate (L/min)	Approximate FiO_2
4	0.35
6	0.50
8	0.55
10	0.60
12	0.65
15	0.70

Note: PaO_2 decreases with age. As an approximate guide, $PaO_2 = 100 - (age \div 3)$

C4 ALVEOLAR GAS EQUATION

$P_AO_2 = PiO_2 (= 710 \times FiO_2) - (P_ACO_2 + 0.8)$

C5 A-a GRADIENT

A-a gradient = $P_AO_2 - P_aO_2$

Normal ranges:

Young   5–15 mmHg

Elderly   15–25 mmHg

Normal A-a gradient = $(age \div 3) - 3$ mmHg

C6 NORMAL VALUES OF PEAK EXPIRATORY FLOW (ADULT MALE)

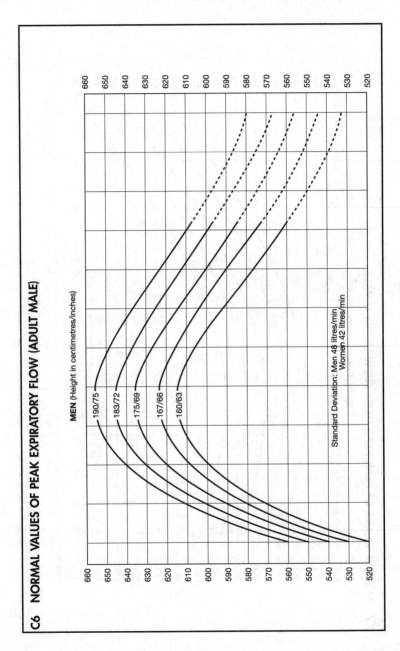

MEN (Height in centimetres/inches)

190/75
183/72
175/69
167/66
160/63

Standard Deviation: Men 48 litres/min
Women 42 litres/min

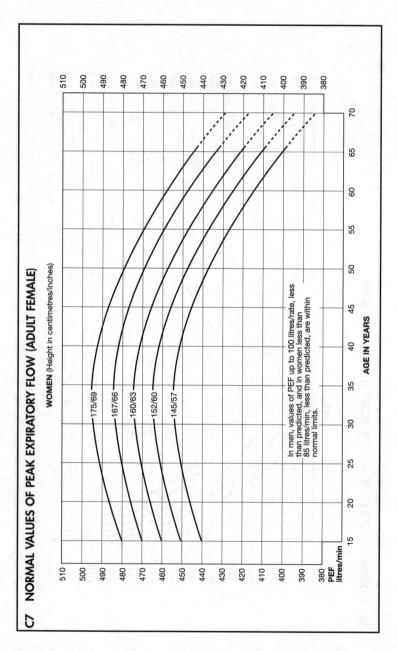

C7 NORMAL VALUES OF PEAK EXPIRATORY FLOW (ADULT FEMALE)

WOMEN (Height in centimetres/inches)

In men, values of PEF up to 100 litres/rate, less than predicted, and in women less than 85 litres/min, less than predicted, are within normal limits.

175/69
167/66
160/63
152/60
145/57

AGE IN YEARS

PEF litres/min

APPENDIX D
Burns

D1 PARKLAND FORMULA

4 mL/kg/ % TBSA burned over 24 hours

where TBSA = total body surface area.

Important
- The 24 hours over which these fluids are given is from the *time of injury*, not the time of presentation.
- Give half the total fluid requirements over first 8 hours, the rest over 16 hours.
- Fluid resuscitation formulas are meant as guides only and patient's haemodynamic status must be monitored continuously (HR, BP, urine output).
- Aim for urine output of >50 mL/h (adult) and ≥1 mL/kg/h (child)

APPENDIX E
Metabolic equations

E1 ANION GAP (AG)

$$AG = (Na^+ + K^+) - (HCO_3^- + Cl^-)$$
$$Normal\ AG = 7 - 12 \pm 2$$

Causes of increased AG acidosis (mnemonic—**MUDPILES**)
- **M**ethanol, **M**etformin
- **U**raemia
- **D**iabetic ketoacidosis
- **P**araldehyde, **P**ropylene glycol
- **I**ron, **I**soniazid
- **L**actic acidosis
- **E**thanol ketoacidosis, **E**thanol
- **S**tarvation ketoacidosis, **S**alicylates

Causes of normal AG acidosis (mnemonic—**USED CARP**)
- **U**reteroenterostomy
- **S**mall bowel fistula
- **E**xtra chloride
- **D**iarrhoea
- **C**arbonic anhydrase deficiency
- **A**ddison's disease
- **R**enal tubular acidosis (type I)
- **P**ancreatic fistula

E2 ACID-BASE DISORDERS FORMULAS: COMPENSATORY MECHANISMS

Metabolic acidosis

$P_{CO2} = (1.5 \times HCO_3) + 8$

Metabolic alkalosis

$P_{CO2} = 40 + [0.7 \times (HCO_{3\ measured} - HCO_{3\ normal})]$

Respiratory acidosis

Acute:	↑ 1 mmol HCO_3 per 10 mmHg ↑ P_{CO2}	]
Chronic:	↑ 3.5 mmol HCO_3 per 10 mmHg ↑ P_{CO2}	] >40 mmHg

Respiratory alkalosis

Acute:	↓ 2 mmol HCO_3 per 10 mmHg ↓ P_{CO2}	]
Chronic:	↓ 5 mmol HCO_3 per 10 mmHg ↓ P_{CO2}	] <40 mmHg

E3 OSMOLAR GAP

Osmolarity = $(2 \times Na^+)$ + glucose + urea

Normal = 275 – 295 mOsm

Osmolar gap = measured osmolarity – calculated osmolarity
Normal ≤10

Causes of increased osmolar gap

Ethanol
Methanol
Ethylene glycol
Isopropyl alcohol

E4 CORRECTION FORMULAE

Corrected Na^+ for glucose = measured Na^+ + [glucose (mmol/L) ÷ 4]

Corrected Ca^{++} for albumin (mmol/L) = measured Ca^{++} (mmol/L) +
[40 – measured albumin (g/L) × 0.02]

APPENDIX F
Tetanus prophylaxis

Tetanus immunisation history	Clean, minor wounds		All other wounds	
	Tetanus toxoid	Tetanus Ig	Tetanus toxoid	Tetanus Ig
Uncertain or <3 doses	Yes	No	Yes	Yes
≥3 doses plus <5 yrs since last dose	No	No	No	No
≥3 doses plus 5–10 yrs since last dose	No	No	Yes	No
≥3 doses plus >10 yrs since last dose	Yes	No	Yes	No

From NHMRC. The Australian immunisation procedures handbook. 5th edn. Canberra: NHMRC; 1994.

APPENDIX G
Cerebrospinal fluid (CSF) studies

CSF studies	Normal	Bacterial	Viral	TB/fungi
Pressure cm H_2O	7–20	↑↑↑	Normal/slight ↑	↑,↑↑↑ in TB
WCC count/mm^3	<5 neonates <30	>200–20,000	<1000	<1000
Predominant cell type	Lymphocytes No polymorphs	Polymorphs (10% lymphocytes)	Lymphocytes	Lymphocytes
Glucose	0.6 × serum 0.8 in neonates	↓	Normal/↑	Normal/↓
Protein	<400 mg/L	↑	Normal/↑	↑
Organisms	0	+ve gram stain in 80%		+ve Indian ink stain with cryptococcal

Correction for a 'bloody' or traumatic tap

Simple contamination adds 1–2 WC for every 1000 RC (unless the blood has an unusually high WCC)

APPENDIX H
Radiology

H1   OTTAWA ANKLE RULES

An ankle X-ray is required if:

There is any pain in the malleolar region and one of the following:

- Bone tenderness at the posterior edge of the distal 6 cm of the fibula or the tip of the lateral malleolus.

OR

- Bone tenderness at the posterior edge of the distal 6 cm of the tibia or the tip of the medial malleolus.

OR

- Inability to weight bear both immediately and in ED.

A foot XR is required if:

There is any pain in the midfoot region and one of the following:

- Bone tenderness over the base of the 5th metatarsal.

OR

- Bone tenderness over the navicular.

OR

- Inability to weight bear both immediately and in ED.

Notes

1. Not applicable to <18 years.

2. Clinical judgment is required for those intoxicated, uncooperative, ↓ sensation in leg or with distracting injuries.

H2   OTTAWA KNEE RULES

- Age >55 years.
- Unable to transfer weight for four steps both immediately after injury and in ED.
- Unable to flex to 90°.
- Tenderness over fibular head.
- Isolated tenderness of patella.

APPENDIX J
Important procedures

J1 CHEST TUBE INSERTION

Insertion sites
5th intercostal space anterior to mid-axillary line on the affected side.
2nd intercostal space in mid-clavicular line on the affected side.*

Size
Use large bore (28–32 Fr) for trauma.

*This is also the site for needle thoracocentesis used in the treatment of life-threatening tension pneumothorax.

J2 INTRAOSSEOUS PUNCTURE

Positioning of patient
Supine with sufficient padding under the knee of the uninjured lower limb, with approximately 30° flexion.

Insertion site
Anteromedial surface of the tibia, approximately one finger-breadth (1–3 cm) below the tubercle.

Method of insertion
Initially at 90°, insert the intraosseous needle through skin and periosteum. After gaining access into bone, direct the needle 45–60° away from the epiphyseal plate (i.e. towards the foot). Use a gentle twisting motion to advance the needle through the bone cortex and into the marrow.

APPENDIX K
Drugs and toxicology

K1 RATIO OF ACUTE EQUIPOTENCY OF OPIOID ANALGESICS

Drug	Oral dose	Parenteral dose
Morphine	30 mg	10 mg
Tramadol	100 mg	80–100 mg
Oxycodone	30 mg	15 mg
Fentanyl	–	150–200 µg
Pethidine	–	75 mg

From St Vincent's Hospital formulary and Australian Medicines Handbook, courtesy of NSW Therapeutic Advisory Group.

K2   RUMACK-MATTHEW NOMOGRAM: PARACETAMOL TOXICITY

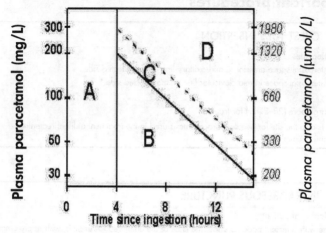

A   Result uninterpretable if sample taken within 4 hours of collection. Repeat collection may be required.

B   Liver damage unlikely.

C   Mild to severe liver damage possible.

D   Severe liver damage likely.

This nomogram is used as a treatment guide. Consider N-acetylcysteine if result falls within area C or D.

Important notes

1. Serum paracetamol is reported in different units from different laboratories. Ensure the correct units are being used before interpreting results with the nomogram. To convert results in μmol/L to mg/L multiply result by 0.151.

2. This nomogram applies only to a single ingestion and is not reliable in the case of chronic overdose (i.e. multiple ingestions over a period of time) or the overdose of multiple substances.

K3 ANTIDOTES

Drug	Antidote
Benzodiazepines	Flumazenil
Beta-blockers	Glucagon
Calcium channel blockers	Calcium chloride
Carbon monoxide	Oxygen
Cyanide	Dicobalt edetate
Digoxin	Digoxin-specific Fabs (Digibind)
Heparin	Protamine
Hydrofluoric acid	Calcium gluconate
Insulin	Dextrose
Isoniazid	Pyridoxine
Methanol, ethylene glycol	Ethanol
Methaemoglobinaemia	Methylene blue
Opiates	Naloxone
Organophosphates	Atropine, pralidoxime
Paracetamol	N-acetylcysteine
Tricyclic antidepressants	Bicarbonate
Warfarin	Vitamin K

APPENDIX L
Drug infusions

L1 N-ACETYLCYSTEINE (NAC) INFUSION: ADMINISTRATION PROTOCOL

Step	Dosage	Duration
1	150 mg/kg IV	Over 15 minutes
2	50 mg/kg IV	Over 4 hours
3	100 mg/kg IV	Over 16 hours

Start with step 1 and continue though to step 3. If after discussion with a toxicologist the infusion needs to be continued after the 20 hours, do so at the dose and rate indicated in step 3.

L2 INOTROPE INFUSIONS: 'RULE OF SIXES'

For adrenaline, noradrenaline and isoprenaline

6 mg in 1000 mL 5% dextrose = 6 µg/mL

∴ 10 mL/h = 1 µg/min

run infusion at 1–20 µg/min = 10–200 mL/hr

For dopamine and dobutamine

6 mg/kg in 1000 mL 5% dextrose = 6 µg/kg/mL

∴ 10 mL/h = 1 µg/kg/min

For dopamine

3–5 µg/kg/min (renal dose) = 30–50 mL/h

>5 µg/kg/min (inotropic dose) = >50 mL/h

For dobutamine

1–20 µg/kg/min = 10–200 mL/h

L3 OTHER DRUG INFUSIONS

Drug	Concentration	Infusion rate	
GTN	50 mg in 500 mL 5% dextrose	Start at 3 mL/h; increase by 3 mL/h every 3–5 min according to pain and BP	
Heparin	15,000 units in 100 mL 5% dextrose	Weight (kg)	Rate (mL/h)
		<54	5
		55–64	6
		65–74	7
		75–84	8
		85–94	9
		>95	10
Amiodarone	Loading dose = 5 mg/kg	Over 20 min (over <3 min if cardiac arrest)	
	15 mg/kg in 500 mL 5% dextrose in GLASS bottle	Over 24 hours	
Octreotide	100 µg in 100 mL 5% dextrose	25 µg/h (25 mL/h)	
Lignocaine	1–1.5 mg/kg loading dose	Bolus over 2–3 min	
	4 g in 500 mL 5% dextrose		
Naloxone	4 mg in 500 mL 5% dextrose or 0.9% saline	25–350 mL/h; titrate to GCS, RR and oxygen saturations	

APPENDIX M
Paediatrics

M1 PAEDIATRIC EMERGENCY DRUGS

Drug	Dose and route of administration
Cardiac arrest	
Adenosine	0.1 mg/kg IV initially (max. 3 mg) ↑ by 0.05 mg/kg to max. 0.3 mg/kg (max 18 mg)
Adrenaline 1:10,000	0.1 mL/kg IV (cardiac arrest) 0.05–0.1 mL/kg IV (anaphylaxis)
Adrenaline 1:1000	0.1 mL/kg via ETT 0.01 mL/kg SC (anaphylaxis)
Adrenaline nebulised 1:1000	0.5 mL/kg/dose (maximum 5 mL)
Amiodarone	5 mg/kg IV (VF)
Atropine	0.02 mg/kg IV (minimum dose 0.1 mg; maximum 0.6 mg)
Calcium chloride 10% (0.7 mmol/mL)	0.2 mL/kg IV (maximum 10 mL)
Calcium gluconate 10% (0.22 mmol/mL)	0.5 mL/kg IV (maximum 20 mL)
Lignocaine 1%	0.1 mL/kg (1 mg/kg)
Naloxone	0.01 mg/kg IV/IM (max. 2 mg)
Sodium bicarbonate (8.4%)	1–2 mL/kg IV
Defibrillation	2 joules/kg, then 2–4 joules/kg, then 4 joules/kg
Miscellaneous	
Amoxycillin	10–25 mg/kg/dose PO/IV/IM q8h 50 mg/kg/dose IV q6h for severe infections
Amoxycillin and clavulanic acid	Dose as for amoxycillin
Cefaclor	10–15 mg/kg/dose PO q8h
Cefotaxime	25 mg/kg/dose IV q12h 50 mg/kg/dose IV (max 2 g) q12h for severe infections
Cefpirome	25–40 mg/kg/dose IV q12h
Ceftriaxone	25 mg/kg/dose IV q12–24h IV/IM 50 mg/kg/dose IV (max. 2 g) for severe infections
Cephalexin	10–25 mg/kg/dose PO q6h
Cephalothin	15–25 mg/kg/dose IV q6h
Cephazolin	10–15 mg/kg/dose IV q6h
Dexamethasone	0.1–0.25 mg/kg PO/IV q6h 0.6 mg/kg IM (max. 12 mg) (severe croup)

M1 (continued)

Drug	Dose and route of administration
Diazepam	0.1–0.2 mg/kg IV 0.5 mg/kg PR
Dicloxacillin	5–10 mg/kg/dose PO/IV/IM q6h 25–50 mg/kg/dose (max. 2 g) IV q6 – 12h for severe infections
Gentamicin (single daily dose)	Neonate 5 mg/kg IV/IM/day One week–10 yrs 8 mg/kg IV/IM/day >10 yrs 7 mg/kg IV/IM stat dose ↓ after initial stat injection
Glucagon (1 unit = 1 mg)	0.5 units if <5 yrs 1 unit if >5 yrs
Glucose	0.5 g/kg = 5 mL/kg IV 10% = 1 mL/kg IV 50%
Hydrocortisone	2–4 mg/kg/dose IV/IM q6h
Midazolam	0.1 mg/kg IV 0.2 mg/kg IM
Morphine	0.1 mg/kg IV 0.2 mg/kg IM
Pancuronium	0.1 mg/kg IV
Penicillin G (benzylpenicillin)	1 mg = 1667 units 30 mg/kg/dose q6h IV 50 mg/kg/dose IV q6h for severe infections
Penicillin V (phenoxymethylpenicillin)	7.5–15 mg/kg/dose PO q6h
Pethidine	0.5–1 mg/kg/dose IV 1–2 mg/kg/dose IM
Phenobarbitone	loading dose = 20–30 mg/kg IM/IV over 30 min maintenance dose = 5 mg/kg (max. 300 mg) PO/IV/IM
Phenytoin	loading dose = 15–20 mg/kg IV (max. 1.5 g) over 1 hour maintenance = 2 mg/kg/dose (max. 100 mg) PO/IV q6 –12h
Prednisolone	1 mg/kg PO daily
Rocuronium	0.6–1.2 mg/kg IV stat then 0.1–0.2 mg/kg IV boluses
Salbutamol (via spacer)	100 µg × 6 puffs if <6 yrs of age 100 µg × 12 puffs if >6 yrs
Suxamethonium Neonate Child	 3 mg/kg/dose IV 2 mg/kg/dose IV double the dose for IM administration
Thiopentone	2–5 mg/kg IV stat
Vecuronium	0.1 mg/kg IV stat

M2 PAEDIATRIC CPR

	Infant (<1 yr)	Small child	Larger child (>8 yrs)
Airway—head tilt position	Neutral	Sniffing	Sniffing
Circulation			
Pulse check	Brachial/femoral	Carotid	Carotid
Compression landmark	One finger-breadth below nipple line	One finger-breadth above xiphisternum	Two finger-breadths above xiphisternum
Technique	Two fingers or two encircling thumbs	One hand	Two hands
Cardiopulmonary ratio	5:1	5:1	15:2
Compression rate	100/minute	100/minute	100/minute
Compression depth	~$\frac{1}{3}$–$\frac{1}{2}$ the depth of chest	~$\frac{1}{3}$–$\frac{1}{2}$ the depth of chest	~$\frac{1}{3}$–$\frac{1}{2}$ the depth of chest

From Mackway-Jones K, ed. Advanced paediatric life support: the practical approach. 3rd edn.
London: BMJ Books; 2001

M3 DEFIBRILLATION AND PADDLE SIZE

Defibrillation
Initially 2 joules/kg, then 2–4 joules/kg, then 4 joules/kg
Paddle size
<10 kg   4.5 cm
>10 kg   4.5 cm or adult size

M4 SELF-INFLATING BAGS

Bag volume	Age group
250 mL	Very small babies only
500 mL	Up to 8 years
1500 mL	>8 years to adults

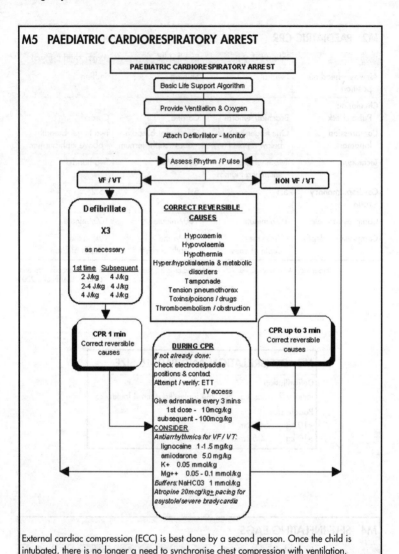

M5 PAEDIATRIC CARDIORESPIRATORY ARREST

PAEDIATRIC CARDIORESPIRATORY ARREST

Basic Life Support Algorithm

Provide Ventilation & Oxygen

Attach Defibrillator - Monitor

Assess Rhythm / Pulse

VF / VT — **NON VF / VT**

Defibrillate

X3

as necessary

1st time	Subsequent
2 J/kg	4 J/kg
2-4 J/kg	4 J/kg
4 J/kg	4 J/kg

CORRECT REVERSIBLE CAUSES

Hypoxaemia
Hypovolaemia
Hypothermia
Hyper/hypokalaemia & metabolic disorders
Tamponade
Tension pneumothorax
Toxins/poisons / drugs
Thromboembolism / obstruction

CPR 1 min
Correct reversible causes

CPR up to 3 min
Correct reversible causes

DURING CPR
If not already done:
Check electrode/paddle positions & contact
Attempt / verify: ETT
IV access
Give adrenaline every 3 mins
1st dose - 10mcg/kg
subsequent - 100mcg/kg
CONSIDER
Antiarrhythmics for VF / VT:
lignocaine 1-1.5 mg/kg
amiodarone 5.0 mg/kg
K+ 0.05 mmol/kg
Mg++ 0.05 - 0.1 mmol/kg
Buffers: NaHCO3 1 mmol/kg
Atropine 20mcg/kg± pacing for asystole/severe bradycardia

External cardiac compression (ECC) is best done by a second person. Once the child is intubated, there is no longer a need to synchronise chest compression with ventilation. Compression should be a firm downwards movement, occupying 50% of each cycle. Commence ECC if the heart rate is <80 bpm in an infant, <60 bpm in a small child, or <40 bpm in a large child.

Adapted from Kilham H, Isaacs D, eds. The New Children's Hospital handbook. Section 3— emergencies. Sydney: Royal Alexandria Hospital for Children; 2000

M6 PAEDIATRIC FORMULAS

1. Formulas for approximate weight (kg) based on age

Age <9 years	$(2 \times age) + 9$
Age >9 years	$3 \times age$
Age <12 months	(age in months ÷ 2) + 4

2. Approximate systolic BP (mmHg) = $80 + (age \times 2)$

3. Formulas for ETT size (appropriate for ages >1 year)

ETT size (mm)	(age ÷ 4) + 4
ETT length (cm) at lips	(age ÷ 2) + 12
ETT length (cm) at nose	(age ÷ 2) + 15

4. Neonate ETT size = 3.0–3.5 mm

5. Pre-term infant ETT size (Adapted from Shann F. Drug doses. 11th edn. Parkville, Victoria: Collective Pty Ltd; 2001)

Weight	ETT size (mm)
<1 kg	2.5 mm
1–3.5 kg	3.0 mm
>3.5 kg	3.5 mm

Note: Uncuffed ETT are preferred until ~8 years of age

M7 PAEDIATRIC VITAL SIGNS: NORMAL RANGES

Age (years)	Heart rate (beats/min)	Systolic BP (mmHg) (breaths/min)	Respiratory rate
<1	110–160	70–90	30–40
1–2	100–150	80–95	25–35
2–5	95–140	80–100	25–30
5–12	80–120	90–110	20–25
>12	60–100	100–120	15–20

Adapted from Mackway-Jones K, ed. Advanced paediatric life support: the practical approach. 3rd edn. London: BMJ Books; 2001

M8 PAEDIATRIC MODIFIED GLASGOW COMA SCORE

Eyes open

Any age	Score
Spontaneously	4
To speech	3
To pain	2
No response	1

Best verbal response

>5 years	2–5 years	0–23 months	Score
Oriented and converses	Appropriate words and phrases	Smiles, coos, cries appropriately	5
Confused	Inappropriate words	Cries but consolable	4
Inappropriate words	Cries and/or screams	Persistent cries and/or screams	3
Incomprehensible sounds	Grunts	Grunts	2
No response	No response	No response	1

Best motor response

>1 year	<1 year	Score
Obeys command	Spontaneously moves	6
Localises pain	Localises pain	5
Flexion-withdrawal	Flexion-withdrawal	4
Flexion-abnormal (decorticate rigidity)	Flexion-abnormal (decorticate rigidity)	3
Extension (decerebrate)	Extension (decerebrate)	2
No response	No response	1

M9 PEAK EXPIRATORY FLOW CHART FOR CHILDREN 5–18 YEARS OF AGE (MALE AND FEMALE)

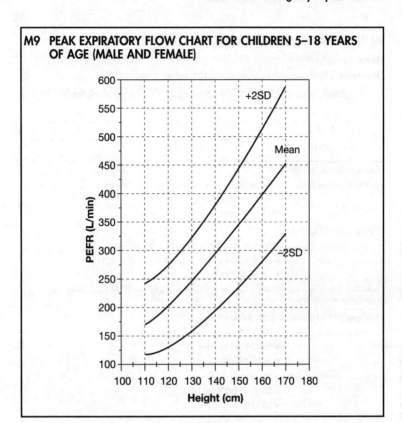

M10 PAEDIATRIC FLUID THERAPY

Bolus: 20 mL/kg IV

Maintenance fluids (usually 4% dextrose + 0.18% normal saline)

Weight in kg	mL/kg/day	mL/kg/hr
0–10 kg	100	4
11–20 kg	50	2
>20 kg	20	1

Example (a) 13 kg child

Maintenance fluids $= (10 \times 100) + (3 \times 50)$ mL/day
$= 1000 + 150$ mL/day
$= 1150$ mL/day

Example (b) 25 kg child

Maintenance fluids $= (10 \times 100) + (10 \times 50) + (5 \times 20)$ mL/day
$= 1000 + 500 + 100$ mL/day
$= 1600$ mL/day

Note: This formula does not include any losses or additional fluid requirements. Add any deficits and ongoing losses to the above.

Example (c) 11 kg child with 5% dehydration

Maintenance fluids $= (10 \times 100) + (1 \times 50)$ mL/day
$= 1000 + 50$ mL/day
$= 1050$ mL/day

Deficit $= 5\% \times 11$ kg
$= 0.05 \times 11\,000$ mL
$= 550$ mL

Total fluids required $= 1050 + 550$ mL/day
$= 1600$ mL/day

Rate of replacement will depend on clinical status of the child. If haemodynamically unstable, some of this total volume may be given faster initially and then slowed over the remaining time in the 24-hour period. Ongoing reassessment of the child's cardiovascular status is always required.

Abbreviations

AAA	Abdominal aortic aneurism
ABCs	The ABCs of resuscitation: airway, breathing, circulation
ABCDE	(In medical retrieval) airway, breathing, cardiovascular, drug therapy, exposure
ABG	Arterial blood gas
ACE	Angiotensin-converting enzyme
ACLS	Advanced cardiac life support
ACTH	Adrenocorticotroph hormones
ADC	AIDS dementia complex
ADH	Antidiuretic hormones
ADL	Activities of daily living
ADT	Adult diphtheria tetanus
AF	Atrial fibrillation
AGE	Arterial gas embolism
AIR	Air, assessment, intervention
ALS	Advanced life support
AMC	Area medical coordinator
AMI	Acute myocardial infarction
AML	Acute myelocytic leukaemia
ANUG	Acute necrotising ulcerative gingivitis
AP	Anteroposterior
APLS	Advanced paediatric life support
APTT	Activated partial thromboplastin time
ARDS	Adult respiratory distress syndrome
ARF	Acute renal failure
ASCOT	A severity characterisation of trauma
ASD	Atrial septal defect
ATLS	Advanced trauma life support
ATN	Acute tubular necrosis
AV	Arteriovenous
AVN	Avascular necrosis
AVNRT	AV nodal re-entry tachycardia
AVRT	AV re-entry tachycardia
AWS	Alcohol Withdrawal Scale
AZT	Zidovudine
BAC	Blood alcohol concentration
bd/bid	Twice daily
BHCG	Beta human chorionic gonadotrophin
BiPAP	Bi-level positive airway pressure
BLS	Basic life support
BNP	Brain natriuretic peptide

BP	Blood pressure
bpm	Beats per minute
BSA	Body surface area
BSL	Blood sugar level
CABG	Coronary artery bypass grafting
CAL	Chronic airflow limitation
CAS	Coloured analogue scale
CBR	Chemical, biological, radiological
CCF	Congestive cardiac failure
CCO	Casualty collecting officer
CCU	Coronary care unit
CHB	Complete heart block
CK	Creatine kinase
CKMB	Creatine kinase isoenzyme
CLL	Chronic lymphocytic leukaemia
CMC	Central medical coordinator
CMV	Cytomegalovirus
CNS	Central nervous system
CO	Carbon monoxide
CO_2	Carbon dioxide
COLD	Chronic obstructive lung disease
COPD	Chronic obstructive pulmonary disease
CPAP	Continuous positive airways pressure
CPK	Creatine phosphokinase
CPP	Cerebral perfusion pressure
CPR	Cardiopulmonary resuscitation
CRAG	Cryptococcal antigen
CRP	C-reactive protein
CSF	Cerebrospinal fluid
CT	Computerised tomogram/tomography
CTG	Cardiotocograph
CTPA	CT pulmonary angiography
CTR	Cardiothoracic ratio
CVA	Cerebrovascular accident
CVP	Central venous pressure
CVS	Cardiovascular system
CXR	Chest X-ray
DC	Direct current
DCI	Decompression illness
DD	Differential diagnoses
DDAVP	Angiovasopressin
DFA	Direct fluorescent antibody
DIC	Disseminated intravascular coagulation
DIP	Distal interphalangeal
DISPLAN	State Disaster Plan
DKA	Diabetes ketoacidosis
DM	Diabetes mellitus
DNA	Deoxyribonucleic acid
DOMS	Director of Medical Services; delayed onset muscle soreness
DPL	Diagnostic peritoneal lavage

DRS	Disability rating scale
DSA	Digital subtraction angiography
DTP	Diptheria/tetanus/pertussis
DTPA	Acellular pertussis vaccine
DTs	Delirium tremens
DVT	Deep vein (venous) thrombosis
EBV	Epstein-Barr virus
ECC	External cardiac compression; emergency control centre
ECF	Extracellular fluid
ECG	Electrocardiogram
ED	Emergency department
EF	Ejection fraction
EEG	Electroencephalogram
EIA	Enzyme immunoassay
ELISA	Enzyme-linked immunosorbent assay
ELS	Emergency life support
EMD	Electromechanical dissociation
EMLA	Trade name for topical anaesthetic
EMST	Emergency management of severe trauma
ENT	Ear, nose, throat
EOC	Emergency operation centre
EPAP	Expiratory positive airway pressure
ERCP	Endoscopic retrograde cholangiopancreatography
ESR	Erythrocyte sedimentation rate
ESWL	Extracorporeal shock-wave lithotripsy
ETT	Endotracheal tube
FAS	Facial affective scale
FAST	Focused assessment with sonography in trauma
FBC	Full blood count
FDI	International Dental Federation (Fédération Dentaire Internationale)
FDP	Fibrin degradation products; flexor digitorum profundus (deep digital flexor)
FDS	Superficial digital flexor
FEV	Forced expiratory volume
FFP	Fresh frozen plasma
FIM	Functional independence measure
FiO$_2$	Fractional inspired oxygen concentration
G&H	Group-and-hold
GHB	Gamma hydroxybutyrate
GCS	Glasgow Coma Score
GOS	Glasgow Outcome Scale
GIT	Gastrointestinal tract
GTN	Glyceryl trinitrate
GVHD	Graft-versus-host disease
HAART	Highly active antiretroviral treatment
HADS	Hospital anxiety and depression scale
HAPE	High-altitude pulmonary oedema
HAV	Hepatitis A virus
Hb	Haemoglobin

HBC	Hepatitis B core antibody
HBO	Hyperbaric oxygen therapy
HBS	Hepatitis B surface antibody
HBV	Hepatitis B virus
HCG	Human chorionic gonadotrophin
HCV	Hepatitis C virus
HDL	High-density lipoprotein
HDV	Hepatitis delta agent
HEV	Hepatitis E virus
HGV	Hepatitis G virus
HHNS	Hyperosmolar hyperglycaemic non-ketotic state
Hib	*Haemophilus influenzae* type b
HIV	Human immunodeficiency virus
HLA	Human leukocyte antigen
HPF	High power field
HR	Heart rate
HSV	Herpes simplex virus
IABC	Intraaortic balloon counterpulsator
IAP	Intraabdominal pressure
ICC	Intercostal catheter
ICP	Intracranial pressure
ICS	Intercellular space
ICU	Intensive care unit
IDC	Indwelling catheter
IDU	Injecting drug user
IHD	Ischaemic heart disease
IM	Intramuscular(ly)
IMI	Intramuscular injection
IMV	Intermittent mandatory ventilation
IN	Intranasal
INH	Isoniazid
INR	International Normalised Ratio (for prothrombin time)
IP	Intraperitoneal
IPAP	Inspiratory positive airway pressure
IPPV	Intermittent positive pressure ventilation
IRED	Infra-red emission detector
ISS	Interstitial space
ITP	Idiopathic thrombocytopenic purpura
IUCD	Intrauterine contraceptive device
IV	Intravenous(ly)
IVC	Inferior vena cava
IVDU	Intravenous drug use
IVI	Intravenous injection
IVP	Intravenous pyelogram
IVS	Intravascular space
JRA	Juvenile rheumatoid arthritis
JVP	Jugular venous pressure
kg	Kilogram
KS	Kaposi's sarcoma
KUB	Kidney-ureter-bladder

L	Litre
LAFB	Left anterior fascicular block
LAP	Left atrial pressure
LCA	Left coronary artery
LBBB	Left bundle branch block
LDL	Low-density lipoprotein
LFT	Liver function test
LIF	Left iliac fossa
LMO	Local medical officer
LMP	Last menstrual period
LMW	Low molecular weight
LOC	Loss of consciousness
LP	Lumbar puncture
LV	Left ventricular
LVF	Left ventricular failure
LVH	Left ventricular hypertrophy
MAC	Mycobacterium avium complex
MAOI	Monoamine oxidase inhibitor
MAP	Mean arterial pressure
MAST	Military antishock trousers
MCH	Mean corpuscular haemoglobin
MCHC	Mean corpuscular haemoglobin concentration
MCP	Metacarpophalangeal
MCU	Micturating cystourethrogram
MCV	Mean corpuscular volume
MET	Mobile emergency teams
MMR	Measles, mumps, rubella
MMSE	Mini-mental state examination
MODF	Multiorgan dysfunction syndrome
MRI	Magnetic resonance imaging
MRSA	Methicillin-resistant *Staphylococcus aureus*
MSU	Midstream urine
MVP	Mitral valve prolapse
NABQI	N-acetylbenzoquinonimine
NAPA	N-acetylprocainamide
NBM	Nil by mouth
NG	Nasogastric
NHL	Non-Hodgkin's lymphoma
NHMRC	National Health & Medical Research Council
NIBP	Non-invasive blood pressure
NMR	Nuclear magnetic resonance
NMS	Neuroleptic malignant syndrome
NNRTI	Non-nucleoside analogue
NPPV	Non-invasive positive pressure ventilation
NRTI	Nucleoside analogue
NRS	Numeric rating scale
NSAID	Non-steroidal anti-inflammatory drug
NTT	Nasotracheal tube
O_2	Oxygen
od	Every day

O&G	Obstetrics and gynaecology
OI	Opportunistic infection
OM	Occipitomental
OPG	Orthopantomogram
OT	Occupational therapy
PA	Posteroanterior
$PaCO_2$	Partial pressure of CO_2 in arterial blood
PAO_2	Partial pressure of oxygen in alveoli
PaO_2	Partial pressure of O_2 in arterial blood
PAWP	Pulmonary artery wedge pressure
PC	Platelet count
PCA	Percutaneous coronary angioplasty
PCP	*Pneumocystis carinii* pneumonia
PCR	Polymerase chain reaction
PE	Pulmonary embolism
PEA	Pulseless electrical activity
PEEP	Positive end-expiratory pressure
PEFR	Peak expiratory flow rate
PGL	Persistent generalised lymphadenopathy
PI	Product information (drugs); protease inhibitor
PID	Pelvic inflammatory disease
PIOPED	Prospective investigation of pulmonary embolism diagnosis
PIP	Proximal interphalangeal
PML	Progressive multifocal leukoencephalopathy
PND	Paroxysmal nocturnal dyspnoea
PO	Per orem (by mouth)
PPE	Personal protective equipment
PPNG	Penicillinase-producing *Neisseria gonorrheae*
PPV	Patency, protection, ventilation
PR	Per rectum (rectally)
PRVC	Pressure-regulated volume control
PSA	Prostate-specific antigen
PSVT	Paroxysmal supraventricular tachycardia
PT	Prothrombin time
PTCA	Percutaneous transluminal coronary angioplasty
PTHrp	Parathyroid hormone related protein
PTP	Pre-test probability
PUVA	Psoralen ultraviolet A therapy
PV	Per vaginam (vaginally)
RA	Radio frequency ablation; rheumatoid arthritis
RAD	Right axis deviation
RAP	Right atrial pressure
RBBB	Right bundle branch block
RBC	Red blood cell(s)
RCA	Right coronary artery
RF	Radio frequency
RNA	Ribonucleic acid
ROM	Range of movement
ROSC	Return of spontaneous circulation
RPFB	Right positive fascicular block

RSV	Respiratory syncytial virus
RTA	Road traffic accident
RVH	Right ventricular hypertrophy
SA	Sinoatrial
SAH	Subarachnoid haemorrhage
SaO2	Arterial oxygen saturation
SBP	Systolic blood pressure
SBT	Skin bleeding time
SC	Subcutaneously
SCIWORA	Spinal cord injury without radiological abnormality
SF-36	A 36-item health survey (Medical Outcomes Study)
SGOT	Transaminase
SIADH	Syndrome of inappropriate antidiuretic hormone secretions
SIDS	Sudden infant death syndrome
SIMV	Synchronised intermittent mandatory ventilation
SIRS	Systemic inflammatory response syndrome
SK	Streptokinase
SLE	Systemic lupus erythematosus
SLS	Sodium lauryl sulphate
SOL	Space-occupying lesion
SSD	Silver sulfadiazine
SSNRI	Serotonin release inhibitor
SSRI	Selective serotonin reuptake inhibitor
SSSS	Staphylococcal scalded skin syndrome
STD	Sexually transmitted disease
SVC	Superior vena cava
SVT	Supraventricular tachycardia
TAC	Tetracaine, adrenaline and cocaine in a gel preparation
TB	Tuberculosis
TBI	Traumatic brain injury
TBSA	Total body surface area
TED	Thromboembolism
TIA	Transient ischaemic attack
TIG	Tetanus immunoglobin
TIPS	Transjugular intrahepatic portosystemic shunt
TLS	Tumour lysis syndrome
TMJ	Temperomandibular joint
TNF	Tumour necrosis factor
TPA	Tissue plasminogen activator
TRISS	Revised Trauma Score and Injury Severity Score combined
TSH	Thyroid stimulating hormone
TSST	Toxic shock syndrome toxin
TT	Thrombin time
U&E	Urea and electrolytes
UEC	Urea/electrolyte/creatinine
UNH	Unfractionated heparin
URTI	Upper respiratory tract infection
UTI	Urinary tract infection

VAS	Visual analogue scale
VDK	Venom detection kit
VDRL	Syphilis test
VEB	Ventricular ectopic beat
VF	Ventricular fibrillation
VP	Ventriculoperitoneal
V/Q	Ventilation perfusion
VSD	Ventricular septal defect
VT	Ventricular tachycardia
WBC	White blood cell(s)
WCC	White (blood) cell count
WHO	World Health Organization
WPW	Wolff-Parkinson-White

Index

Index

Index

Index

Index

Index

Index